Photoaging

BASIC AND CLINICAL DERMATOLOGY

Series Editors

ALAN R. SHALITA, M.D.

Distinguished Teaching Professor and Chairman
Department of Dermatology
State University of New York
Health Science Center at Brooklyn
Brooklyn, New York

DAVID A. NORRIS, M.D.

Director of Research
Professor of Dermatology
The University of Colorado
Health Sciences Center
Denver, Colorado

1. Cutaneous Investigation in Health and Disease: Noninvasive Methods and Instrumentation, *edited by Jean-Luc Lévêque*
2. Irritant Contact Dermatitis, *edited by Edward M. Jackson and Ronald Goldner*
3. Fundamentals of Dermatology: A Study Guide, *Franklin S. Glickman and Alan R. Shalita*
4. Aging Skin: Properties and Functional Changes, *edited by Jean-Luc Lévêque and Pierre G. Agache*
5. Retinoids: Progress in Research and Clinical Applications, *edited by Maria A. Livrea and Lester Packer*
6. Clinical Photomedicine, *edited by Henry W. Lim and Nicholas A. Soter*
7. Cutaneous Antifungal Agents: Selected Compounds in Clinical Practice and Development, *edited by John W. Rippon and Robert A. Fromtling*
8. Oxidative Stress in Dermatology, *edited by Jürgen Fuchs and Lester Packer*
9. Connective Tissue Diseases of the Skin, *edited by Charles M. Lapière and Thomas Krieg*
10. Epidermal Growth Factors and Cytokines, *edited by Thomas A. Luger and Thomas Schwarz*
11. Skin Changes and Diseases in Pregnancy, *edited by Marwali Harahap and Robert C. Wallach*
12. Fungal Disease: Biology, Immunology, and Diagnosis, *edited by Paul H. Jacobs and Lexie Nall*
13. Immunomodulatory and Cytotoxic Agents in Dermatology, *edited by Charles J. McDonald*
14. Cutaneous Infection and Therapy, *edited by Raza Aly, Karl R. Beutner, and Howard I. Maibach*
15. Tissue Augmentation in Clinical Practice: Procedures and Techniques, *edited by Arnold William Klein*
16. Psoriasis: Third Edition, Revised and Expanded, *edited by Henry H. Roenigk, Jr., and Howard I. Maibach*
17. Surgical Techniques for Cutaneous Scar Revision, *edited by Marwali Harahap*
18. Drug Therapy in Dermatology, *edited by Larry E. Millikan*
19. Scarless Wound Healing, *edited by Hari G. Garg and Michael T. Longaker*
20. Cosmetic Surgery: An Interdisciplinary Approach, *edited by Rhoda S. Narins*
21. Topical Absorption of Dermatological Products, *edited by Robert L. Bronaugh and Howard I. Maibach*

22. Glycolic Acid Peels, *edited by Ronald Moy, Debra Luftman, and Lenore S. Kakita*
23. Innovative Techniques in Skin Surgery, *edited by Marwali Harahap*
24. Safe Liposuction, *edited by Rhoda S. Narins*
25. Psychocutaneous Medicine, *edited by John Y. M. Koo and Chai Sue Lee*
26. Skin, Hair, and Nails: Structure and Function, *edited by Bo Forslind and Magnus Lindberg*
27. Itch: Basic Mechanisms and Therapy, *edited by Gil Yosipovitch, Malcolm W. Greaves, Alan B. Fleischer, and Francis McGlone*
28. Photoaging, *edited by Darrell S. Rigel, Robert A. Weiss, Henry W. Lim, and Jeffrey S. Dover*

ADDITIONAL VOLUMES IN PREPARATION

Vitiligo: Problems and Solutions, *edited by Torello Lotti and Jana Hercogova*

Photodamaged Skin, *edited by David J. Goldberg*

Photoaging

edited by

Darrell S. Rigel
New York University School of Medicine
New York, New York, U.S.A.

Robert A. Weiss
Johns Hopkins University School of Medicine
Baltimore, Maryland, U.S.A.

Henry W. Lim
Henry Ford Health System
Detroit, Michigan, U.S.A.

Jeffrey S. Dover
Yale University School of Medicine
New Haven, Connecticut,
and
Dartmouth Medical School
Hanover, New Hampshire, U.S.A.

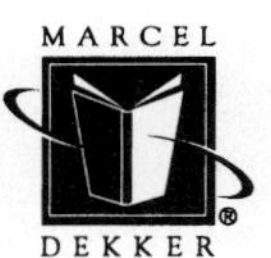

Marcel Dekker, Inc.   New York • Basel

Library of Congress Cataloging-in-Publication Data
A catalog record for this book is available from the Library of Congress.

ISBN: 0-8247-5450-6

This book is printed on acid-free paper.

Headquarters
Marcel Dekker, Inc., 270 Madison Avenue, New York, NY 10016, U.S.A.
tel: 212-696-9000; fax: 212-685-4540

Distribution and Customer Service
Marcel Dekker, Inc., Cimarron Road, Monticello, New York 12701, U.S.A.
tel: 800-228-1160; fax: 845-796-1772

Eastern Hemisphere Distribution
Marcel Dekker AG, Hutgasse 4, Postfach 812, CH-4001 Basel, Switzerland
tel: 41-61-260-6300; fax: 41-61-260-6333

World Wide Web
http://www.dekker.com

The publisher offers discounts on this book when ordered in bulk quantities. For more information, write to Special Sales/Professional Marketing at the headquarters address above.

Current printing (last digit):
10 9 8 7 6 5 4 3 2 1

PRINTED IN CANADA

Series Introduction

Over the past decade, there has been a vast explosion in new information relating to the art and science of dermatology as well as fundamental cutaneous biology. Furthermore, this information is no longer of interest only to the small but growing specialty of dermatology. Scientists from a wide variety of disciplines have come to recognize both the importance of skin in fundamental biological processes and the broad implications of understanding the pathogenesis of skin disease. As a result, there is now a multidisciplinary and worldwide interest in the progress of dermatology.

With these factors in mind, we have undertaken to develop this series of books specifically oriented to dermatology. The scope of the series is purposely broad, with books ranging from pure basic science to practical, applied clinical dermatology. Thus, while there is something for everyone, all volumes in the series will ultimately prove to be valuable additions to the dermatologist's library.

The latest addition to the series, edited by Drs. Rigel, Weiss, Lim, and Dover, is both timely and pertinent. The authors are well known authorities in the field of photoaging. We trust that this volume will be of broad interest to scientists and clinicians alike.

Alan R. Shalita
SUNY Health Science Center
Brooklyn, New York

Foreword

Photoaging is an exceedingly broad field that embraces disciplines as diverse as photomedicine and photobiology to surgical light-based therapy. In this book, the entire electromagnetic spectrum from its effect on the skin to harnessing this energy to treat the skin is presented by experts in the field. Dermatologists, who synthesized the existing knowledge and skills from a variety of disciplines and applied them to the skin, write about the recent advancements. Each editor is the leading representative of a portion of the field. By working together, they master the full spectrum of photoaging.

Dermatologists understand the enormous importance of the scientific basis of photomedicine to dermatology. The positive aspects of the usage of ultraviolet radiation to treat skin disease with phototherapy and photochemotherapy (PUVA) have given millions of people with skin diseases a better quality of life. In this book, Drs. Rigel, Lim, Weiss and Dover bring together the negative story of the effect of ultraviolet energy on the skin, photoaging that sets the stage for photodamage, and photocarcinogenesis. The authors deal with issues that are important to the medical practitioner in a practical and sensible way with the medical and surgical approach to repair of photodamage.

Physicians who study photoaging wish to apply the knowledge of the pure basic scientists to enhance the ability to diagnose, prevent, and improve photoaging. This text provides a comprehensive review of the field and imaginatively moves forward to explore new topics such as photoaging in patients with skin of color. As society has evolved over the last hundred years, the "farmer's and sailor's skin" associated with occupational solar exposure has become the "sun worshipper's skin" of recreational exposure with indoor and outdoor light. Youths and young adults concerned about their appearance often deliberately tan to have the "healthy glow" of a life of outdoor leisure activities on the beach, the boat, the golf course, the tennis court, or by the pool. The individual's concern about their appearance continues throughout life; thus, the changes of photoaging become a concern with psychosocial consequences. With the demographic change influencing the adult population of the United States as the "baby boomer" generation enters their 50s, photoaging will continue to be a concern based upon the unprotected sun exposure of their youth in the 1950s. In the 1950s and 1960s, effective forms of sunscreens were not available and the pervasive attitude was to glorify tanning. For this generation, medical and surgical treatment of photoaging is an important psychosocial concern and a way to treat photodamaged skin that may evolve into skin cancer.

This book brings credit to its editors, its authors and its publishers and offers the reader the opportunity to use the information to help many patients. One can go through this book without a specific order just to pick up a fact, good advice, or a different perspective. It will become an instant resource for the busy surgeon planning a procedure or the harassed clinician trying to remember which topical agent is better to use in people of color. It clearly guides and assists clinicians in their selection of the best treatment for their patients by examining the benefits, limitations, and challenges of each technique and modifying the treatment program to the patient's expectations.

June K. Robinson, MD
Director, Division of Dermatology
Professor of Medicine and Pathology
Loyola University Medical Center
Maywood, Illinois, U.S.A.

Preface

One of the most dynamic changes that our society is currently undergoing is the aging of the population. This evolution has lead to a marked change in the way that people view themselves and an increased desire to improve their appearance.

The primary extrinsic factor associated with an aging appearance is exposure to ultraviolet radiation whether from natural sources (sunlight) or artificial sources (tanning salons). It is clear that acute and chronic exposure over time leads to exacerbations of photoaging-associated problems.

Photoaging can be described as a continuum—from the earliest changes of mild dyschromias and telangectasias to deep rhytids and loss of elasticity. Because of the rapidly increasing demand for treating signs of photoaging, a multitude of medical, surgical, and cosmetic approaches have been developed and significant new therapies are being released on almost a monthly basis. Dermatologic surgeons remain at the forefront of these research and development efforts with dozens of new treatment modalities being released each year.

To that end, we have tried to make this text represent the most up to date comprehensive review of the causes and management of photoaging-related problems written by recognized world authorities in this area. From basic science to specific "how to" application of techniques, this text has been designed as a resource to help the practitioners interested in this field be the best that they can be.

Several specific events have made the need for a textbook of this type to add to our knowledge of the photoaging process even more critical. The effects of photoaging may not be seen until later in life. Therefore, protection efforts against photoaging such as sunscreen usage must begin early. The newer formulations and prevention strategies are comprehensively reviewed in this text.

Also, this text presents the dramatically evolving therapeutic approaches in the field. Less then a decade ago the mainstay of therapy consisted of surgery requiring general anesthesia, deeply ablative lasers, and painful deep peels. Advances have led to equal or more effective superficial or non-ablative therapies that put our patients at less risk for complications, delivering equal or better results.

In addition, we realize that the photoaging process is not limited to those with lighter skin phenotypes. Even those with Fitzpatrick skin types V and VI can experience signs of photoaging and newer approaches related to treating these persons are also reviewed.

Finally, with the rapid advances that are occurring in all aspects of this field, we attempted to assess what the future may bring with a "future directions" section in each chapter.

We hope that you will find this text to be useful and a reference in your management of photoaging patients.

Darrell S. Rigel, MD
Robert A. Weiss, MD
Henry W. Lim, MD
Jeffery S. Dover, MD

Contents

Contributors

Murad Alam Northwestern University, Chicago, Illinois, U.S.A.

Christophe Antille Dermatology Department, Geneva University Hospital, Geneva, Switzerland

Alastair Carruthers University of British Columbia, Vancouver, British Columbia, Canada

Jean Carruthers University of British Columbia, Vancouver, British Columbia, Canada

Henry H. Chan Division of Dermatology, Department of Medicine, Queen Mary Hospital, Pokfulam, Hong Kong

John Z. S. Chen New York University School of Medicine, New York, New York, U.S.A.

Soyun Cho Department of Dermatology, University of Michigan, Ann Arbor, Michigan, U.S.A.

Jinho Chung Department of Dermatology, Seoul National University, Seoul, Korea

William P. Coleman Department of Dermatology, Tulane University Health Sciences Center, New Orleans, Louisiana, U.S.A.

Alpesh Desai Manhattan Beach Skin and Laser Institute, Manhattan Beach, California, U.S.A.

Nicole M. DeYampert Department of Dermatology, St. Luke's-Roosevelt Hospital Center, New York, New York, U.S.A.

Lisa M. Donofrio Yale University, New Haven, Connecticut, and Tulane University, New Orleans, Louisiana, U.S.A.

Jeffrey S. Dover Yale University School of Medicine, New Haven, Connecticut, and Dartmouth Medical School, Hanover, New Hampshire, U.S.A.

A. Fourtanier L'Oréal Recherche, Clichy, France

Marjan Garmyn Department of Dermatology, University Hospital Sint Rafael, Leuven, Belgium

Roy G. Geronemus New York University School of Medicine, New York, New York, U.S.A.

Richard G. Glogau University of California, San Francisco, California, U.S.A.

David J. Goldberg Skin and Laser Surgery Specialists of NY/NJ, Mount Sinai School of Medicine, and Fordham University School of Law, New York, New York, U.S.A.

Mitchel P. Goldman La Jolla Spa MD, La Jolla, and University of California, San Diego, California, U.S.A.

Rebat M. Halder Department of Dermatology, Howard University College of Medicine, Washington, D.C., U.S.A.

Karen F. Han Department of Dermatology, Palo Alto Medical Foundation, Palo Alto, California, U.S.A.

Jeffrey T. S. Hsu SkinCare Physicians of Chestnut Hill, Chestnut Hill, Massachusetts, U.S.A.

Sewon Kang Department of Dermatology, University of Michigan, Ann Arbor, Michigan, U.S.A.

Henry W. Lim Department of Dermatology, Henry Ford Health System, Detroit, Michigan, U.S.A.

Gary D. Monheit Department of Dermatology, University of Alabama at Birmingham, Birmingham, Alabama, U.S.A.

Ronald L. Moy Dermatologic Surgery, West Los Angeles VA Medical Center, Los Angeles, California, U.S.A.

Lawrence S. Moy Manhattan Beach Skin and Laser Institute, Manhattan Beach, California, U.S.A.

D. Moyal L'Oréal Recherche, Clichy, France

Walter K. Nahm University of California, San Diego School of Medicine, San Diego, and Dermatologic Surgery, West Los Angeles VA Medical Center, Los Angeles, California

Rhoda S. Narins New York University, New York, New York, U.S.A.

Mark Steven Nestor Center for Cosmetic Enhancement, Aventura, and University of Miami School of Medicine, Florida, U.S.A.

Georgianna M. Richards Department of Dermatology, Howard University College of Medicine, Washington, D.C., U.S.A.

Darrell S. Rigel Department of Dermatology, New York University School of Medicine, New York, New York, U.S.A.

Adam M. Rotunda Dermatologic Surgery, West Los Angeles VA Medical Center, Los Angeles, California, U.S.A.

Jean-Hilaire Saurat Dermatology Department, Geneva University Hospital, Geneva, Switzerland

Adriana N. Schmidt Dermatologic Surgery, West Los Angeles VA Medical Center, Los Angeles, California, U.S.A.

Olivier Sorg Dermatology Department, Geneva University Hospital, Geneva, Switzerland

Susan C. Taylor Department of Dermatology, College of Physicians and Surgeons, Columbia University, New York, New York, U.S.A.

Laura Thomas Department of Dermatology, Henry Ford Health System, Detroit, Michigan, U.S.A.

Joost Van den Oord Department of Morphology and Molecular Pathology, University Hospital Sint Rafael, Leuven, Belgium

Margaret A. Weiss Johns Hopkins University School of Medicine, Baltimore, Maryland, U.S.A.

Robert A. Weiss Johns Hopkins University School of Medicine, Baltimore, Maryland, U.S.A.

1

Why Does the Skin Age?

Intrinsic Aging, Photoaging, and Their Pathophysiology

Jinho Chung *Seoul National University, Seoul, Korea*

Soyun Cho / Sewon Kang *University of Michigan, Ann Arbor, Michigan, U.S.A.*

- Reduced capacity of the antioxidant defense system in aged human skin results in age-associated oxidative stress and contributes to intrinsic aging.
- Increased matrix metalloproteinase (MMP) and decreased procollagen expressions involving mitogen-activated protein kinase signal-transduction pathways are central to the pathophysiology of intrinsic skin aging.
- Ultraviolet (UV)-induced generation of reactive oxygen species activates multiple signaling pathways.
- UV-induced activation of signaling pathways activator protein 1 and nuclear factor κ B results in induction of MMPs that degrade collagen.
- Smoking and estrogen deficiency are independent risk factors that exacerbate intrinsic aging in human skin.

Aging is a process perhaps best defined as decreased maximal function and reserve capacity in all body organs, resulting in an increased likelihood of disease and death. With age, the biochemical compositions of tissues change, physiological capacity is progressively reduced, the ability to respond adaptively to environmental stimuli is diminished, and the susceptibility to disease is increased. Aging is widely known to be the consequence of a genetic program and of cumulative environmental damage (1–3).

Like all other tissues, skin unavoidably ages, a process than affects the function and appearance of the skin. Skin aging is a degenerative process whereby alterations from the passage of time (chronological/intrinsic aging) are superimposed with effects produced by environmental factors (e.g., sun, heat, pollution, smoking). Among the extrinsic factors, solar ultraviolet (UV) irradiation is the most significant, and consequently the most studied. Premature skin aging that occurs from excessive exposure to solar UV light is referred to as photoaging. In this chapter, we review recent advances in our understanding of skin aging, giving emphasis to intrinsic and photoaging.

MECHANISMS OF AGING

Several theories on the causes of aging have been proposed. Most remain controversial as the fundamental molecular mechanisms proposed for aging have been difficult to prove in humans. Historically, theories on aging have been largely divided into genetically programmed mechanisms and a free radical-mediated damage mechanism. Before focusing on skin aging, we will briefly review these two views.

Genetically Programmed Mechanisms

This group of theories proposes that aging is a genetically programmed process. It is supported by the observation that the maximum lifespan is highly species specific. For example, the maximum lifespan for humans is 30 times that of mice. In addition, studies that have compared the longevity of monozygotic and dizygotic twins and non-twin siblings have shown that monozygotic twins are also remarkably similar in this respect.

Longevity Genes

Over the past two decades, many genes that alter the rate of aging have been identified in yeast, nematode worms, and fruit flies. Some of them affect both the average and maximum lifespan (4). These gene products function in diverse ways, such as modulating stress response, sensing nutritional status, increasing metabolic capacity, and silencing genes that promote aging. In the nematode (*Caenorhabditis elegans*), mutants with an increased lifespan have been found to possess genes that alter stress resistance (particularly in response to UV light), signal transduction, or metabolic activity (5).

Genetic analysis of longevity in mammals has not been as revealing. However, immune loci in mice and humans have been implicated in long-lived subjects (4), and a number of mitochondrial DNA polymorphisms have also been associated with longevity (6).

The Role of Telomeres in Aging

Of the many hypotheses that have been generated to explain the process of cellular aging, presently the most favored is the telomere hypothesis. This hypothesis proposes that the proliferation-dependent, continuous shortening of the telomeres (specific structures at the ends of chromosomes) plays a role in setting the internal biologic clock. Increasing cumulative population doublings of normal human fibroblasts is associated with telomeric shortening (7). Moreover, telomeric length determined directly from tissues in vivo was found to be inversely related to the individual's physiologic age, in that it was shorter in cells from older persons than in those from younger adults (7,8). Cells from patients with premature aging syndromes like Werner's syndrome (WS) and progeria also have been shown to have short telomere length (9). In germ line and tumor cells, however, a specific ribonucleoprotein complex, telomerase, exists. Telomerase is able to synthesize telomeric sequences de novo and thereby counteract telomeric shortening. Telomerase is composed of an RNA component (hTR), which acts as an anchor and template for the telomeric DNA, a catalytic subunit (hTERT), which catalyzes the addition of nucleotides to the end of the telomere, and a number of associated proteins, the functions of which remain poorly understood (10).

Telomerase activity can also be detected in certain normal tissues. In general telomerase is active during fetal development in all tissues, though its expression is inhibited at a certain stage of development. Only in permanently or periodically regenerative tissues, such as the hematopoietic system or the epidermis of the skin, is telomerase expression maintained (11). Compared to tumor cells, however, these tissues exhibit little telomerase activity, and during in vivo aging and in vitro cultivation, the telomeres shorten (12). On the other hand, it has been convincingly demonstrated that introduction of exogenous hTERT, thereby expressing telomerase in otherwise negative cells, causes the elongation of telomeres and an extension of lifespan (13).

Accelerated Aging Syndromes

Several human genetic diseases, including WS, Hutchinson-Gilford syndrome, and Down's syndrome, display some features of accelerated aging (14). WS is an autosomal recessively inherited disease (15). WS patients prematurely develop arthrosclerosis, glucose intolerance, and osteoporosis. They also manifest the more directly associated symptoms of aging, such as early graying, loss of hair, skin atrophy, and menopause. The gene responsible for WS has been localized to chromosome 8 (16), and encodes a protein that appears to be a helicase (17). This is an enzyme involved in DNA unwinding, and is therefore needed in DNA replication and repair.

Hutchinson-Gilford syndrome is an extremely rare, autosomal-recessive disease in which features characteristics of aging develop within several years of birth (15). These include wrinkled skin, a stooped posture, and growth retardation. Patients suffer from advanced atherosclerosis, and usually die of myocardial infarction by the age of 30.

People with Down's syndrome have trisomy or a translocation involving chromosome 21 (14,15) and suffer from the early onset of vascular disease, glucose intolerance, hair loss, and degenerative diseases of the bones and joints. In addition, they have an increased incidence of cancer.

Free-Radical Theory of Aging

The free-radical theory of aging was initially proposed about half century ago. Primarily to explain the biological aging processes, Harman suggested that most aging changes are due to molecular damage caused by free radicals (18). Free radicals are either atoms or molecules that possess an unpaired electron, and are therefore highly reactive. Aerobic metabolism generates the superoxide radical, which is metabolized by superoxide dismutases to form hydrogen peroxide and oxygen (19). Hydrogen peroxide can be converted to an extremely reactive hydroxyl radical. These oxygen-derived species can react with macromolecules including DNA and proteins. It has been proposed that reactive oxygen species (ROS) contribute significantly to the somatic accumulation of mitochondrial DNA mutations (20). Since mitochondria do not contain any repair mechanism to remove bulky DNA lesions, the mutation frequency of mitochondrial DNA (mtDNA) is approximately 50-fold higher than nuclear DNA (21). As a result of accumulated damage, the aged cell has reduced antioxidant capacity, further exacerbating ROS-mediated damage and the aged phenotype (22).

Related to the free-radical theory of aging is caloric restriction (CR). Defined as a significant reduction in calorie intake without essential nutrient deprivation, CR is a major research area in biological gerontology. The life-extending action of CR has been found to occur in both genders of many different strains of rats and mice, in hamsters, and in nonmammalian species, such as the fish and flies (23–25). In addition, the restriction of food intake delays and slows the progression of a variety of age-associated diseases, including neoplasia, and maintains many physiological processes in a youthful state to a very advanced age. Although the mechanism of this effect is poorly understood, CR is presumed to act by reducing the oxidative damage that occurs secondary to ROS generation by the cellular metabolism (26,27). Interestingly, in the muscle and brain of mice, caloric restriction either completely or partially prevents age-related changes in gene expression.

INTRINSIC SKIN AGING

Intrinsic skin aging is characterized primarily by functional alterations rather than by gross morphological changes in the skin. Chronologically aged skin appears dry and pale with fine wrinkles. It displays a certain degree of laxity and is prone to a variety of benign neoplasms. Histologically, the most consistent change associated with intrinsic aging is a flattening of the dermal-epidermal junction. Also, progressive decreases in melanocyte and Langerhans cell density occur. The dermis displays loss of extracellular matrix and increased levels of collagen-degrading metalloproteinases, loss of fibroblasts and vascular network, and, in particular, a loss of the capillary loops that occupy the dermal papillae (28,29).

The skin is constantly exposed to ROS from the environment, including air, solar radiation, ozone, or other airborne pollutants. The normal metabolism also produces ROS, primarily via the mitochondrial respiratory chain wherein excess electrons are donated to molecular oxygen to generate superoxide anions. Accumulated ROS have been suggested to play important roles in the intrinsic aging of human skin in vivo (30). Moreover, ROS levels increase with aging owing to the reduced activities of antioxidant defense enzymes.

An intimately interlinked network regulates the skin's antioxidant defense system. It is becoming increasingly clear that antioxidants interact in a complex fashion such that changes in the redox status or in the concentration of one component may affect the levels and capacity of other components in the system (31–33). Thus, a comprehensive and integrated antioxidant skin defense mechanism is considered to be crucial in protecting the skin from ROS, and consequently preventing the skin aging process.

Rhie et al. (34) demonstrated decreased activities of catalase and nonenzymatic antioxidants in the dermis of aged human skin in vivo. This reduced capacity of the antioxidant defense system is believed to be the cause of age-associated oxidative stress. Consequently, ROS such as hydrogen peroxide may increase and accumulate in aged skin, further contributing to skin aging in vivo (34).

Skin Wrinkling and Intrinsic Aging

It is estimated that collagen content of the dermis decreases by 1% per year throughout adult life. The molecular mechanisms of collagen deficiency during natural skin aging result from increased matrix metalloproteinase (MMP) expression and a concomitant reduction in collagen synthesis (35). With increasing age, levels of MMP-1, 2, 9, and 12 increase. On the other hand, procollagen mRNA expression in aged skin is significantly lower than in young skin (35,36).

Recent studies indicate that the mitogen-activated protein (MAP) kinase signal-transduction pathways play an important role in regulating a variety of cellular functions (37,38), including cell growth (39,40), MMP expression (41), and type I procollagen synthesis (42,43). Three distinct but related families of MAP kinases exist: extracellular signal-regulated kinase (ERK), c-Jun amino-terminal kinase (JNK), and p38 MAP kinase. Although ''cross-talk'' exists between pathways, the ERK pathway primarily mediates cellular responses to growth factors (39), whereas the JNK and p38 pathways primarily mediate cellular responses to cytokines and physical stress (39,44,45). It has been suggested that the dynamic balance that exists between the growth factor-activated ERK and the stress-activated JNK and p38 pathways may be important in regulating cell survival versus apoptosis (39).

Downstream effectors of the MAP kinases include several transcription factors, which include Elk-1, Ets, CREB, c-Fos, and c-Jun. c-Jun and c-Fos heterodimerize to form the activator protein 1 (AP-1) complex. Phosphorylation of c-Jun by JNK stimulates AP-1 transactivation activity (46). Binding of activated AP-1 to its response element induces the expressions of numerous genes, including certain members of the MMP family (i.e., collagenase, stromelysin, and 92-kd gelatinase) (47). MMPs specifically degrade connective tissue proteins such as collagen and elastin in the skin. AP-1 has also been shown to negatively regulate type I procollagen gene expression (48). This inhibition appears to result from its interference with the induction of procollagen transcription by transforming growth factor β (TGF-β).

It has been demonstrated in vivo that the ERK pathway activity is reduced, whereas c-Jun kinase (JNK and p38) pathway activity is activated, in intrinsically aged human skin compared with young skin (49). This higher c-Jun kinase activity in intrinsically aged skin is responsible for the increased expression of c-Jun, which leads to functional AP-1 activation, resulting in increased MMP expression and decreased procollagen expression. Reduced procollagen synthesis coupled with enhanced matrix degradation by MMPs are responsible for atrophic skin that characterizes intrinsically aged human skin.

PHOTOAGING

Fine and coarse wrinkles, dyspigmentations, sallow color, dry texture, and loss of tone in habitually sun-exposed skin characterize the photoaged phenotype (50). Recent advances in photobiology have provided substantial insight into the process by which UV irradiation causes disruption of dermal extracellular matrix. This emerging information reveals that chronological aging and photoaging share fundamental molecular pathways. Photoaging, like chronological aging, is a cumulative process that is superimposed on intrinsic aging. However, unlike chronological aging, which depends solely on the passage of time, photoaging depends mainly on the degree of sun exposure and skin pigment, preferentially affecting individuals with fair skin who have outdoor lifestyles and who live in sunny climates (51).

Pathophysiology of Photoaging

UV irradiation of human skin activates a complex sequence of specific molecular responses that damage skin connective tissue. To exert its biological effects, molecules in the skin called chromophores must absorb UV, and the absorbed energy must be converted into chemical reactions. Depending on the chromophore, absorbed energy may cause direct chemical modification of the chromophore itself, or the energy may be transferred from the chromophore to another molecule, which undergoes chemical modification. UVA light primarily acts indirectly through generation of ROS, which subsequently can put forth a multitude of effects such as lipid peroxidation, activation of transcription factors, and generation of DNA-strand breaks. While UVB light can also generate ROS, its main mechanism of action is the direct interaction with DNA via induction of DNA damage; i.e., cross-linking of adjacent pyrimidines (52). Photoaging is mediated by direct UV absorption and ROS-mediated photochemical reactions.

The cellular machinery that mediates UV damage to human skin connective tissue includes cell surface receptors, protein kinase signal-transduction pathways, transcription factors, and MMPs. Based on the available data on human subjects to date, the following model of photoaging is proposed. First, UV irradiation causes activation of cytokine and growth factor receptors on the surface of keratinocytes and dermal cells, via stimulation of distinct tyrosine kinase activities, and initiates downstream signal-transduction pathways (51). Epidermal growth factor, interleukin (IL) 1, and tumor necrosis factor α (TNF-α) receptors are activated within minutes following UV exposure in human skin in vivo. The mechanism(s) of receptor activation by UV irradiation are not well understood.

Generation of ROS is one of the earliest measurable UV responses in human skin. In less than 30 minutes following UV irradiation, the hydrogen peroxide level more than doubles in human skin (53). This generation of hydrogen peroxide after UV exposure is distinct from photochemical generation of ROS. Similar to phagocytes, human keratinocytes express nicotinamide adenine dinucleotide phosphate (NADPH) oxidase, which catalyzes the reduction of molecular oxygen to superoxide anion. It has been recently demonstrated that NADPH oxidase is a major enzymatic source of hydrogen peroxide production following UV irradiation in human keratinocytes (51). Hydrogen peroxide can rapidly generate other ROS, such as the hydroxyl radical. Both direct chemical oxidation of cellular components (i.e., DNA, proteins, and lipids) and activation of cellular machinery, both caused by UV-induced oxidative stress, act in concert to cause photoaging.

ROS seem to be crucial for MAP kinase-mediated signal transduction (54,55) that leads to AP-1 induction. UV irradiation activates protein kinase-mediated signaling pathways that converge in the nucleus of cells to induce c-Jun. The induced c-Jun heterodimerizes with constitutively expressed c-Fos to form activated complexes of the transcription factor AP-1. Consistent with these signaling events, the induction of c-Jun protein in human skin trails MAP kinase activation (56). In the dermis and epidermis, AP-1 induces expression of MMPs collagenase (MMP-1), stromelysin 1 (MMP-3), and 92-kd gelatinase (MMP-9), which degrade collagen and other proteins that comprise the dermal extracellular matrix (57–59). Transcription factor AP-1 also interferes with collagen gene expression in human dermal fibroblasts. UV irradiation also activates the transcription factor nuclear factor κ B (NF-κB) (60) that amplifies the expression of 92-kd gelatinase, but more importantly, NF-κB stimulates transcription of proinflammatory cytokine genes, including IL-1β, TNF-α, IL-6, and IL-8, and adhesion molecules including intercellular adhesion molecule 1 (61). NF-κB recruits neutrophils, thereby introducing preformed neutrophil collagenase (MMP-8) into UV-irradiated skin. Collectively, these MMPs degrade skin collagen and thus impair the structural integrity of the dermis.

In addition to degrading mature dermal collagen, UV irradiation impairs ongoing collagen synthesis, mainly through down-regulation of type I and III procollagen gene expression (62), leading to acute collagen loss in skin. Two mechanisms contribute to reduced procollagen gene expression: the induction of AP-1 and subsequent AP-1–mediated transcriptional repression, and down-regulation of type II TGF-β with resultant loss of TGF-β responsiveness (63).

This sequence of events can be viewed as a wound response to UV trauma (64). Following injury from any cause, including UV, a repair process is engaged. Induction of tissue inhibitors of metalloproteinases (65), for example, would be a part of this compensatory response acting to limit matrix degradation. Although very efficient, the repair of a UV-induced wound is not perfect, resulting in a minute defect called a solar scar. The accumulation of invisible solar scars caused by imperfect repair occurs with multiple exposures to UV light over many years. Eventually, at some point, the sum total of invisible scars crosses the clinical threshold, and the scars become visible. These visible scars are believed to be the cause of the dermal component of photoaging.

The Role of Damaged Collagen in Skin Aging

It has been demonstrated that exposure of cultured fibroblasts from either photodamaged or sun-protected skin to partially degraded type I collagen (produced by in vitro treatment of collagen with a mixture of MMPs from human skin) inhibits procollagen synthesis (66). Among collagen fragments, not small ones but larger breakdown fragments of type I collagen negatively regulate its synthesis, suggesting that the high-molecular-weight fragments of type I collagen serve as negative regulators of type I collagen synthesis and that further degradation of MMP-1–cleaved collagen by MMP-9 can alleviate this inhibition (51). Thus, UV-induced MMPs damage the dermis by two related mechanisms: direct degradation of collagen and indirect inhibition of collagen synthesis by MMP-generated collagen degradation products. Since aged skin, similar to photoaged skin, contains elevated levels of partially degraded collagen, the inhibitory effects of collagen fragments found in photoaged skin are also likely to be operative in aged skin and are superimposed on an intrinsic decline in collagen synthetic activity (51). The role of MMP-damaged collagen in inhibiting new collagen synthesis in vivo is not known. However, since the rate of collagen synthesis is proportional to the level of mechanical tension (67,68), we speculate that damaged collagen fibrils are more pliable than native fibrils. As fibroblasts interact with damaged collagen fibrils, the cells experience less resistance and therefore less mechanical tension, resulting in reduced procollagen synthesis.

Mitochondrial DNA in Photoaging

Recent evidence indicates that mtDNA mutations may also be involved in the process of photoaging. It has been demonstrated that chronically sun-exposed, clinically photodamaged skin has a higher mutation frequency of mtDNA than sun-protected skin, with several large-scale deletions of mtDNA in photoaged skin (69–71). A possible link for the involvement of ROS in the generation of the most frequent mtDNA deletion, common deletion, has been provided recently in vitro, where a time- and dose-dependent increase of the common deletion was demonstrated in normal human fibroblasts when repetitively exposed for 3 weeks to sublethal doses of UVA (72). In the same study, it was revealed that this UVA-induced mtDNA mutagenesis was mediated by singlet oxygen. There was a close correlation between the existence of the common deletion and a decrease in mitochondrial function as well as expression of MMP-1 that is causally involved in photoaging, while its tissue-specific inhibitor remained unaltered (52). However, more studies are needed to strengthen the link between mtDNA mutations and the process of photoaging.

SMOKING AND HORMONES

Before closing, two other factors that contribute to skin aging need to be mentioned. It is known that smoking causes premature aging and wrinkling of the face in white (73) and Asian skins (74). Premature wrinkling increases with increased pack-years of smoking. In studies that included white and Asian subjects, heavy smokers (>50 pack-years) were 2.3 –5.5 times more likely to be wrinkled than nonsmokers (73–75). When histories of smoking and excessive sun exposure coexist, the effects of smoking on wrinkling are multiplicative. Chung et al. (76) reported that the combined effect of sun exposure and smoking was synergistic and reported an 11-fold increased risk of wrinkling in sun-exposed smokers versus nonsmokers with a lower level of sun exposure. Yin et al. (76) also reported that subjects with a high pack-year (>30 pack-years) and sun-exposure (>2 hr/day) history in the Japanese people had a 22 times higher risk of developing severe skin wrinkling than subjects who had never smoked and had been less exposed to the sun (<2 hr/day). These studies suggest that cigarette smoking is an important risk factor in the development of skin aging. Furthermore, the detrimental effects of smoking are also synergistic to those induced by aging and sun exposure.

Recently, Chung et al. (74) found that compared with Korean men, Korean women have an increased risk of developing facial wrinkles. Ernster et al. (73) also reported that white women showed a 28-fold increased risk of developing wrinkles with age, compared with a 11.4-fold risk for white men. The reasons why women are more prone to develop wrinkles remain to be elucidated. Several studies have suggested that skin collagen content declines because of hypoestrogenism after menopause (77–79). The significantly decreased skin collagen content in postmenopausal women caused by estrogen deficiency may accelerate or aggravate skin wrinkling due to natural aging and photoaging. Various endocrinological changes such as menstruation, pregnancy, lactation, menopause, history of hormone replacement therapy, etc. may also affect the collagen metabolism in the dermis, contributing to the development of facial wrinkles in women.

Climacteric skin aging is an entity distinct from intrinsic aging and photoaging. Hypoestrogenism has been implicated in many diseases such as osteoporosis and cardiovascular disease in postmenopausal women, and may be involved in the skin aging processes. It is well known that the amount of skin collagen declines in the years following menopause (77–80). Moreover, menopause-related reductions in skin collagen occur at a faster rate during the initial postmenopausal years; approximately 30% is lost in the first 5 years after the menopause (81). The average rate of loss of skin collagen is 2.1% per postmenopausal year (82). However, this menopause-related collagen decrease is not limited to skin, but also occurs in bone and in the urinary tract, thus contributing to the pathogenesis of osteoporosis and stress incontinence. In addition, this postmenopausal decrease in skin collagen content due to estrogen deficiency may aggravate facial wrinkle formation in postmenopausal women.

Based on our data, the risk of wrinkling is significantly greater in men than in women up to the age of 50, after which facial wrinkling starts to accelerate in women. After 70 years of age, Korean women exhibit significantly more severe facial wrinkling than Korean men (personal observation). These observations suggest that in postmenopausal women, hypoestrogenism may contribute more to the decrease in skin collagen than chronological aging.

CONCLUSIONS

Photoaging and intrinsic aging are caused largely by a disruption of finely orchestrated molecular mechanisms that maintain the structural integrity of skin. Two critical mediators of skin aging are the transcription factor AP-1 and AP-1–regulated MMPs. UV irradiation of human skin invokes a complex sequence of events that causes damage to the dermal matrix. Mapping of the UV signaling cascade that leads to MMP induction has identified several potential targets for photoaging prevention strategies. According to the photoaging model described earlier, UV induction of c-Jun is crucial in causing the destruction of the dermal matrix. Therefore, any method of interrupting the UV-induced c-Jun response is likely to prevent photoaging. Topical tRA, which is known to repair photodamage, also blocks UV induction of c-Jun, a key component of AP-1 that is required for MMP expression, thus preventing photoaging. Similar to UVA-induced MMP induction, the generation of mtDNA mutations is due to production of singlet oxygen, indicating that substances with ROS-quenching potential may be utilized to prevent photoaging of human skin.

REFERENCES

1. Kirkwood TB, Cremer T. Cytogerontology since 1881: a reappraisal of August Weismann and a review of modern progress. Hum Genet 1982; 60:101–121.
2. Harman D. Free radical theory of aging. Mutat Res 1992; 275:257–266.
3. Finch CE, Tanzi R. Genetics of aging. Science 1997; 278:407–411.
4. Jazwinsk SM. Longevity, genes, and aging. Science 1996; 273:54–59.
5. Murakami S, Johnson TE. A genetic pathway conferring life extension and resistance to UV stress in *Caenorhabditis elegans*. Genetics 1996; 143:1207–1218.
6. Ross OA, McCormack R, Curran MD, Duguid RA, Barnett YA, Rea IM, Middleton D. Mitochondrial DNA polymorphism: its role in longevity of the Irish population. Exp Gerontol 2001; 36:1161–1178.
7. Harley B, Futcher AB, Greider CW. Telomeres shorten during ageing of human fibroblasts. Nature 1990; 345:458–460.
8. Allsopp RC, Vaziri H, Patterson C, Goldstein S, Younglai EV, Futcher AB, Greider CW, Harley CB. Telomere length predicts replicative capacity of human fibroblasts. Proc Natl Acad Sci U S A 1992; 89:10114–10118.
9. Schulz VP, Zakian VA, Ogburn CE, McKay J, Jarzebowicz AA, Edland SD, Martin GM. Accelerated loss of telomeric repeats may not explain accelerated replicative decline of Werner syndrome cells. Hum Genet 1996; 97:750–754.
10. Prescott JC, Blackburn EH. Telomerase: Dr Jekyll or Mr. Hyde. Curr Opin Genet Dev 1999; 9:368–373.
11. Bachor C, Bachor OA, Boukamp P. Telomerase is active in normal gastrointestinal mucosa and not up-regulated in precancerous lesions. J Cancer Res Clin Oncol 1999; 125:453–460.
12. Lindsey J, McGill NI, Lindsey LA, Green DK, Cooke HJ. In vivo loss of telomeric repeats with age in humans. Mutat Res 1991; 256:45–48.
13. Bodnar AG, Ouellette M, Frolkis M, Holt SE, Chiu CP, Morin GB, Harley CB, Shay JW, Lichtsteiner S, Wright WE. Extension of life-span by introduction of telomerase into normal human cells. Science 1998; 279:349–352.
14. Turker MS, Martin GM. Genetics of human disease, longevity and aging. In: Hazzard WR, Blass JP, Ettinger WH Jr, Halter JB, Eds. Principles of Geriatric Medicine and Gerontology. 4th ed.. London: McGraw-Hill, 1999:21–44.
15. Brown WT. Genetic diseases of premature aging as models of senescence. Annu Rev Gerontol Geriatr 1990; 10:23–42.

16. Goto M, Rubenstein M, Weber J, Woods K, Drayna D. Genetic linkage of Werner's syndrome to five markers on chromosome 8. Nature 1992; 355:735–738.
17. Yu CE, Oshima J, Fu YH, Wijsman EM, Hisama F, Alisch R, Matthews S, Nakura J, Miki T, Ouais S, Martin GM, Mulligan J, Schellenberg GD. Positional cloning of the Werner's syndrome gene. Science 1996; 272:258–262.
18. Harman D. Aging: a theory based on free radical and radiation chemistry. J Gerontol 1956; 11:298–300.
19. Fridovich I. Superoxide dismutases. An adaptation to a paramagnetic gas. J Biol Chem 1989; 264:7761–7764.
20. Linnane AW, Zhang C, Baumer A, Nagley P. Mitochondrial DNA mutation and the ageing process: bioenergy and pharmacological intervention. Mutat Res 1992; 275:195–208.
21. Richter C. Oxidative damage to mitochondrial DNA and its relationship to ageing. Int J Biochem Cell Biol 1995; 27:647–653.
22. Harman D. Aging: overview. Ann N Y Acad Sci 2001; 928:1–21.
23. Merry BJ, Holehan AM. Onset of puberty and duration of fertility in rats fed a restricted diet. J Reprod Fertil 1979; 57:253–259.
24. Holehan AM, Merry BJ. The experimental manipulation of ageing by diet. Biol Rev Camb Philos Soc 1986; 61:329–368.
25. Sohal RS, Weindruch R. Oxidative stress, caloric restriction, and aging. Science 1996; 273: 59–63.
26. Lee CK, Klopp RG, Weindruch R, Prolla TA. Gene expression profile of aging and its retardation by caloric restriction. Science 1999; 285:1390–1393.
27. Youngman LD, Park JY, Ames BN. Protein oxidation associated with aging is reduced by dietary restriction of protein or calories. Proc Natl Acad Sci U S A 1992; 89:9112–9116.
28. Yaar M, Gilchrest BA. Skin aging: postulated mechanisms and consequent changes in structure and function. Clin Geriatr Med 2001; 17:617–630.
29. Yaar M, Eller MS, Gilchrest BA. Fifty years of skin aging. J Invest Dermatol Symp Proc 2002; 7:51–58.
30. Kawaguchi Y, Tanaka H, Okada T, Konishi H, Takahashi M, Ito M, Asai J. The effects of ultraviolet A and reactive oxygen species on the mRNA expression of 72-kDa type IV collagenase and its tissue inhibitor in cultured human dermal fibroblasts. Arch Dermatol Res 1996; 288:39–44.
31. Packer JE, Slater TF, Willson RL. Direct observation of a free radical interaction between vitamin E and vitamin C. Nature 1979; 278:737–738.
32. Martensson J, Meister A, Mrtensson J. Glutathione deficiency decreases tissue ascorbate levels in newborn rats: ascorbate spares glutathione and protects. Proc Natl Acad Sci U S A 1991; 88:4656–60.
33. Lopez-Torres M, Thiele JJ, Shindo Y, Han D, Packer L. Topical application of alpha-tocopherol modulates the antioxidant network and diminishes ultraviolet-induced oxidative damage in murine skin. Br J Dermatol 1998; 138:207–215.
34. Rhie G, Shin MH, Seo JY, Choi WW, Cho KH, Kim KH, Park KC, Eun HC, Chung JH. Aging- and photoaging-dependent changes of enzymic and nonenzymic antioxidants in the epidermis and dermis of human skin in vivo. J Invest Dermatol 2001; 117:1212–1217.
35. Varani J, Warner RL, Gharaee-Kermani M, Phan SH, Kang S, Chung JH, Wang ZQ, Datta SC, Fisher GJ, Voorhees JJ. Vitamin A antagonizes decreased cell growth and elevated collagen-degrading matrix metalloproteinases and stimulates collagen accumulation in naturally aged human skin. J Invest Dermatol 2000; 114:480–486.
36. Chung JH, Seo JY, Choi HR, Lee MK, Youn CS, Rhie G, Cho KH, Kim KH, Park KC, Eun HC. Modulation of skin collagen metabolism in aged and photoaged human skin in vivo. J Invest Dermatol 2001; 117:1218–1224.
37. Waskiewicz AJ, Cooper JA. Mitogen and stress response pathways: MAP kinase cascades and phosphatase regulation in mammals and yeast. Curr Opin Cell Biol 1995; 7:798–805.

38. Robinson MJ, Cobb MH. Mitogen-activated protein kinase pathways. Curr Opin Cell Biol 1997; 9:180–186.
39. Xia Z, Dickens M, Raingeaud J, Davis RJ, Greenberg ME. Opposing effects of ERK and JNK-p38 MAP kinases on apoptosis. Science 1995; 270:1326–1331.
40. Rosette C, Karin M. Ultraviolet light and osmotic stress: activation of the JNK cascade through multiple growth factor and cytokine receptors. Science 1996; 274:1194–1197.
41. Gum R, Wang H, Lengyel E, Juarez J, Boyd D. Regulation of 92 kDa type IV collagenase expression by the jun aminoterminal kinase- and the extracellular signal-regulated kinase-dependent signaling cascades. Oncogene 1997; 14:1481–1493.
42. Davis BH, Chen A, Beno DW. Raf and mitogen-activated protein kinase regulate stellate cell collagen gene expression. J Biol Chem 1996; 271:11039–11042.
43. Chen A, Beno DW, Davis BH. Suppression of stellate cell type I collagen gene expression involves AP-2 transmodulation of nuclear factor-1-dependent gene transcription. J Biol Chem 1996; 271:25994–25998.
44. Ham J, Babij C, Whitfield J, Pfarr CM, Lallemand D, Yaniv M, Rubin LL. A c-Jun dominant negative mutant protects sympathetic neurons against programmed cell death. Neuron 1995; 14:927–939.
45. Verheij M, Bose R, Lin XH, Yao B, Jarvis WD, Grant S, Birrer MJ, Szabo E, Zon LI, Kyriakis JM, Haimovitz-Friedman A, Fuks Z, Kolesnick RN. Requirement for ceramide-initiated SAPK/JNK signalling in stress-induced apoptosis. Nature 1996; 380:75–79.
46. Whitmarsh AJ, Davis RJ. Transcription factor AP-1 regulation by mitogen-activated protein kinase signal transduction pathways. J Mol Med 1996; 74:589–607.
47. Fisher GJ, Datta SC, Talwar HS, Wang ZQ, Varani J, Kang S, Voorhees JJ. Molecular basis of sun-induced premature skin ageing and retinoid antagonism. Nature 1996; 379:335–339.
48. Chung KY, Agarwal A, Uitto J, Mauviel A. An AP-1 binding sequence is essential for regulation of the human alpha2(I) collagen (COL1A2) promoter activity by transforming growth factor-beta. J Biol Chem 1996; 271:3272–3278.
49. Chung JH, Kang S, Varani J, Lin J, Fisher GJ, Voorhees JJ. Decreased extracellular-signal-regulated kinase and increased stress-activated MAP kinase activities in aged human skin in vivo. J Invest Dermatol 2000; 115:177–182.
50. Kligman AM. Early destructive effects of sunlight on human skin. JAMA 1969; 210: 2377–2380.
51. Fisher GJ, Kang S, Varani J, Bata-Csorgo Z, Wan Y, Datta S, Voorhees JJ. Mechanisms of photoaging and chronological skin aging. Arch Dermatol 2002; 138:1462–1470.
52. Berneburg M, Plettenberg H, Krutmann J. Photoaging of human skin. Photodermatol Photoimmunol Photomed 2000; 16:239–244.
53. Duell EA, Kang S, Voorhees JJ. Endogenous antioxidant enzyme activities in human skin are decreased by four but not one exposure to ultraviolet light [abstr]. J Invest Dermatol 1999; 112:657.
54. Lo Y, Cruz T. Involvement of reactive oxygen species in cytokine and growth factor induction of c-Fos expressions in chondrocytes. J Biol Chem 1995; 270:11727–11730.
55. Whisler RL, Goyette MA, Grants IS, Newhouse YG. Sublethal levels of oxidant stress stimulate multiple serine/threonine kinases and suppress protein phosphatases in Jurkat T cells. Arch Biochem Biophys 1995; 319:23–35.
56. Fisher GJ, Talwar HS, Lin JY, Lin P, McPhillips F, Wang Z, Li X, Wan Y, Kang S, Voorhees JJ. Retinoic acid inhibits induction of c-Jun protein by ultraviolet radiation that occurs subsequent to activation of mitogen-activated protein kinase pathways in human skin in vivo. J Clin Invest 1998; 101:1432–1440.
57. Karin M, Liu ZG, Zandi E. AP-1 function and regulation. Curr Opin Cell Biol 1997; 9:240–246.
58. Angel P, Szabowski A, Schorpp-Kistner M. Function and regulation of AP-1 subunits in skin physiology and pathology. Oncogene 2001; 20:2413–2423.

59. Fisher GJ, Voorhees JJ. Molecular mechanisms of photoaging and its prevention by retinoic acid: ultraviolet irradiation induces MAP kinase signal transduction cascades that induce AP-1-regulated matrix metalloproteinases that degrade human skin in vivo. J Invest Dermatol 1998; 3(suppl):S61–S68.
60. Senftleben U, Karin M. The IKK/NF-κB pathway. Crit Care Med 2002; 30(suppl 1):S19–S26.
61. Yamamoto Y, Gaynor RB. Therapeutic potential of inhibition of the NF-κB pathway in the treatment of inflammation and cancer. J Clin Invest 2001; 107:135–142.
62. Fisher GJ, Datta S, Wang ZQ, Lin XY, Quan T, Chung JH, Kang S, Voorhees JJ. c-Jun-dependent inhibition of cutaneous procollagen transcription following ultraviolet irradiation is reversed by all-trans retinoic acid. J Clin Invest 2000; 106:663–670.
63. Quan T, He TY, Voorhees JJ, Fisher GJ. Ultraviolet irradiation blocks cellular responses to transforming growth factor-β by down regulating its type-II receptor and inducing Smad7. J Biol Chem 2001; 276:26349–26356.
64. Kang S, Fisher GJ, Voorhees JJ. Photoaging: pathogenesis, prevention, and treatment. Clin Geriatr Med 2001; 17:643–659.
65. Fisher GJ, Wang ZQ, Datta SC, Varani J, Kang S, Voorhees JJ. Pathophysiology of premature skin aging induced by ultraviolet light. N Engl J Med 1997; 337:1419–1428.
66. Varani J, Spearman D, Perone P, Fligiel SE, Datta SC, Wang ZQ, Shao Y, Kang S, Fisher GJ, Voorhees JJ. Inhibition of type I procollagen synthesis by damaged collagen in photoaged skin and by collagenase-degraded collagen in vitro. Am J Pathol 2001; 158:931–942.
67. Lambert C, Colige A, Lapiere C, Nusgens B. Coordinated regulation of procollagens I and III and their post-translational enzymes by dissipation of mechanical tension in human dermal fibroblasts. Eur J Cell Biol 2001; 80:479–485.
68. Kessler D, Dethlefsen S, Haase I, Plomann M, Hirche F, Krieg T, Eckes B. Fibroblasts in mechanically stressed collagen lattices assume a ''synthetic'' phenotype. J Biol Chem 2001; 279:36575–36585.
69. Yang JH, Lee HC, Lin KJ, Wei YH. A specific 4977-bp deletion of mitochondrial DNA is human ageing skin. Arch Dermatol Res 1994; 286:386–390.
70. Berneburg M, Gattermann N, Stege H, Grewe M, Vogelsang K, Ruzicka T, Krutmann J. Chronically ultraviolet-exposed human skin shows a higher mutation frequency of mitochondrial DNA as compared to unexposed skin and the hematopoietic system. Photochem Photobiol 1997; 66:271–275.
71. Birch-Machin MA, Tindall M, Turner R, Haldane F, Rees JL. Mitochondrial DNA deletions in human skin reflect photo- rather than chronologic aging. J Invest Dermatol 1998; 110: 149–152.
72. Berneburg M, Grether-Beck S, Kürten V, Ruzicka T, Briviba K, Sies H, Krutmann J. Singlet oxygen mediates the UVA-induced generation of the photoaging-associated mitochondrial common deletion. J Biol Chem 1999; 274:15345–15349.
73. Ernster VL, Grady D, Miike R, Black D, Selby J, Kerlikowske K. Facial wrinkling in men and women, by smoking status. Am J Public Health 1995; 85:78–82.
74. Chung JH, Lee SH, Youn CS, Park BJ, Kim KH, Park KC, Cho KH, Eun HC. Cutaneous photodamage in Koreans: influence of sex, sun exposure, smoking, and skin color. Arch Dermatol 2001; 137:1043–1051.
75. Kadunce DP, Burr R, Gress R, Kanner R, Lyon JL, Zone JJ. Cigarette smoking: risk factor for premature facial wrinkling. Ann Intern Med 1991; 114:840–844.
76. Yin L, Morita A, Tsuji T. Skin aging induced by ultraviolet exposure and tobacco smoking: evidence from epidemiological and molecular studies. Photodermatol Photoimmunol Photomed 2001; 17:178–183.
77. Brincat M, Moniz CJ, Studd JW, Darby A, Magos A, Emburey G, Versi E. Long-term effects of the menopause and sex hormones on skin thickness. Br J Obstet Gynaecol 1985; 92:256–259.
78. Brincat M, Moniz CF, Kabalan S, Versi E, O'Dowd T, Magos AL, Montgomery J, Studd JW. Decline in skin collagen content and metacarpal index after the menopause and its prevention with sex hormone replacement. Br J Obstet Gynaecol 1987; 94:126–129.

79. Brincat M, Versi E, Moniz CF, Magos A, de Trafford J, Studd JW. Skin collagen changes in postmenopausal women receiving different regimens of estrogen therapy. Obstet Gynecol 1987; 70:123–127.
80. Castelo-Branco C, Duran M, Gonzalez-Merlo J. Skin collagen changes related to age and hormone replacement therapy. Maturitas 1992; 15:113–119.
81. Brincat M, Kabalan S, Studd JW, Moniz CF, de Trafford J, Montgomery J. A study of the decrease of skin collagen content, skin thickness, and bone mass in the postmenopausal woman. Obstet Gynecol 1987; 70:840–845.
82. Brincat M, Studd J. Skin and menopause. In: Whitehead MI, Studd JWW, Eds. The Menopause. Oxford: Blackwell Scientific Publications, 1988:24–42.

2

Acute and Chronic Effects of UV on Skin

What Are They and How to Study Them?

D. Moyal / A. Fourtanier *L'Oréal Recherche, Clichy, France*

- Ultraviolet (UV) B-induced erythema peaks at 6–24 hours, whereas erythema induced by UVA may be observed from 2–24 hours.
- UVA induces immediate pigment darkening (at 0–2 hr) and persistent pigment darkening (which can last several hours to days after exposure).
- Delayed tanning can be induced by both UVA and UVB; it becomes visible within 3 days.
- UV exposure suppresses immunity; UVA plays an active role in photoimmunosuppression.
- There is a strong association between sun exposure and the development of nonmelanoma skin cancer; the role of sunlight in melanoma is less clearly defined.

Acute and repeated sun exposure provoke short-term as well as long-term effects on skin, ranging from sunburn and suntan to the development of skin aging and skin cancer. The various types of sun damage have been defined clinically and histologically, and in the last 10 years knowledge of the underlying molecular and cellular events has increased.

Laboratories studies have enabled a better understanding of the differences between the effects due to ultraviolet (UV) B (290–320 nm) and UVA (320–400 nm) radiation. This has been possible because of the enormous progress made in UV simulation, dosimetry, and spectrophotometry. With reconstructed human skin models, it has also become possible to study the effects of radiation on the epidermis and on the dermis and to elucidate mechanisms.

This chapter begins with a few basic principles of photobiology and will be followed by a review of the different types of photodamage ranging from erythema to photocarcinogenesis. Some experimental methods used to reproduce and to study the effects of UV radiation on the skin will be described.

BASIC PRINCIPLES OF PHOTOBIOLOGY

Solar UV Radiation

The electromagnetic spectrum emitted by the sun ranges from the very short cosmic rays to the very long radio waves and beyond. About 9% of solar radiation is in the form of UV radiation. Most of the photocutaneous changes that occur are due to UV radiation. There are three categories of UV radiation. UVC rays, which are the shortest in wavelength, extend from 100 to 290 nm. No wavelengths shorter than 290 nm reach the earth's surface, primarily because of filtration by the ozone layer. In contrast, UVB rays (290–320 nm) reach the earth's surface and are responsible for most of the cutaneous photobiological events. UVA (320–400 nm) rays pass through window glass and have been divided into UVA1 (340–400 nm) and UVA2 (320–340 nm) categories.

Because of the elliptical orbit of the earth around the sun, the distance between the sun and the earth varies by about 3.4% over the year. This results in a variation in intensity of about 7% and in slightly higher levels of UV radiation in summers in the southern compared to the northern hemisphere. The quality (spectrum) and the quantity (intensity) of terrestrial UV radiation vary with the elevation of the sun above the horizon, or solar altitude. The solar altitude depends on the time of the day, day of year, and geographical location (latitude and longitude). On a summer's day, the UV energy received (daily dose) on the surface of the earth comprises approximately 3.5% UVB and 96.5% UVA (1).

Examples of how UVB and UVA irradiances vary along a clear summer's day and how UVB and UVA daily doses vary throughout the year in Sophia Antipolis (south of France) are shown in Figures 1 and 2, respectively.

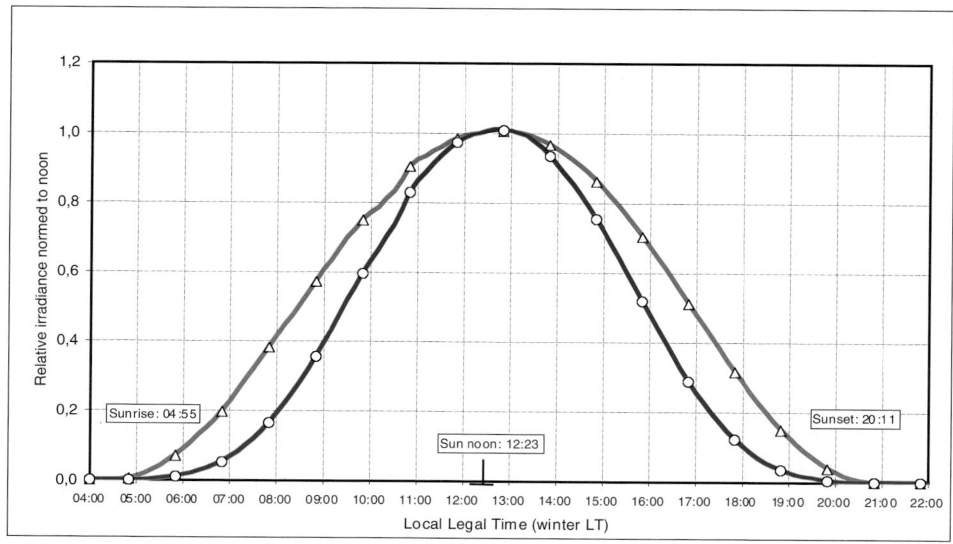

Figure 1 Sun UVB (○) and UVA (Δ;) relative irradiance versus time, during a clear June day in Sophia Antipolis, France (43°38′ N-7°3′E).

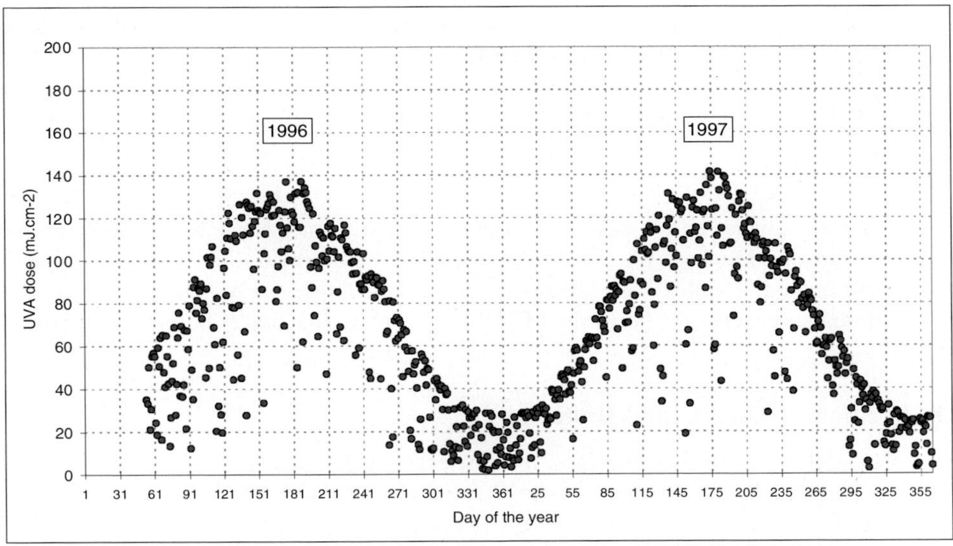

Figure 2 Cumulated daily UVA dose throughout 2 years measured at Sophia Antipolis, France (43°38′ N-7°3′E).

UV Radiation and Skin

Of the UVB radiation reaching the skin, 70% is absorbed by the stratum corneum, 20% reaches the viable epidermis, and only 10 % reaches the upper part of the dermis. UVA radiation is absorbed partly by the epidermis, but 20% to 30% of this radiation reaches the deep dermis. Thus, UVA rays are more penetrating than UVB rays. The major chromophores that determine the depth of penetration are nucleic acids, aromatic amino acids, and melanin.

SIMULATION OF UV RADIATION FOR LABORATORY STUDIES

Solar UV Simulation

The relevance and reliability of all laboratories studies depend on having a UV source that reproduces as closely as possible the UV emission spectra of the sun at ground level. Of course, the output and stability of the source have to be higher than those of the sun for practical reasons and reproducibility.

Today, more and more investigations are conducted with UV solar simulators equipped with a xenon arc source. This lamp has a smooth continuous emission spectrum that may match the UV solar ones provided correct filtering systems are added in the light beam. By fitting this source with a Schott WG 320 filter of appropriate thickness (between 1 and 2 mm), UVC and short UVB radiation can be eliminated to mimic the ozone effect. This source also emits visible and infrared radiation that can be reduced or cut off by other optical filters (Schott UG11 or UG5 filters of 1-mm or 3-mm thickness) and/or dichroic mirrors.

From the same light source it is also possible to obtain the total UVA spectrum (UVA1 and UVA2: 320–400 nm) or long UVA (UVA1: 340–400 nm) by using a WG 335/3 mm or a WG 365/1 mm Schott filter instead of the WG 320. A UG11 filter may be added depending on whether the short visible is to be rejected.

Radiometry

The spectral irradiance of the source received on the test surface has to be measured before each experiment. The best way to do this is to use a calibrated double-monochromator spectroradiometer, coupled with adequate integral calculation. However, routine control of the irradiance is generally performed with broadband sensors and radiometers or thermopiles.

UV Irradiance, Doses, and Units

Energetic radiant intensities received on the test surface (irradiance) are expressed by photobiologists in watts per square meter (W/m^2) or derived unit (mW/cm^2). The energetic exposure dose is equal to the energetic irradiance multiplied by the exposure time in seconds and expressed in joules per square meter (J/m^2).

It must be noticed that the same UV energetic dose delivered by two different UV simulator spectra to the same subject can result in different biological effects, depending on the product of the emission spectrum of the source and the action spectra of the biological damage considered. Therefore, biological study reports and publications must always include the emission spectra of the UV sources used. Excellent papers have reviewed this subject (1–3).

UV ERYTHEMA AND PIGMENTATION

In this section, we will discuss the erythemal and tanning effects of UVA and UVB radiation as observed visually and quantified by colorimetric measurements (L*a*b* color space) (4). L^* represents the lightness (or luminance) of the skin, on a scale of 0 (black) to 100 (white); a^* represents the red component of the skin; and b^* represents the yellow component of the skin.

Erythema

Erythema (sunburn) is an acute cutaneous inflammatory reaction associated with redness that follows excessive exposure to UV radiation. Erythema is readily visible by noninvasive methods and can be monitored over time. It is used as the end-point for many photobiological studies.

The erythema reaction to UV radiation depends on the waveband range. UVA has been broken down into two bands because of the increased erythemogenic activity of UVA2 compared to UVA1. The relative effectiveness of different wavelengths in producing erythema, called the action spectrum, shows that erythemal effectiveness declines considerably with increasing wavelengths. Figure 3 gives the relative action spectrum of erythema at 24 hours after exposure, according to the CIE-1987 standard (5).

UVB-induced erythema is a delayed response. It reaches its peak at 6–24 hr depending on dose (6). Its intensity is dose dependent (Fig. 4). This erythema fades over a day or longer, depending on the dose and on the skin type (7). For skin type I, it may last

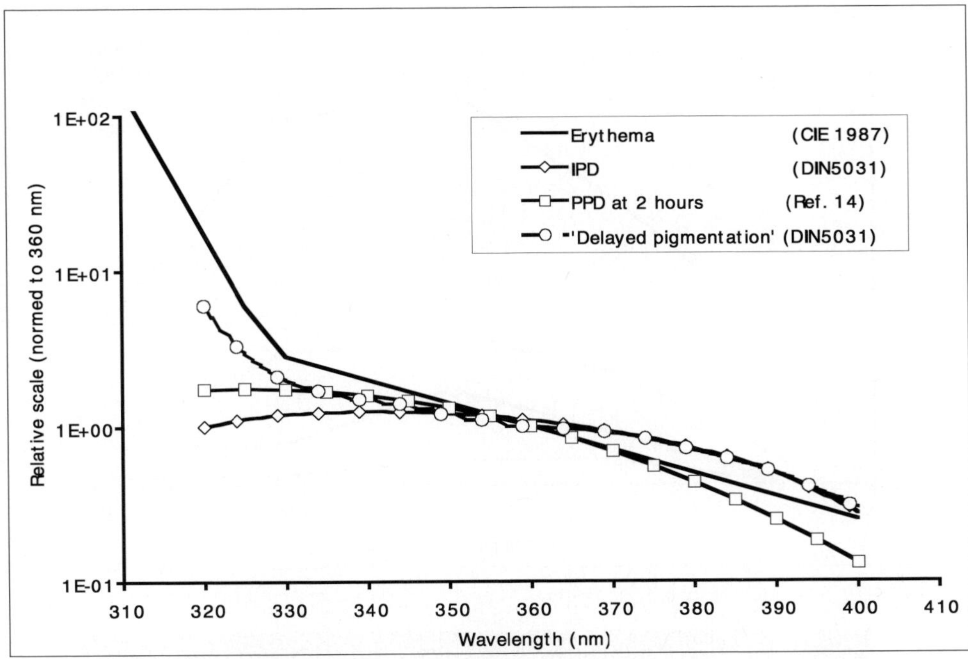

Figure 3 Action spectra of the various responses of the skin to UV exposure: erythema, transient immediate pigment darkening (IPD), persistent pigment darkening (PPD), and delayed pigmentation (neomelanization).

longer compared to skin type III or IV (8). Although the final reaction is an increase in redness of the skin, the time course and the dose response of erythema of UVB and UVA wavebands is different. UVA radiation is 1000-fold less effective than UVB in producing skin erythema. UVA induced erythema contributes towards at least 15% of the total sunlight-induced erythema and is an immediate reaction already present at the end of the irradiation period (9). Care should be taken by appropriate means not to confuse the actinic UVA erythema with the immediate erythema induced by heat load due to the infrared radiation that is usually present to some extend in UV sources. Actinic UVA erythema fades partly within 2 hours. However, for high UVA doses on skin type I, persistent erythema is observed from 2 to 24 hours (Fig. 5). Immediate and persistent UVA erythema is easily inducible with relatively low UVA doses (10–30 J/cm^2) on very fair skin (skin type I). Conversely, higher UVA doses (>30 J/cm^2) are necessary to induce erythema on darker skin (skin type III and IV). In this case, UVA erythema is mixed with persistent pigment darkening response (10).

The time course of UVA induced erythema is similar to that of the persistent pigment-darkening reaction. The presence of oxygen is required for both reactions, whereas UVB-induced erythema is oxygen independent (11). These observations suggest that UVA- and UVB-induced erythema involve different chromophores (12).

The smallest dose causing a minimally perceptible erythema with well-defined borders on the site of irradiation 24 hr after irradiation is called the minimal erythema dose

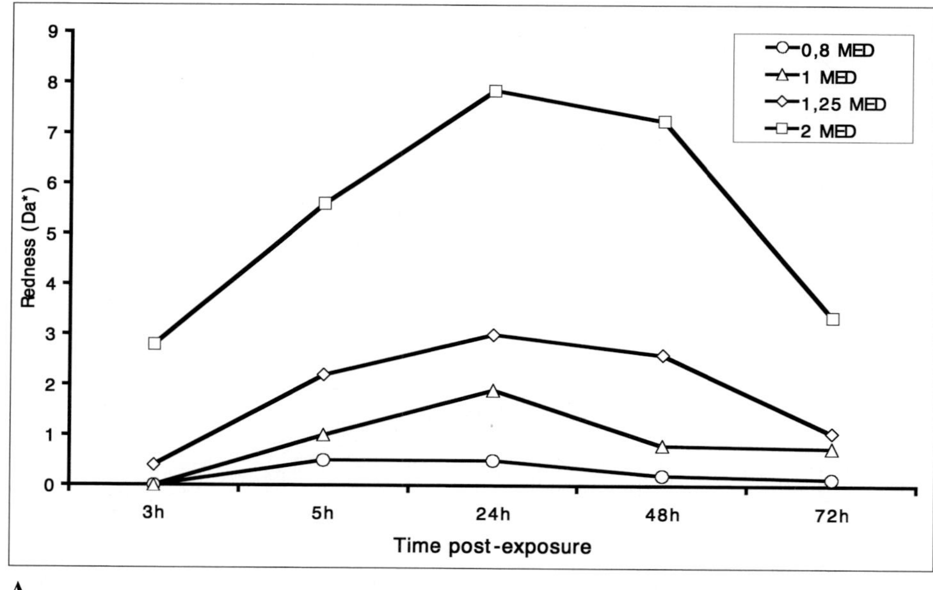

A

B

Figure 4 (a) Erythema dose response and kinetic for UVB radiation in skin type I/II volunteers, and (b) clinical aspect 24 hr after exposure from 0.6 MED to 2 MED with a 1.25 progression.

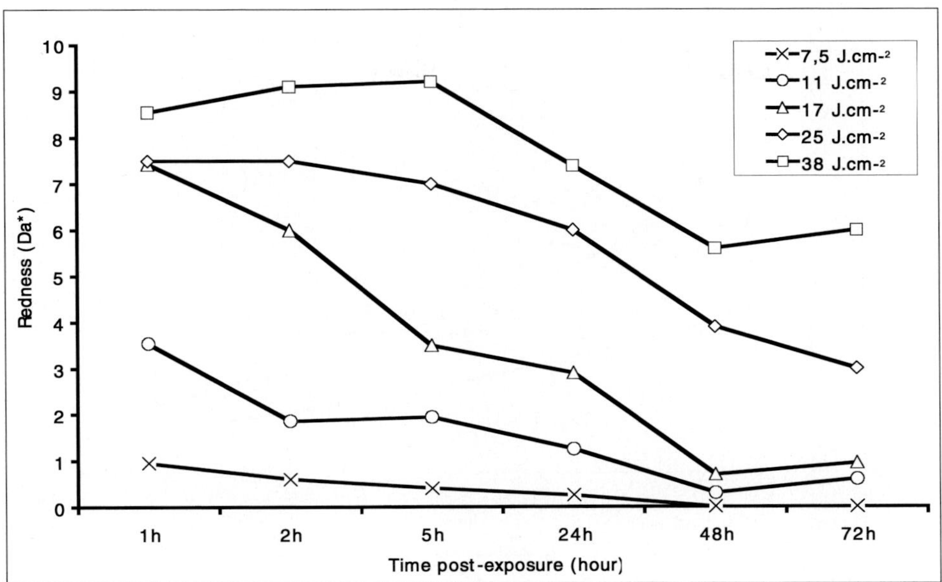

Figure 5 Erythema dose response and kinetic for UVA radiation in skin type I/II volunteers.

(MED). This biological value obviously varies from one subject to another depending on skin phototype, skin color typing, and anatomical sites. Constitutional pigmentation is well described in the L* vs. b* colorimetric plane (13). Skin color categories have been defined according to the so-called individual typology angle (ITA°), which is calculated by the following formula:

$$ITA^\circ = \text{Arctangent}((L^* - 50)/b^*) \times 180/3.14$$

The values proposed for the angles of skin categories boundaries are:

Very light skin > 55° > Light skin > 44° > Intermediate skin > 28° > Mat/Tan skin >10°

Figure 6 illustrates the relationship between skin color typing defined by the ITA° values and MED values determined on the back of volunteers 24 hr after exposure to solar simulator (xenon arc lamp complying with Colipa recommendations) (unpublished results, 2003). As shown on this figure, the MED values decrease when ITA° values increase.

Pigmentation

The skin pigmentation response following exposure to sunlight comprises an immediate tanning reaction and the delayed formation of new melanins. The tanning response of human skin depends on the wavelength of radiation.

During a short single exposure to UVA radiation in skin types III or IV, a dark-bluish pigmentation ($\Delta L^* << 0$, $\Delta b^* < 0$, $\Delta a^* > 0$) develops with doses smaller than 6 J/cm^2 (14). This phenomenon named immediate pigment darkening (IPD) is transient and fades in about 2 hr after the end of exposure. IPD has been attributed to the photo-oxidation of pre-existing melanins and melanin precursors (9).

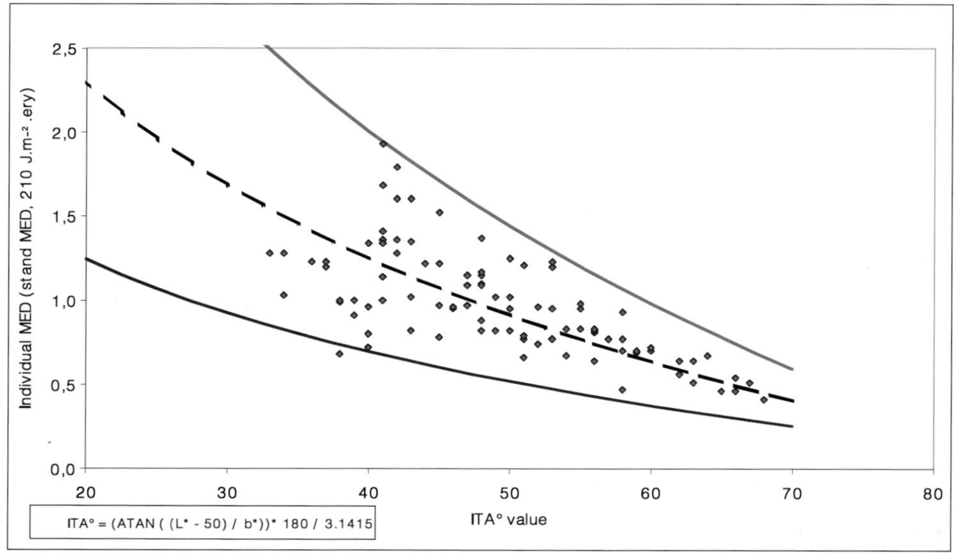

Figure 6 MED versus ITA° in skin type I, II, and III volunteers.

For UVA doses higher than about 10 J/cm^2, a stable residual pigmentation named persistent pigment darkening (PPD) is observed after the transient part of IPD has faded away (Fig. 7) (14) . Although induced with different dose ranges, both IPD and PPD phenomena result from an immediate UVA effect. While various UVA doses are applied to skin (phototypes II–IV), an immediate grey-blue pigmentation develops, reaching its maximum at end of exposure. Then, the transient part of this pigmentation (IPD) quickly fades away. If the UVA dose was sufficient a persistent part (PPD) may last for several hours or days.

The UVA dose required to induce a minimal PPD is about 15 J/cm^2 and represents a little less than the amount received in 1 hr of exposure to a quasi-zenithal sun. Figure 3 gives the relative action spectra of IPD (15) as observed immediately at the end of exposure and PPD as observed 2 hr after exposure (14).

Through colorimetric follow-up, the color of the residual PPD pigmentation cannot be confused with that of the delayed pigmentation resulting from neomelanization (Fig. 8), because the latter occurs with a typical brown (dark yellow) color, similar to basic melanins, and only in the following conditions: after UVA induced erythema on dark skin (phototypes III–V) with UVA doses higher than 60 J/cm^2; on very fair skin (phototype I) with UVA doses higher than 15 J/cm^2; or after successive UVA exposures on all phototypes even by suberythemogenic doses (16,17) but cumulating a sufficient dose. Colorimetric follow-up clearly confirmed that neomelanization starts with a 3-day delay after UVA exposure.

UVB-induced erythema is followed by pigmentation. There is no pigmentation production after UVB exposure unless there is a preceding erythema response. Whereas the time courses of UVA and UVB erythema differ markedly from each other, the time courses of UVA and UVB delayed tanning, though induced with very different UV energetic

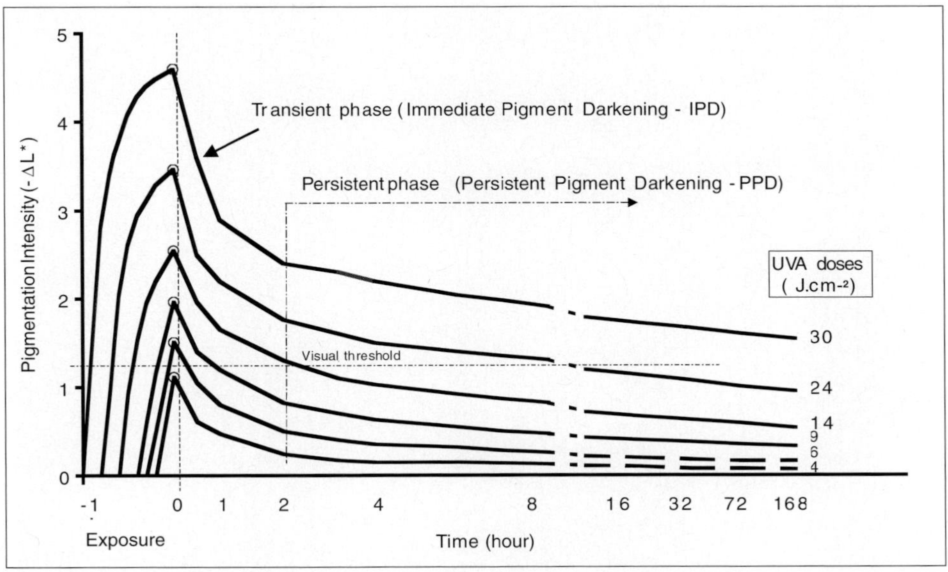

Figure 7 Kinetic and dose-effect of immediate pigment darkening (IPD) and persistent pigment darkening (PPD) skin response.

doses, are similar. Delayed tanning becomes visible within 3 days after exposure. The action spectrum for tanning observed 7 days after exposure is broadly similar to that for erythema (Fig. 3) (15).

Melanization acquired by cumulative UVA exposure appears to be much more longer lasting (several months or even a year) than that acquired with UVB exposure. This difference is probably due to the more basal localization of UVA-induced pigment. UVB-induced melanization disappears with epidermal turnover within a month.

DNA DAMAGE

The adverse effects of solar radiation are mostly attributed to the DNA damage. Cellular DNA directly absorbs UVB, and this absorption causes lesions at the pyrimidine bases, which become covalently linked and distort the DNA helix. These lesions are cyclobutane-pyrimidine dimers (CPDs), 6-4 photoproducts (6-4 PPs), and Dewar isomers (formed by photoisomerization of 6-4 PPs). The CPDs are the most abundant and probably the most cytotoxic lesions as they block transcription and replication. If they are not repaired, they can lead to misreading of the genetic code and cause mutations and cell death.

UVA radiation also damages the DNA but less than UVB radiation. UVA damage is induced indirectly, through absorption by other endogenous chromophores that release reactive forms of oxygen. These free radicals alter the purines or cause strand breaks. The most abundant UVA-induced DNA lesion, 8-hydroxy-2′deoxyguanosine (8-OHdG), is highly mutagenic if not repaired (18).

Fortunately, the cells have several mechanisms to repair the DNA lesions. First they are halted in their replicative cycle to allow extra time for repair. The *p53* gene product

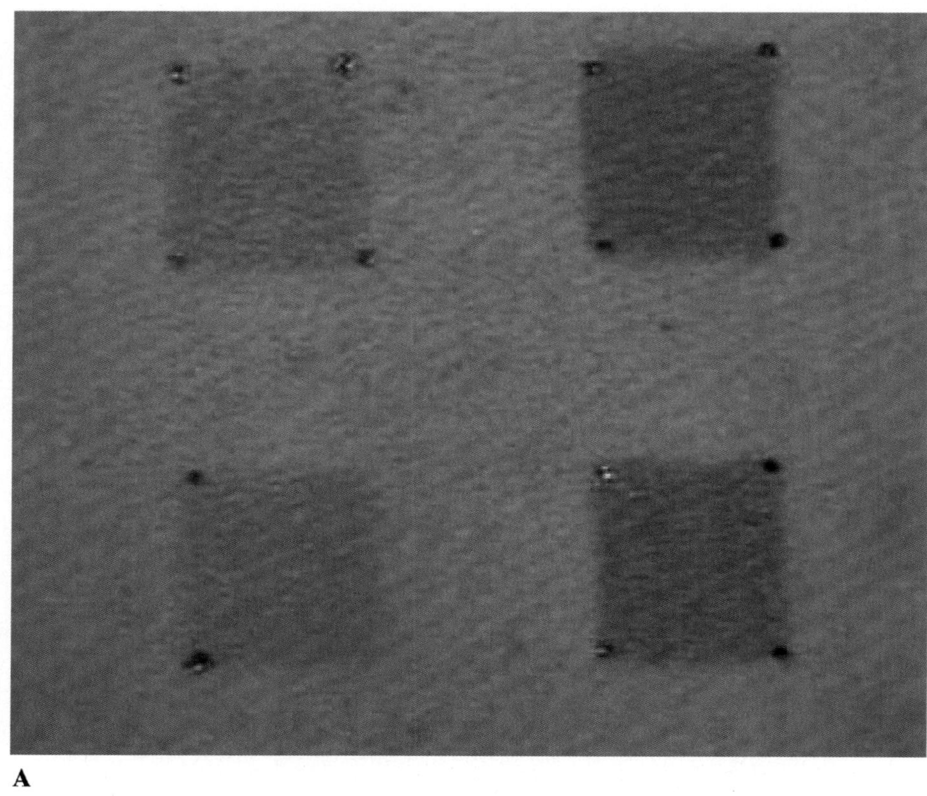

A

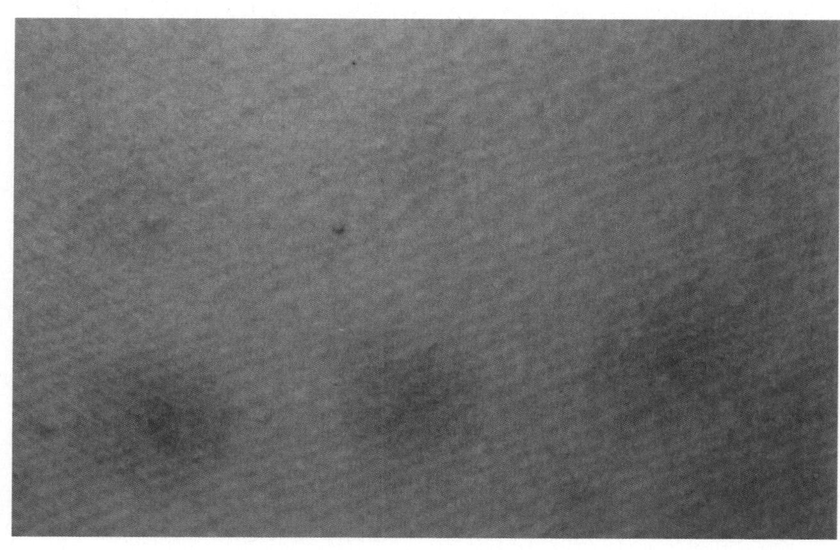

B

Figure 8 Clinical aspect of (a) neomelanization and (b) persistent pigment darkening reaction.

appears to play an important role in this arrest. Moreover, the p53 protein may force the cell to undergo apoptosis if the cell is overly damaged and the risk of gene mutation becomes too great (19). The apoptotic cells induced by UV in the epidermis (Fig. 9) are called sunburn cells (SBC) (20–22).

The most frequent repair mechanism used by the cells is called excision repair. Altered bases or nucleotides are removed and replaced by new, undamaged elements. The enzymes involved in this repair system are glycosylases, endonucleases, and polymerases. Photoreactivation, the other repair mechanism, involves only one enzyme, photolyase, which reverses the damage using the energy of light. Photolyase seems to be absent or nonfunctional in humans. However, it has recently been shown that topical application of this enzyme on human skin repairs the CPDs induced by UV radiation (23).

DNA damage can induce mutations in oncogenes and tumor-suppressor genes. These mutations may lead to gene dysfunction. For example, UV-induced *p53* tumor suppressor

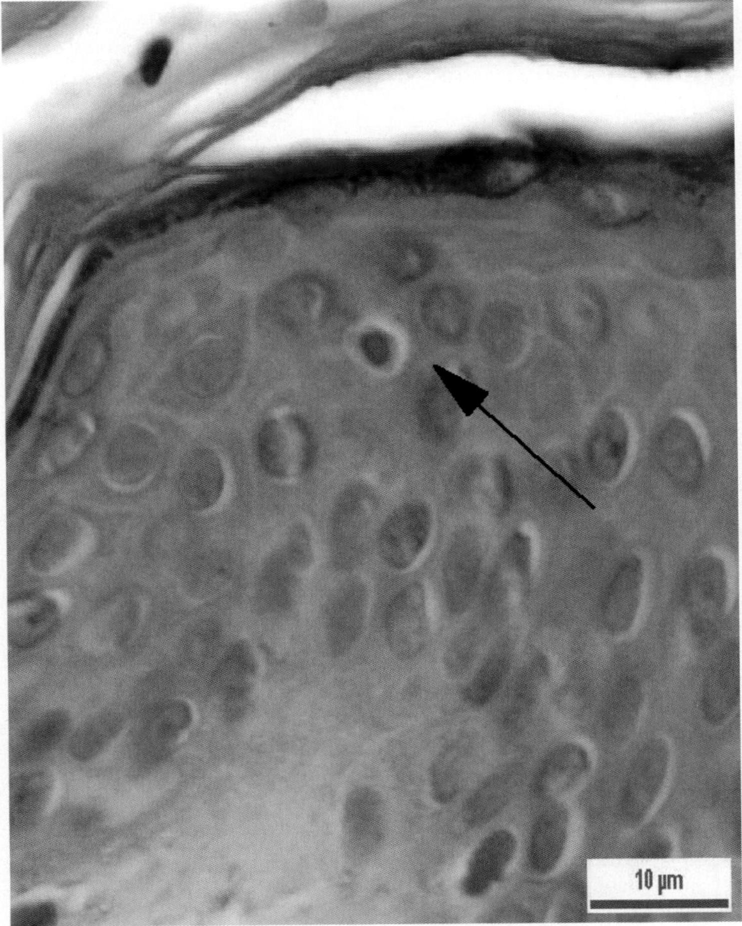

Figure 9 A sunburn cell (SBC) originally described on the basis of its pyknotic nucleus and shrunken and eosinophilic cytoplasm.

gene mutations alter the p53 protein function, facilitate further mutations in other cancer genes, and enhance tumor development. *p53* mutations at dipyrimidine sites are found in a majority of human skin carcinomas.

Several methods exist for quantifying DNA damage and repair. A recent method is an in vitro test called the comet assay (24). This test analyses the number of breaks induced in the DNA by UV exposure or by the DNA repair enzymes in single cells. This assay can be performed with keratinocytes, fibroblasts, or melanocytes (25). DNA lesions and p53 deposition are currently evaluated on skin sections using lesion-specific antibodies or p53 antibodies and immunofluorescence or immunoperoxidase techniques (Fig. 10).

In vivo studies on human volunteers may be difficult to set up, particularly when biopsies have to be done. It has been shown that it is possible to reconstruct human skin *in vitro* with a living dermal equivalent and a fully differentiated epidermis (26). Using this model, it has been possible to show that UVB radiation induces the formation of SBC and CPD in the DNA of epidermal cells (27), and that UVA radiation induces apoptosis of fibroblasts, located in the upper dermis, and secretion of collagenase I, a matrix-degrading enzyme, in the culture medium (28). This skin model appears to be a useful tool for studying the effects of UV radiation *in vitro*. The recent success of introduction of melanocytes and Langerhans cells (LC) in the reconstructed epidermis should contribute to the improvement of the model (29,30).

PHOTOIMMUNOSUPPRESSION

It is well established that UV exposure can suppress immunity. This phenomenon is called photoimmunosuppression. Accumulating evidence indicates that photoimmunosuppres-

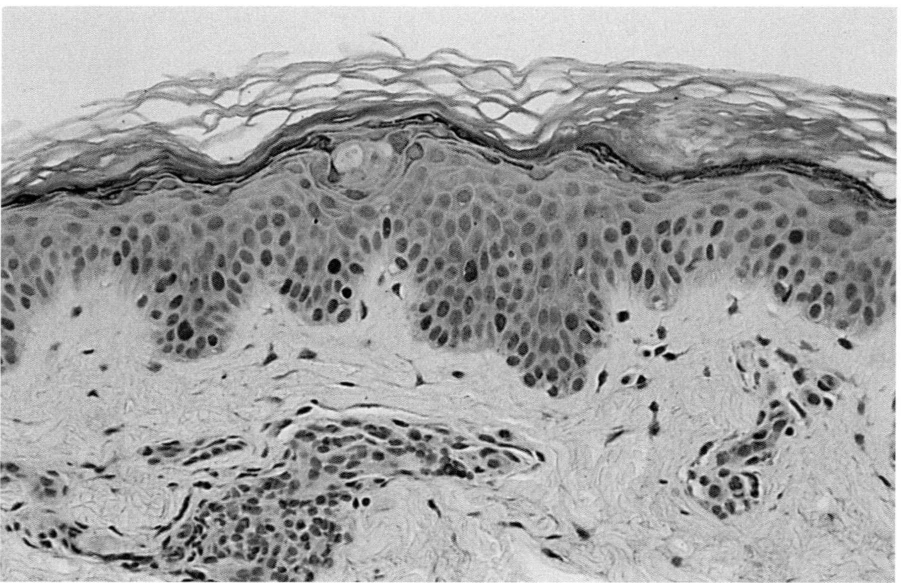

Figure 10 p53 protein accumulation visualized by dense brown-red nuclear coloration in UV-exposed human epidermis.

sion plays an important role in the development of skin cancer, increases the incidence and the severity of infections and viral diseases, and decreases vaccine effectiveness.

The sequence of events leading to this immune-suppression phenomenon has been extensively studied in the last 10 years. The initiating events seem to be DNA damage and *trans* to *cis* urocanic acid isomerization. As a result of these alterations, various cytokines, histamine, and neuropeptides are produced. These mediators act on different skin and blood cell populations. Some LC migrate from skin to the lymph nodes, whereas others are altered and become ineffective or undergo apoptosis (31). Macrophages invade the dermis. In the lymph nodes, LC depress the T helper 1 lymphocytes that are required for tumor growth and intracellular infection controls. In contrast, the T helper 2 lymphocytes are only slightly affected. The production of some cytokines, like interleukin (IL) 10 (an immunosuppressive one), are enhanced, whereas others, like IL-12 (an immunostimulating one), are decreased (32). A consequence of this phenomenon is the suppression of hypersensitivity responses to allergens or haptens.

These reactions have been used to study the effect of UV exposure on the immune system in humans. It has been shown that a single suberythemal dose of solar simulated radiation (0.25 or 0.5 MED) suppresses the induction of the contact hypersensitivity response (CHS) to dinitrochlorobenzene by 50% to 80% (33). Skin types I and II show a twofold to threefold greater sensitivity than skin types III and IV for the same biological UV dose. This observation may explain the difference in skin cancer susceptibility between the two subpopulations (33).

It seems that slightly higher acute solar simulated radiation dose or repeated suberythemal doses are requested to suppress established immune response, like delayed-type hypersensitivity (DTH) response to recall antigens (34) or CHS to nickel (35).

Recent studies have emphasized the role of UVA in immunosuppression. UVA suppressed the CHS induction and elicitation response (35,36) as well as the elicitation of DTH to recall antigens (34). Sunscreen studies have provided indirect evidence of the significant role of UVA in immunosuppression, and have shown that protection of the immune system is improved when UVA absorption is high (37–39).

PHOTOAGING

Repeated insults to the skin by UV radiation result in a phototrauma called photoaging or dermatoheliosis. Photoaging differs significantly from intrinsic aging, although both may occur simultaneously.

Clinically photoaged skin is characterized by roughness, fine and coarse wrinkling, mottled hyperpigmentation evidenced by lentigines or freckles, laxity, sallowness, and telangiectasias. All these alterations can be evaluated by noninvasive methods.

The decrease of smoothness can be evaluated by friction measurements. As smoothness is also a consequence of loss of lipids, moisture, and altered desquamation, other devices can also be used. These include:

- the Sebumeter®, which quantifies skin surface lipids;
- the Corneometer®, which determines the humidity level of the stratum corneum by measuring the electrical capacitance; and
- the Evaporimeter®, which measures the transepidermal water loss, an assessment of the ability of the horny layer to retain water in the skin (i.e., the quality of the barrier).

Wrinkles and changes in cutaneous microrelief are characteristics of photoaged skin. Various noninvasive methods have been developed to investigate the density and the depth of furrows and wrinkles from skin replicas or directly on skin in vivo (40).

Skin color, hypopigmentation, and hyperpigmentation can be assessed using colorimetric measurements. However, it is sometimes difficult to differentiate very small lentigines or pigmented spots from skin background color. New techniques based on the use of CCD camera or spectrocolorimetry can be used to obtain the absorbance spectra of the skin and to qualify pigmentary changes.

To assess the change in elasticity of the skin, different techniques have been developed. The more common ones are based on the following principles: a deformation is applied to the skin and the force generated by this distortion is measured as a function of time (relaxation process), or a force is applied on the skin surface and the resulting deformation is measured as a function of time. These measurements are done in the axis of the skin surface or perpendicular to it (elevation) (41).

As photoaging is characterized by hypertrophy, skin thickness measurements have been often used to assess photoaging. High-frequency ultrasonography has revealed a subepidermal nonechogenic band (SENEB) just below the basement membrane (Fig. 11). The thickness of the SENEB correlates with the severity of photodamage. The SENEB is due to a decrease in the echogenicity of the upper dermis, generated by an alteration of collagen and elastin fibers and by the accumulation of glycosaminoglycans in a water-rich ground substance (41).

It is also possible to measure epidermal thickness by confocal microscopy. The more recent devices allow a precision on the order of the micrometer. In addition, these confocal microscopes allow the visualization of melanosomes migrating towards the skin surface via the dendrites of melanocytes and alteration induced by chronic sun exposure in the process of pigment transfer (42).

PHOTOCARCINOGENESIS

There is strong evidence supporting the direct role of sunlight exposure in the development of skin cancers, especially nonmelanoma skin cancers (NMSC) like squamous cell carcinoma (SCC) and basal cell carcinoma (BCC). These skin cancers occur most frequently on the head, neck, arms, and hands, areas frequently exposed to sun. Lightly pigmented

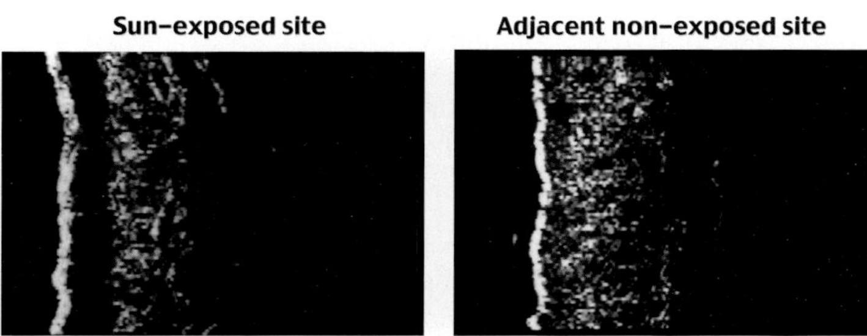

Figure 11 High-resolution ultrasonogram of the low neck in an elderly woman showing a SENEB in the sun-exposed site.

individuals (skin types I or II) are more prone to NMSC than those with deeply pigmented skin. Persons with occupational or recreational outdoor exposure, as well as those living at latitudes close to the equator, have higher incidence rates. BCC is the most common skin cancer in whites, accounting for about 75% of all skin tumors, whereas SCC is less frequent, accounting for about 20% of all skin cancers (43).

Lesions called actinic keratoses (AK) or solar keratoses are precursors of SCC. About 5% to 20% of these lesions progress to SCC. BCC arises de novo, which means there is no known precursor lesion.

Unlike NMSC, cutaneous malignant melanoma (CMM) is not associated with chronic occupational or recreational sun exposure and appears less than 25% of the time on sun-exposed body sites. CMM is frequently seen on the upper back in men and on the lower leg in women. For these reasons, it is still unclear how UV contributes to the induction and pathogenesis of these lesions. CMM accounts for about 5% of all skin tumors, but its incidence has been rising extremely rapidly (43). Risk factors for melanomas include a combination of constitutional predisposition (nevi, freckles, fair skin types), intense exposure, and frequent sunburn during childhood.

It is difficult to evaluate the effect of UV exposure on skin cancer induction and progression in humans. These lesions take years to develop, and frequency and the intensity of sun exposure as well as the nature of the UV radiation spectrum received are extremely difficult, if not impossible, to evaluate. At the present time, there is not enough scientific and epidemiological evidence for all types of skin cancer to support the essential role of UV. There is a very strong relationship for SCC, and a less strong relationship for BCC. Melanoma is even more problematic as some melanomas are unrelated to UV exposure. Epidemiological studies are often biased, based on questionnaire or interview and therefore on the subject's memory.

Animal models are useful for studying UV-induced carcinogenesis. Unfortunately, at present a good model is only available for SCC and AK. This model is the hairless mouse. For melanoma, different models have been developed, such as transgenic or knockout mice, but there a lot of work still needs to be done. To date, no melanoma induced in an animal has mimicked precisely all the features of human melanoma. A promising model is the development of UV-induced melanoma in hepatocyte growth factor and scattered factor transgenic mice (44–47).

CONCLUSION

This chapter has reviewed the evidence that UV radiation inflicts deleterious effects on skin. UV radiation causes DNA damage, erythema, pigmentation, and immunologic alterations. Phototrauma insults progress over decades to clinical and histological changes that characterize photoaging. Ultimately, photodamage may lead to photocarcinogenesis.

REFERENCES

1. Diffey BL. What is light. Photodermatol Photoimmunol Photomed 2002; 18:68–74.
2. Gasparro FG, Brown DB. Photobiology 102: UV sources and dosimetry—the proper use and measurement of photons as a reagent. J Invest Dermatol 2000; 114:613–616.
3. Chardon AM, Christiaens FJ, Dowdy JC, Sayre RM. Variation of sunscreen efficacy using solar spectrum and solar simulators [abstr 107], 8th Meet European Society of Photobiology, Granada, Spain, September 3–8, 1999.

4. Commission Internationale de l'Eclairage: Colorimetry. 2nd ed. Publication CIE No., 1986: 15–2.
5. McKinlay AF, Diffey BL. A reference action spectrum for ultraviolet induced erythema in human skin. CIE J 1987; 6:17–22.
6. Farr PM, Diffey BL. The erythemal response of human skin to ultraviolet radiation. Br J Dermatol 1985; 113:65.
7. Fitzpatrick TB. The validity and practicality of sun-reactive skin types I through VI. Arch Dermatol 1988; 124:869–871.
8. Kollias N, Malallah Y, Al-Ajmi H, Baqer A, Johnson B, Gonźlez S. Erythema and melanogenesis action spectra in heavily pigmented individuals as compared to fair-skinned Caucasians. Photodermatol Photoimmunol Photomed 1996; 12:183–188.
9. Kaidbey K, Kligman A. The acute effects of long-wave ultraviolet radiation on human skin. J Invest Dermatol; 1978; 72:253–256.
10. Chardon A, Moyal D. Immediate and delayed pigmentary responses to solar UVA radiation (320–400 nm). In: Ortonne JP, Ballotti R, Eds. Mechanisms of Suntanning. London: Martin Dunitz, 2002:315–325.
11. Auletta M, Gange W, Tan O, Matzinger B. Effect of cutaneous hypoxia upon erythema and pigment responses to UVA, UVB and PUVA (8-MOP + UVA) in human skin. J Invest Dermatol 1986; 6:649–652.
12. Anders A, Altheide HJ, Knalmann M, Tronnier H. Action spectrum for erythema in humans investigated with dye lasers. Photochem Photobiol 1995; 61:200–205.
13. Chardon A, Crétois I, Hourseau C. Skin colour typology and suntanning pathways. Int J Cosmet Sci 1991; 13:191–208.
14. Chardon A, Moyal D, Hourseau C. Persistent pigment darkening response as a method for evaluation of UVA protection assays. In: Lowe N, Shath N, Pathak M, Eds. Sunscreens: Development, Evaluation and Regulatory aspects. 2nd ed.: Marcel Dekker, 1996:559–582.
15. Deutsche Norm: Strahlungsphysik im optischen Bereich und Lichttechnik—Teil 10: Photobiologisch wirksame Strahlung, Grösen, Kurzziechen und Wirkungsspektrum. DIN 5031-10, 1996.
16. Seité S, Moyal D, Richard S, de Rigal J, Lévêque JL, Hourseau C, Fourtanier A. Effects of repeated suberythemal doses of UVA in human skin. Eur J Dermatol 1997; 7:203–209.
17. Bech-Thomsen N, Ravnborg L, Wulf HC. A quantitative study of the melanogenesis effect of multiple suberythemal doses of different ultraviolet radiation sources. Photodermatol Photoimmunol Photomed 1994; 10:53–56.
18. Sinha RP, Häder DP. UV-induced DNA damage and repair: a review. Photochem Photobiol Sci 2002; 1:225–236.
19. Woods DB, Vousden KH. Regulation of p53 function. Exp Cell Res 2001; 264:56–66.
20. Sheehan JM, Young AR. The sunburn cell revisited: an update on mechanistic aspects. Photochem Photobiol Sci 2002; 1:365–377.
21. Murphy G, Young AR, Wulf HC, Kulms D, Schwarz T. The molecular determinants of sunburn cell formation. Exp Dermatol 2001; 10:155–160.
22. Kulms D, Schwarz T. Molecular mechanisms of UV-induced apoptosis. Photodermatol Photoimmunol Photomed 2000; 16:195–201.
23. Stege H, Roza L, Vink AA, Grewe M, Ruzicka T, Grether-Beck S. Enzyme plus light therapy to repair DNA damage in ultraviolet-B-irradiated human skin. Clin Exp Photodermatol 2000; 97:1790–1795.
24. Tice RR. The single cell gel/comet assay: a microgel electrophoretic technique for the detection of DNA damage and repair in individual cells. In: Philips DH, Venett S, Eds. Environmental Mutagenesis. Oxford: Bios, 1995:315–339.
25. Marrot L, Belaidi JP, Meunier JR, Perez P, Agapakis-Causse C. The human melanocyte as a particular target for UVA radiation and an endpoint for photoprotection assessment. Photochem Photobiol 1999; 69:686–693.

26. Asselineau D, Bernard BA, Bailly C, Darmon M. Retinoic acid improves epidermal morphogenesis. Dev Biol 1989; 133:322–335.
27. Bernerd F, Asselineau D. Successive alteration and recovery of epidermal differentiation and morphogenesis after specific UVB-damages in skin reconstructed in vitro. Dev Biol 1997; 183:123–138.
28. Bernerd F, Asselineau D. UVA exposure of human skin reconstructed in vitro induces apoptosis of dermal fibroblasts: subsequent connective tissue repair and implications in photoaging. Cell Death Differ 1998; 5:792–802.
29. Régnier M, Staquet MJ, Schmitt D, Schmidt R. Integration of Langerhans cells into a pigmented reconstructed human epidermis. J Invest Dermatol 1997; 109:510–512.
30. Duval C, Régnier M, Schmidt R. Distinct melanogenic response of human melanocytes in mono-culture, in co-culture with keratinocytes and in reconstructed epidermis, to UV exposure. Pigment Cell Res 2001; 14:348–355.
31. Seité S, Zucchi H, Moyal D, Tison S, Compan D, Christiaens F, Gueniche A, Fourtanier A. Alterations in human epidermal Langerhans cells by ultraviolet radiation: quantitative and morphological study. Br J Dermatol 2003; 148:291–299.
32. Schwarz T. Photoimmunosuppression. Photodermatol Photoimmunol Photomed 2002; 18: 141–145.
33. Kelly DA, Young AR, McGregor JM, Seed PT, Potten CS, Walker SL. Sensitivity to sunburn is associated with susceptibility to ultraviolet radiation-induced suppression of cutaneous cell-mediated immunity. J Exp Med 2000; 191:561–566.
34. Moyal D, Fourtanier A. Broad-spectrum sunscreens provide better protection from the suppression of the elicitation phase of delayed type hypersensitivity response in humans. J Invest Dermatol 2001; 117:1186–1192.
35. Damian DL, Barnetson RSC, Halliday GM. Low-dose UVA and UVB have different time-courses for suppression of contact hypersensitivity to a recall antigen in humans. J Invest Dermatol 1999; 112:939–944.
36. LeVee GJ, Oberhelman L, Anderson T, Koren H, Cooper KD. UVAII exposure of human skin results in decreased immunization capacity, increased induction of tolerance and a unique pattern of epidermal antigen-presenting cell alteration. Photochem Photobiol 1997; 65: 622–629.
37. Wolf P, Hoffmann C, Grinschgl S, Quehenberger F, Kerl H. Human *in vivo* immune protection factors of sunscreens containing chemical UV filters measured in UV dose response studies in the local contact hypersensitivity model [abstr]. J Invest Dermatol; 2001:117.
38. Damian DL, Halliday GM, Taylor CA, Barnetson RSC. Broadspectrum sunscreens provide greater protection against ultraviolet-radiation-induced suppression of contact hypersensitivity to a recall antigen in humans. J Invest Dermatol 1997; 109:146–151.
39. Moyal DD, Fourtanier AM. Efficacy of broad-spectrum sunscreens against the suppression of elicitation of delayed-type hypersensitivity responses in humans depends on the level of ultraviolet A protection. Exp Dermatol 2003; 12:153–159.
40. Akazaki S, Imokawa G. Mechanical methods for evaluating skin surface architecture in relation to wrinkling. J Dermatol Sci 2001; 27(suppl1):S5–S10.
41. Lévêque JL. Quantitative assessment of skin aging. Geriatr Dermatol 2001; 17:673–689.
42. Corcuff P, Chaussepied C, Madry G, Hadjur C. Skin optics revisited by in vivo confocal microscopy: melanin and sun exposure. J Cosmet Sci 2001; 52:91–102.
43. Diepgen TL, Mahler V. The epidemiology of skin cancer. Br J Dermatol 2002; 146(suppl 61): 1–6.
44. Ortonne JP. From actinic keratosis to squamous cell carcinoma. Br J Dermatol 2002; 146(suppl 61):20–23.
45. Lacour JP. Carcinogenesis of basal cell carcinomas : genetics and molecular mechanisms. Br J Dermatol 2002; 146(suppl 61):17–19.

46. Ortonne JP. Photobiology and genetics of malignant melanoma. Br J Dermatol 2002; 146(suppl 61):11–16.
47. Noonan FP, Dudek J, Merlino G, DeFabo EC. Animal models of melanoma: an HGF/SF transgenic mouse model may facilitate experimental access to UV initiating events. Pigment Cell Res 2003; 16:16–25.

3

Clinical and Histological Changes of Photoaging

Marjan Garmyn / Joost Van den Oord *University Hospital Sint Rafael, Leuven, Belgium*

- Photoaging represents a superimposition of chronic cumulative photodamage on the intrinsic aging process and affects both epidermis and dermis.
- Chronic photodamage of the epidermis results in pigment changes and benign, premalignant, and malignant hyperproliferations.
- Epidermal changes of photoaging reflect deregulated growth and predisposition to photocarcinogenesis.
- The dermis in photoaged skin demonstrates loss of collagen, dermal elastosis, and reduction in fibrillin-rich microfibrils.
- Dermal changes of photoaging result in decreased skin strength and elasticity and increased wrinkling.

Photoaging describes those clinical histological and physiological changes that occur in the habitually sun-exposed skin of older individuals and represents a superimposition of chronic cumulative photodamage on the innate of intrinsic aging process. Chronological aging, or intrinsic aging, affects the skin in a manner similar to other organs and can best be defined as a loss of maximal functional capacity in tissues and organs throughout the body. This intrinsic aging has only a minor impact on the appearance of skin, while it has important functional implications. Most of the unwanted changes in skin appearance that occur with age are due to the process of photoaging. It has been estimated that photoaging accounts for more than 90% of the skin's age-associated cosmetic problems, which in turn dramatically impact an individual's self-esteem (1).

Photoaged skin is clearly distinguishable from intrinsically aged skin. Intrinsically aged skin or skin that has not been chronically exposed to sunlight is characterized by generalized fine wrinkling, dry and thin appearance, seborrheic keratosis, and other benign hyperproliferations such as cherry angiomas (also known as senile hemangiomas). Photoaged skin has a leathery appearance and demonstrates often-deep wrinkling, loss of resilience, increased fragility, and reduced wound healing. The damaging effects of solar ultraviolet (UV) radiation on the dermis cause most of these attributes (1–4). Pigment changes (so-called age spots, diffuse hyperpigmentations, and hypomelanosis guttata) are due to the damaging effects of UV radiation on the epidermis. An important consequence of damaging effects of sunlight on skin is the propensity of photoaged epidermis to develop malignancies, reflected by the high prevalence of premalignant and malignant skin lesions (1,5,6).

Because the features of photoaging appear only on chronically sun-exposed skin, their distribution may vary according to dress and hairstyle. Skin type profoundly influences the clinical picture of photoaging. At the one extreme are the fair-skinned individuals with freckles in early childhood. After chronic sun exposure, telangiectasia and fine wrinkling develop in these persons, followed later on by actinic keratoses, which in the long run may evolve into invasive squamous cell carcinoma. Their skin also demonstrates irregular pigmentation, including areas of depigmentation. Ultimately the skin becomes very atrophic. In contrast, diffuse hyperpigmentation initially tends to develop in darker-skinned individuals, and later on these persons develop discrete permanent areas of hyperpigmentation, also called lentigines (caused by changes in the epidermal pigmentary system). Changes in the elastic tissue, termed elastosis, can also subsequently develop in these persons, giving the skin a coarse leathery quality or very deep furrowing (1).

Photoaging is the result of chronic cumulative sun damage that occurs year after year. When UV radiation in sunlight hits the skin, part of it is scattered and reflected in the stratum corneum, and part is transmitted. The depth of penetration depends on the wavelength. Both UVB and UVA within the solar spectrum contribute to this process of photoaging. Most of the shorter but relatively more powerful UVB (290–320 nm) wavelengths are absorbed in the epidermis, and only 10% penetrates beyond this barrier, even in persons with fair skin. These shorter wavelengths affect the keratinocytes and melanocytes within the epidermis; however, the small part that reaches the dermis also has important effects on this compartment of skin since it is more energetic than UVA. The UVA wavelengths penetrate deeper into the dermis and interact with epidermal keratinocytes, melanocytes, and dermal fibroblasts. More specifically, about 50% of incident UVA radiation traverses the epidermis and reaches a depth of 0.1 to 0.2 mm in the papillary dermis (7). Because of its obligatory link to chronic cumulative sun exposure, photoaging will be even of greater concern in the future, given the expected extended lifespan, more spare time, and excessive sun exposure from natural sunlight or tanning devices

Photoaging affects the epidermis and dermis at the morphological level. The epidermis shows a variability in thickness, atypia of keratinocytes and melanocytes, and loss of Langerhans cells. These changes reflect deregulated growth and predisposition to photocarcinogenesis, which is clinically visible as pigment changes, benign hyperproliferative skin lesions, premalignant lesions, and malignant skin tumors. The dermis demonstrates loss of collagen, dermal elastosis, and a reduction in fibrillin rich microfibrils, which results in decrease in skin strength and elasticity, and increased wrinkling. In this chapter, the clinical and histological aspects of chronic cumulative photodamage of the epidermis and dermis and possible underlying mechanisms are discussed.

CLINICAL AND HISTOLOGICAL CHANGES DUE TO CUMULATIVE UV DAMAGE TO THE EPIDERMIS

Pigment Changes and Benign Hyperproliferations

The so-called *age spot* is an important sign of chronic photodamage and represents different entities. The most common variant is the lentigo senilis, or senile lentigo, which represents a pigmented macule in chronically sun-exposed skin. It appears mainly in white patients between the fourth and sixth decade of life. Since chronic cumulative sun exposure is the cause of these lesions, one finds them on those parts of the body that are chronically exposed to sunlight: the face, extensor aspects of the forearms, and the back of the hands. Lentigines seniles are sharply but irregularly outlined and vary in color from yellow-brown to dark brown. The size may range from a few millimeters to several centimeters (Fig. 1). These lentigines seniles are due to an increase in the melanin content inside keratinocytes, and may or may not be associated with melanocytic hyperplasia (8). They are usually numerous and may be accompanied by adjacent patchy hypopigmentation, which involves a decrease in the number of melanocytes, associated with a reduction in the production of mature melanosomes. This results a mottled appearance of the skin (9). On histology, senile lentigo characteristically shows elongated, bulb-like and hyper-pigmented rete ridges that on extension and branching may result in a reticulate pattern (Fig. 2) (10). The number of melanocytes in the bulb-like regions is increased, and these cells contain large melanosome complexes (11); in the papillary dermis, melanophages may be quite numerous. Senile lentigo may occasionally evolve into lentigo maligna (12).

The main differential diagnosis of senile lentigo is *reticulate* or *flat seborrheic keratosis*. These lesions are sometimes clinically indistinguishable from senile lentigines. They appear, like senile lentigines, on sun-exposed areas of skin in middle-aged individuals, and vary in color from light to dark brown. In contrast to the usual seborrheic keratosis, they exhibit a smooth surface. It is a matter of debate whether a reticulate seborrheic keratosis can evolve from a senile lentigo (10). On histology, there is a reticulate type of acanthosis with interlacing thin strands of basaloid cells that often are pigmented. Seborrheic keratosis and senile hemangioma are examples of benign hyperproliferations of keratinocytes and capillary blood vessels, respectively; however, they do not exclusively occur on chronically sun-exposed skin and are as such also a clinical aspect of intrinsic aging.

Premalignant and Malignant Hyperproliferations

Actinic keratosis can be considered as the premalignant lesion of the keratinocyte. Actinic keratoses are seen on chronically sun-exposed areas, especially the dorsal aspects of the hands, the face (forehead, nose, cheeks, temples, vermilion border, lower lip), ears (in males), vertex (in balding males), and neck (sides). They present clinically as discrete scaly hyperkeratotic rough-surfaced areas, usually less than 1 cm in diameter, with an adherent hyperkeratotic scale that is removed with difficulty and pain (Fig. 3). These lesions may be erythematous, skin colored, yellow-brown, or brown. Often there is a reddish tinge. They are predominantly seen in individuals with skin types I and II, less often in those with skin types III and IV, and almost never in patients with skin types V or VI. Since chronically cumulative sun exposure is the cause of these lesions, they are seen predominantly in outdoor workers and outdoor sportsmen. Actinic keratoses may

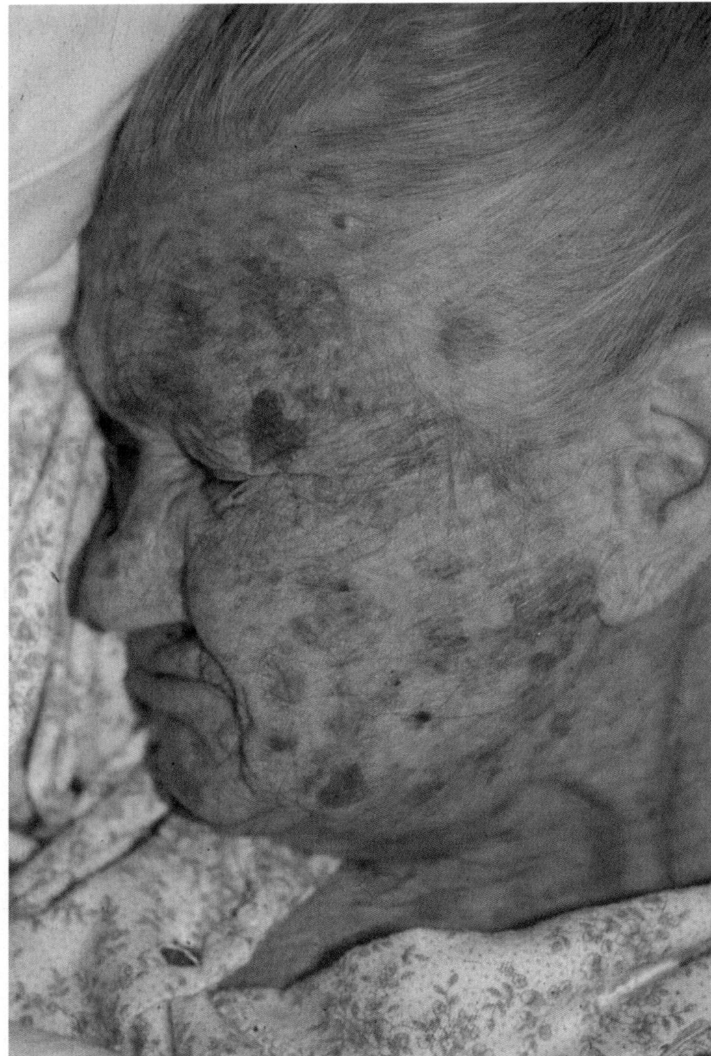

Figure 1 A patient with lentigines seniles. The face is covered with lentigines seniles, sharply but irregularly outlined pigmented maculae that vary in color from yellow brown to dark brown. Note also the yellowish thickening and the coarse leathery quality and deep furrowing of the skin, which are typical photoaging-associated changes in darker-skinned persons.

regress spontaneously, but in general they remain for years. The incidence of squamous cell carcinoma developing from preexisting solar keratoses is not known.

On histological assessment, the epidermis is usually thickened due to irregular downward, budlike growth of basal keratinocytes that show variable nuclear and cellular atypia including nuclear hyperchromasia, prominent nucleoli, and an altered nucleocytoplasmic index. The suprabasal cells show normal maturation except in bowenoid actinic keratosis,

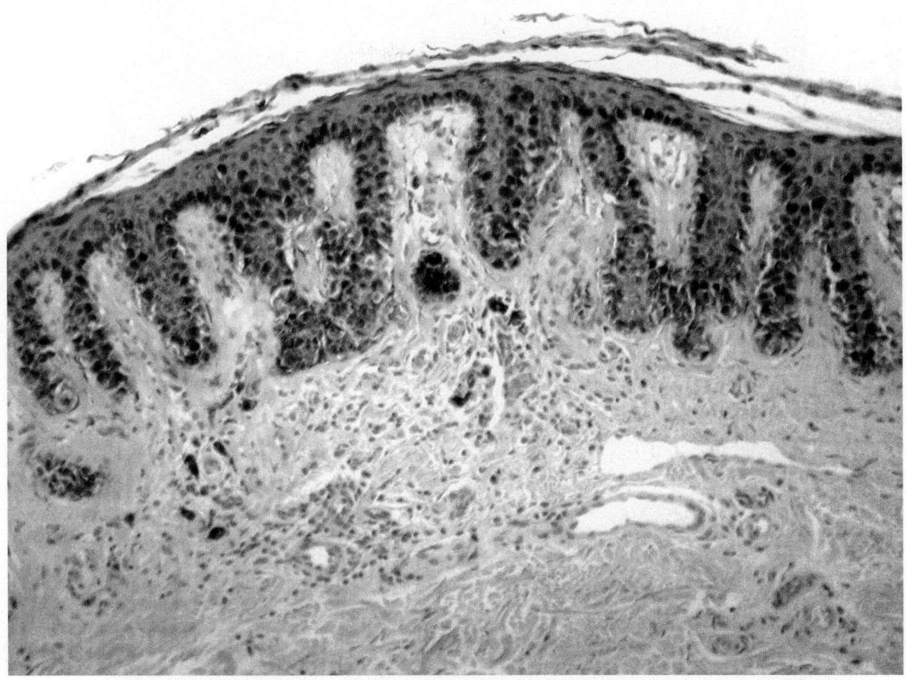

Figure 2 Solar lentigo showing delicate acanthosis, hyperpigmentation of basal keratinocytes, increased numbers of melanocytes, and some melanophages in the papillary dermis.

in which cellular atypia is found over the full thickness of the squamous epithelium. The lesion is invariably covered by a focal parakeratotic layer (Figs. 4a–c) (13). Histological variants include the atrophic type in which the epidermis is markedly thinned; the acantholytic type in which the atypical basal cells are separated from the overlying stratum spinosum by a cleft (Fig. 4d); the hypertrophic/hyperplastic form in which irregular psoriasiform hyperplasia and some papillomatosis accompanies minimal atypia in the basal cell layer; the pigmented variant in which keratinocytes are heavily loaded with melanin, and the dermis contains numerous melanophages; and finally the lichenoid type in which a superficial bandlike mononuclear cell infiltrate results in vacuolopathy and variable apoptosis of single keratinocytes (Fig. 4e). In all types of actinic keratosis, the dermis shows actinic elastosis and a variable mononuclear inflammatory infiltrate.

There has been debate whether actinic keratosis represents a truly neoplastic lesion. Ackerman considers actinic keratosis a de novo squamous cell carcinoma and not a premalignant lesion (14), but this is seemingly in contradiction with the finding that these lesions may remain unchanged over several years or even may regress (15) and rather infrequently transform into invasive squamous cell carcinoma (16). Person et al. (17) suggested that actinic keratosis represents a lesion of initiated tumor cells that require a second ''hit'' to become truly neoplastic.

Morbus Bowen (or *Bowen's disease*) is a carcinoma in situ of the epidermis. Morbus Bowen can arise on exposed skin, and is then caused by chronic cumulative sun exposure.

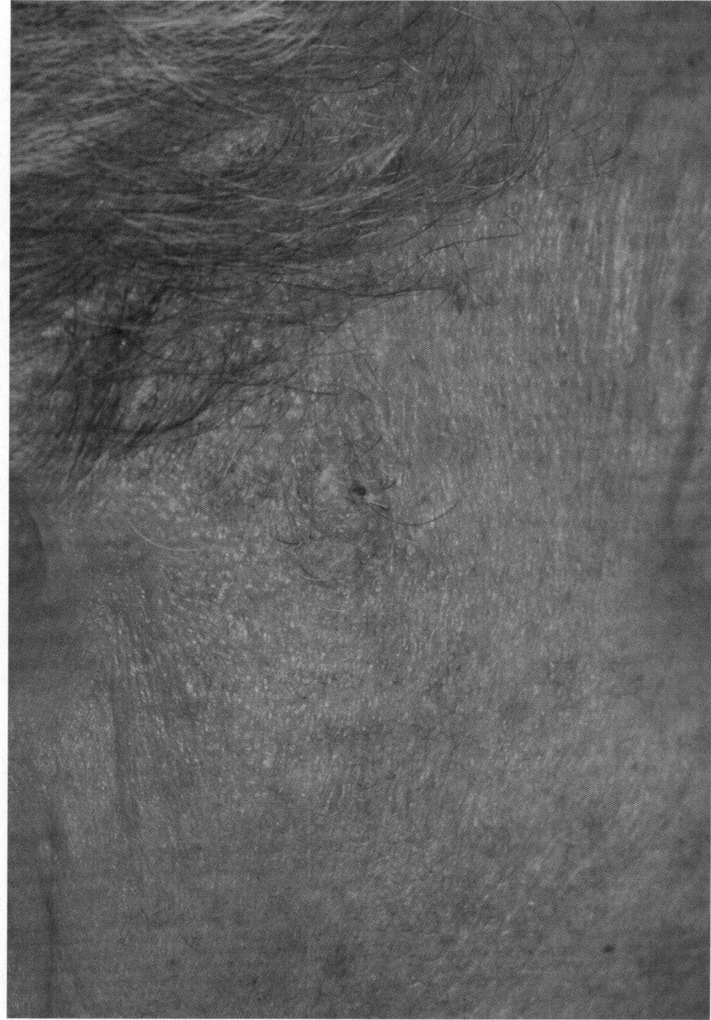

Figure 3 Actinic keratosis. A solitary lesion with adherent ''rough'' hyperkeratotic scale is seen on the temple.

The lesion appears as a slowly enlarging erythematous macule, with sharp border and little or no infiltration. There is usually slight scaling and some crusting. On histological examination, the epidermis shows full-thickness atypia and disordered maturation, which may extend into the epithelium of hair follicles and eccrine ducts. Keratinocytes show suprabasal mitotic figures, dyskeratosis, multinucleation, and severe nuclear atypia. Parakeratosis is usually present (Fig. 4f). Histological variants include a form with psoriasiform hyperplasia of the epidermis; an atrophic variant that is often covered by a thickened orthokeratotic or parakeratotic horny layer; a verrucous type characterized by papillomatosis and hyperkeratosis; a pigmented variant with melanin accumulation in neoplastic

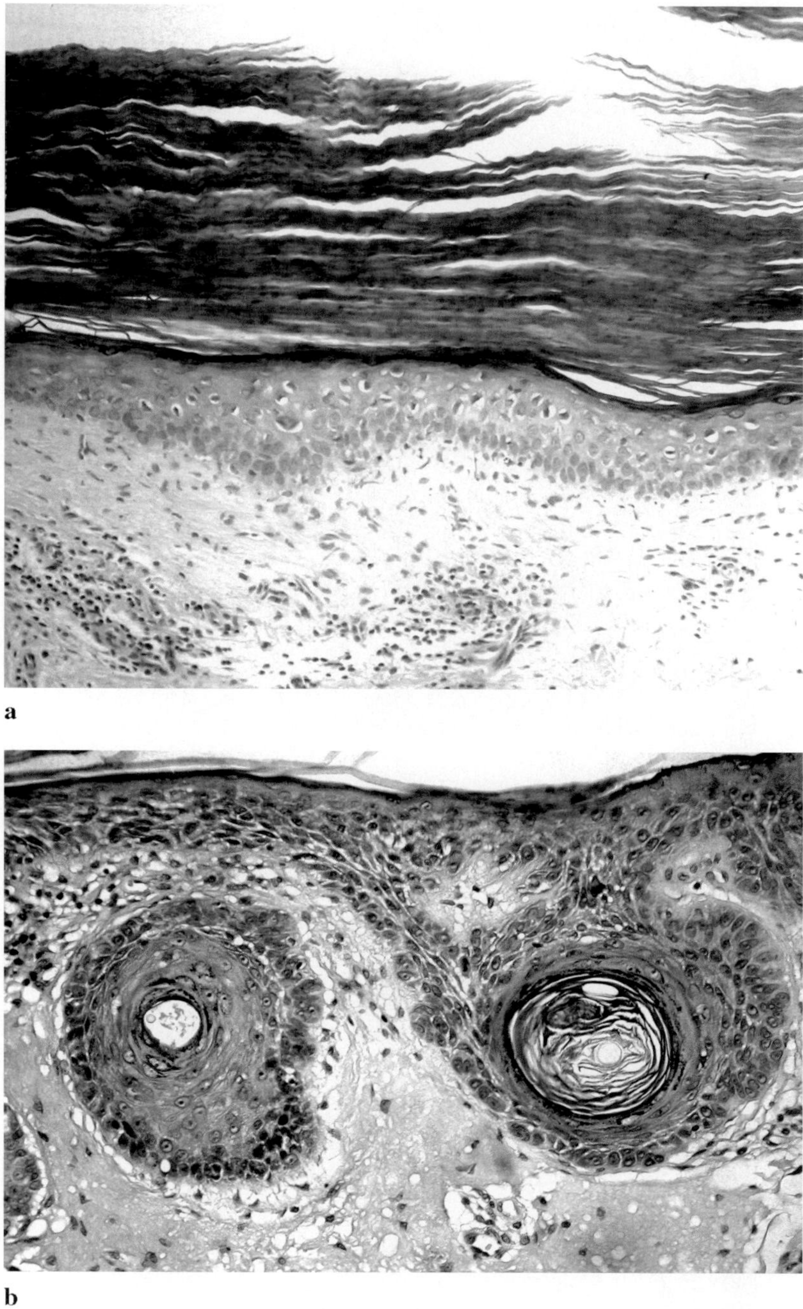

Figure 4 (a) Actinic keratosis showing mild nuclear pleomorphism in the epidermis and a thick, parakeratotic horny layer. (b) The atypical basal keratinocytes extend around the hair follicles. (c) Actinic keratosis covered by a thick hyperkeratotic scale (cornu cutaneum). (d) Actinic keratosis of the acantholytic type showing mild acantholysis between atypical basal keratinocytes and suprabasal cell layers. (e) Actinic keratosis of the lichenoid type showing discrete atypia in the basal keratinocytes and an underlying bandlike mononuclear infiltrate. (f) Actinic keratosis of the bowenoid type showing nuclear atypia throughout all layers of the epidermis.

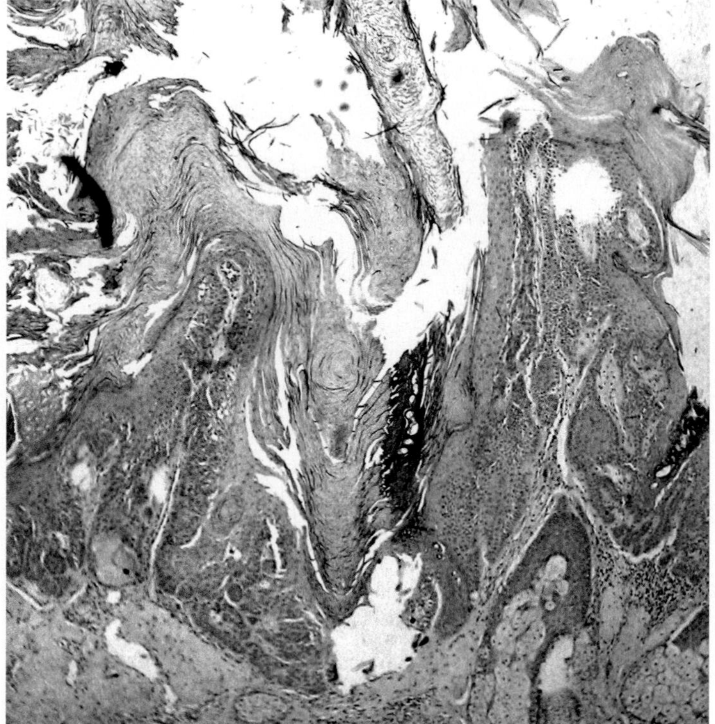

c

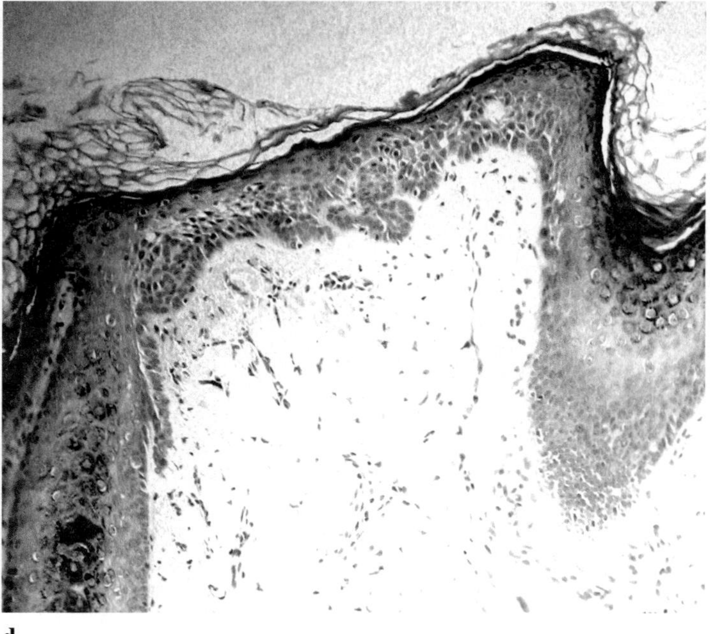

d

Figure 4 Continued.

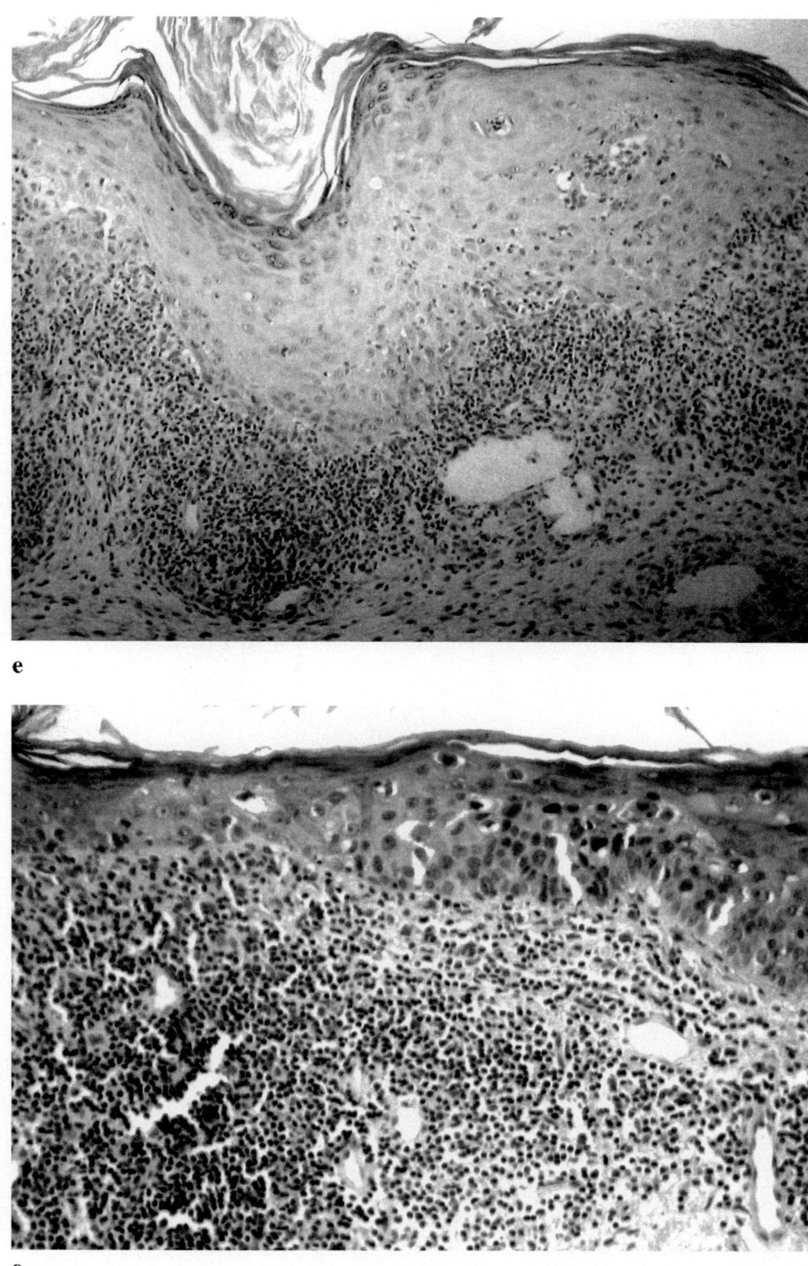

e

f

Figure 4 Continued.

keratinocytes and in dermal macrophages; and a pagetoid variant in which single atypical keratinocytes spread out horizontally in the epidermis, adjacent to classical Bowen's disease. The underlying dermis in all types shows a variable mononuclear inflammatory infiltrate and increased numbers of blood vessels (18).

Actinically induced invasive squamous cell carcinoma is a malignant tumor of epidermal keratinocytes that arises on sun-exposed skin and may develop from an actinic keratosis. The tumor presents as an indurated papule, plaque, or nodule with an adherent thick keratotic scale. When eroded or ulcerated, the lesion may have a crust in the center and a firm hyperkeratotic elevated margin. This type of sun-induced squamous cell carcinoma develops on sun-exposed skin, such as the face (cheeks, nose, lips, tips of the ears, preauricular areas), scalp, and dorsa of the hands. The lesions occur predominantly in fair-skinned individuals (phototypes I and II). The skin surrounding these lesions shows signs of photodamage, including irregular pigmentation, wrinkling (mostly fine), and actinic keratoses (Fig. 5). Squamous cell carcinoma on sun-exposed skin, regardless of whether it arises from actinic keratosis, usually shows signs of differentiation, clinically presenting as tumors that are firm or hard on palpation, which are signs of keratinization. Histologically, nests of atypical squamous cells arise from the epidermis and extend into the dermis (Fig. 6). The

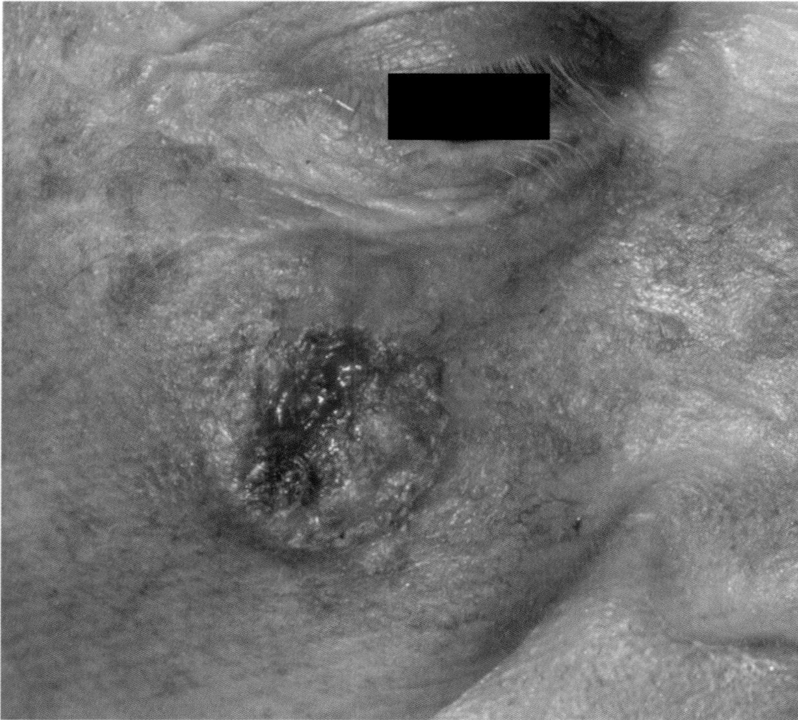

Figure 5 Squamous cell carcinoma on the right cheek. An ulcerating plaque with crust in the center and a firm hyperkeratotic elevated margin is shown. The surrounding skin demonstrates irregular pigmentations, fine wrinkling, telangiectasia, and atrophic changes, all of which are typical photoaging-associated changes in fair-skinned persons.

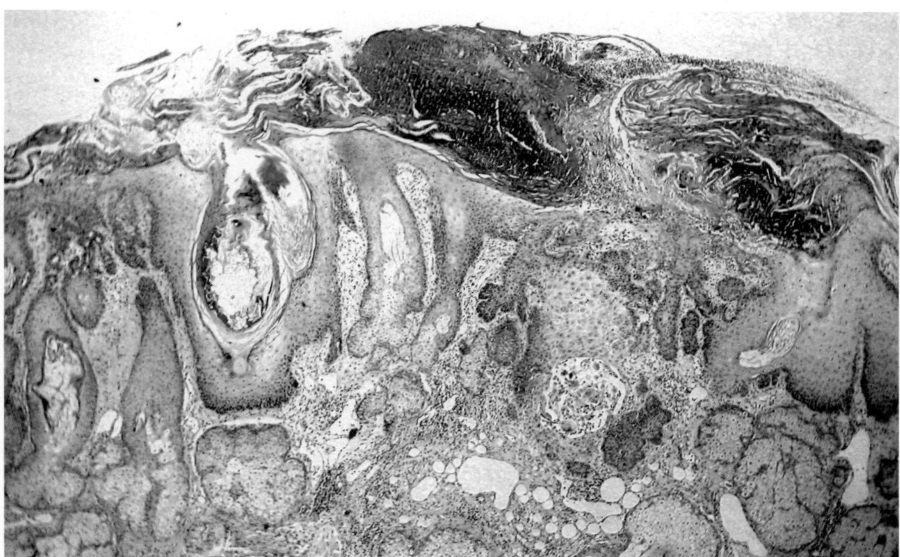

Figure 6 Actinic keratosis (left) with invasive squamous cell carcinoma (right).

polygonal cells have abundant pink cytoplasm and a large nucleus with prominent nucleolus. Dyskeratotic cells as well as horn pearls are usually found when the neoplasm arises from actinic keratosis; the invasive squamous cell carcinomas that originate from Bowen's disease are usually less differentiated. The neoplasm invades in the form of thin strands into the deep dermis and subcutis, as well as along nerve sheaths and blood vessel walls (Fig. 7). At the periphery, a variable lymphocytic host response is seen, and some tumors evoke a desmoplastic response. Histological variants include spindle cell squamous carcinoma, which arises almost exclusively in sun-damaged skin and may be misdiagnosed as atypical fibroxanthoma or amelanotic melanoma. On immunohistochemistry, the neoplastic cells may coexpress vimentin and cytokeratin. The acantholytic or pseudoglandular/adenoid squamous cell carcinoma shows extensive acantholysis resulting in ''gland-like'' spaces in the center of tumor nests; this variant usually arises from an acantholytic type of actinic keratosis. Rare variants of squamous cell carcinoma include the pigmented, clear-cell, signet-ring cell, pseudovascular, mucin-producing, inflammatory, infiltrative, and desmoplastic types.

Basal cell carcinoma (BCC) is the most common type of skin cancer. This malignant tumor of the keratinocyte is locally invasive, aggressive, and destructive, but does not have the capacity to metastasize. BCC arises only from epidermis that has a capacity of developing (hair) follicles. Therefore, BCC does not develop on the vermilion border of the lips or on genital mucosa. The commonest type is the nodular type, which is characterized by a translucent or pearly papule or nodule, sometimes with a central ulceration (Fig. 8). White-skinned persons with poor tanning capacity (phototypes I and II) and albinos are highly susceptible to develop BCC with prolonged sun exposure. UV radiation certainly has a role it the development of BCC, albeit not an exclusive one. In addition, there is also discussion whether short intensive sun exposure (sunburn) rather than chronic

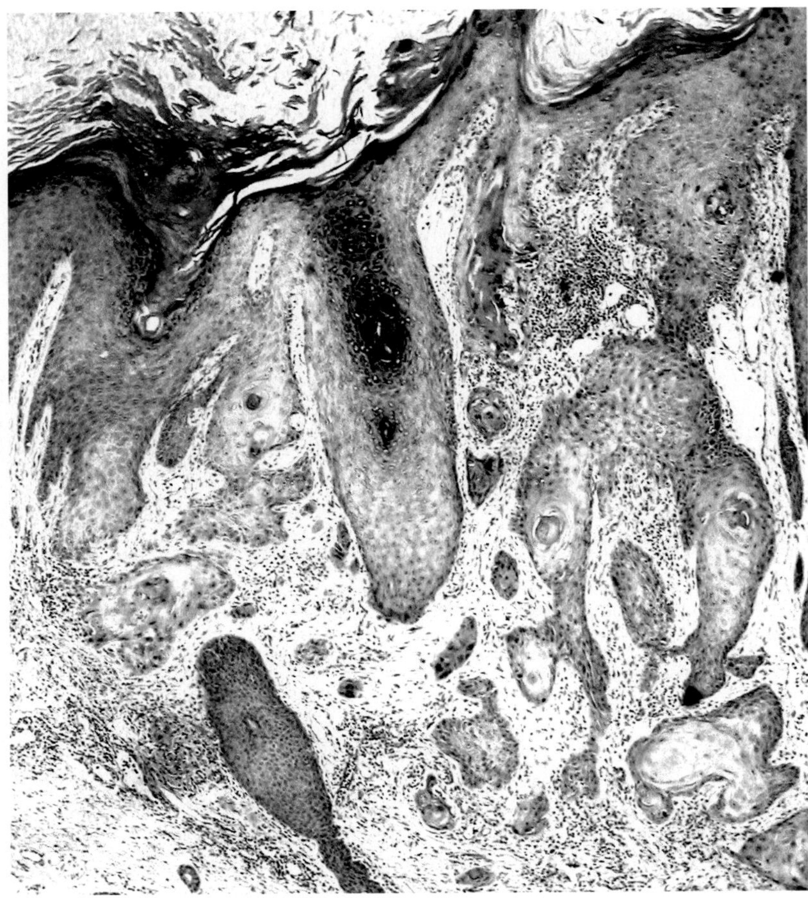

Figure 7 Superficially invasive squamous cell carcinoma showing spiky strands of atypical keratinocytes invading an actinically damaged dermis.

cumulative sun exposure plays the major role in the development of BCC. A recent study found a discordance between facial wrinkling and the presence of BCC.(19).

On histological assessment, BCCs consist of nests and strands of small, basaloid cells; at the periphery of the nests, the nuclei of the basaloid cells show palisading, whereas in the center the neoplastic cells are haphazardly arranged and show mitotic figures and apoptosis, despite their expression of the antiapoptotic bcl-2 protein (Fig. 9). The adjacent dermis shows solar elastosis and a mononuclear inflammatory infiltrate. Some BCCs may arise from a subtype of actinic keratosis, but the immunohistochemical profile of the basaloid cells suggests that this type of carcinoma originates from the matrix cells of the hair follicle. Various morphological subtypes have been described, depending on the size or aspect of the tumor nests (solid or nodular, micronodular, cystic, pigmented, and adenoid types), patterns of differentiation within the tumor nests (keratotic, infundibulocystic, and basosquamous types), localization of the nests (superficial or multifocal type), pattern of invasion or host response (infiltrating type, sclerosing type, and fibroepithelioma).

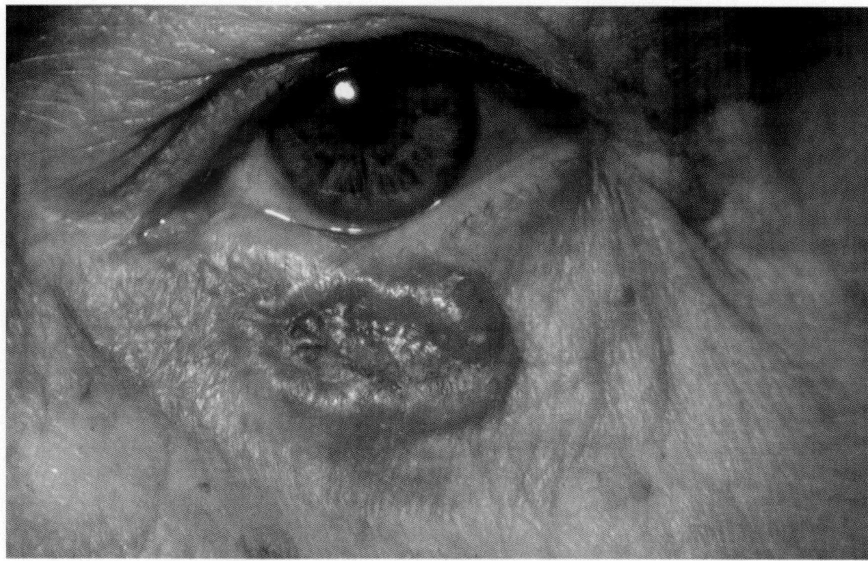

Figure 8 Basal cell carcinoma showing a typical pearly edge and central ulceration.

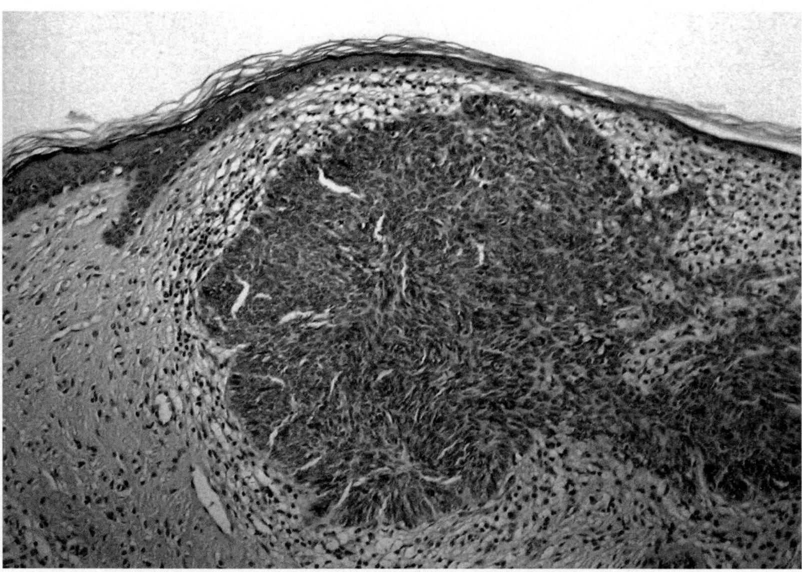

Figure 9 Nodular basal cell carcinoma consisting of a dermal collection of basal cells surrounded by mononuclear inflammatory cells.

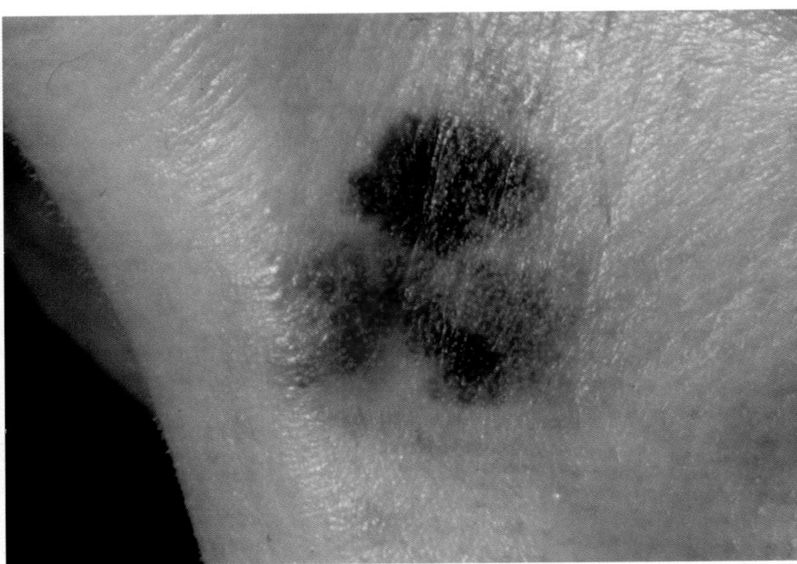

Figure 10 Lentigo maligna on the nose. Shown is a uniformly flat macule, irregularly pigmented with striking variations in hues of brow and black, and with irregular borders.

Regarding melanocytic neoplasia, photoaged skin is often riddled by atypical intraepidermal proliferations of melanocytes, frank lentiginous malignant melanoma in situ also called *lentigo maligna in situ* (precarcinomatous lesion of the melanocyte) and *lentigo malignant melanoma* (invasive malignant tumor of the melanocyte).

Lentigo maligna presents as a uniformly flat macule that is irregularly pigmented with striking variations in hues of brown and black irregular borders, often with a notch. Often they have a ''geographic'' shape with inlets and peninsulas. Their size may vary from approximately 3 to 20 cm (Fig. 10). On histological assessment, single and nested melanocytes with variable nuclear atypia and mitotic activity are found in the basal cell layer of a usually atrophic epidermis, and show variable pagetoid spread. Some of the melanocytes in the basal cell layer show multinucleation and have prominent dendritic processes (the so-called starburst giant cell) (20). The atypical melanocytes may extend into the basal cell layer of pilosebaceous units over a variable distance (Fig. 11). In the underlying dermis, profound elastosis is seen, as well as a mononuclear inflammatory infiltrate and scattered melanophages. There is disagreement whether lentigo maligna should be regarded as a dysplastic lesion or as a truly in situ melanoma. Flotte and Mihm (21) discern two types of lesions on the basis of subsequent clinical follow-up analyses: a lesion without propensity to proceed toward invasive melanoma (i.e., the so-called lentigo maligna), and a precursor of invasive melanoma (i.e., malignant melanoma in situ, lentigo maligna type). Both lesions differ with regard to the degree of junctional nesting, crowding and confluence, pagetoid spread, atypia, and adnexal involvement. These morphological differences are likely to be reflected in functional differences; it has been shown that in some cases of lentigo maligna, expression of certain matrix metalloproteinases is minimal or absent, which may explain the lack of invasiveness (22).

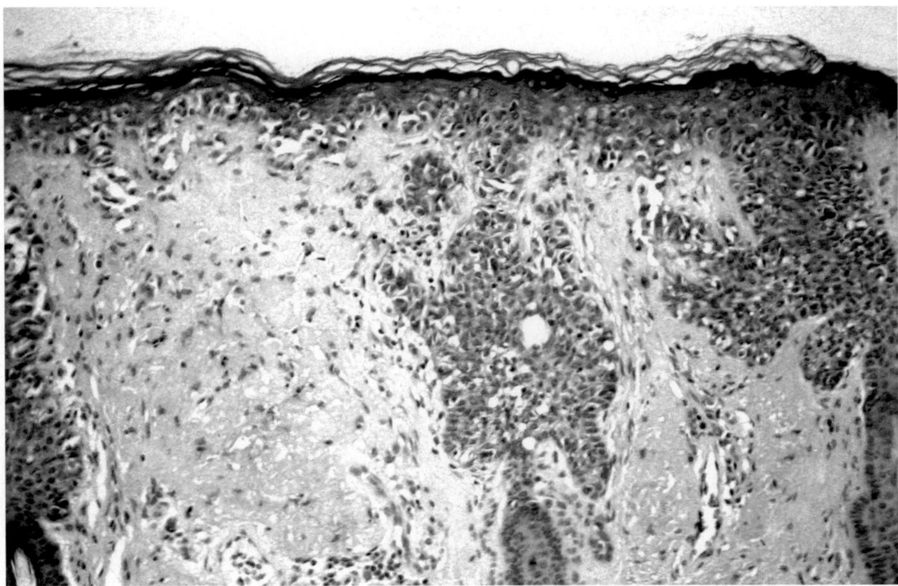

Figure 11 Lentigo maligna. Atypical melanocytes are present in a lentiginous pattern at the dermoepidermal junction, and extend into the basal layer of hair follicles.

A *lentigo malignant melanoma* develops in an in situ lentigo maligna. The clinical presentation is initially the same as lentigo maligna in situ, plus the development of gray areas (indicating focal regression) or blue areas (indicating dermal pigment, melanocytes, or melanin), or papules and nodules. Lentigo maligna and lentigo malignant melanoma present as a single isolated pigmented lesion on chronically sun-exposed areas, such as the forehead, nose, cheeks, neck, forearms, and dorsa of the hands. The areas surrounding the tumor show other signs of chronic photodamage including actinic keratosis, lentigines seniles, telangiectasia, and thinning of the skin. In lentigo malignant melanoma, an invasive component has evolved that may be epithelioid or spindled. The presence or absence of invasion is sometimes difficult to assess, particularly when the lentigo maligna shows extensive involvement of adnexal structures; immunohistochemistry for melanocytic markers may be helpful.

Pathogenic Mechanism

The epidermal changes that are characteristic of photoaging reflect deregulated growth and predisposition to photocarcinogenesis. Different mechanisms may contribute to these processes, including an age-associated decrease in repair capacity (23–25), changed expression of differentiation-associated genes and growth-regulatory genes in chronically photodamaged skin cells (26,27), and finally UV-induced mutations in proto-oncogenes and tumor-suppressor genes. The impact of UV on gene mutation has been clearly shown for the characteristic point mutations in p53, so-called UV signature mutations. The p53 mutation is the most frequently found mutation in sun-induced skin cancer, and is found not only in squamous cell carcinomas but also in actinic keratosis and even in normal appearing sun-damaged skin, indicating that p53 mutation is an early event (28–30).

It appears that at least a combination of an activated oncogenic pathway and inactivated tumor-suppressor pathway is needed for a skin cancer to arise (31). Changes in surrounding dermal matrix, the transformed cells' local environment, and/or diminished immunosurveillance with age may also contribute (5). Hence, keratinocytes in actinic keratosis show nuclear accumulation of mutated p53 (UV-signature p53 mutations) (32) and may show mutational activation of *ras* genes (33), features that are consistent with genuine neoplastic proliferation. Transition into invasive squamous cell carcinoma would be accompanied by inactivation of the tumor suppressor p16 (INK4a) (34), alterations in cadherins and catenins (35), and loss of human mismatch repair (hMSH2) gene function (36). In addition, upregulation of several matrix metalloproteinases (37) and alterations in the immunodefense mechanisms (38) are associated with the development of invasive squamous cell carcinoma. In BCC, the PTHC gene is often mutated, leading to consistent activation of the mitogenic Hedgehog pathway (39). This mutation often occurs in combination with a mutated (UV-signature) p53 tumor-suppressor gene (28). The equivalent early mutation required for malignant conversion of melanocytes has not been identified. Germline p16 mutations are frequently found in familial melanomas and atypical nevi in these kindreds, but p16 signature mutations are only reported occasionally in sporadic melanomas (5,40–42).

CLINICAL AND HISTOLOGICAL CHANGES DUE TO CUMULATIVE UV DAMAGE TO THE DERMIS

Increased Wrinkling, Decreased Elasticity and Decreased Skin Strength

Intrinsically aged skin is smooth and shows fine wrinkles and wrinkles due to gravitational or conformational forces. In contrast, photoaged skin often shows deep wrinkles and has a leathery yellow appearance. This coarse leathery quality of skin and deep furrowing and deep wrinkle formation is predominantly due to the process of dermal elastosis, and is predominantly seen in darker-pigmented white patients (phototypes II and IV). The Favre-Racouchot sign (Fig. 12), which consists of deep furrowing, nodular elastic changes, comedones, and keratinous cysts; and cutis rhomboidalis nuchae (Fig. 13), or chronic sun damage of the neck with furrows arranged in a typical rhomboidal pattern, also belongs to this type of photoaging. Damaging effects of UV on the dermis is also greatly responsible for increased skin fragility, blister formation, decreased wound healing, and vascular changes, including telangiectasia.

Both intrinsic and photoinduced aging processes have quantitative and qualitative effects on collagen and elastic fibers in the skin (43). The histological hallmark of dermal photodamage is the accumulation of so-called elastotic material, termed solar or actinic elastosis. The dermis also demonstrates loss of collagen, a focal dermal perivascular infiltrate, and a narrow band of apparent sparing (Grenz zone) just below the epidermis

In sun-protected skin, elastic fibers in the papillary dermis appear as thin structures that run perpendicular to the dermoepidermal junction and that connect the basal lamina to the dermal elastic tissue. These fibers are composed of microfibrils without a central core of elastin and are termed oxytalan fibers. They subsequently branch to form a horizontal network in the upper reticular dermis where they contain small amounts of elastin (so-

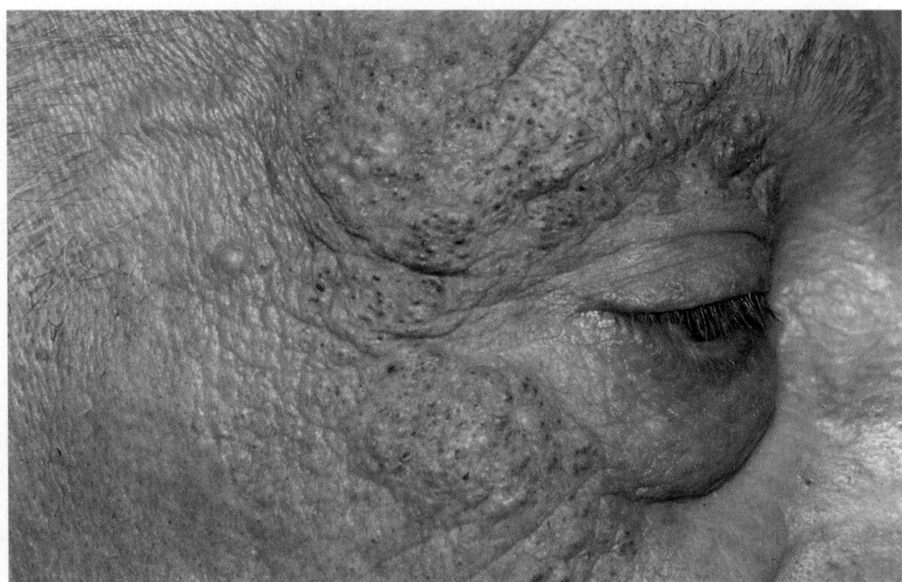

Figure 12 Favre-Racouchot is characterized by deep furrowing, nodular elastotic changes, comedones, and keratinous cysts.

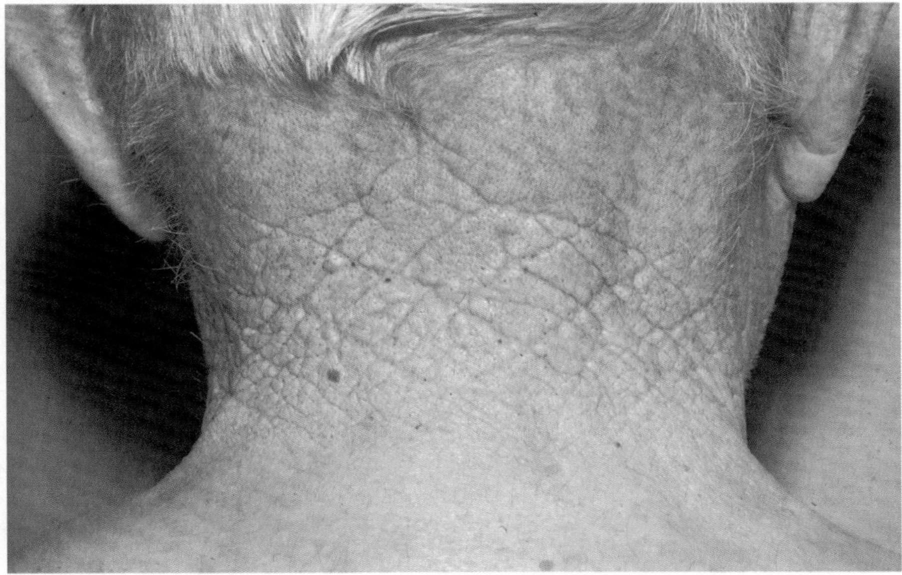

Figure 13 Cutis rhomboidalis nuchae. Chronic photodamage of the neck is shown. The furrows are arranged in a typical rhomboidal pattern.

called elaunin fibers). Still deeper in the dermis are the fully mature elastic fibers, composed of structural glycoproteins arranged around a core of elastin (44). With age, the newly formed fibers are rather loosely assembled (45), together with a loss of fibers in the superficial dermis and a degradation of deeply located mature fibers (46); ultrastructurally, fragmentation of the fibers may result in the formation of lacunae and cystic spaces (47).

In sun-damaged skin, the mid-dermis shows massive accumulation of abnormal elastic tissue, a process known as solar or actinic elastosis. This elastotic material is mainly derived from elastic fibers, as is evident from the positive staining with Verhoeff-van Gieson stain, but is accompanied by small amounts of type I and IV collagen as well as procollagen type III (48), fibronectin, and various proteoglycans and glycosaminoglycans, and macromolecules such as versican and decorin that accumulate on the elastotic material (49). Collagen type VII is usually reduced (50), whereas several matrix metalloproteinases are increased and participate in the remodelling of the elastotic material (51). On histological analysis, the process starts with an increase of slightly thickened elastic fibers in the papillary dermis; with time, thickened, curled, and fragmented fibers accumulate in the papillary and reticular dermis in the form of basophilic material (45) that may assume a homogeneous appearance. Capillaries, embedded in this material, become telangiectatic. On electronmicroscopic analysis, the thickened microfibrils have an irregular, fuzzy outline and are more electron dense; finally, the material becomes granular and disrupted, and electron-lucent areas appear (45).

In addition, intrinsically aged and photoaged skin both show an age-dependent reduction in the size of blood vessels in the skin, but only photoaged skin exhibits significantly reduced numbers of dermal vessels, particularly in areas that display extensive stromal changes (52). Recent ultrastructural data indicate that the photodamaged microvascular system is characterized by the coexistence of regressive changes and angiogenesis (52).

Pathogenic Mechanisms

Studies by the Uitto et al. (53–55) have shown that elastin gene expression is enhanced in sun-damaged skin owing to enhanced promotor activity of the elastin gene. UV can activate the elastin promotor in transgenic mice, and this may by one of the mechanisms by which chronic sun damage induces dermal elastosis. Thus, although the synthesis of elastin is increased, skin shows inelasticity and has a leathery appearance. This paradoxical situation can be explained by the fact that fibrillin and elastin fibers do not assemble into functional elastic and fibrillin fibers. Instead, elastotic material is ultrastructurally disorganized and functionally deficient. This accumulation of elastotic material is accompanied by concomitant degeneration of surrounding collagenous network. The mean concentration of collagen as determined by hydroxyproline assay is diminished in photoaged skin. The synthesis of collagen type I, the major structural component of dermal connective tissue, is diminished in chronically photodamaged skin (56). Collagen type I provides tensile strength and stability to the skin. In addition to decreased synthesis, direct damage or increased degradation can be the cause of decreased collagen and decreased procollagen I in chronically photodamaged skin. Indeed, dermal fibroblasts as well as the inflammatory infiltrate that surrounds cells in photoaged skin have the enzymatic capacity to degrade the extracellular matrix, including collagen. The mediators of this collagen breakdown are the matrix metalloproteinases (MMPs). It has been shown that MMP expression and activity are increased after UVB and UVA irradiation (4,57). In addition, studies in mast cell-deficient mice have shown that the products of mast cells either directly or indirectly increase elastin production by fibroblasts (58), and an ultrastructural study has shown marked qualitative and quantitative ultrastructural differences in Langerhans cells between photodamaged and intrinsically aged skin (59).

Reactive oxygen species (ROS) play a major role in the pathogenesis of photoaging of the dermis. ROS are generated following absorption of photons (UVB and UVA) by endogenous photosensitizers. Increased ROS production results in the depletion or damage of enzymatic and nonenzymatic antioxidant defense mechanisms. A recent study has shown that photoaged skin demonstrates depletion of antioxidant enzymes and accumulation of protein oxidation (60).

These ROS are also involved in the described photodamage of the dermal connective tissue. Indeed, ROS can enhance tropoelastin mRNA levels, directly destroy interstitial collagen, inactivate tissue inhibitor of metalloproteinase, and induce the synthesis and activation of MMPs (4).

REFERENCES

1. Gilchrest BA. Clinical features of photoageing differ from those of intrinsic ageing. J Dermatolog Treat 1996; 7:S5–S6.
2. Scharffetter-Kochanek K, Brenneissen P, Wenk J, Herrmann G, Ma W, Kuhr L, Meewes C, Wlashek M. Photoaging of the skin from phenotype to mechanisms. Exp Gerontol 2000; 35: 307–316.
3. Ma W, Wlaschek M, Tantcheva-Poor I, Schneider LA, Naderi L, Razi-Wolf Z, Schuller J, Scharffetter-Kochanek K. Chronological ageing and photoageing of the fibroblasts and the dermal connective tissue. Clin Exp Dermatol 2001; 26:592–599.
4. Wlaschek M, Tancheva-Poor I, Nader L, Ma W, Alexander Schneider L, Razi-Wolf Z, Schuller J, Scharffetter-Kochanek K. Solar UV irradiation and dermal photoaging. J Photochem Photobiol B 2001; 63:41–51.
5. Yaar M, Gilchrest BA. Ageing and photoageing of keratinocytes and melanocytes. Clin Exp Dermatol 2001; 26:583–591.
6. Yaar M, Gilchrest BA. Aging versus photoaging: postulated mechanisms and effectors. J Invest Dermatol Symp Proc 1998; 3:47–51.
7. Gilchrest Ba. Actinic injury. Annu Rev Med 1990; 41:199–210.
8. Nikkels A, Mosbah T, Pierard-Franchimont C, de la Brassinne M, Pierard GE. Comparative morphometric study of eruptive PUVA-induced and chronic sun-induced lentigines of the skin. Anal Quant Cytol Histol 1991; 13:23–26.
9. Holzle GE. Pigmented lesions as a sign of photodamage. Br J Dermatol 1992; 127:48–50.
10. Mehregan GE. Lentigo senilis and its evolutions. J Invest Dermatol 1975; 65:429–433.
11. Montagna W, Hu F, Carlisle K. A reinvestigation of solar lentigines. Arch Dermatol 1980; 116:1151–1154.
12. Stern JB, Peck GL, Haupt HM. Malignant melanoma in xeroderma pigmentosum: search for a precursor lesion. J Am Acad Dermatol 1993; 28:591–594.
13. Bhawan J. Histology of epidermal dysplasia. J Cutan Aging Cosm Dermatol 1988; 1:95–103.
14. Heaphy MR, Ackerman AB. The nature of solar keratosis: a critical review in historical perspective. J Am Acad Dermatol 2000; 43:138–150.
15. Frost C, Williams G, Green A. High incidence and regression rates of solar keratoses in a Queensland community. J Invest Dermatol 2000; 115:273–277.
16. Glogau RG. The risk of progression to invasive disease. J Am Acad Dermatol 2000; 42: 523–524.

17. Person JR. An actinic keratosis is neither malignant nor premalignant: It is an initiated tumor. J Am Acad Dermatol 2003; 48:637–638.
18. Strayer DS, Santa Cruz DJ. Carcinoma in situ of the skin: a review of histopathology. J Cutan Pathol 1980; 7:244–259.
19. Brooke Griffiths. Discordance between facial wrinkling and the presence of basal cell carcinoma. Arch Dermatol 2001; 137:751–754.
20. Cohen LM. The starburst giant cell is useful for distinguishing lentigo maligna from photodamaged skin. J Am Acad Dermatol 1996; 35:962–968.
21. Flotte TJ, Mihm MC. Lentigo maligna and malignant melanoma in situ, lentigo maligna type. Hum Pathol 1999; 30:533–536.
22. van den Oord JJ, Paemen L, Opdenakker G, Peeters C. Expression of gelatinase B and the extracellular matrix metalloproteinase-inducer EMMPRIN in benign and malignant pigment cell lesions of the skin. Am J Pathol 1997; 151:665–670.
23. Wei Q. Effect of aging on DNA repair and skin carcinogenesis: a minireview of population-based studies. J Investig Dermatol Symp Proc 1998; 3:19–22.
24. Moriwaki S, Ray S, Tarrone RE, Kraemer KH, Grossman L. The effect of donor age on the processing of UV-damaged DNA by cultured human cells: reduced DNA repair capacity and increased DNA mutability. Mutat Res 1996; 364:117–23.
25. Gad GF, Yaar M, Eller MS, Nehal US, Gilchrest BA. Mechanisms and implications of the age-associated decrease in DNA repair capacity. FASEB J 2000; 14:1325–1334.
26. Gilchrest BA, Garmyn M, Yaar M. Aging and photoaging affect gene expression in cultured human keratinocytes. Arch Dermatol 1994; 130:82–86.
27. Garmyn M, Yaar M, Boleau N, Backendorf C, Gilchrest B. Effect of aging and habitual sun exposure on the genetic response of cultured human keratinocytes to solar-simulated irradiation. J Invest Dermatol 1992; 99:743–748.
28. Ziegler A, Leffell DJ, Kunala S, Sharma HW, Gailani M, Simon JA, Halperin AJ, Baden HP, Shapiro PE, Bale AE, Brash DE. Mutation hotspots due to sunlight in the *p53* gene of nonmelanoma skin cancers. Proc Natl Acad Sci U S A 1993; 90:4216–4420.
29. Brash DE, Rudolph JA, Simon JA, Lin A, McKenna GJ, Baden HP, Halperin AJ, Ponten J. A role for sunlight in skin cancer: UV-induced *p53* mutations in squamous cell carcinomas. Proc Natl Acad Sci U S A 1991; 88:10124–10128.
30. Jonason AS, Kunula S, Price GJ, Restifo RJ, Spinelli HM, Persing JA, Leffell DJ, Tarrone RE, Brash DE. Frequent clones of p53-mutated keratinocytes in normal human skin. Proc Natl Acad Sci U S A 1996; 93:14025–14029.
31. De Gruijl FR. Photocarcinogenesis: UVA vs. UVB radiation. Skin Pharmacol Appl Skin Physiol 2002; 15:316–320.
32. Park WS, Lee HK, Lee JY, Yoo NJ, Kim CS, Kim SH. p53 mutations in solar keratosis. Hum Pathol 1996; 27:1180–1184.
33. Spencer JM, Kahn SM, Jiang W, Deleo VA, Weinsteine IB. Activated ras genes occur in human actinic keratoses, premalignant precursors to squamous cell carcinomas. Arch Dermatol 1995; 31:796–800.
34. Mortier L, Marchetti P, Delaporte E, Martin de Lasalle E, Piette F, Formstecher P, Polakowska R, Danze PM. Progression of actinic keratosis to squamous cell carcinoma of the skin correlates with deletion of the 9p21 region encoding the p16(INK4a) tumor suppressor. Cancer Lett 2002; 176:205–214.
35. van Ruissen F, Jansen BJ, de Jongh GJ, Van Vlijmen-Willems IM, Schalkwijk J. Differential gene expression in premalignant human epidermis revealed by cluster analysis of serial analysis of gene expression (SAGE)libraries. FASEB J 2002; 16:246–248.
36. Liang SB, Furihata M, Takeuchi T, Sonobe H, Ohtsuki Y. Reduced human mismatch repair protein expression in the development of precancerous skin lesions to squamous cell carcinoma. Virchows Arch 2001; 439:622–627.

37. Tsukifuji R, Tagawa K, Hatamochi A, Shinkai H. Expression of matrix metalloproteinase-1, -2 and -3 in squamous cell carcinoma and actinic keratosis. Br J Cancer 1999; 80:1087–1091.
38. Tucci MG, Offidani A, Lucarini G, Simonelli L, Amatti S, Cellini A, Biagini G, Ricotti G. Advances in the understanding of malignant transformation of keratinocytes: an immunohistochemical study. J Eur Acad Dermatol Venereol 1998; 10:118–124.
39. Dahmane N, Lee J, Robins P, Heller P, Ruiz i Altaba A. Activation of the transcription factor Gli1 and the sonic hedgehog signalling pathway in skin tumours. Nature 1997; 389:876–881.
40. Bataille V. Genetics of familial and sporadic melanoma. Clin Exp Dermatol 2000; 25:464–470.
41. Herbst RA, Gutzmer R, Matiaske F, Mommert S, Kapp A, Weiss J, Arden KC, Cavenee WK. Further evidence for ultraviolet light induction of CDKN2 (p16INK4) mutations in sporadic melanoma in vivo. J Invest Dermatol 1997; 108:950.
42. Peris K, Chimenti S, Fargnoli MC, Valeri P, Kerl H, Wolf P. UV fingerprint CDKN2a but no p14ARF mutations in sporadic melanomas. J Invest Dermatol 1999; 112:825–826.
43. El-Domyati M, Attia S, Saleh F, Brown D, Birk DE, Gasparro F, Ahmad H, Uitto J. Intrinsic aging vs. photoaging: a comparative histopathological, immunohistochemical, and ultrastructural study of skin. Exp Dermatol 2002; 11:398–340.
44. Cotta-Pereira G, Rodrigo FG, Bittencourt-Sampaio S. Oxytalan, eulaunin, and elastic fibers in the human skin. J Invest Dermatol 1976; 66:143–148.
45. Braverman IM, Fonferko E. Studies in cutaneous aging. I. The elastic fiber network. J Invest Dermatol 1982; 78:434–443.
46. Takema Y, Yorimoto Y, Kawai M, Imokawa G. Age-related changes in the elastic properties and thickness of human facial skin. Br J Dermatol 1994; 131:641–648.
47. Tsuji T, Hamada T. Age-related changes in human dermal elastic fibres. Br J Dermatol 1981; 105:57–63.
48. Chen VL, Fleischmaier R, Schwartz E, Palaia M, Timple R. Immunochemistry of elastotic material in sun-damaged skin. J Invest Dermatol 1986; 87:334–337.
49. Bernstein EF, Underhill CB, Hahn PJ, Brown DB, Uitto J. Chronic sun exposure alters both the content and distribution of dermal glycosaminoglycans. Br J Dermatol 1996; 135:255–262.
50. Craven NM, Watson REB, Jones CJP, Shuttleworth CA, Kielty CM, Griffiths CE. Clinical features of photodamaged skin are associated with a reduction in collagen VII. Br J Dermatol 1997; 137:344–350.
51. Saarialho-Kere U, Kerkelä E, Jeskanen L, Hasan T, Pierce R, Starchner B, Randasoja R, Ranki A, Oikarinen A, Vaalamo M. Accumulation of matrilysin (MMP-7) and macrophage metalloelastase (MMP-12) in actinic damage. J Invest Dermatol 1999; 113:664–672.
52. Chung JH, Yano K, Lee MK, Youn CS, Seo JK, Kim KH, Cho KH, Eun HC, Detmar M. Differential effects of photoaging vs intrinsic aging on the vascularization of human skin. Arch Dermatol 2002; 138:1437–1442.
53. Bernstein EF, Chen YQ, Tamai K, Shepley KJ, Resnik KS, Zhang H, Tuan R, Mauviel A, Uitto J. Enhanced elastin and fibrillin gene expression in chronically photodamaged skin. J Invest Dermatol 1994; 103:182–186.
54. Bernstein EF, Brown DB, Urbach F, Forbes D, Del Monaco M, Wu M, Katchman SD, Uitto J. Ultraviolet radiation activates the human elastin promoter in transgenic mice: a novel in vivo and in vitro model of cutaneous photoaging. J Invest Dermatol 1995; 105:269–273.
55. Uitto J, Bernstein EF. Molecular mechanisms of cutaneous aging: connective tissue alterations in the dermis. J Invest Dermatol Symp Proc 1998; 3:41–44.
56. Talwar HS, Griffiths CE, Fisher GJ, Hamilton TA, Voorhees JJ. Reduced type I and type III procollagens in photodamaged adult human skin. J Invest Dermatol 1995; 105:285–290.
57. Fisher GJ, Wang ZQ, Datta SC, Varani J, Kang S, Voorhees JJ. Pathophysiology of premature skin aging induced by ultraviolet light. N Engl J Med 1997; 337:1419–1428.
58. Gonzalez S, Moran M, Kochevar IE. Chronic photodamage in skin of mast cell-deficient mice. Photochem Photobiol 1999; 70:248–253.

59. Toyoda M, Bhawan J. Ultrastructural evidence for the participation of Langerhans cells in cutaneous photoaging processes: a quantitative comparative study. J Dermatol Sci 1997; 14: 87–100.
60. Sander CS, Chang H, Salzmann S, Muller CS, Ekanayake-Mudiyanselage S, Elsner P, Thiele JJ. Photoaging is associated with protein oxidation in human skin in vivo. J Invest Dermatol 2002; 118:618–625.

4

Photoaging in Patients of Skin of Color

Rebat M. Halder / Georgianna M. Richards *Howard University College of Medicine, Washington, DC, U.S.A.*

- All races are subject to photoaging.
- The clinical features of photoaging in Asians are primarily discrete pigmentary changes, tactile roughness, and coarse and fine wrinkling.
- In African Americans, photoaging appears primarily in lighter-complexioned individuals and may not be apparent until the late fifth or sixth decades of life.
- Photoaging is the third most common dermatologic diagnosis in Hispanic patients treated in a dermatology private practice.
- Not previously described as being common in Asians and fair-skinned Hispanics, wrinkling is a major clinical manifestation of photoaging.

INTRODUCTION

Asians

People of skin of color comprise the majority of the world's population. These include Asians who can be subdivided into East Asians (Chinese, Japanese, Koreans), Southeast Asians (Indonesians, Malaysians, Singaporeans, Thais, Cambodians, Vietnamese), and South Asians (Bangladeshis, Indians, Pakistanis, Sri Lankans). Those from East Asia tend to be lighter in skin color, although Koreans are more brown skinned than Chinese or Japanese. Southeast Asians are brown in skin color. East Asians and Southeast Asians are of Mongoloid ethnic background. South Asians are of Caucasian ethnic background but have brown to dark-brown skin.

Hispanics

Hispanics are another large group comprising individuals of skin of color. There are European Hispanics, who are of Caucasian ethnic origin and lighter in skin color. However, a large number of Hispanics worldwide are brown skinned. Some Hispanics can be of mixed ancestry, having Caucasian and Native Indian heritage. There are also some Hispanics with black heritage. The geographical areas for brown-skinned Hispanics include North America, Mexico, Central and South America, and the Caribbean.

Blacks

Blacks are also a large group of people of skin of color. For the purposes of discussion in this chapter, the term black includes those from the African continent, African Americans, and Afro-Caribbeans. Thus, the term skin of color includes an extremely heterogeneous group of peoples. Patients of skin of color can be anywhere within Fitzpatrick's skin phototype III to VI. With this wide range of skin colors, patients of skin of color vary considerably in their response to sunlight, sun exposure, and ultimately photodamage and photoaging.

All Races Are Susceptible to Photoaging

In general, all races are susceptible to photoaging (1). However, it is clear that those who fall within Fitzpatrick's skin phototype IV to VI are less susceptible, most likely owing to the photoprotective role of melanin (2,3). It has been shown that the mean protective factor (PF) for ultraviolet (UV) B for black epidermis is 13.4 as compared to 3.4 for white epidermis (4). The mean UVB transmission by black epidermis is 5.7% compared to 29.4% for white epidermis. For UVA, the mean PF of black epidermis is 5.7, which is significantly higher than that of white epidermis (1.8) (4). Thus, the mean UVA transmission by black epidermis is 17.5% compared to 55.5% for white epidermis, meaning that about three to four times more UVA reaches the upper dermis of whites than that of blacks. The main site of UV filtration in white skin is the stratum corneum, whereas in black skin it is the malpighian layers (4). The malpighian layers of black skin remove twice as much UVB radiation as the stratum corneum (4). For UVA, possibly greater removal of radiation occurs in black malpighian layers (4). Other factors besides melanin may be responsible for natural photoprotection. However, no major differences in the thickness or composition of the epidermal layers have been demonstrated between the two racial groups (4,5), and it is likely that these observed differences in transmission of UVB and UVA are mainly due to melanin (4). Although these studies were performed on black skin, the data can probably be extrapolated to most persons of Fitzpatrick's skin types IV to VI.

PHOTOAGING IN EAST AND SOUTHEAST ASIANS

The largest number of studies on photoaging in patients of skin of color conducted to date have included East and Southeast Asians (Chinese, Japanese, Koreans, Malaysians, Singaporeans, and Thais) (1,6–10). In these regions of the world, photoaging is common because of geographical proximity to the equator (1).

Discrete Pigmentary Changes

The clinical features of photoaging in East and Southeast Asians are primarily discrete pigmentary changes. These include actinic lentigines; flat, pigmented seborrheic keratoses and mottled hyperpigmentation (Fig. 1). Solar-induced facial melasma is more common

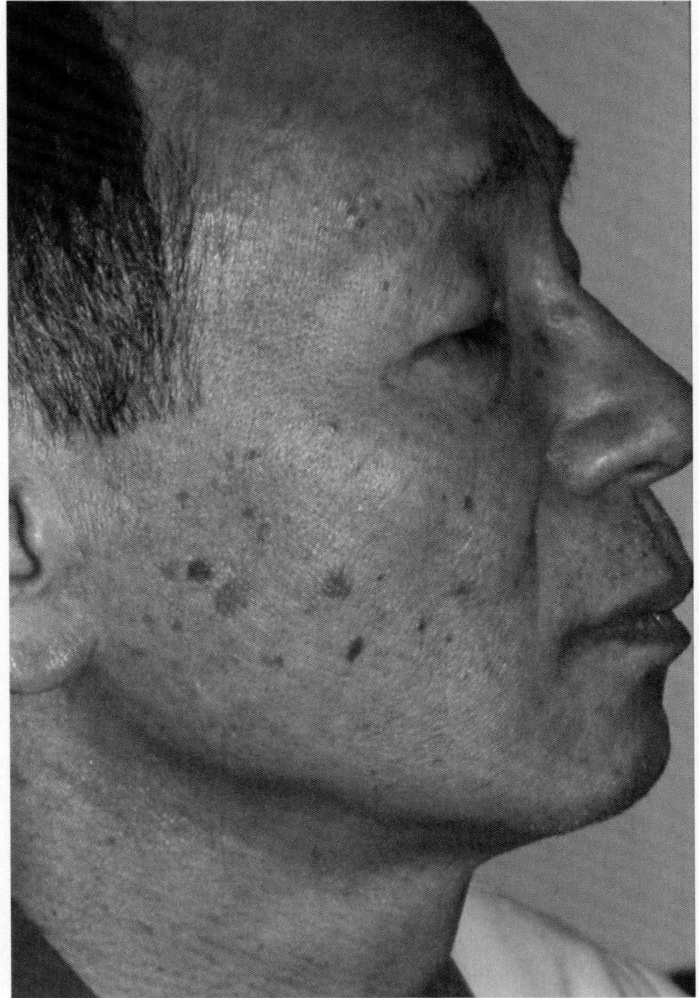

Figure 1 Photoaging in an Asian patient characterized by flat pigmented seborrheic keratoses, actinic lentigines, and mottled hyperpigmentation. Fine wrinkling is present.

in this group than in whites and should be considered a form of actinic dyspigmentation in this instance (1). In Asian cultures, the standard of beauty is flawless facial skin, uniform in color and texture (1,6,7); thus, the pigmentary changes of photoaging become significant cosmetic problems. In a study of 61 Thai subjects of whom 80% were women, Kotrajaras and Kligman (7) found unexpected histological findings of photodamage. Most of the subjects were Fitzpatrick's type IV. However, Thailand is in a tropical zone with approximately 12 hours of continuous sunshine almost year round. Because the population makes little effort to protect their skin from excessive sun exposure, the clinical signs of photoaging appear in Thais by age 40 (7). Skin biopsy specimens were taken from the cheek over the lateral zygomatic process, avoiding lesional skin such as lentigos or keratoses.

There was an extraordinary degree of dermal photodamage, which was found in practically all of the subjects older than 50 years. Even subjects in their 30s showed a surprising degree of actinic damage. The epidermis of those subjects older than 50 years showed atrophy, atypia, and dysplasia (7). There was poor polarity and disorderly differentiation, and the quantity of melanin in the keratinocytes was high. Basilar keratinocytes had dense clusters of highly melanized melanosomes. Subepidermal melanophages, which were found in most subjects in this study, were often numerous, large, packed with pigment, and sometimes scattered throughout the reticular dermis. This pigment dumping is a characteristic feature of darkly pigmented races after various chemical and physical traumas (7).

Dermal Changes

Dermal changes were severe in the group of patients studied (7). There was marked elastosis presenting as twisted fibers, in various stages of amorphous degeneration. This finding in older Thai individuals was almost equivalent to that of end-stage photodamaged white skin with the amorphous degeneration and twisted fibers described (7). Elastotic tissue almost completely replaced the collagen network.

Wrinkling

A study by Griffiths et al. (1) that consisted of 45 photoaged Asian patients (23 Chinese, 22 Japanese) indicated that wrinkling was not a prominent feature of photoaging in Asian skin. Histological diagnoses of photoaging in this patient group included seborrheic keratoses, benign keratoses (seborrheic keratosis without horn-cyst formation), actinic lentigo, and solar elastosis.

The largest study to date of Asian patients with photoaging was done by Goh et al. (6), and included over 1500 patients of skin type III or IV who were of Singaporean (of Chinese ancestry), Indonesian, or Malaysian background and between the ages of 30 and 50 years. The main features of photoaging included hyperpigmentation, tactile roughness, and coarse and fine wrinkling .

A more recent study by Chung et al. (9), however, indicates that wrinkling may be a major feature of photoaging in Asians. In this study, which was limited only to Koreans aged 30 to 92 years (236 men and 171 women), seborrheic keratosis was the major pigmentary lesion associated with photoaging in men, whereas in women it was hyperpigmented macules. The number of hyperpigmented macules and seborrheic keratoses increased with each decade of age ($P < 0.05$). In those 60 years and older, seborrheic keratosis was more common in men than in women ($P < 0.001$). In those 50 years and older, hyperpigmented macules were found more frequently in women than in men ($P < 0.01$). The most striking feature of the study by Chung et al. (9) was the finding of moderate to severe wrinkling associated with photodamage that becomes apparent at about age 50 years in Koreans. Women tended to have more severe wrinkling, and the risk of developing wrinkling was higher in women (prevalence odds ratio, 3.7). This was also the first study to demonstrate a relationship between cigarette smoking and wrinkling in Asians, which has previously been demonstrated in white subjects (11–14). In the study by Chung et al. (9), a history of cigarette smoking of 0 to 0.9 pack-years was reported by 194 subjects, and 213 subjects reported a smoking history of 1 to 120 pack-years. After controlling for age, sex, and sun exposure, an association between cigarette smoking and wrinkling showed a significant trend with increasing pack-years. There was also an association between exposure to the sun and development of wrinkling. Sun exposure of more than 5 hours per day was associated with a 48-fold increased risk for wrinkling, compared with 1 to 2 hours per day.

There was also seen a combined effect of sun exposure and cigarette smoking in Koreans. Sun exposure of more than 5 hours per day and a smoking history of more than 30 pack-years were associated with a 4.2 fold increased risk of wrinkling, compared with a 2.2-fold increase for nonsmokers with 1 to 2 hours of daily sun exposure. In another recent study by Chung et al. (10), which was also limited to Koreans, 21 subjects (12 men, nine women)— three subjects for each decade of life from the third to ninth—were evaluated to quantify the effects of photoaging on cutaneous vascularization over time. Previous studies on photoaged skin have focused for the most part on end-stage dermal vascular changes. Punch biopsy specimens were taken from chronically sun-exposed skin (crow's feet area of the face). Immunostaining was done with a specific antibody for the CD31 antigen (platelet endothelial cell adhesion molecule) and was examined using computer-assisted morphometric analysis.

Degenerative Matrix Changes

Chung et al. (10) found that photoaged skin showed significantly reduced numbers of dermal vessels, in particular in the subepidermal areas that had extensive matrix damage. There was an inverse relationship between vessel numbers and age of the subject in photodamaged skin. The investigators concluded that in Korean skin, chronic photodamage results in a gradual decrease in the number and size of dermal vessels over decades of sun exposure, most likely because of degenerative changes of the dermal extracellular matrix. This is an interesting study as it was done in Koreans of skin type V only. A similar study has not yet been conducted in white patients.

Another recent study on photoaging in Asians was conducted by Kwon et al. (15). A total of 303 Korean brown-skinned men aged 40–70 years were examined for seborrheic keratoses, one of the signs of photoaging in Asians. The mean overall prevalence of seborrheic keratoses was 88.1%. The prevalence of seborrheic keratoses increased considerably, from 78.9% at 40 years to 93.9% at 50 years and 98.7% in those older than 60 years. The keratoses were considerably more frequent on sun-exposed areas, with the majority of lesions concentrated on the face and the dorsa of the hands. The size of each lesion also became significantly larger with each decade of life. The estimated area covered by seborrheic keratosis per percentage body surface area on sun-exposed areas was 5.7, 11.2, and 18.3 times greater than partially exposed areas at ages 40, 50, and 60 years, respectively (15). More than 6 hours per day of lifetime cumulative sunlight exposure was found to have 2.28 times higher risk of seborrheic keratoses than less than 3 hours of daily sun exposure. The authors concluded that seborrheic keratoses are common in Korean men aged 40–70 years, and that aging and cumulative sunlight exposure are both independent contributory factors (15).

PHOTOAGING IN BLACKS

Photoaging occurs in blacks, but is presently uncommon. Although unusual, it is more often seen in African Americans rather than in Africans or Afro-Caribbeans. This may be because African Americans are often a heterogenous mixture of African, Caucasian, and Native American ancestry. Published studies on photoaging in blacks have been limited to African Americans. Thus, this section will focus on photoaging in the African American population. In an earlier portion of this chapter, data were presented on the efficient filtering capacity of black skin for UVA and UVB compared to white skin due mainly to increased levels of melanin in black skin.

In African Americans, photoaging appears primarily in lighter-complexioned individuals within this group and may not be apparent until the late fifth or sixth decades of life (16). Clinically, the features of photoaging in African Americans are fine wrinkling and mottled pigmentation (Fig. 2.) In a study by Montagna and Carlisle (17) of 19 black and 19 white females who had lived in Tucson, Arizona for 2 or more years, there were few histological findings of photoaging in blacks. Biopsy specimens were taken from the malar eminences of the subjects. Histological findings showed that in white sun-exposed skin the stratum lucidum was usually distorted, whereas black sun-exposed rarely showed any evidence of alteration in the stratum lucidum. In addition, the stratum lucidum remained compact and unaltered in black sun-exposed skin regardless of age, whereas in white sun-exposed skin it was swollen and distinctly cellular.

Oxytalan fibers were found in the papillary dermis of sun-exposed skin of 50-year-old black subjects, but these fibers were usually lacking in sun-exposed skin of white persons of the same age. Oxytalan fibers were found in the facial skin of white subjects who were in their 20s and early 30s, but they seemed to disappear in the sun-exposed skin of persons age 40 years or older. No solar elastosis was seen in specimens of black sun-exposed skin. Older black subjects appeared to have an increase in the number and thickness of elastic fibers that separated the collagenous fiber layer in the reticular dermis. Single-stranded elastic fibers in younger subjects resembled braids in older (>50 years) subjects. The distribution and amount of elastic fibers in the sun-exposed skin of a 45-year-old light-skinned black woman resembled those in white sun-exposed skin (17).

The facial skin of black women in the study had elastic fibers that stained (hematoxylin and Lee) differently than those of white skin. Photodamaged white skin showed only elastic fibers in the papillary and reticular dermis, which stained pink, and the wide ribbon-like fibers in the intermediate dermis stained blue (18). All dermal elastic fibers in black

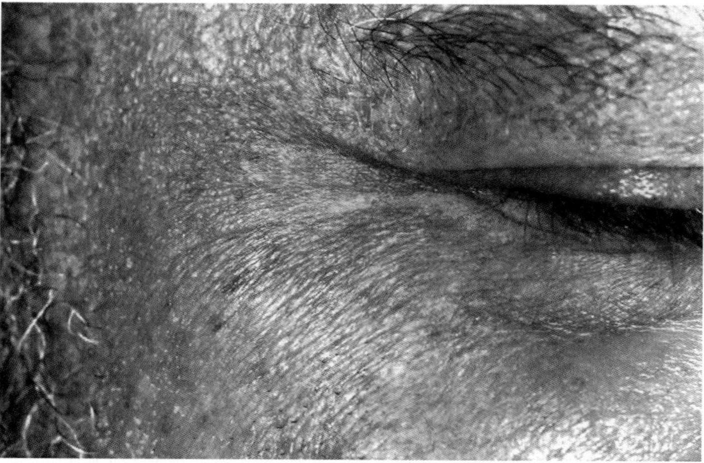

Figure 2 Photoaging in a fair-skinned African American patient characterized by mottled hyperpigmentation and fine wrinkling.

sun-exposed skin stained pink, similar to the sun-protected skin of white individuals. The staining of the elastic fibers in a light-skinned 45-year-old black woman was similar to that observed in white subjects (17).

Protection Against Wrinkling by Melanin in Black Skin

The majority of the white women aged 45 to 50 years in Montagna and Carlisle's study (17) had wrinkles beside the lateral canthi of the eyes and at the corners of the mouth, whereas none of the black women showed any obvious wrinkles. Long-term sun exposure to black skin resulted in only minor changes compared to the profound alterations present in sun-exposed white skin. The presence of greater number of melanosomes and their distribution in black skin likely protects the epidermis from photodamage (17).

One key factor in the dermal photodamage of white skin is the presence of elastotic material (18). Elastotic tissue, once it is formed, is constantly resorbed and replaced with other elastotic tissue and large collagenous fiber bundles. This results in shrinkage and reduction of the dermal volume. This process occurs less precipitously in the facial skin of young and middle-aged black women (17).

The presence of abundant fiber fragments in black skin could be due to degradation products in addition to newly synthesized fibers. The fiber fragments, hypertrophied multinucleated fibroblasts, and macrophages are numerous in black skin. These histological characteristics represent active biosynthesis degradation and turnover, and may be responsible for the clean appearance of black dermis compared to the damaged dermis of sun-exposed white skin.

PHOTOAGING IN HISPANICS

There are no studies in the literature that specifically address photoaging in Hispanics. However, Sanchez (19) found that photoaging was the third most common dermatological diagnosis in 1000 Hispanic patients treated in a dermatology private practice, accounting for 16.8% of visits.

Photoaging in European and fair-skinned Hispanics most likely occurs in the same frequency and degree as in whites, so that the clinical manifestation is primarily wrinkling rather than pigmentary alterations. Wrinkling appears at the same age that it would appear in whites. Darker skinned Hispanics, that are type IV and V, and live in hot tropical climates such as Mexico, Central America, or South America will have clinical manifestations of photoaging that are similar to those of South Asians and African Americans. These manifestations include fine wrinkling and mottled pigmentation occurring in the late fourth through sixth decades of life. However, with many years of occupational sun exposure, there are some darker-skinned Hispanics that have marked deep wrinkling. No histological studies that specifically address photoaging in Hispanics could be located in the literature.

SUMMARY AND CONCLUSIONS

Protective Effect of Melanin

Photoaging in skin of color has variable presentations. Asians and fair-skinned Hispanics do experience wrinkling, a clinical manifestation that was not previously described as being common in these populations. Wrinkling is not as common a manifestation of photoaging in blacks, South Asians, or darker-skinned Hispanics. In general, melanin still gives protection against photodamage in patients of color. Within most pigmented racial groups, it is the lighter-colored individuals that show evidence of photodamaged skin. Pigmentary manifestations of photoaging are common in skin of color and include seborrheic keratosis, actinic lentigines, mottled hyperpigmentation, and solar-induced facial melasma.

Increased Unprotected Sun Exposure

A significant component of photoaging in patients of skin of color may be related to the fact that many of these persons live in sunny, hot, tropical areas. It has been previously accepted that increased skin melanin affords protection against photoaging. However, since both clinical and histological studies have shown that photoaging is a global problem, it may be that there are other factors that contribute to the degree of photodamage observed in patients of skin of color. It has been shown that many patients of skin of color do not protect themselves with sunscreen when exposed to the sun (20–22). Many times this is by choice, as patients of skin of color often do not believe or understand that they need sun protection when involved in either occupational or recreational sun exposure. Studies have shown that sunscreen use is less prevalent in African American and Hispanic populations than among whites (20,21). Hispanics, however, use sunscreen more frequently than African Americans.

Recreational Activities

Patients of skin of color worldwide now engage in recreational activities that involve sun exposure. These activities were previously engaged in primarily by white populations, and include water and snow skiing, tennis, golf, and sunbathing on the beach. With access to these activities, many patients of skin of color do not use sun protection and may be exposed to the sun for prolonged periods (22). If public education concerning sun exposure and proper protection for this segment of the population is not available, the number of photodamaged patients of skin of color will increase.

The reasons why patients of color are prone to photoaging are not completely known. Even though the efficient UV filtering capacity of pigmented skin was described earlier in the chapter, it may be that high UV exposure overwhelms the filtering capacity of melanin in hot sunny climates (7). Many patients of skin of color live in sunny and hot areas of the world. The question of whether infrared radiation also contributes to photodamage should be addressed. In addition, there is evidence that chronic exposure to natural or artificial heat sources can lead to histological changes resembling those induced by UV radiation, including elastosis and carcinoma (23). Finally, an animal study has shown that infrared radiation can potentiate the photodamaging effects of UV radiation (24).

REFERENCES

1. Griffiths CE, Goldfarb MT, Finkel LJ, Roulia V, Bonawitz M, Hamilton TA, Ellis CN, Voorhees JJ. Topical tretinoin treatment of hyperpigmented lesions associated with photoaging in Chinese and Japanese patients: a vehicle-controlled trial. J Am Acad Dermatol 1994; 30: 76–84.
2. Pathak MA, Fitzpatrick TB. The role of natural photoprotective agents in human skin. In: Fitzpatrick TB, Pathak MA, Harber LC, Seiji M, Kukita A, Eds. Sunlight and Man. Tokyo: University of Tokyo Press, 1974:725–750.

3. Kligman AM. Solar elastosis in relation to pigmentation. In: Fitzpatrick TB, Pathak MA, Harber LC, Seiji M, Kukita A, Eds. Sunlight and Man. Tokyo: University of Tokyo Press, 1974:157–163.
4. Kaidbey KH, Agin PP, Sayre RM, Kligman AM. Photoprotection by melanin: a comparison of black and Caucasian skin. J Am Acad Dermatol 1979; 1:249–260.
5. Weigand DA, Haygood C, Gaylor JR. Cell layers and density of negro and Caucasian stratum corneum. J Invest Dermatol 1974; 62:563–568.
6. Goh SH. The treatment of visible signs of senescence: the Asian experience. Br J Dermatol 1990; 122:105–109.
7. Kotrajaras R, Kligman AM. The effect of topical tretinoin on photodamaged facial skin: the Thai experience. Br J Dermatol 1993; 129:302–309.
8. Griffiths CE. Assessment of topical retinoids for the treatment of Far-East Asian skin. J Am Acad Dermatol 1998; 39:S104–S107.
9. Chung JH, Lee SH, Youn CS, Park BJ, Kim KH, Park KC, Cho KH, Eun HC. Cutaneous photodamage in Koreans. Arch Dermatol 2001; 137:1043–1051.
10. Chung JH, Yano K, Lee MK, Youn CS, Seo JY, Kim KH, Cho KH, Eun HC, Detmar M. Differential effects of photoaging vs intrinsic aging on the vascularization of human skin. Arch Dermatol 2002; 138:1437–1442.
11. Daniell HW. A study in the epidemiology of ''crow's feet''. Ann Intern Med 1971; 75:873–880.
12. Kadunce DP, Burr R, Gress R, Kanner R, Lyon JL, Zone JJ. Cigarette smoking: risk factor for premature facial wrinkling. Ann Intern Med 1991; 114:840–844.
13. Ernster VL, Grady D, Miike R, Black D, Selby J, Kerlikowske K. Facial wrinkling in men and women, by smoking status. Am J Public Health 1995; 85:78–82.
14. Smith JB, Fenske NA. Cutaneous manifestations and consequences of smoking. J Am Acad Dermatol 1996; 34:717–732.
15. Kwon OS, Hwang EJ, Bae JH, Park HE, Lee JC, Youn JI, Chung JH. Seborrheic keratosis in the Korean males: causative role of sunlight. Photodermatol Photoimmunol Photomed 2003; 19:73–80.
16. Halder RM. The role of retinoids in the management of cutaneous conditions in blacks. J Am Acad Dermatol 1998; 39(2 Pt. 3):S98–S103.
17. Montagna W, Carlisle K. The architecture of black and white facial skin. J Am Acad Dermatol 1991; 24:929–937.
18. Montagna W, Kirchner S, Carlisle K. Histology of sun-damaged human skin. J Am Acad Dermatol 1989; 21:907–918.
19. Sanchez MR. Cutaneous disease in Latinos. Derm Clin. In press.
20. Hall HI, Jones SE, Saraiya M. Prevalence and correlates of sunscreen use among US high school students. J Sch Health 2001; 71:453–457.
21. Friedman LC, Bruce S, Weinberg AD, Cooper HP, Yen AH, Hill M. Early detection of skin Cancer: racial/ethnic differences in behaviors and attitudes. J Cancer Educ 1994; 9:105–110.
22. Halder RM, Bridgeman-Shah S. Skin cancer in African Americans. Cancer 1995; 15(suppl 2):667–673.
23. Kligman LH. Intensification of ultraviolet-induced dermal damage by infra-red radiation. Arch Dermatol 1982; 272:229–238.
24. Kligman AM. Aging, light and heat. In:. Psoralens in Cosmetics and Dermatology. Proceedings of the International Symposium (SIR). Paris: Pergamon Press, 1981:57–64.

5

Photoaging and Aging Skin

Richard G. Glogau *University of California, San Francisco, California, U.S.A.*

- Photoaging is related to intrinsic and ultraviolet-induced factors.
- Clinical findings in photoaging have direct histologic correlates.
- A systematic classification of patient photoaging types facilitates the matching of appropriate therapy to a given patient situation and is the basis for rationale selection of rejuvenation techniques.
- Combination minimally invasive therapy will continue to complement traditional resurfacing and surgical techniques to treat the aging appearance of the face and reverse the signs of photoaging.
- Problems associated with photoaging are increasing and will continue to increase due to evolving population demographics.

Currently, one person in the United States turns 50 years old every 8 seconds. The baby boomers are aging, and the phenomenon of the aging appearance looms large in consumer conscience. The sustained post-World War II period of economic growth ended in the heady bubble of high-tech expansion and stock market collapse with downsizing added to the social strains of divorce and remarriage. A corresponding boom in media communications, iconographic images, and retail advertising parallel wider acceptance of cosmetic rejuvenation and wider availability of such services. The preoccupation with appearance also dovetails with the renewed emphasis on health and fitness, and the burgeoning consumer market of products promoting wellness.

Medical response to this consumer-driven demand has not been stagnant. In the past two decades a logarithmic explosion of medical and surgical techniques has occurred. Many techniques, such as liposuction surgery, were unimaginable only two decades ago, and now number among the most common cosmetic procedures performed in the United

States in the last year. Laser surgery appears poised to overtake the field in sheer number of cases performed. And the last 2 years have seen the introduction of botulinum toxin as the cosmetic agent of the moment, poised to sell over U.S.$600 million in the domestic market this year.

One of the physiological aging processes that now afflicts the entire baby boomer generation is photoaging. With the increase in post-World War II leisure time, the increasing availability of automobile and air travel, and an increased emphasis on fitness and outdoor activity, the baby boomers spent their formative years in the 1950s and 1960s out in the sun, without the benefit of currently available sunscreens. Early years of ''baby oil and iodine,'' skimpier clothing, and the oxymoronic desire of the physically fit to acquire a ''healthy tan'' have produced steadily rising rates of skin cancer and premature aging skin. While there are certainly intrinsic aging factors that combine with certain external factors, such as gravity, that are unrelated to ultraviolet exposure, cumulative exposure to sun remains the largest single factor in aging skin and is responsible for most of the unwanted aesthetic effects that plague this population moving into their 50s.

MOLECULAR MECHANISMS IN PHOTOAGING SKIN

The current understanding of molecular mechanisms in photoaging has been nicely reviewed by the investigators at the University of Michigan under Dr. John Voorhees (1). There appears to be a convergence of molecular pathways involved in the intrinsic and ultraviolet-induced skin aging. Ultraviolet light activates cell-surface cytokines and growth factor receptors on keratinocytes and fibroblasts such as epidermal growth factor (EGF), interleukin (IL), and tumor necrosis factor alpha (TNF-α) within 15 minutes of exposure to twice the minimal erythema dose. These activated receptors stimulate intracellular signals that induce transcription factor AP-1, which stimulates matrix metalloproteinase (MMP) genes and inhibits procollagen gene expression. MMP breaks down collagen and other proteins that constitute the extracellular matrix. This damaged protein accumulates and produces the characteristic thickened upper dermis that we recognize clinically as solar elastosis and wrinkles.

The primary pathway of photochemical response to ultraviolet light in human skin is the production of reactive oxygen species such as superoxide anion, peroxide, and singlet oxygen, which in turn remove phosphate groups from the tyrosine phosphatase receptors, leading to a net increase in receptor phosphorylation and, hence, activation of receptors (EGF, IL, TNF-α). Photoaged skin accumulates degraded, disorganized collagen fibrils and reduced production of type I and type III procollagen. All-*TRANS* retinoic acid induces type I and type III procollagen, the precursor to collagen and new fibrils, which improves the appearance of photoaged skin (2–5).

HISTOLOGICAL CORRELATES OF AGING SKIN

Clinical signs of photoaging of the skin include rhytids, lentigines, keratoses, telangiectasia, loss of translucency, loss of elasticity, and sallow color (6). From the clinician's viewpoint, the microscopic differences between sun-exposed skin and normal undamaged skin give indications of how rejuvenation procedures could potentially normalize the microscopic appearance of sun-damaged skin.

Montagna et al.'s classic histological studies (7,8) using 2.0-μm-thick specimens embedded in glycolmethacrylate have shown the sun-damaged epidermis to be characterized by a compact and laminated or gelatinous stratum corneum without clear transition to the underlying stratum lucidum. The epidermis shows evidence of atypical keratinocytes and dysplasia,, vacuolization of epidermal cells, scattered cell necrosis, and a noticeable loss of Langerhans cells. Change in vertical polarity in epidermal cells and irregularity of the epidermal cell alignment is characteristic of chronically sun-damaged skin.

The dermis shows homogenization of the upper papillary dermal ground substance, often termed elastosis, with formation of amorphous masses and breakage of fibers. There is an increase in reticulin fibers, and often mast cells and macrophages with coarse granules are present. The collagen substance in the upper dermis appears to be destroyed over time and gradually replaced by the amorphous material that stains poorly and is frequently associated with an increase in reticulin fibers in and around the amorphous material. The amount of elastotic material and associated fibrorhexis or fiber breakdown can be quite large and is probably responsible for the fine wrinkle formation seen in sun-damaged skin.

CLASSIFICATION OF PHOTOAGING TO FACILITATE PATIENT SELECTION

Matching appropriate therapy to a given patient situation is the basis for rationale selection of rejuvenation techniques. A systematic classification of patient photoaging types that combines photoaging with the impact of muscle movement in the face has been developed by the author (9,10). The scale facilitates discussion of therapies for photodamaged skin and the aging face and permits rational comparisons of therapies and clinical results. An alternative visual grading systems for cutaneous photodamage is also available and recommended for reference (11).

While other areas, such as the upper chest, dorsal hands, and extensor forearms, may also be areas of concern, as a practical matter, facial aging is what brings the patient to the clinician. In the author's scale, patients are classified as photoaging type I through IV (Table 1), depending on the degree of facial wrinkling and expression lines that have appeared.

Younger patients, usually those in their 20s, have only the earliest signs of photoaging, manifest as a loss of evenness of color, but they have no wrinkles or lines, even when the face is animated in conversation (Fig. 1, type I). These patients are categorized as type I (no wrinkles). They generally wear little or no makeup since they do not require it for either color or lines.

As the patient ages, wrinkles begin to appear, at first only when the face is in motion (Fig. 1, type II). Visible expression lines first appear parallel and lateral to the nasolabial fold, the corners of the mouth, the eyes, the zygomatic arch, and malar eminences. These patients are usually in their early 30s and look unlined when their face is at rest. However, as soon as they begin to talk, the lines appear. They frequently use makeup to hide the irregularity in color and sallow tones that result from the chronic sun exposure. Premalignant actinic keratoses are usually not visible, but the characteristic roughness can often be palpated with light touch. These patients are classified as type II (wrinkles on motion).

As aging proceeds, lines persist even when the face is at rest (Fig. 1, type III). By the time patients are in their 40s, there are expression lines visible at the corners of the eyes known as crow's feet, as well as lines parallel to the corners of the mouth, lines radiating down from the lower eyelids onto the malar cheeks, and across the upper and lower lip. Makeup use is now problematic since it can still help with the irregular photodamaged color in these patients, but tends to accentuate the appearance of the lines.

Table 1 Glogau Photoaging Classification

Type I: No wrinkles
- Early photoaging
  - Mild pigmentary changes
  - No keratoses
  - Minimal wrinkles
- Patient age: 20s or 30s
- Minimal or no makeup

Type II: Wrinkles in motion
- Early to moderate photoaging
  - Early senile lentigines visible
  - Keratoses palpable but not visible
  - Parallel smile lines beginning to appear
- Patient age: late 30s or 40s
- Usually wears some foundation

Type III: Wrinkles at rest
- Advanced photoaging
  - Obvious dyschromia, telangiectasia
  - Visible keratoses
  - Wrinkles even when not moving
- Patient age: 50s or older
- Always wears heavy foundation

Type IV: Only wrinkles
- Severe photoaging
  - Yellow-gray color of skin
  - Prior skin malignancies
  - Wrinkled throughout, no normal skin
- Patient age: sixth or seventh decade
- Can't wear makeup— "cakes and cracks"

Source: Ref. 10 (with the permission of Health Management Publications, King of Prussia, PA).

Premalignant actinic keratoses are frequently visible as well as palpable. These patients appear lined even when their face is at rest, and are classified as type III (wrinkles at rest).

As photoaging continues, the wrinkles gradually cover the most of the facial skin, usually by the sixth or seventh decade of life, but earlier in more severe cases (Fig. 1, type IV). Many of these patients have already had one or more skin cancers. Makeup is completely impractical since it gives the appearance of cracked mud when applied to a surface riddled with lines and creases. These patients really have no unwrinkled skin anywhere on their face, and are classified as type IV (only wrinkles).

Patients must also be categorized according to their Fitzpatrick sun-reactive skin type (12). This classification (Table 2) gives a very good indication of risk for potential dyschromia following epidermal/papillary dermal injury and the likelihood of developing postinflammatory hyperpigmentation during the short-term postoperative period, and the potential for permanent hypopigmentation resulting from destruction of melanocytes.

The implication of the Fitzpatrick scale is that there is a range of possible responses of the pigmentary system, not only to sunlight, but to peeling agents as well. The typical

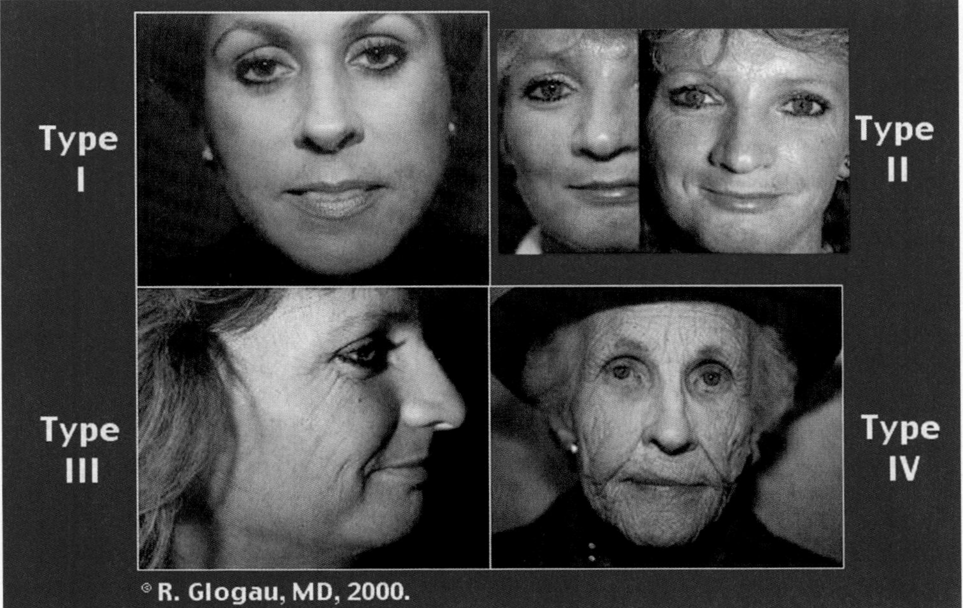

Figure 1 Type I: no wrinkles. The skin is uniform in color and there is an absence of lines, even at the corners of the eyes and mouth. Type II: wrinkles on motion. When the face is at rest (left), the patient appears similar to the type I patient. However, when the face is animated by expression (right), many parallel lines appear, first at the corners of the mouth, then parallel to the nasolabial folds, then at the corners of the eyes, and finally over the malar cheeks. Type III: wrinkles at rest. This patient clearly shows the parallel lines seen with animation in type II, except they are now present when the face is at complete rest. Type IV: only wrinkles. The perioral skin in particular is likely to demonstrate the total replacement of normal skin with minute, rhomboid, and geometric rhytids, which are clearly seen in this patient. The entire face shows similar rhytids on close inspection.

Table 2 Fitzpatrick's Sun-Reactive Skin Types

Skin type	Skin color	Tanning response
I	White	Always burn, never tan
II	White	Usually burn, tan with difficulty
III	White	Sometimes mild burn, tan average
IV	Brown	Rarely burn, tan with ease
V	Dark brown	Very rarely burn, tan very easily
VI	Black	No burn, tan very easily

pale-skinned, light-haired, light-eyed type I patient can be expected to go through the deep resurfacing without fear of either postinflammatory hyperpigmentation or dyschromia secondary to permanent hypopigmentation. Type IV skin, such as that typified by the dark, deep-olive skin of Hispanics or Asians with dark hair and dark eyes, may develop significant postinflammatory hyperpigmentation with medium to deep types of resurfacing and is at some risk for depigmentation from deeper peels.

As a general rule, patients with Fitzpatrick skin types I through III will tolerate resurfacing without significant risk of color change. While resurfacing may be undertaken in Fitzpatrick skin types IV through VI, the risk of pigmentary change is certainly high enough that the patient should be warned that there is can be color change in the treated skin. The skin tone of patients with Fitzpatrick type II or III skin and significant degrees of skin bronzing from chronic sun damage may appear to lighten following resurfacing techniques since chronic sun-damaged skin is replaced with new, undamaged skin. This is widely misunderstood to be loss of color when, in fact, it is merely replacement of chronically sun-damaged skin tones with normal skin color.

Combination therapies can provide optimal improvement in appearance. At one end of the therapeutic spectrum, topical medical therapy utilizing agents like tretinoin, tazarotene, alpha-hydroxy acids, hydroquinones, and fluorouracil can inhibit or reverse ultraviolet-associated changes in aging skin. At the other end of the therapeutic spectrum, rhytidectomy, blepharoplasty, brow lift, and suction-assisted lipectomy often provide dramatic results in facial rejuvenation by correcting laxity removing excess subcutaneous fat and skin and muscle redundancy.

Botulinum toxin can dramatically lessen movement associated expression lines in the face (13,14), converting the Glogau type III to type II or even type I. Clinicians now can directly address the movement-associated expression lines in the aging face by using chemodenervation as a rejuvenative technique separate and parallel to the photodamaged quality of the skin.

Chemical peeling, laser resurfacing, and dermabrasion are focused on resurfacing the skin itself, giving an improved texture irrespective of underlying soft tissue or bony changes. Resurfacing techniques specifically target the epidermal and dermal components of photoaging, and while the results are frequently more dramatic than cold steel surgery, it is very important that the physician be able to identify what components of the aged appearance need to be addressed, particularly in discussing the aging face.

Is the main problem photodamage of the skin, movement of the muscles and laxity of fascia, change in volume of fat, or a combination of all three factors? To achieve significant cosmetic improvement, each component must be analyzed separately and a judgment made as to the relative contribution that each makes to the aging appearance. The therapeutic solution should be tailored to the individual components of aging, balancing risk and benefits ratios of each therapy against the patient's desires and expectations.

A common mistake is to offer the patient rhytidectomy when the overwhelming problem is aging secondary to photodamage, movement, or volume changes in the face. Put more simply, the doctor "redraped" when he/she should have "resurfaced" (laser/peeling), "relaxed" (botulinum toxin), or "refilled" (soft-tissue fillers). The aesthetic effects of a superficial musculoaponeurotic system face lift are complementary to those obtained by resurfacing, botulinum toxin, or fillers. While the interventions may be complementary, they do not equally address the component problems of the aging face and should not be promoted as such.

Patients with photoaging type I are not suitable candidates for deep resurfacing, nor are patients with photoaging type IV likely to be well served by superficial techniques. The art in resurfacing comes in managing the type II and type III patients as one chooses between the techniques available. Certainly many, if not most, of the type III patients get dramatic improvement from deep peeling or laser resurfacing, but what degree of improvement can they routinely achieve with medium-depth techniques? Likewise the type II patients are not really in need of deep resurfacing, and may not be willing to suffer the morbidity of even the medium-depth peels. Can they be improved with superficial peeling, perhaps done repetitively, and if so, to what degree? And what role do so-called nonablative techniques using intense pulsed light, monochromatic laser light, light-emitting diode lights, and radio-frequency tightening play in managing these patients?

FUTURE OUTLOOK

Temporary and permanent alterations in color remain the most significant limiting risk factors in rejuvenation techniques in general, and will continue to be a major reason to use standard classification schemes for patient selection to facilitate comparison of various techniques. It is appropriate to match the rejuvenation technique to the degree of photoaging, balancing risk and morbidity against the anticipated benefit. The use of combination minimally invasive techniques with topical therapy, botulinum toxin, fillers, and non-ablative light and laser therapy will become an even more important supplement and substitute to traditional resurfacing and surgical techniques to treat the aging appearance of the face and reverse the signs of photoaging.

REFERENCES

1. Fisher GJ, Kang S, Varaniy J, Bata-Csorgo Z, Wan Y, Datta S. Mechanisms of photoaging and chronological skin aging. Arch Dermatol 2002; 138:1462–1470.
2. Griffiths CE, Voorhees JJ. Topical retinoic acid for photoaging: clinical response and underlying mechanisms. Skin Pharmacol 1993; 6(suppl 1):70–77.
3. Kligman AM. Topical retinoic acid (tretinoin) for photoaging: conceptions and misperceptions. Cutis 1996; 57:142–144.
4. Kligman LH. Preventing, delaying, and repairing photoaged skin. Cutis 1988; 41:419–420.
5. Griffiths CE, Russman AN, Majmudar G, Singer RS, Hamilton TA, Voorhees JJ. Restoration of collagen formation in photodamaged human skin by tretinoin (retinoic acid). N Engl J Med 1993; 329:530–535.
6. Balin AK, Pratt LA. Physiological consequences of human skin aging. Cutis 1989; 43:431–436.
7. Montagna W, Carlisle K, Kirchner S, Epidermal and dermal histological markers of photodamaged human facial skin [poster exhibited at the 1988 AAD meeting, Washington, DC], Richardson-Vicks, Shelton, CT, 1988.
8. Montagna W, Kirchner S, Carlisle K. Histology of sun-damaged human skin. J Am Acad Dermatol 1989; 21(5 Pt 1):907–918.
9. Glogau RG. Aesthetic and anatomic analysis of the aging skin. Semin Cutan Med Surg 1996; 15:134–138.
10. Glogau RG. Chemical peeling and aging skin. J Geriatr Dermatol 1994; 2:30–35.
11. Griffiths CE. The clinical identification and quantification of photodamage. Br J Dermatol 1992; 127(suppl 41):37–42.

12. Fitzpatrick TB. The validity and practicality of sun-reactive skin types I through VI. Arch Dermatol 1988; 124:869–871.
13. Carruthers JD, Carruthers JA. Treatment of glabellar frown lines with C. botulinum-A exotoxin. J Dermatol Surg Oncol 1992; 18:17–21.
14. Carruthers J, Carruthers A. Botulinum toxin (Botox) chemodenervation for facial rejuvenation. Facial Plast Surg Clin North Am 2001; 9:197–204.

6

Photoprotection

Henry W. Lim / Laura Thomas *Henry Ford Health System, Detroit, Michigan, U.S.A.*

Darrell S. Rigel *New York University School of Medicine, New York, New York, U.S.A.*

- A regular regimen of photoprotection is effective in reducing subsequent clinical photodamage and skin cancer.
- Broad-spectrum coverage is important.
- The ideal sunscreen should provide broad-spectrum ultraviolet (UV) A and B coverage, have good substantivity and photostability, and be cosmetically acceptable.
- To optimally protect the skin from the acute and chronic effects of UV radiation, a combination of behavior modification and the use of photoprotective devices and agents is needed (avoidance of the midday sun, clothing, and sunscreens).

Proper photoprotection is an integral part of the management of photoaging. Much of this is behavioral, such as minimizing exposure to sunlight during the peak hours of 10 AM to 4 PM, seeking shade, and the use of broad-brim hat and ultraviolet (UV)-protective eyewear (1). Sunscreen and UV-protective clothing are integral part of this strategy, and will be covered in this chapter.

SUNSCREEN

History

Although there is some evidence to suggest that people were already using zinc cream to prevent sunburn, the first documented use of sunscreen occurred in 1928 with the introduction of an emulsion composed of benzyl salicylate and benzyl cinnamate in the United States. Then, in the 1930s, a south Australian chemist by the name of H. A. Milton Blake formulated a protective agent containing 10% salol (phenyl salicylate) (2). By 1935, protective lotions containing quinine oleate and quinine bisulfate appeared in the United States (3). L'Oréal's founder, E. Schueller, introduced the first commercially available sunscreen product in 1936 (4).

During World War II (1939–1945), large numbers of U.S. servicemen in the Pacific theater were exposed to the adverse effects of the tropical sun. Severe sunburn imposed a serious problem. At the time, the military issued red petrolatum as a sunscreen. In the 1940s, dermatologists began prescribing 2–5% *p*-aminobenzoic acid (PABA) in aqueous cream or in 70% alcohol (5). Patented in 1943, PABA led the way for the development of numerous derivatives (3). In 1947, sensitization to glyceryl PABA was first reported (6).

At the annual meeting of the Dermatological Association of Australia in Melbourne, the consensus was that PABA allergy occurred so frequently that it should no longer be used as a sunscreen (5). The result was a gradual withdrawal of PABA from the market. In the 1970s, the PABA-free'' label began appearing on sunscreen containers.

In 1972, the U.S. Food and Drug Administration (FDA) reclassified sunscreens from cosmetics to over-the-counter (OTC) drugs, and applied more stringent labeling requirements. Johnson & Johnson developed the first waterproof sunscreen, Coppertone®, in 1977, and quickly followed with a product containing polyanhydride resin, PA-18, as the agent imparting water resistance. In 1978, the *Federal Register* published the established guidelines for the formulation and evaluation of sunscreens marketed in the United States (7). These guidelines were re-evaluated in 1988 and further revised in 1993 and 1999 (8,9). By the late 1970s, the FDA declared sunscreens as safe and effective in helping to prevent skin cancer, alleviate premature aging of the skin, and prevent sunburn (10). The sun protective factor (SPF) numbering system (2–15) was also introduced. The SPF is defined as the ratio of the minimal erythema dose (MED) of sunscreen-protected skin over the MED of unprotected skin. For SPF testing, sunscreen is to be applied at 2 mg/cm^2. The cosmetic industry began to add sunscreens to various skin care cosmetics, carefully avoiding claims that would place the products clearly in the drug category (11).

The 1980s continued to be a sun-loving time, and companies continued to capitalize on safety and technological enhancements. Coppertone developed the first UVA/UVB sunscreen. Sunscreens continued to be incorporated into more and more cosmetics. Because of the growing incidence of skin cancer, the American Academy of Dermatology (AAD) became the first medical society to start a public education campaign on skin cancer prevention. The AAD educated people on the proper use of sunscreen and of the long-term consequences of early childhood sunburn on the development of cancer (12). During this same time, the sunscreen industry produced sunscreens with higher SPFs. In 1981, Skin Cancer Foundation started its ''Seal of Recommendation'' program for sunscreens. In 1988, the AAD coined the phrase ''there is no safe way to tan.''

Beginning in the 1990s, the sunscreen industry offered products that provided protection against UVA and UVB radiation. Sunscreens were incorporated into a widening range of consumer products, including daily-use cosmetics (13). Foundation makeup with sunscreen provides full-spectrum UVA protection achieved through high pigment content and inorganic particulates. Coppertone premiered a new sun-care specialty line for outdoor sports enthusiasts called Coppertone Sport Ultra Sweatproof Dry Lotion®. The sport-type sunscreen products were designed to hold the sunscreen actives in place to prevent spreading. Shade UVA Guard Lotion®, SPF 15, was introduced in 1993, delivering the broadest UV protection available in the United States. It was also the first PABA-free sunscreen formulation in the country to use the UVA absorber Parsol® 1789. On May 12, 1993, the Tentative Final Sunscreen Monograph was published, outlawing claims such as those relating to aging and wrinkling.

Currently available products offer excellent protection from UVB and, to a more variable extent, from UVA; therefore, the regular use of sunscreens should offer protection against sunburn as well as photoaging (Table 1). It should be noted, however, that unlike in many other countries, no standardized guidelines on the measurement and labeling of UVA protection of sunscreen are currently available in the United States; therefore, UVA protection of sunscreens sold in the United States varies considerably. It has been demonstrated that in humans, sunscreen's protection against UV-induced immunosuppression was more that 50% lower than protection against sunburn, which is most likely because UVA is relatively more immunosuppressive than it is erythemogenic (14).

The particulate sunscreens have gained popularity during the last decade owing to their low toxicity potential and the effectiveness of the particulates (15). On May 21, 1999, the FDA published its Final Sunscreen Monograph (9). The FDA proposed SPF 30 as the upper limit for SPF labeling (12). Products with SPF values more than 30 may be labeled as ''30 plus'' or ''30+''. Permissible labeling claims are limited to the prevention of sunburn. Extended wear claims of a specific number of hours of protection are no longer allowed (12). Because UVA protection of sunscreen was not specifically addressed in the 1999 FDA monograph, on February 4, 2000, the AAD sponsored a consensus conference on the UVA protection of sunscreens (16). The recommendations from this conference have been submitted to the FDA for their consideration. Following response by the FDA of all the comments received, the revised version of the Final Sunscreen Monograph is scheduled to be released on December 31, 2004.

Photoprotective Effects

Sunscreens have been shown to have protective effects in terms of the development of nonmelanoma skin cancer (17), but the relationship between the protection of sunscreens and the development of melanoma is more complex (18). Studies have shown persons who ''regularly'' use sunscreens may have a lower, unchanged, or higher risk of subsequently developing melanoma. These results vary because the existing studies relating the use of sunscreen to skin cancer prevention are retrospective and suffer from one or more of the

Table 1 Biological Properties of UV

UV	Wavelength range (nm)	Comments
UVC	200–290	Germicidal. Not present in sunlight reaching the surface of the earth.
UVB	290–320	Sunburn, photoimmunosuppression. Sunscreens with high SPF are effective against the erythemogenic effect of UVB.
UVA2	320–340	Photoaging, photoimmunosuppression, Protection against immunosuppression can be best achieved with broad-spectrum sunscreens.
UVA1	340–400	

flaws typically associated with the retrospective approach. A recent meta-analysis of multiple studies in this area concluded that no specific conclusions could be drawn, but that sunscreens should still be recommended as part of an overall sun protection regimen (19) since no harmful effects have been documented.

Sunscreens are designed to protect against the development of sunburn, and the data linking regular use of sunscreen to protection from sunburn leading to the minimization of photoaging are stronger. Recent studies have shown that the regular use of high-SPF broad-spectrum sunscreens protects against photodamage at the cellular level. A study using previously unexposed buttocks skin exposed 5 days per week for 6 weeks to 1 MED of solar simulated radiation per exposure confirmed in vivo that an appropriate full-UV-spectrum product significantly reduced the skin damage induced by solar UV radiation, demonstrating the benefit of daily photoprotection (20). A subsequent study evaluated daily use of a sunscreen and found that this regimen reduces the skin damage produced by UV exposure compared with intermittent use of equal or higher SPF products. The daily application of sunscreens in appropriate quantities was found to reduce the harmful effects of solar UV radiation on skin (21).

However, compliance is essential to obtain the maximal benefit of regular sunscreen use. Compliance is maximized when there is a belief that a person is at risk by a behavior and that a change in behavior can lower that risk. The use of a UV camera, which demonstrates current photodamage significantly, increased intentions to use sunscreen in the future (22). A combination of UV photo and photoaging information resulted in substantially lower reported sunbathing and other photoprotective efforts (22).

Finally, sunscreens must be used appropriately to be effective in photoprotection. The effectiveness of sunscreens begin to degrade at 2 hours, and therefore should be reapplied regularly within that interval (23).

Structure-Activity Relationship

Sunscreens reduce or prevent UV-induced erythema in ways that are chemical, physical, and biological (24). Chemically, the compounds absorb the UV radiation to prevent the radiation from damaging viable tissue. Physically, a UV blocker would predominantly reflect the UV radiation. Although still theoretical, biological sunscreens would allow the sunscreen to reduce inflammation either by blocking the biological inflammatory response or by enhancing biological repair. The 1999 FDA sunscreen monograph indicates that the terms ''organic'' and ''inorganic'' should replace ''chemical'' and ''physical,'' respectively (9).

The FDA currently approves 16 category I sunscreens, of which 14 are organic and two are inorganic (25) (Table 2). Protective wavelengths of filters commonly used in the United States and other countries are listed in Table 3. In the United States, new UV filters must go through New Drug Application to FDA, a process that is costly and time consuming. European countries have established the European Cosmetics and Perfumery Trade Association (COLIPA) to regulate the sunscreen industry, simplifying the process for approving new products (26). COLIPA is a task force that was formed to address the various concerns associated with sunscreens such as UV source, application techniques, and number of volunteers for testing.

Current Terminology

- Sun protection factor (SPF): The dose of UV radiation (290–400 nm) required to produce 1 MED on protected skin after application of 2 mg/cm^2 of product

Table 2 FDA-Approved Sunscreens: Category I

Organic sunscreens		
UVB filters	UVA filters	Inorganic sunscreens
p-Aminobenzoic acid (PABA)	Oxybenzone (benzophenone-3)	Titanium dioxide
Padimate O (octyldimethyl PABA)		
	Sulisobenzone (benzophenone-4)	Zinc oxide
Octisalate (octyl salicylate; ethylhexyl salicylate)	Dioxybenzone (benzophenone-8)	
Homosalate		
	Avobenzone (Parsol 1789)	
Trolamine salicylate		
	Meradimate (menthyl anthranilate)	
Cinoxate		
Octinoxate (octyl methoxycinnamate)		
Octocrylene		
Ensulizole (phenylbenzimidazole sulfonic acid)		

divided by the dose of UV radiation to produce 1 MED on unprotected skin. The Austrian scientist Franz Greiter originally proposed this concept (27). Because UVB is the erythemogenic portion of UV, SPF is primarily a reflection of protection against the acute effect of UVB. Protection against UVA is not well quantified by SPF.

- Water-resistant: Maintains the SPF level after two 20-minute periods of water immersion.
- Very water-resistant: Maintains the SPF level after four 20-minute periods of water immersion.
- Broad-spectrum or full-spectrum: Provides UVB, UVA2, and UVA1 coverage.
- Extinction coefficient (ε): This is a reflection of the efficiency of electron delocalization in a molecule; the more efficient the electron delocalization, the higher the extinction coefficient. Chemicals with a high extinction coefficient are more efficient in absorbing the energy of the harmful UV radiation than chemicals with a lower extinction coefficient.
- Efficacy: The ability to protect the skin against UV-induced burning, or SPF (24).
- Substantivity: The ability to remain on or in the skin.

Organic Sunscreens

UVB Filters

PABA AND P-AMINOBENZOATE DERIVATIVES. *p*-Aminobenzoate was one of the first sunscreens to be widely available and was commonly used in the 1950s and 1960s in the United States. In 1943, PABA was the first sunscreen to receive patent protection. An UVB chemical sunscreen with an absorption maxima at 296 nm, it penetrates the stratum

Table 3 Current Common Sunscreen Agents and Their UV-Protective Wavelengths

Sunscreen	Range of protection (nm)	Maximal effect of protection (nm)
PABA and PABA esters		
PABA	260–313	283
Glyceryl PABA	260–313	297
Padimate A	290–315	309
Padimate O	290–315	311
Salicylates		
Octisalate (octyl salicylate)	260–310	307
Homosalate	290–315	306
Trolamine salicylate	269–320	298
Cinnamates		
Cinoxate	270–328	290
Octinoxate (octyl methoxycinnamate)	280–310	311
Octocrylene	287–323	303
Etocrylene	296–383	303
Benzophenones		
Oxybenzone	270–350	290–325
Sulisobenzone	250–380	286–324
Dioxybenzone	206–380	284–327
Dibenzoylmethanes		
Avobenzone (butylmethoxy-dibenzoylmethane; Parsol 1789)	310–400	358
Meradimate (menthyl anthranilate)	200–380	336
Terephthalylidene dicamphor sulfonic acid (Mexoryl® SX)	310–400	345
Anisotriazine: bis-ethylhexyloxyphenol methoxyphenyl triazine (Tinosorb® S)	320–395	343

corneum and bonds with the epidermis proteins through hydrogen bonds (28). Because it bonds with the epidermis, PABA demonstrates increased durability through perspiration and washing (28). PABA was originally supplied to pharmacists as a white or slightly yellowish crystalline powder that darkened when exposed to air or light.

Reports cast doubt on its safety as a sunscreen as a result of it being a possible contact allergen (29). Because of its potential to cause sensitization, PABA is now rarely used as a sunscreen. PABA was found to cross-react with both benzoic acid and *p*-phenylenediamine (30). The PABA-free claim became more popular owing to increasing concerns about toxicity, resulting in further decline of PABA usage.

Other drawbacks also led to the decreased use of PABA. It was found to produce off-color skin tones as the amines tend to oxidize rapidly in air (31). The PABA sunscreen can stain clothing, especially synthetics and fiberglass, a popular component of sailboats. Boat shop owners often would not rent sailboats to people wearing PABA-based sunscreen because of the staining that often occurred. Another drawback to the use of PABA in sunscreens is its crystalline physical state that constrains cosmetic formulations. It also exhibits dramatic solvent effects that influence the efficacy of the sunscreen by shifting absorption from 293 nm in nonpolar solvents to 266 nm in polar solvents (31). PABA is also sensitive to pH changes.

PABA DERIVATIVES. All PABA derivatives are UVB chemical sunscreens, popular in the 1950s and 1960s, and many are still used in sunscreen formulations.

Glyceryl PABA is currently approved for use in Europe (32), but was removed from the FDA-approved list of sunscreens (25). It is a creamy white powder that was designed to prevent the chemical reactions prevalent with PABA. However, the compound is still a solid and is more water-soluble (31). The first case of sensitization to PABA was reported in 1947 (6). Many of the cases of glyceryl PABA sensitization showed uniform strong reactions to benzocaine, suggesting that the sensitization may be due to the presence of impurities in the glyceryl PABA (33). This has since been confirmed (34–38). Impurities such as glyceryl di-*p*-aminobenzoate, traces of PABA, and glyceryl tri-*p*-aminobenzoate were also found in the sunscreen. Glyceryl PABA was reported to be irritating to the skin and may cause allergic contact dermatitis (28).

Ethyl-4-*bis*(hydroxypropyl)aminobenzoate is another PABA derivative that is approved in Europe under the trade name Amerscreen P. It has drawbacks similar to those of glyceryl PABA: partial water solubility and relative insolubility in cosmetic formulations.

Padimate A or amyldimethyl PABA is a PABA derivative. It was responsible for several phototoxic reactions and is now banned in Europe and is not among the FDA-approved sunscreens.

Padimate O (octyldimethyl PABA) is the most widely used PABA derivative and is approved by the FDA. Identified by the trade name of Escalol® 507, it is a potent UVB absorber. It has a much lower potential for staining then PABA and has a lower risk of causing adverse reactions. Padimate O is also a liquid instead of a crystalline solid; however, it is subject to solvents effects. In nonpolar solvents its absorption is 300 nm compared to 316 nm in polar solvents, both well within the UVB range.

SALICYLATES. Salicylates were the first UV filters used in sunscreen preparations. These relatively weak UVB chemical sunscreens were used for more than 50 years and were supplanted by the more efficient PABA and cinnamate derivatives. Salicylates are mostly used to augment other UVB absorbers and have an excellent safety profile. They are stable compounds with a low extinction coefficient, and are not subject to solvent effects. Salicylates have a safe record in that they are nonsensitizing. They are also excellent solubilizers of other traditionally nonsoluble cosmetic ingredients, including oxybenzone and avobenzone (13).

Octisalate, formerly known as octyl salicylate (ethylhexyl salicylate), is a salicylate that has been approved by the FDA and enjoys the most positive exposure in sunscreen formulations. Octisalate incorporates the 2-ethylhexyl grouping: 2-ethylhexyl p-methoxycinnamate, 2-ethylhexyl dimethyl *p*-aminobenzoate, and 2-ethylhexyl-cyano-3, 3-diphenyl acrylate (31). This product is used in many formulations because of its incorporation into cosmetic formulations, aesthetics, stability, emoliency, and non–water solubility. It is insoluble in water and other aqueous formulations. Octisalate, however, has been reported to cause photocontact dermatitis (30).

Homosalate (homomenthyl salicylate) is very popular in the United States. It is used as the standard sunscreen agent in the testing of SPFs. Part of its continuing popularity is attributed to the fact that it rarely causes photodermatitis or contact dermatitis.

Trolamine salicylate, formerly called triethanolamine salicylate, is another FDA-approved sunscreen used in the United States. It is mostly used for water-soluble sunscreens to help increase the SPF of a cosmetic formulation owing to their substantivity to the skin. These products are also used in hair preparations as a sun-protective agent. Trolamine salicylate has been found to cause photocontact dermatitis (30).

Other salicylates that have not been approved by the FDA include benzyl salicylate, potassium salicylate, amyl salicylate, *p*-isopropylphenyl salicylate, and 4-isopropylbenzyl salicylate.

CINNAMATES. Cinnamates are UVB chemical sunscreens that absorb wavelengths of about 305 nm (31). They are the most potent UVB absorbers and have improved over the years. The major disadvantage of cinnamates is their lack of substantivity (39). Because they do not bind to skin, their durability depends on the vehicle in which they are prepared. Cinnamates have the added advantage over PABA because they are nonstaining and are rarely reported to cause contact dermatitis. There are few reports of photosensitivity and phototoxicity. Benzylcinnamate was reported to be one of the earliest sunscreens used in combination with benzyl salicylate. This sunscreen is no longer in use today.

Cinoxate and octyl methoxycinnamate are the cinnamates currently approved by the FDA. Cinoxate is much more common in Europe than in the United States. Octinoxate (formerly known as octyl methoxycinnamate, Parsol MCX, and 2-ethylhexyl-*p*-methoxycinnamate) is the most widely used sunscreen agent in the United States because of its excellent absorption in the UVB range. The decreased water solubility of octinoxate makes it suitable for most waterproof sunscreen formulations. It also has a reasonable degree of photostability. Diethanolamine methoxycinnamate is an agent that is used mostly in hair applications. It is used in water-soluble applications with the diethanolamine salt (31).

CAMPHOR DERIVATIVES. Camphor derivatives are bicyclic compounds with high extinction coefficient; they are not approved for use in the United States. Camphor derivatives are extremely stable to photodegradation (40). Most are UVB chemical sunscreens that absorb in the 290–300 nm range, with a notable exception of terephthalylidene dicamphor sulfonic acid (Mexoryl® SX), which is a broad UVA absorber available in Europe and other parts of the world. Mexoryl SX has been shown to prevent UVA produced histochemical alterations in the skin associated with photoaging (41).

MISCELLANEOUS COMPOUNDS. Octocrylene is a UVB filter with relatively low extinction coefficient. It can improve the water resistance of many preparations. Lately, it has become more commonly used with avobenzone since it can stabilize the photodegradation of the latter.

Ensulizole, formerly known as phenylbenzimidazole sulfonic acid, or 2-phenylbenzimidazole-S-sulfonic acid, is a water-soluble, FDA-approved UVB filter. However, it is not commonly used in the United States.

Digalloyl trioleate, a UVB absorber, was removed from the 1999 FDA list of approved sunscreens along with lawsone with dihydroxyacetone. Lawsone with dihydroxyacetone is an artificial tanning accelerator, but the mixture acts as a barrier to UV rays.

UVA Filters

BENZOPHENONES. Benzophenones were the most commonly used UVA organic sunscreens in the past 15 years. These sunscreens absorb both UVB and a significant part of the UVA spectrum. They are dibenzoylmethane derivatives with two aromatic ketone rings (28). Staining does not occur with the benzophenones and they cause fewer allergic reactions than PABA (30). Benzophenones are added to compounds fairly easily, and are therefore often found in broad-spectrum sunscreen formulations mixed with other sunscreen agents. However, there are certain drawbacks to the use of benzophenones. More allergic reactions were reported with the use of oxybenzone when compared to PABA (42). Sensitization to oxybenzone and dioxybenzone has also been reported (43).

The FDA currently approves the use of oxybenzone (benzophenone-3) in the United States under the trade name Eusolex® 4360 or Uvinul® M-40. It is the most commonly used benzophenone. It is used primarily as a UVA absorber and to boost the SPF values in combination with other UVB absorbers. Oxybenzone has been reported to cause a significant amount of photocontact dermatitis and contact dermatitis. A recent study found that the most common UV filter photoallergen was to oxybenzone (44). Oxybenzone was found to be the second leading cause of allergic contact reactions next to benzophenone-10 in the same study from England (44).

The FDA also approved sulisobenzone (benzophenone-4) and dioxybenzone (benzophenone-8) for use in the United States. Reported cases of contact dermatitis, allergic contact urticaria, and photocontact reactions are associated with dioxybenzone (benzophenone-8).

DIBENZOYLMETHANES. Dibenzoylmethanes are substituted diketones with high extinction coefficient but low photostability. Parsol 1789 (avobenzone), a member of the dibenzoylmethane family, was approved in the United States for use as UVA chemical sunscreen. It provides no protection against UVB. Avobenzone and inorganic sunscreen zinc oxide are two of the latest ingredients in sunscreens to be approved by the FDA in its 1999 monograph. Avobenzone has been used extensively in Europe for much longer. There has been some reported sensitivity to avobenzone, but it was discovered that this was due to the cross-reactivity to isopropyl dibenzoylmethane. Allergy to pure avobenzone is rare (45). Avobenzone can lose up to 36% of efficacy in the first hour of sun exposure, and it can cause photodegradation of octinoxate (octyl methoxycinnamate), the most frequently used UVB filter (31,46). Photostability of avobenzone can be achieved in the presence of octocrylene, a UVB filter.

Eusolex 8020 (isopropyl dibenzoylmethane) was previously available in Europe, but has never been approved in the United States. In the 1980s, its use declined owing to the finding of a high incidence of adverse photosensitivity with the combination of isopropyl dibenzoylmethane with methylbenzylidene camphor by coupled reactions. The production of Eusolex 8020 was discontinued in 1993.

ANTHRANILATE. Anthranilates are derivatives of aminobenzoates. Meradimate, formerly known as menthyl anthranilate, is another FDA-approved UVA filter. It is not widely used in the United States.

UVA and UVB Filters

MISCELLANEOUS COMPOUNDS. A benzylidene derivative, Mexoryl SX (terephthalylidene dicamphor sulfonic acid, absorption maxima: 345 nm), and a triazole derivative, Mexoryl XL (drometrizole trisiloxane, absorption maxima: 345 nm), are two photostable filters with good UVA absorption; Mexoryl XL is also a good UVB filter. Mexoryl SX/XL-containing sunscreen has been shown to be effective in suppressing the development of UV-induced lesions of lupus erythematosus, and the development of lesions in patients with polymorphous light eruption (47,48). Both are available worldwide; however, in the United States, both are pending the FDA approval at the time of this writing (17).

Tinosorb® S (*bis*-ethylhexyloxyphenol methoxyphenyl triazine, absorption maxima: 343 nm) and Tinosorb M (methylene *bis*-benzotriazolyl tetramethylbutylphenol, absorption maxima: 359 nm) are two new sunscreens developed by Ciba Specialty Chemicals that are currently being used in many parts of the world (Europe, Asia, and Central and South America); they are not yet approved by the FDA in the United States. Both are photostable and have absorption in the UVB and UVA range. Tinosorb S is an UVA absorber that is compatible with other UV filter, photostable, and oil soluble. Tinosorb M is the only organic UV absorber consisting of microfine particles; therefore, its UV-protective properties consist of absorption, reflection, and scattering. It is available as a 50% aqueous dispersion.

Neo Heliopan® AP (disodium phenyl dibenzimidazole tetrasulfonate) is a new water-soluble UVA filter (absorption maximum: 335 nm) that has been included in the approved list of UV filters by the European Scientific Committee. It is not available in the United States.

Inorganic Sunscreens

Early on, inorganic sunscreens (previously known as physical sunscreens), such as pigmentary or nonmicronized forms of zinc oxide, were used because of their proven effectiveness in reducing sunburn; however, their use did result in chalky white discoloration of the skin on application. Red (veterinarian) petrolatum is a semirefined form of petrolatum and was used by troops in the World War II. This product can make a person appear red and greasy, leading to its declined use (30). Talc was also used around that time as a physical sunscreen.

With the development of the micronized form titanium dioxide, this product is enjoying renewed popularity as an inorganic sunscreen. Pigmentary titanium dioxide has a mean particle size between 150 and 300 nm, appearing white and opaque. The micronized form has a mean size of 20 to 150 nm (49), making it optically more transparent and cosmetically more acceptable by consumers. The smaller particle size also allows it to the better attenuate UVB. It protects through a combination of UV reflection and absorption. Micronized titanium dioxide provides good coverage of the UVB and part of the UVA2 and UVA1 (290–360 nm). No irritant or sensitization reactions have been reported.

Another inorganic sunscreen that protects through a combination of UV reflection and absorption is microfine zinc oxide (50,51). Similar to the advances made with titanium dioxide, microfine zinc oxide has a particle size of less than 200 nm, which minimizes visible light scattering, making the particles relatively transparent. This agent offers excellent UVB, UVA2, and UVA1 (excluding 380–400 nm) protection; the protection in the UVA range is broader than that of micronized titanium dioxide. No irritant or sensitization reactions have been reported with zinc oxide. An added benefit of this product is that it may be applied to inflamed, skin barrier-compromised (nonintact) skin, and is approved for diaper rash treatment.

The current popularity of the above two products is the result of particulate technology creating fine submicron particles to reduce the whitening effect on the skin (28). At this small particle size, the particles attenuate UV light predominantly by absorption similar to an organic sunscreen (13). The particles are still large enough to stop entry into the skin (52).

Both metal oxides are crystalline semiconductors that can produce oxygen free radicals at their surface when exposed to UV radiation. Photoreactivity can be markedly diminished when the particles are coated, usually with dimethicone or with silica (51). Therefore, when prepared properly, titanium dioxide and zinc oxide are extremely photostable and safe.

Clinical Reactions to Sunscreens

The most common sunscreen agent causing an allergic reaction is PABA. It has been estimated that 3–7% of the U.S. population is PABA sensitive (53). Both contact and photoallergic reactions have been reported. Benzophenone sensitization has been estimated at 1–2%. Other organic sunscreen agents also can cause contact reactions.

By far, the most common sunscreen reaction is due to ''sensitive'' skin. It is estimated that up to one in three persons using sunscreens will at some time complain about sunscreens irritating their skin. Complaints include subjective signs such as stinging, burning, and itching, as well as objective findings such as urticaria, acnegenicity, and pustulgenicity. The most effective method for alleviating these findings is to choose an alternative sunscreen from a different chemical family or with a different base.

True sunscreen reactions need to be both patch and photopatch tested to determine whether the reaction is merely allergic or possibly light related. Use of too low a concentration of the testing materials may produce a false-negative result.

Systemic Photoprotectants

Ideally, using a photoprotective agent should be as easy as taking a pill. There are a few promising systemic therapies that may eventually be used to prevent sunburn. Because reactive oxygen species can be generated following UV exposure, the use of oral antioxidants has been evaluated. It was shown that combination of high-dosage oral antioxidants (L-ascorbic acid and alpha-tocopherol) resulted in a modest increase in the MED (54,55). Beta carotene, a quencher of reactive oxygen species, has been used for decreasing the photosensitivity in patients with erythropoietic protoporphyria (13). An extract of *Polypodium leucotomos*, a tropical fern plant, has been shown to have immunomodulatory and antioxidant properties; it could provide photoprotection as measured by an associated increased immediate pigment darkening dose, MED, and minimal phototoxic dose following oral and topical administration in human volunteers (56). Antimalarials such as hydroxychloroquine are used to decrease the photosensitivity in patients with diseases such as polymorphous light eruption, cutaneous lupus erythematosus, and solar urticaria; their mechanism(s) of action is not clear (13).

CLOTHING

Ultraviolet Protection Factor

The UV protection factor (UPF) is the most commonly used measurement of the photoprotectiveness of fabrics. It was first developed and used in Australia and New Zealand in 1996, and it has now been incorporated in the standards used in Europe and the United States (57–60). In the determination of UPF, a solar simulator is used as a light source, and the amount of UV transmitted over a wavelength range of 290 to 400 nm is recorded by a spectrophotometer. UPF is defined as the ratio of the effective UV irradiance calculated in the absence and in the presence of fabric. The irradiance is weighted against the erythemal action spectrum; therefore, UPF is heavily influenced UVB. Fabric with high UPF indicates that it has good UVB protection, however, it may have also significant UVA transmission.

While UPF was designed as an in vitro measurement, this term has also been used as a reflection of protection afforded by fabric on UV-induced erythema on skin in vivo. In this in vivo determination, UPF is the ratio of the MED in the presence or absence of fabric (61,62). SPF, a standard term used in assessing the protectiveness of sunscreen, has been used by some investigators as a synonym to in vivo UPF.

Factors Affecting UPF

There are several factors that affect UPF (Table 4). This subject has been well reviewed by Hoffman et al. (63).

- Type of fibers: Polyester fabrics have high UPF, followed by fabrics made of nylon, wool and silk. Cotton, viscose, rayon, and linen usually have a low UPF (64).
- Cover factor: This is defined as the area cover by yarns in a given area; it is a reflection of the porosity of the fabric. Tightly knitted materials, or heavy fabrics, would have high UPF (65).
- Color/dye: Fabrics with dark color (e.g., black, dark blue) have a higher UPF compared to those with light color such as pink or yellow; the difference in the UPF may be threefold or higher (66)
- Stretch: The UPF decreases when the fabric is stretched. It has been demonstrated that the UPF of women's stockings decreased by more than eightfold when stretched 30% from their original size (67).
- Wetness: For cotton, the presence of water in the interstices of the fabric increases UV transmission, resulting in a decrease in the UPF. However, for linen, viscose, and polyester, wetness increases the UPF (68).
- Washing/laundering: First wash of a fabric generally results in an increase in the UPF because of shrinkage (66).
- Chemical treatment: Bleaching of cotton and silk removes the natural UV-absorbing pigments present in these fabrics, which results in a decrease in UPF (69). Incorporation of UV absorbers (e.g., titanium dioxide, Rayosan®, optical brightening agent) during the manufacturing process increases the UPF. Tinosorb FD (stilbene disulfonic acid triazine derivative) is a laundry treatment manufactured by Ciba Specialty Chemicals and marketed in the United States as Rit Sun Guard. It gets incorporated into the fibers during the laundering process; one

Table 4 Factors Affecting UPF

Type of fibers
Cover factor/porosity
Color/dye
Stretch
Wetness
Washing/laundring
Chemical treatment
UV/heat exposure

Modified from Ref. 63.

treatment could last for 20 launderings. It has been shown to produce a fourfold increase the UPF (66).

- Ultraviolet radiation/heat: Extensive exposure to UV radiation or heat causes degradation of the fibers, hence a decrease in UPF.

CONCLUSION

To optimally protect the skin from the acute and chronic effects of UV radiation, a combination of behavior modification and the use of photoprotective devices and agents is needed. Public education on photoprotection is an important part of the strategy. Continued research to develop better sunscreens is also necessary. An ideal sunscreen should provide broad-spectrum UVB and UVA coverage, have good substantivity and photostability, and be cosmetically acceptable. Regulatory agencies need to consider an appropriate method to assess the UVA protection of sunscreen and clothing, and to assess protection against immunosuppression.

REFERENCES

1. Lim HW, Cooper K. The health impact of solar radiation and prevention strategies. Report of the Environment Council, American Academy of Dermatology. J Am Acad Dermatol 1999; 41:81–99.
2. Groves GA. The sunscreen industry in Australia: past, present, and future. In: Lowe NJ, Shaath NA, Pathak MA, Eds. Sunscreens. New York: Marcel Dekker, 1997:227–240.
3. Safer and More Successful Suntanning. Consumers Guide. New York: Wallaby Pocketbooks, 1979:31–33.
4. Rebut D. The sunscreen industry in Europe: past, present, and future. In: Lowe NJ, Shaath NA, Pathak MA, Eds. Sunscreens. New York: Marcel Dekker, 1997:215–226.
5. Mackie BS, Mackie LE. The PABA Story. Aust J Dermatol 1999; 40:51–53.
6. Sulzberger MB, Kanof A, Baer RL. Sensitization by topical application of sulfonamides. J Allergy 1947; 18:92.
7. Sunscreen products for over-the-counter use. Fed Regist 1978:43L28269.
8. Sunscreen drug products for over-the-counter human use; tentative final monograph: proposed rule. Fed Regist 1993; 58:28194–28302.
9. Food and Drug Administration. Sunscreen drug products for over-the-counter human use: final monograph; final rule. Fed Regist 1999; 64:27666–27693.
10. Sikes R. The history of suntanning: a love/hate affair. J Aesthetic Sci 1998; 1:6–7.
11. Murphy EG. Regulatory aspects of sunscreens in the United States. In: Lowe NJ, Shaath NA, Pathak MA, Eds. Sunscreens. New York: Marcel Dekker, 1997:201–214.
12. Gasparro FP. Sunscreens, skin photobiology, and skin cancer: the need for UVA protection and evaluation of efficacy. Environ Health Perspect 2000; 108:71–78.
13. DeBuys HV, Levy SB, Murray JC, Madey DL, Pinnell SR. Modern approaches to photoprotection. Dermatol Clin 2000; 18:577–590.
14. Kelly DA, Seed PT, Young AR, Walker SL. A commercial sunscreen's protection against ultraviolet radiation-induced immunosuppression is more than 50% lower than protection against sunburn in humans. J Invest Dermatol 2003; 120:65–71.
15. Fairhurst D, Mitchnick MA. Particulate sun blocks: general principles. In: Lowe NJ, Shaath NA, Pathak MA, Eds. Sunscreens. New York: Marcel Dekker, 1997:313–352.
16. Lim H W, Naylor M, Hönigsmann H, Gilchrest BA, Cooper K, Morison W, DeLeo VA, Scherschun L. American Academy of Dermatology Consensus Conference on UVA protection of sunscreens: summary and recommendation. J Am Acad Dermatol 2001; 44(3):505–508.

17. Green A, Williams G, Neale R, Hart V, Leslie D, Parsons P, Marks GC, Gaffney P, Battistutta D, Frost C, Lang C, Russell A. Daily sunscreen application and betacarotene supplementation in prevention of basal-cell and squamous-cell carcinomas of the skin: a randomised controlled trial. Lancet 1999; 354:723–729.
18. Rigel DS, Naylor M, Robinson J. What is the evidence for a sunscreen and melanoma controversy?. Arch Dermatol 2000; 136:1447–1449.
19. Huncharek M, Kupelnick B. Use of topical sunscreens and the risk of malignant melanoma: a meta-analysis of 9067 patients from 11 case-control studies. Am J Public Health 2002; 92: 1173–1177.
20. Seite S, Colige A, Piquemal-Vivenot P, Montastier C, Fourtanier A, Lapiere C, Nusgens B. A full-UV spectrum absorbing daily use cream protects human skin against biological changes occurring in photoaging. Photodermatol Photoimmunol Photomed 2000; 16:147–155.
21. Phillips TJ, Bhawan J, Yaar M, Bello Y, Lopiccolo D, Nash JF. Effect of daily versus intermittent sunscreen application on solar simulated UV radiation-induced skin response in humans. J Am Acad Dermatol 2000; 43:610–618.
22. Mahler HI, Kulik JA, Gibbons FX, Gerrard M, Harrell J. Effects of appearance-based interventions on sun protection intentions and self-reported behaviors. Health Psychol 2003; 22: 199–209.
23. Rigel DS, Chen T, Appa Y. Sunscreens and UV protection [abstr], American Academy of Dermatology Annual Meeting, Washington, DC, March 2–7, 2001.
24. Caswell M. Sunscreen formulation and testing. Allured Cosmet Toil Mag 2001; 116:48–60.
25. Chemical and physical characteristics of sunscreen constituents. In: Vainio H, Bianchini F, Eds. IARC Handbooks of Cancer Prevention. Lyon, France: International Agency for Research on Cancer, 2001:17–21.
26. Ferguson J. European guidelines (COLIPA) for evaluation of sun protection factors. In: Lowe NJ, Shaath NA, Pathak MA, Eds. Sunscreens. New York: Marcel Dekker, 1997:513–526.
27. Diffey B. Has the sun protection factor had its day?. BMJ 2000; 320:176–177.
28. Roelandts R. Shedding light on sunscreens. Clin Exp Dermatol 1998; 23:147–157.
29. Kligman AM. The identification of contact allergens by human assay: III. The maximization test: a procedure for sunscreening and rating contact sensitizers. J Invest Dermatol 1966; 47: 393–409.
30. Nelson O'Donoghue M. Sunscreen: the ultimate cosmetic. Dermatol Clin 1991; 9:99–104.
31. Shaath NA. Evolution of modern sunscreen chemicals. In: Lowe NJ, Shaath NA, Pathak MA, Eds. Sunscreens. New York: Marcel Dekker, 1997:3–34.
32. Liem DH, Hilderink LTH. UV absorbers in suncosmetics 1978. Int J Cosmet Sci 1979; 1: 341–361.
33. Fisher AA. Sunscreen dermatitis due to glyceryl PABA: Significance of cross-reactions to this PABA ester. Cutis 1976; 18:495.
34. Bruze M, Fregert S, Gruvberger B. Occurrence of para-aminobenzoic acid and benzocaine as contaminants in sunscreen agents of para-aminobenzoic acid type. Photodermatology 1984; 1:277.
35. Bruze M, Gruvberger B, Thune P. Contact and photocontact allergy to glyceryl para-aminobenzoate. Photodermatology 1988; 5:162.
36. Fisher AA. Dermatitis due to benzocaine present in sunscreens containing glyceryl PABA (Escalol 106). Contact Derm 1977; 3:170.
37. Hjorth N, Wilkinson D, Magnusson B, Bandmann HJ, Maibach H. Glyceryl *p*-aminobenzoate patch testing in benzocaine-sensitive subjects. Contact Derm 1978; 4:46–48.
38. Kaidbey KH, Allen H. Photocontact dermatitis to benzocaine. Arch Dermatol 1981; 117:77.
39. Nelson O'Donoghue M. Sunscreen: one weapon against melanoma. Dermatol Clin 1991; 9: 789–793.
40. Kao Corp. German patent 3,411,636, 1983.

41. Seite S, Moyal D, Richard S, de Rigal J, Leveque JL, Houseau C, Fourtanier A. Mexoryl SX: a broad absorption UVA filter protects human skin from the effects of repeated suberythemal doses of UVA. J Photochem Photobiol B Biol 1998; 44:69–76.
42. Lenique P, Machet L, Vaillant L, Bensaid P, Muller C, Khallouf R, Lorette G. Contact and photocontact allergy to oxybenzone. Contact Dermatitis 1992; 26:177–181.
43. Ferguson J, Collins P. Photoallergic contact dermatitis to oxybenzone. Br J Derm 1994; 131: 124–129.
44. Darvay A, White IR, Rycroft RJG, Jones AB, Hawk JLM, McFadden JP. Photoallergic contact dermatitis is uncommon. Br J Dermatol 2001; 145:597–601.
45. Schauder S, Ippen H. Contact and photocontact sensitivity to sunscreens: review of a 15-year experience and of the literature. Contact Derm 1997; 37:221–232.
46. Sayre RM, Dowdy JC. Photostability testing of avobenzone. Cosmet Toil 1999; 114:85–91.
47. Stege H, Budde MA, Grether-Beck S, Krutmann J. Evaluation of the capacity of sunscreens to photoprotect lupus erythematosus patients by employing the photoprovocation test. Photodermatol Photoimmunol Photomed 2000; 16:256–259.
48. Moyal D, Binet O, Richard A, Rougier A, Hourseau C. Prevention of polymorphous light eruption by a new sunscreen: need for a high UVA protecting factor. J Eur Acad Dermatol Venereol 1999; 12(suppl 2):s317.
49. Anderson MW, Hewitt JP, Spruce SR. Broad-spectrum physical sunscreens: titanium dioxide and zinc oxide. In: Lowe NJ, Shaath NA, Pathak MA, Eds. Sunscreens. New York: Marcel Dekker, 1997:353–398.
50. Pinnell SR, Fairhurst D, Gillies R, Mitchruck MA, Kollias N. Microfine zinc oxide (Z-Cote) is a superior sunscreen ingredient to microfine titanium dioxide. Dermatol Surg 2000; 26: 309–314.
51. Mitchnick MA, Fairhurst D, Pinnell SR. Microfine zinc oxide (Z-Cote) as a photostable UVA/UVB sunblock agent. J Am Acad Dermatol 1999; 40:85–90.
52. Lademann J, Weigmann H, Rickmeyer C, Barthelmes H, Schaefer H, Mueller G, Steny W. Penetration of titanium dioxide microparticles in a sunscreen formulation into the horny layer and the follicular orifice. Skin Pharmacol Appl Skin Physiol 1999; 12:247–256.
53. Fotiades J, Soter NA, Lim HW. Results of evaluation of 203 patients for photosensitivity in a 7.3-year period. J Am Acad Dermatol 1995; 33:597–602.
54. Eberlein-Konig B, Placzek M, Przybilla B. Protective effect against sunburn of combined systemic ascorbic acid (vitamin C) and d-alpha-tocopherol (vitamin E). J Am Acad Dermatol 1998; 38:45–48.
55. Fuchs J, Kern H. Modulation of UV-light-induced skin inflammation by D-alpha-tocopherol and L-ascorbic acid: a clinical study using solar stimulated radiation. Free Radic Biol Med 1998; 25:1006–1012.
56. Gonzalez S, Pathak MA, Cuevas J, Villanubia VG, Fitzpatrick TB. Topical or oral administration with an extract of *Polypodium leucotomos* prevents acute sunburn and psoralen-induced phototoxic reactions as well as depletion of Langerhans cells in human skin. Photodermatol Photoimmunol Photomed 1997; 13:50–60.
57. Sun protective clothing: evaluation and classification, Standards Australia International Ltd, Sydney, New South Wales, Australia/New Zealand Standard (AS/NZS) 4399, Marcel Dekker, 1996.
58. CEN: The European Committee for Standardization. Textiles: solar UV protective properties: methods of test for apparel fabrics. Brussels: CEN: Stassart, 1999:rEN 13758.
59. American Association of Textile Chemists and Colorists. Transmittance or blocking of erythemally weighted ultraviolet radiation through fabrics. AATCC 1998:183.
60. American Society of Testing and Materials. Guide to labeling of UV protective textiles. ASTM D6603-00 Standard, 2000.
61. Stanford DG, Georgouras KE, Pailthorpe M. Rating clothing for sun protection: current status in Australia. J Eur Acad Dermatol Venereol 1997; 8:12–17.

62. Gies HP, Roy CR, Holmes G. Ultraviolet radiation protection by clothing: comparison of in vivo and in vitro measurements. Radiat Protect Dosimetr 2000; 91:247–250.
63. Hoffmann K, Laperre J, Avermaete A, Altmeyer P, Gambichler T. Defined UV protection by apparel textiles. Arch Dermatol 2001; 137:1089–1094.
64. Davis S, Capjack L, Kerr N, Fedosejevs R. Clothing as protection from ultraviolet radiation: which fabric is most effective?. Int J Dermatol 1997; 36:374–379.
65. Pailthorpe M. Textile and sun protection: the current status. Aust Text 1994; 14:54–66.
66. Wang SQ, Kopf AW, Marx J, Bogdan A, Polsky D, Bart RS. Reduction of ultraviolet transmission through cotton T-shirt fabrics with low ultraviolet protection by various laundering methods and dyeing: clinical implications. J Am Acad Dermatol 2001; 44:767–774.
67. Kimlin MG, Parisi AV. Meldrum LR. Effect of stretch on the ultraviolet spectral transmission of one type of commonly used clothing. Photodermatol Photoimmunol Photomed 1999; 15: 171–174.
68. Gambichler T, Hatch KL, Avermaete A, Altmeyer P, Hoffmann K. Influence of wetness on the ultraviolet protection factor (UPF) of textiles: in vitro and in vivo measurements. Photodermatol Photoimmunol Photomed 2002; 18:29–35.
69. Crew PC, Kachmann S, Beyer AG. Influences on UVR transmission of undyed woven fabrics. Text Chem Color 1999; 31:17–26.

7

Retinoids, Other Topical Vitamins, and Antioxidants

Olivier Sorg / Christophe Antille / Jean-Hilaire Saurat
Geneva University Hospital, Geneva, Switzerland

- The two main theories of aging—genetic and damage-accumulation theories—converge on the general theory of oxidative stress.
- The predominant environmental factor that accelerates human skin aging is ultraviolet (UV) irradiation from the sun.
- The biochemical actions of UV radiation on the skin are induction of oxidative stress, DNA damage, and modulation of signal transduction.
- Topical retinoic acid has been shown to improve the clinical signs of photoaging; however, due to its irritant action, research is focused on a nonirritant retinoid that would retain the beneficial actions of retinoic acid.
- Since oxidative stress plays a crucial role in aging process, topical antioxidants should be helpful in preventing photoaging. Among them, the endogenous vitamins C and E are the most promising, although α-hydroxy acids and plant antioxidants have an interesting potential. Ideally, a combination of various antioxidants acting in synergy would be the best way to use topical antioxidants to treat and prevent photoaging.

GENERAL THEORIES OF AGING

Aging is a complex, general process affecting all living organisms that leads to death. The changes observed throughout the life that oppose the infinite preservation of the characteristics acquired during development define aging. As a natural, ineluctable process, aging cannot be prevented, but it can be accelerated by environmental conditions. Thus the purpose of the research on aging is to understand the mechanisms of chronological (intrinsic) and extrinsic aging in order to decrease the influence of environmental conditions that worsen natural aging. Two general theories explain intrinsic aging: genetic theories and theories about the accumulation of cellular damages.

Genetic Theories of Aging

According to genetic theories, aging is a continuation of development—a diminution of cellular proliferation in favor of their differentiation (1,2). A fully differentiated organism is able to perform very elaborated actions, but this is realized to the detriment of the renewal of tissues, and leads to general aging. According to this theory, aging is thus a natural ineluctable process encoded by genes. Moreover, according to neodarwinism, the power of natural selection to favor beneficial genes declines with the age at which they affect adult fitness, since young adults represent the largest contributors to succeeding generations. Thus, aged individuals who have already cared for their offspring can keep defective genes without any consequences for the evolution of the species. Genetics clearly makes a considerable contribution to what is perceived as the aging process. Generally speaking, genes that are beneficial in early life can be deleterious in later life and vice versa. For instance, studies with various invertebrates demonstrated the existence of genes that regulate lifespan, but such individuals with mutated genes and a longer lifespan often give rise to descendants with reduced early-life fitness components. One of the main genes involved in aging is that encoding telomerase (3,4). Telomeres are specialized structures found at the ends of the chromosomes in eukaryotic cells, and are required for complete replication of chromosomal DNA, but due to their function, their length is decreased during chromosomal DNA replication. Thus, after a limited number of cellular divisions, there is a complete loss of telomeres and cells stop dividing, a condition incompatible with life (5). An RNA-enzyme, telomerase, which is present in germinal cells but not in most somatic ones, replaces the lost telomeric repeats at the ends of chromosomes. Thus telomeres appear as a biological clock of aging, and their preservation in germinal cells is required for the perpetuation of the species (6,7). However, an infinite number of replication cycles, which is not necessary for the evolution of the species, would necessarily produce cancers (4,8,9). In summary, genetic theories of aging tell us that (1) aging is a natural ineluctable process required for the survival of the species, (2) the latter does not take advantage of a very long lifespan, and (3) a longer lifespan will be associated with more cancers.

Damage-Accumulation Theories of Aging

The theories of accumulation of cellular damages explain aging by the accumulation of the alterations of proteins, lipids, glucides, DNA, and other biomolecules that the organism cannot repair or eliminate. Among these theories, that involving aging due to free radicals was introduced in 1956 by Denham Harman (10), and many studies have confirmed the involvement of oxidative stress in aging processes (11–16). Similarly, other random processes produce alterations of tissues that accumulate with time: DNA cross-links during mitoses and other DNA damages (17), protein misfolding, protein glycation (18), and unavoidable membrane damages lead to organic dysfunction (12). The organism possesses various enzymatic and nonenzymatic systems to repair damaged endogenous molecules: antioxidants prevent and attenuate oxidative stress, whereas enzymes such as proteases, phospholipases, and acetyltransferases eliminate oxidized proteins and lipids. More complex systems involving many proteins detect then repair damaged DNA (19). When cellular damage is too high, cells are eliminated by apoptosis and replaced by new ones. Finally, the natural metabolic activity produces ''metabolic waste'' that the organism cannot always eliminate properly. These catabolites are oxidized molecules that can become oxidants for other ones if they are not eliminated. Generally speaking, the organism adapts to any situation by preventing undesirable reactions and repairing damaged molecules and tissues, but with a success that never reach 100%. For this reason, the very few undesirable reactions that escape the prevention and repair systems accumulate little by little, and will irremediably end up becoming deleterious after a long period of time (20–22). Thus, in conclusion, genetic and damage-accumulation theories of aging converge on the general theory of oxidative stress (23,24).

SKIN AGING: PHOTOAGING

Human skin, like all other organs, undergoes chronological aging. This ineluctable process involves a series of biological processes such as oxidative stress, DNA damage, and telomere shortening, and leads to a progressive inability of the skin to regenerate properly (5,21). Skin aging is characterized histologically by irregularly dispersed melanocytes, elastosis, reductions and alterations in collagen, and accumulation of a variety of lipid-derived pigments such as chromolipoids and lipofuscins. These histological changes manifest clinically by fine and coarse wrinkling, roughness, dryness, laxity, sallowness, pigmentary mottling, telangiectasia, actinic keratosis, and, finally, preneoplastic and neoplastic alterations (25–28). In addition, skin is in direct contact with the environment and therefore undergoes all consequences of environmental damage. The predominant environmental factor that accelerates human skin aging is UV irradiation from the sun. This sun-induced skin aging, called photoaging, is a cumulative process that depends primarily on the degree of sun exposure and skin phototype. During the last decade, substantial progress has been made in understanding cellular and molecular mechanisms of chronological aging and photoaging. In particular, it appears that chronological aging and photoaging, considered in the past as distinct processes, share fundamental molecular pathways. These new insights regarding convergence of intrinsic and extrinsic aging provide exciting new opportunities for the development of new antiaging therapies (29–33). As mentioned above, such new treatments would at best counteract the influence of extrinsic aging (photoaging), but won't affect the progression of chronological aging.

Biochemical Actions of UV in the Skin

The condition allowing UV radiation to interact with the skin is the presence of chromophores, which absorb the energy from UV and resituate it under physical or biochemical reactions. The main cutaneous chromophores of sunlight are DNA, urocanic acid, aromatic amino acids, retinoids, carotenoids, bilirubin, flavins, hemoglobin, melanins, and NAD(P)H (34). Absorption of sunlight by these chromophores can activate various biochemical pathways, as discussed below in some details.

Oxidative Stress

Any biochemical activity leads to oxidation and reduction reactions, i.e., in electron transfers between molecules. The main biological oxidant is molecular oxygen, present in all tissues. It is stabilized after having received four electrons and four protons, which gives water. This electron transfer is sequential, and the superoxide radical anion

($\cdot O_2^-$) is produced during any reduction of molecular oxygen. However, this intermediate does not produce always water, and can give rise to more oxidant intermediates, collectively referred to as reactive oxygen species (ROS) such as hydrogen peroxide (H_2O_2) or hydroxyl radical (•OH). These ROS can react with any biomolecule and produce alterations and the destruction of biological tissues. The organism possesses enzymatic and nonenzymatic systems able to trap these ROS and counteract their deleterious effects (Fig. 1, Box 1) (12,35–37). However, if the production of ROS exceeds the capacity of the organism to neutralize them, then a condition of oxidative stress occurs and the organism's integrity can no longer be preserved.

The skin can receive oxygen by dermal vessels, as well as by direct contact with the epidermis. The latter is also directly exposed to sunlight, in particular UV radiation, which can induce an oxidative stress by activating the enzyme NADPH oxidase or by promoting lipid peroxidation (Fig. 2, Box 2) (38). Thus the skin is potentially exposed to oxidative stress when receiving UV radiation from the sun (39).

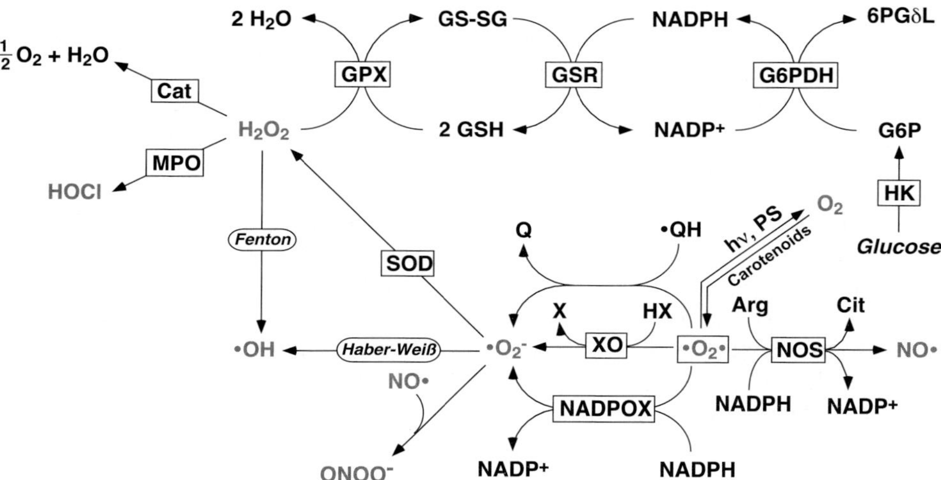

Figure 1 Production and destruction of ROS in the organism. Reactive oxygen species are in gray; enzymes involved in ROS production or scavenging are within rectangular frames. The two reactions involving transition metals are within oval frames. Abbreviations used for enzymes are as follows: CAT, catalase; GPX, glutathione peroxidase; GSR, glutathione reductase; G6PDH, glucose 6-phosphate dehydrogenase; HK, hexokinase; MPO, myeloperoxidase; NADPHOX, NADPH oxidase; NOS, nitric oxide synthetase; SOD, superoxide dismutase; XO, xanthine oxidase; ROS : H_2O_2, hydrogen peroxide; HOCl, hypochlorous acid; NO, nitric oxide; $\cdot O_2 \cdot$, molecular oxygen (biradical, triplet or ground state); O_2, singlet oxygen (nonradical, activated state); $\cdot O_2^-$, superoxide; •OH, hydroxyl radical; $ONOO^-$, peroxynitrite; other abbreviations: Arg, L-arginine; Cit, L-citrulline; hν, photon; NADP(H), nicotinamide dinucleotide phosphate, oxidized ($^+$) or reduced (H) form; G6P, glucose 6-phosphate; 6PGδL, 6-phosphoglucono-deltalactone; GSH, glutathione (reduced); GS-SG, glutathione (oxidized); HX, hypoxanthine; PS, photosensitizer; Q, ubiquinone; •QH, ubiquinol radical (semiquinone); X, xanthine; XO, xanthine oxidase.

Box 1 Production and destruction of ROS in the organism (see Fig. 1).
The predominant production of ROS starts with the partial reduction of molecular oxygen (a biradical) to superoxide. This can be enzymatic, catalyzed by the enzymes NADPH oxidase from activated neutrophils (201) or by xanthine oxidase, or nonenzymatic (e.g., by the oxidation of ubiquinol radical semiquinone to ubiquinone). Superoxide is normally transformed to oxygen and hydrogen peroxide by the enzyme superoxide dismutase; however, depending on the microenvironment, it can partially reduce hydrogen peroxide—a reaction giving rise to the hydroxyl radical—or react with nitric oxide to produce peroxynitrite. Hydrogen peroxide can be converted to hypochlorite by myeloperoxidase, or reduced to water by catalase; it can also undergo a dismutation to oxygen and water, a reaction catalyzed by glutathione peroxidase, to the detriment of glutathione. The latter is recycled by glutathione reductase to the detriment of NADPH, which is recycled by glucose 6-phosphate dehydrogenase after glucose has been phosphorylated by hexokinase. Thus glucose allows the regeneration of reductant cofactors in the scavenging system of ROS. Nitric oxide, which is both an ROS and an intercellular messenger, is produced during a complex reaction involving arginine and NADPH, and catalyzed by nitric oxide synthetase. Finally, molecular oxygen (a biradical, triplet state) can be activated to singlet oxygen after absorption of visible light by a photosensitizer such as a porphyrin; singlet oxygen is a much more reactive oxidant than triplet oxygen, in particular toward double bonds. Carotenoids and other molecules possessing a highly conjugated system can deactivate a singlet oxygen to a triplet one. The other ROS—hydrogen peroxide, hydroxyl radical, and peroxynitrite—can oxidize most of biological molecules, which would lead to cell and tissue dysfunction and then to cell death and tissue necrosis if no efficient system existed to scavenge these reactive intermediates before they can destroy vital molecules.

Box 2 Induction of oxidative stress by UV radiation in the skin (see Fig. 2)
Ultraviolet rays may induce an oxidative stress in the skin by two distinct pathways. Ultraviolet radiation can induce the release of mediators of inflammation (202), then activated leucocytes produce the radical anion superoxide, a reaction catalyzed by the enzyme NADPH oxidase (201,203). Superoxide then undergoes a dismutation to oxygen and hydrogen peroxide—a reaction catalyzed by superoxide dismutase—and hydrogen peroxide is converted to hypochlorite by myeloperoxidase (Fig. 1, Box 1). All the ROS produced following activation of NADPH oxidase generate an oxidative stress. Alternatively, UV rays can remove a proton and an electron from lipid molecules, especially polyunsaturated ones, giving rise to lipid radicals (204). These lipid radicals react easily with molecular oxygen, which is a biradical, leading to the formation of lipid peroxides and new lipid radicals. This accumulation of lipid peroxides and radicals can disrupt cellular membranes and oxidize other biomolecules.

DNA Damage

DNA absorbs UV rays with a maximum at 260 nm, corresponding to the absorption maximum for the bases purines and pyrimidines. This wavelength corresponds to UVC range, and is not received by the sun at the earth surface. However, the absorption at 300

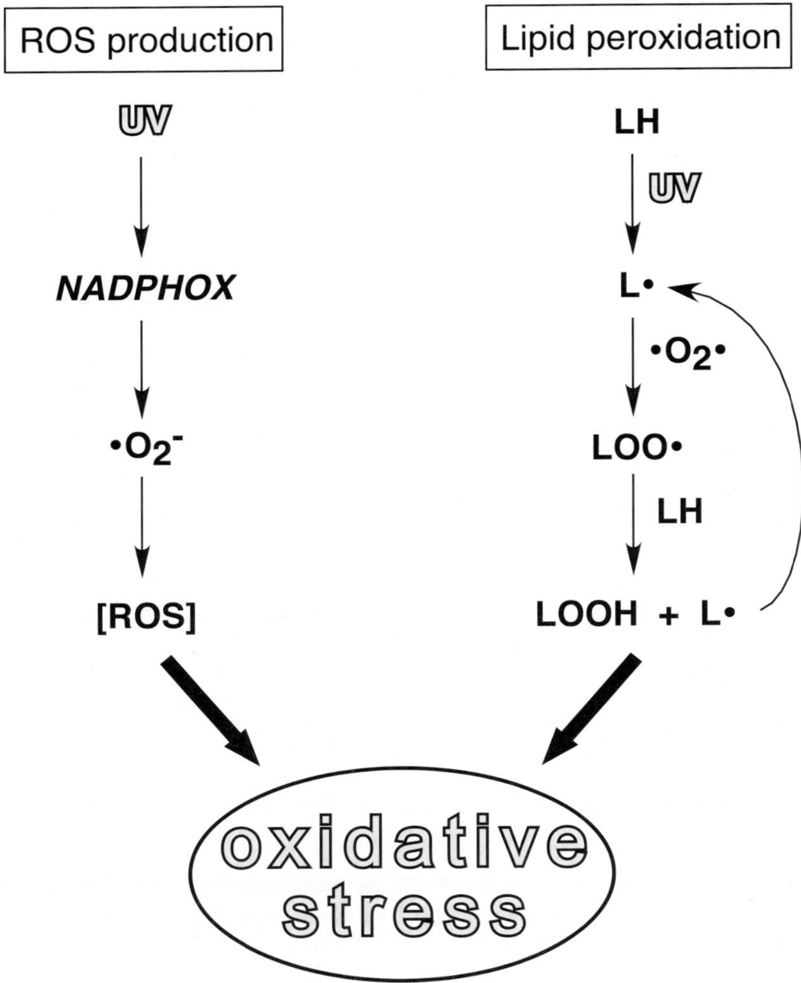

Figure 2 Induction of oxidative stress by UV in the skin. Abbreviations used: LH, lipid molecule; L·, lipid radical; LOOH, lipid hydroperoxide; LOO·, lipid peroxyradical; NADPHOX, NADPH oxidase; $\cdot O_2^-$, superoxide.

nm is still important, and the skin can receive this wavelength, in the UVB range, during exposure to the sun. This explains why DNA photoproducts such as the pyrimidine-(6-4)-pyrimidone photoproduct and thymidine dimers can be found in epidermal DNA following solar simulated light (Fig. 3A) (40–43). Another DNA alteration following UV exposure is the oxidation of 2′-deoxyguanosine into 8-oxo-2′-deoxyguanosine (Fig. 3B). This modified purine is an oxidation product, and requires the formation of reactive oxygen species; however, this oxidation takes place in response to UV, and thus is found in epidermal DNA following UV exposure (44–46). Although these DNA alterations are efficiently detected and repaired by a complex enzymatic system, if the rate of formation of these photoproducts surpasses the rate at which they can be repaired (19,47,48), biological consequences can be expected, including erythema, inflammation, cutaneous immunosuppression, DNA mutations, cancer initiation, or apoptosis (49). For this reason, any topical treatment able to prevent the formation of these photoproducts or to improve their reparation could be useful for the prevention of long-term consequences of sun exposure, such as skin cancers and photoaging.

Modulation of Signal Transduction

Although the primary chromophores are still unknown, UV can modulate membrane receptor-coupled signal transduction in a manner that is independent of the presence of their usual ligands (29,50–52) (Fig. 4). Thus UV can activate the transcription factor activator protein-1 (AP-1), normally activated by the transduction cascades triggered by receptor tyrosine kinases or G protein-coupled receptors (53,54). In keratinocytes and fibroblasts, AP-1 activates the genes encoding matrix metalloproteinases (54–56), whereas in fibroblasts, it represses the expression of procollagen (57). UV also activates the transduction signaling pathways of inflammatory cytokine receptors, leading to activation of the transcription factor nuclear factor κB (NF-κB), which in turns activates the genes encoding inflammatory cytokines; these cytokines can increase the mentioned transduction signaling pathways by binding to their receptors, and promote ROS formation (58–60). Finally, UV represses the signaling pathways of transforming growth factor-β (TGF-β), a growth factor that promotes differentiation, extracellular matrix deposition, and apoptosis. Taken together, these cellular effects elicited by UV lead to collagen degradation, inhibition of collagen synthesis, inflammation and oxidative stress, and decrease the ability of damaged cells to be eliminated by apoptosis.

TREATMENT AND PREVENTION OF PHOTOAGING

In the previous section, we described the different biochemical pathways that can be modulated by UV radiation. To prevent the deleterious actions of UV, the first approach obviously consists of avoiding UV exposure. However, despite its efficiency, this solution is usually incompatible with many outdoor professional and recreational activities. Thus the next approach is to protect the skin from UV radiation. This can be achieved by wearing clothes in such a way that any part of the body is covered by weighty material. This solution is still not fulfilling when running or working during sunny and hot journeys. Moreover, many people go to sunny places to take advantage of the sun. Thus there is a definite need for a solution that would counteract the deleterious actions of UV radiation to the skin in spite of sun exposure. The use of topical sunscreens, a solution chosen by many people for several decades, has been shown to be effective in certain conditions, but is not totally satisfying for the following reasons: (i) to be efficient, sunscreens have to be applied quite often; thus people have to remember to apply the sunscreen regularly during outdoor activity, the consumption of the sunscreen is high, and a great amount of exogenous substances penetrates into the skin; (ii) most of the sunscreens used until recently efficiently filter UVB radiation—the most biologically active part of sunlight—but are relatively transparent to UVA radiation; the latter, although much less potent in inducing biological effects, represents more than 95% of the UV radiation received by the sun at the earth surface, and is involved in various cutaneous reactions, including oxidative stress (61,62), DNA damage (63,64), immunosuppression (65), nonenzymatic signal transduction (66,67), photoaging (68), and carcinogenesis (69,70), thereby demonstrating the

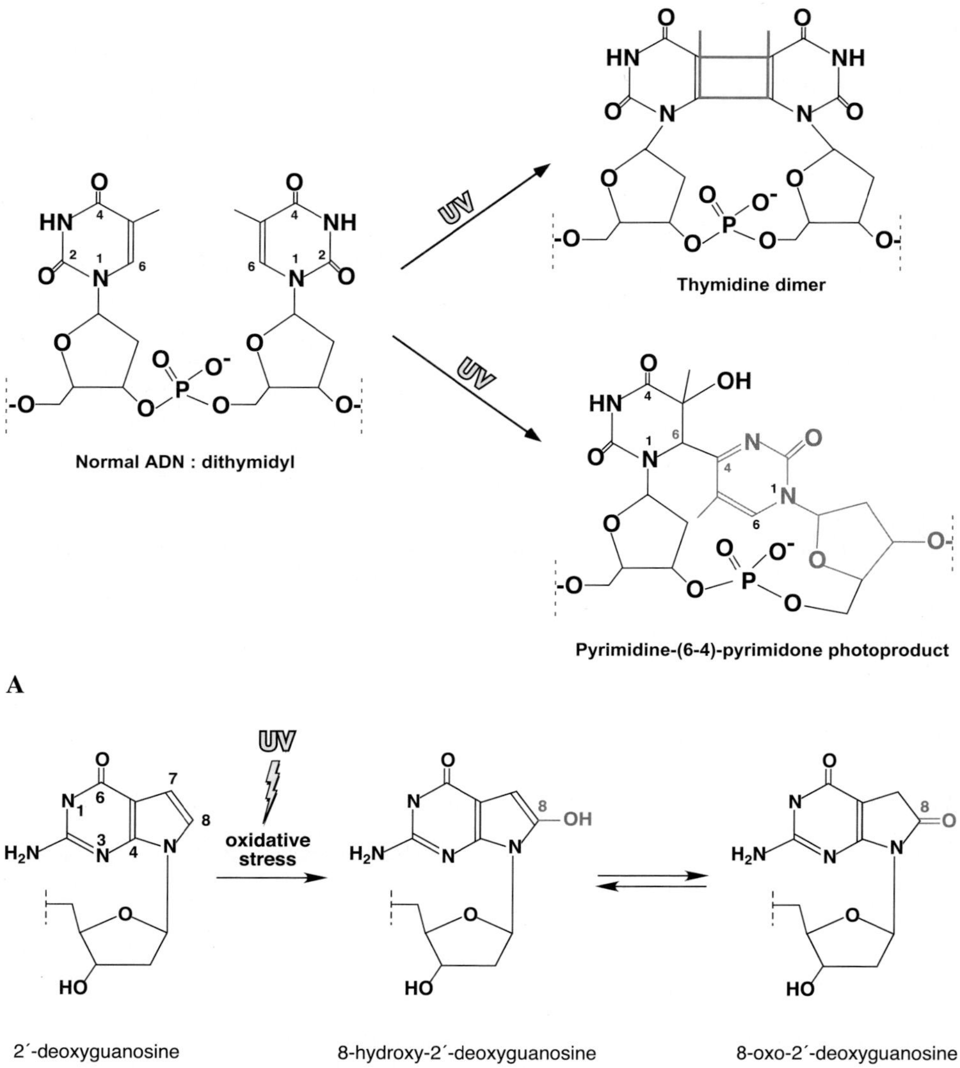

UV

UV

Thymidine dimer

Normal ADN : dithymidyl

Pyrimidine-(6-4)-pyrimidone photoproduct

A

UV

oxidative stress

2´-deoxyguanosine

8-hydroxy-2´-deoxyguanosine

8-oxo-2´-deoxyguanosine

B

Figure 3 UV-induced DNA damage. (A) A DNA sequence containing two successive pyrimidine bases (thymine, cytosine) can give rise to two kinds of photoproducts: a dimer of thymidine or a pyrimidine-(6–4)-pyrimidone adduct. (B) In response to UV radiation, ROS can be generated to oxidize the guanine base into 8-hydroxyguanine or 8-oxoguanine.

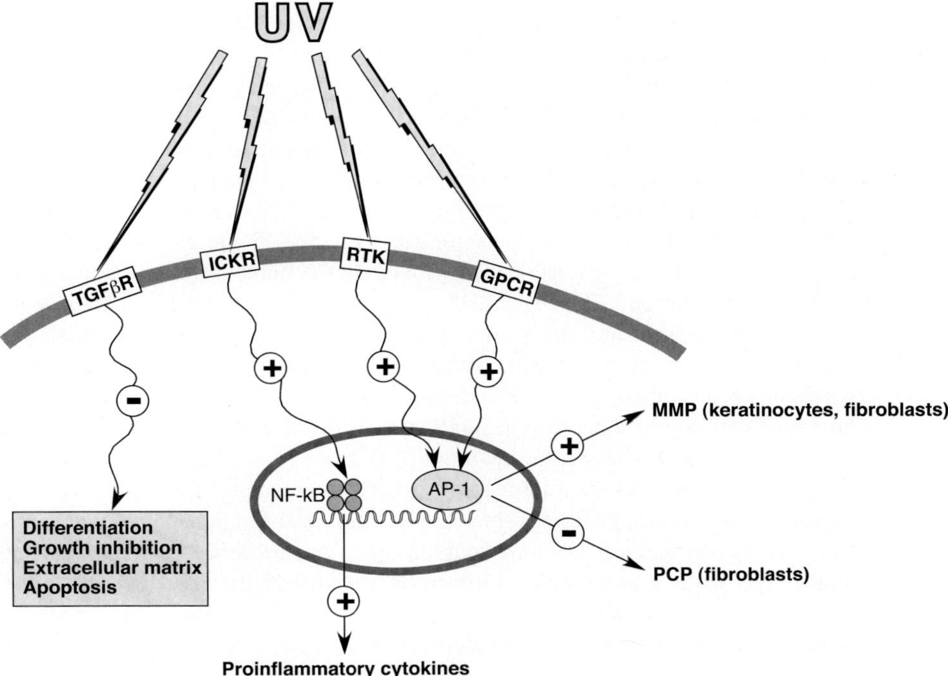

Figure 4 Modulation of signal transduction by UV light. Ultraviolet radiation can modulate the signal transduction pathways of various families of membrane-bound receptors. The receptor tyrosine kinases (RTK) and G-protein-coupled receptors (GPCR) are linked to signal transduction pathways that may lead to activator protein-1 (AP-1) activation. Inflammatory cytokine receptors (ICKR) mediate the activation of nuclear factor κB (NF-κB). Activation and inhibition of signal transduction pathways are indicated by plus and minus symbols, respectively. Other abbreviations used: MMP, matrix metalloproteinases; PCP, procollagen promoters; TGF-βR, transforming growth factor-β receptor.

need for efficient UVA photoprotection (71); (iii) commercially available sunscreens have been tested for their physical absorption properties, but much less is known about their long-term safety, their photostability, and the cutaneous effects of the energy absorbed during UV exposure. For these reasons, and in particular since oxidative stress is the common denominator of the conditions leading to the development of photoaging, much attention is now focusing on the potential benefits provided by the use of topical natural substances that possess antioxidant properties, or can improve the natural defense of the organism against the biological actions elicited by UV radiation (30,72).

Retinoids

Biochemistry of Retinoids

Vitamin A (all-*trans*-retinol; retinol) and its naturally occurring and synthetic derivatives are collectively referred to as retinoids. The main sources of vitamin A are retinyl esters (animal fat, mammal liver, fish), carotenoids (vegetables), and retinol (egg yolk). These precursors are converted to retinol in the small intestine; retinol is then esterified to fatty acids and stored in the liver (73,74). The biologically active forms of vitamin A are all-*trans*- and 9-*cis*- retinoic acids, which are produced by oxidation of retinol to retinal and then to retinoic acids. The latter bind to various isoforms of nuclear receptors (RAR-α, -β, -γ and RXR-α, -β, -γ), then the ligand-receptor complexes modulate gene expression either directly as transcription factors by binding to specific DNA sequences (RARE), or indirectly by repressing the transcription factor AP-1 (75,76). By activating RARE and repressing AP-1, retinoids are powerful agents mediating cellular differentiation and repressing cellular proliferation (77) (Fig. 5). Human epidermis and dermis contain about 1 nmol/g of total vitamin A (retinol and retinyl esters), as well as much lower concentrations of retinoic acids ($\leq$ 20 pmol/g) (78–82). Although the biological function of cutaneous vitamin A is still unclear, increasing evidence suggest a role of vitamin A in the control of epidermis renewal, due to its ability to modulate cell proliferation and differentiation (83–85). Effectively, the RARE sequences control the expression of genes involved in cellular differentiation, whereas the transcription factor AP-1 mediates signals from growth factors, oncogenes, and tumor promoters that activate cell proliferation. In the epidermis, however, these two antagonistic actions are coupled, since the proliferation of keratinocytes from the basal layer lead to an increase in the number of differentiated cells in the upper layers. It is therefore not surprising that retinoids induce both an epidermal acanthosis and an increase of the number of differentiated keratinocytes.

Topical Retinoids in the Treatment of Photoaged Skin

The application of topical retinoids loads the epidermis with large amounts of retinoids. In humans, topical retinoic acid (86,87), retinol (80,88), and retinyl palmitate (89) have been shown to induce a manifold increase of the epidermal concentration of the applied retinoid. In the hairless mouse, we analyzed the metabolism of topical retinoids and showed that retinoic acid, retinol, retinal, and retinyl palmitate dramatically increased both total epidermal vitamin A (retinol and retinyl esters) and the applied retinoid (90). Although topical retinoids penetrate easily through the epidermis, many studies performed in humans or other mammals reported no significant increase of plasma retinoids after topical application of natural or synthetic retinoids (91–94); theoretically, this would indicate that topical retinoids are not teratogenic; however, owing to the high teratogenic actions of systemic retinoids, topical retinoids are not recommended during pregnancy. Thus topical retinoids have powerful therapeutic potential in the treatment of a various diseases. However, nonselective retinoids that indiscriminately activate many or all of the different retinoid receptors and their signaling pathways will invariably produce beneficial as well as adverse effects. Therefore, current and future retinoid research should be directed toward new retinoid drugs with sufficient receptor or function selectivity that only those biological systems relevant to a specific disease would be affected (95).

Photoaging is the consequence of long term UV-induced damage to the skin and is characterized, among other things, by inhibition of keratinocyte turnover (due to TGF-β repression) and upregulation of AP-1–driven matrix metalloproteinases (see Modulation of Signal Transduction and Fig. 4). Topical retinoids promote proliferation of basal keratinocytes and extracellular matrix synthesis by restoring TGF-β–signaling pathways and inhibiting AP-1 activity, and thus are the candidates of choice in treating photoaging. The three main candidates are described below.

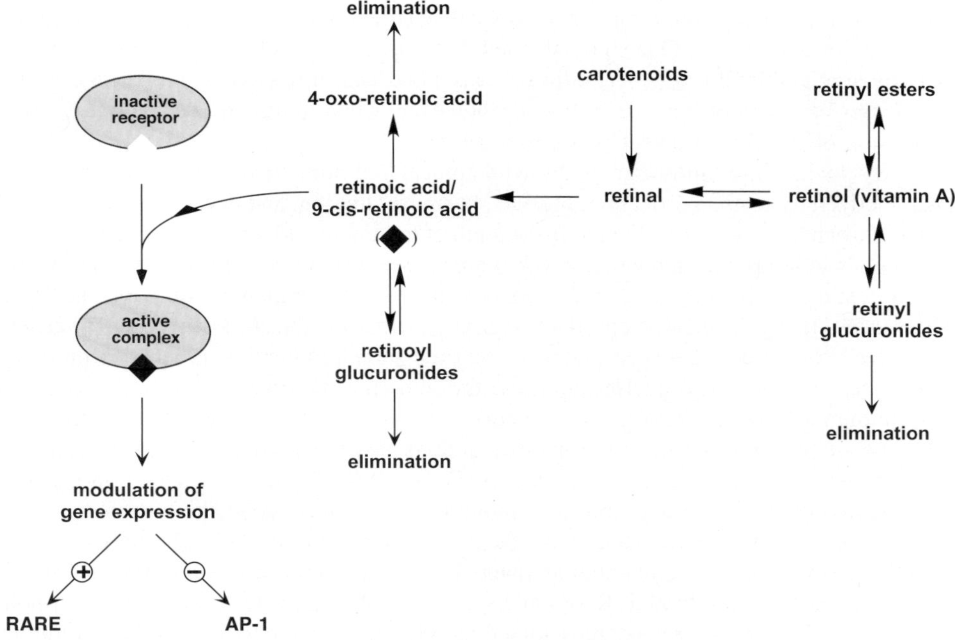

Figure 5 Biochemistry of vitamin A. Vitamin A (retinol), retinyl esters, and carotenoids are present in the diet. Retinol and carotenoids are converted to retinal, then retinal is oxidized to retinoic acids, the biologically active forms of vitamin A. Vitamin A and its metabolites are eliminated either by oxidation or by conjugation to glucuronate. Retinoic acids can bind to the nuclear receptors RAR or RXR, and then the ligand-receptor complexes modulate gene expression by activating RARE DNA sequences or inhibiting the transcription factor AP-1.

Retinoic Acid. As described previously, photodamaged skin is characterized by fine and coarse wrinkling, rough texture, sallow color, and irregular pigmentation. The potential effects of tretinoin (retinoic acid) on photodamaged skin were first observed by Kligman et al. (25) in postadolescent women treated for persistent acne. These investigators found that long-term use of tretinoin led to an improvement in skin wrinkling and roughness. Subsequently, numerous controlled studies have clearly demonstrated that once-daily topical application of retinoids, particularly 0.05% tretinoin, improves fine and coarse wrinkling and lightens actinic lentigines and mottled hyperpigmentation (96–101). 13-*cis* retinoic acid (isotretinoin) showed similar results in a study involving 776 patients treated over a 36-week period (102). Histological findings of tretinoin application to the skin include (i) compaction of the stratum corneum, (ii) epidermal hyperplasia (acanthosis), (iii) correction of atypia (e.g., actinic keratosis), (iv) dispersion of melanin granules, (v) increased dermal collagen synthesis, and (vi) angiogenesis. These findings explain the smoother skin, the rosy glow, the decreased blotchy pigmentation, and the diminished fine lines and wrinkles observed following long-term topical treatment with tretinoin. It generally takes 3–6 months of daily application to appreciate significant clinical improvement. There is no correlation between the clinical efficacy of tretinoin and the level of irritation; therefore it is not advisable to use high concentrations (0.1%) to achieve a good clinical result. Equally impressive results were obtained with 0.025% or 0.05% tretinoin with less irritation (103). One study showed that improvement observed during 48 weeks of daily application of 0.05% tretinoin was sustained with thrice-weekly applications and to a lesser extent with once-daily dosing; however, when treatment was stopped, some regression of the clinical benefits occurred (96).

By far the most limiting factor with topical tretinoin treatment is skin irritation characterized by erythema, scaling, pruritus, burning, stinging, and dryness. This so-called retinoid dermatitis occurs within the first month of treatment and tends to recede thereafter. It responds to temporary reduction in the frequency or amount of retinoid application and to application of moisturizers. Although pharmaceutical companies focus on the large differences among the different products regarding irritation, the clinically observed differences are often greater between patients using the same products than between products (104). Desquamation and peeling translate the hyperproliferative response of epidermis to tretinoin mediated by RARs, but erythema does not seem to be receptor mediated (88). Although no photoallergic or phototoxicity reactions have been proved for topical retinoids, many patients note a decreased tolerance to UV radiation shortly after sun exposure, but infrared radiation (heat) rather than UV radiation may contribute to this response.

RETINALDEHYDE. Retinaldehyde, the precursor of retinoic acid, was shown to be as effective as tretinoin in treating photodamage, and had a better tolerance profile (105,106). Retinaldehyde does not bind to RARs and selectively delivers low concentrations of retinoic acid (107). A comparative study including 357 female patients who applied tretinoin 0.05%, retinaldehyde 0.05%, or placebo compared the tolerance of retinoic acid and retinaldehyde with that of vehicle. The frequency of side effects at 12 months was lower with retinaldehyde (1%) than with retinoic acid (9%) (108). It has been hypothesized that topical retinaldehyde reduces the side effects of retinoic acid (e.g., irritation) through a more controlled delivery of the biologically active retinoic acid to target cells from a less irritant precursor reservoir confined to the stratum corneum, thereby limiting the ''overload'' of retinoic acid in the skin, which may be related, at least in part, to cutaneous irritation (109,110). Theoretically, retinol, a precursor of retinaldehyde and retinoic acid, could also be useful in treating photoaging. However, although it is widely used in cosmetic formulations for this purpose, topical retinol has not been proven effective in treating photoaging, maybe because of the slow transformation into retinaldehyde and retinoic acid.

TAZAROTENE. Tazarotene is a receptor-selective retinoid (RAR-β, and-γ) that has been used in the treatment of patients with psoriasis, acne vulgaris, and photoaging. It normalizes keratinocyte differentiation, reverses keratinocyte hyperproliferation, and has anti-inflammatory effects. A recent study showed that 0.1% tazarotene produced a statistically significant improvement of photodamage. The first effects were seen on pigment changes to be followed by fine wrinkles, tactile roughness and coarse wrinkling. Adverse events include primarily of irritation, peeling, erythema, dryness, burning, and itching, and were noted in 30–40% of patients during the first 24 weeks of treatment (111).

Ultraviolet Radiation Exposure and Safety of Topical Retinoids

Exposure to UV radiation decreases the epidermal vitamin A content (retinol and retinyl esters) in human and mouse skin (62, 81). Topical delivery of retinoids counteract this UV-induced depletion (90,112). A recent human study analyzed the expression of RAR and RXR nuclear receptors in normal skin, actinic keratoses, and squamous cell carcinoma. Expression was decreased early in sun-exposed skin (112,113), and the decrease was more pronounced as the stage progressed from actinic keratosis to squamous cell carcinoma (113).

The use of topical retinoids, especially retinoic acid in a context of sun exposure, remains controversial. We demonstrated that retinyl palmitate exerts a filter effect in human skin in vivo (205). In vitro experiments showed that, in certain conditions, natural retinoids have pro-oxidant abilities that could be carcinogenic. Retinol and retinaldehyde caused cellular DNA cleavage and induced 8-oxo-deoxyguanosine formation in HL-60 cells. They also induced Cu(II)-mediated DNA damage in DNA fragments (114). Retinoic acid also has a role in regulating the skin immune system. Topical retinoic acid prevents UV light from reducing the density of Langerhans cells and dendritic epidermal cells in mouse skin (115).

A retrospective study including 61 patients who applied 0.05% retinaldehyde during a 6-month to 142-month period evaluated the safety of long-term application of retinal in terms of photocarcinogenesis. The finding clearly showed that long-term use of topical retinaldehyde was not associated with a higher risk of actinic keratoses or nonmelanoma skin cancers. However, patients who applied retinaldehyde daily were less inclined to develop actinic keratosis than those who applied it irregularly (116). Topical retinoids display both pro-oxidative and antioxidative properties and anticarcinogenic or procarcinogenic activities in different in vivo and in vitro models, but it is interesting to note that human studies have shown both prevention or no effect of topical retinoids on nonmelanoma skin cancers (117–120). Altogether actual data suggest that topical retinoids are not procarcinogenic and may even be effective for chemoprevention, especially in early phases of carcinogenesis, for reduction of the incidence of actinic keratosis and inhibition of progression to squamous cell carcinoma (121–125).

Antioxidants

A Need for Antioxidants

When talking about the need to protect the skin from sun-induced damage, everybody thinks immediately about sunscreens, the "gold standard" for photoprotection. However, recent developments have demonstrated the limited efficiency of sunscreens for the following reasons (126). First, sunscreens usually efficiently filter UVB (290–320 nm), but no one product provides excellent protection over the whole UVA range (320–400 nm), and UVA radiation can induce most of the biochemical pathways that lead to photoaging. Second, the sun protection factor (SPF) of sunscreens is determined in laboratories using a concentration of 2 mg/cm^2, but controlled studies have shown that most people apply sunscreens at a rate of 0.5 mg/cm^2 or less (127,128). This is important, because SPF is not linearly proportional to the concentration; in particular, at an application of 0.5 mg/cm^2, no sunscreen provides more than threefold protection (127). Third, UV-induced DNA damage and immunosuppression are still present at suberythemal levels of irradiation. Finally, the components of sunscreens, as well as their photoproducts—which are often free radicals—are absorbed by the skin and may cause harm to the epidermis (129,130). However, oxidative stress has been shown to be the cornerstone of the biochemical pathways leading to photoaging (see Oxidative Stress). As described above (see Oxidative Stress and Fig. 1), human cells, particularly those in the epidermis, possess an efficient antioxidant system, including enzymatic and nonenzymatic reductants that are able to deactivate ROS and to reduce oxidized molecules such as lipid peroxides. These endogenous antioxidant defenses are able to counteract the deleterious effects of occasional oxidative stress of moderate magnitude, but in the case of chronic or severe oxidative stress, they reach their limit and irremediable tissue damage is unavoidable. Thus, since sunscreens are not the panacea for the photoprotection of the skin, oxidative stress plays a central role in photodamage, and endogenous antioxidants can be saturated during chronic or excessive oxidative stress, topical antioxidants appear as an exciting alternative to sunscreens in preventing photoaging and other types of skin damage induced by acute or long-term sun exposure (37,82,126,131,132).

Topical Antioxidants

Low-molecular-weight antioxidants were shown to be efficient in preventing oxidative stress in various models (62,133–135). Although antioxidants can be supplied to the skin through diet and oral supplementation, physiological processes related to absorption, solubility, transport, and metabolism limit the amount of the active form that can be delivered to the skin. Direct application therefore has the advantage of targeting the antioxidants to the area where they are needed, provided they are applied in a formulation that is able to prevent their deactivation by undesirable oxidation and to facilitate their absorption into the skin.

ENDOGENOUS ANTIOXIDANTS. The main advantages provided by endogenous antioxidants over exogenous ones are their very low toxicity—since they are natural components of the organism—and the existence of recycling pathways. This is important because an antioxidant that has done its job (to reduce an oxidant intermediate) becomes an oxidant itself, and in the case of its accumulation, it could contribute to oxidative stress instead of counteracting it. Furthermore, in order to maintain their efficiency, antioxidants have to be recycled to their reduced state, or eliminated from the organism and replaced by new ones. Thus vitamin E, the first endogenous antioxidant that prevents lipid peroxidation, once oxidized to a radical by a free radical, can be recycled by other antioxidants (126,136,137) (Fig. 6).

Vitamin E (tocopherols). Vitamin E is the major endogenous lipophilic antioxidant, and its main biological function is to prevent lipid peroxidation of biological membranes. It consists of eight naturally occurring tocopherols: α-tocopherol accounts for about 90% of tissue vitamin E, and the remaining 10% being essentially γ-tocopherol. δ-Tocopherol, because of its poor intestinal absorption, is not represented in the constitutive skin vitamin E content; however, it displays the highest biological activity in vitro and can be used topically, since all tocopherols, lipophilic compounds with a polar functional group, penetrate easily to the skin. Since vitamin E is able to stop a radical chain reaction, a high load in epidermal vitamin E would prevent epidermal damage induced by UV radiation (82,138,139). In particular, in mouse skin, topical α-tocopherol was shown to prevent UV-induced free radical formation (140), to protect endogenous epidermal antioxidants and prevent lipid peroxidation (82,141), and to prevent UV-induced systemic immunosuppression (142).

Until now, most scientific studies aimed at assessing the potential benefit of topical vitamin E have been performed in animals. Although many people use cosmetics containing tocopherols, very few human studies have been conducted. It should be noted, however, that although many cosmetics contain tocopheryl acetate or other tocopheryl esters, these compounds have no direct antioxidant properties, and are not tocopherol precursors owing to the lack of adequate esterases in the skin (143,144). However, when δ-tocopherol is covalently linked to D-glucose and then applied to the skin, free δ-tocopherol can be delivered to the epidermis, indicating the presence of a glucocerebrosidase in human

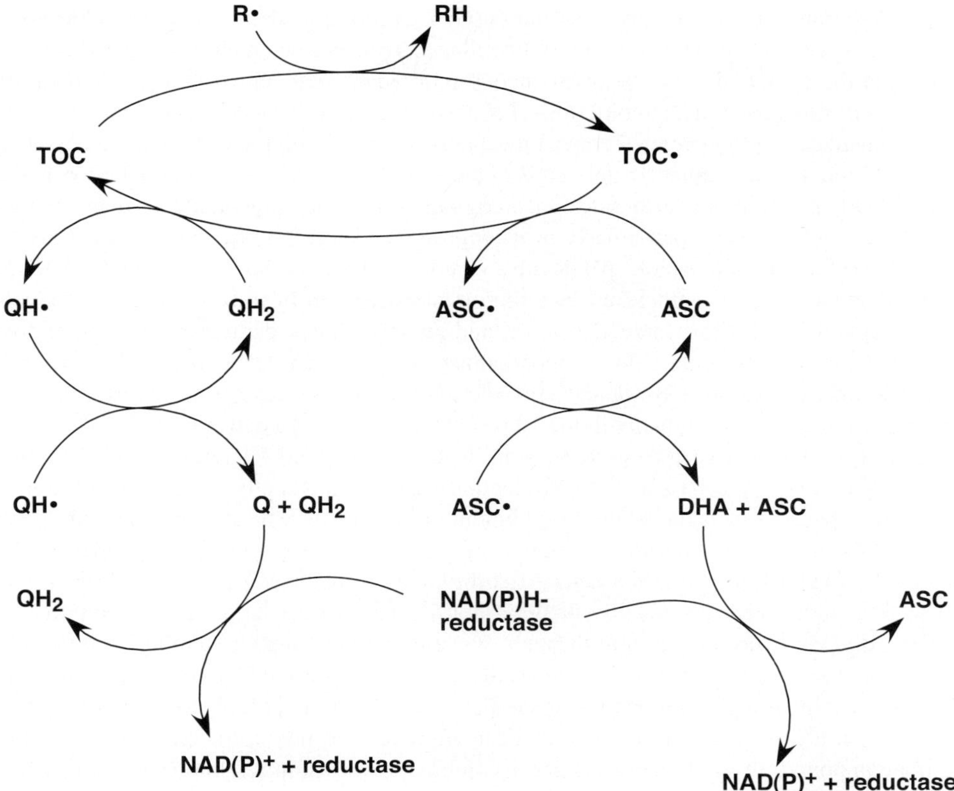

Figure 6 Interacting network of nonenzymatic endogenous antioxidants. Vitamin E (tocopherol, TOC) reduces a free radical (R·), produced during oxidative stress, to its natural form (RH), and becomes a radical itself (TOC·). The latter can be recycled to vitamin E by vitamin C (ascorbate, ASC) or ubiquinol (QH_2), leading to the formation of their respective radicals semidehydroascorbate (ASC·) or ubisemiquinone (QH·). Two ASC· radicals dismutate to ascorbate (ASC) and dehydroascorbate (DHA); two QH· radicals dismutate to ubiquinol (QH_2) and ubiquinone (Q). Finally, the oxidized forms dehydroascorbate and ubiquinone are reduced to ascorbate and ubiquinol, respectively, by NADH- or NADPH-dependent reductases.

epidermis (D. Redoules, personal communication). In hairless mice exposed to long-term suberythemal UVB doses, Bissett et al. reported that a topical application of α-tocopherol (5%) in combination with ascorbate (5%) or a photoprotective sunscreen on mouse skin prior to suberythemal UVB exposure was effective in preventing photoaging, as assessed by skin wrinkling and histological alterations (epidermal thickening, dermal infiltrate, collagen damage) (145,146). In humans, however, an extensive review of the literature revealed that the clinical efficacy of α-tocopherol alone in protection from distinct photodermatoses including photoaging is largely unproven (147–149), and a combination of various antioxidants is a more promising way to prevent photodamage because of the possible synergism between them, such as the well-known recycling of vitamin E by vitamin C (150).

Vitamin C (ascorbic acid). Vitamin C (L-ascorbic acid) is a water-soluble, low-molecular-weight antioxidant required for collagen synthesis and maintenance of the redox status of the cells, and is the major cutaneous antioxidant, with a predominant localization in the aqueous phase of the epidermis (126,151). When taken orally, even with massive supplementation, physiological control mechanisms limit the amount that can be absorbed in the blood and subsequently delivered to the skin (152). Thus topical application is the only way to increase skin ascorbate concentrations. As a polar reagent, it does not penetrate easily through the skin, particularly in its deprotonated form, which occurs at pH above 3.5; however, at more acidic pH levels, vitamin C has no electric charge, and when formulated in adequate vehicle, a 15% solution increases significantly ascorbate skin levels in 3 days (153). Various animal (mouse and swine) studies demonstrated a protective action of topical ascorbic acid in photodamage (146,154,155), whereas only very few studies aimed at examining topical ascorbic acid in human have been reported to date (156). Among these, a study involving 10 patients who applied a newly formulated vitamin C complex consisting of 10% ascorbic acid (water soluble) and 7% tetrahexyldecyl ascorbate (lipid soluble) to half of the face demonstrated a statistically significant difference in clinical scoring of facial wrinkles, although no difference was shown in pigmentation (157). The modest photoprotective action of topical ascorbate may be explained by its difficulty to penetrate the skin and its instability in aqueous vehicles, and lipophilic ascorbate derivatives such as succinyl or phosphoryl esters appear as promising compounds owing to their easier penetration through the skin and their higher stability in lipophilic vehicles (158–160). As for topical antioxidants in general, topical ascorbic acid alone is not very useful as a photoprotective agent, but in combination with photoprotective agents or other antioxidants, such as vitamin E, it improves the photoprotective action of the latter compounds (154). In hairless mice, a combination of vitamin E linoleate, nordihydroguaradinic acid, and magnesium-ascorbyl phosphate significantly decreased the formation of sunburn cells produced following long-term UVB exposure (161). In humans, a combination of ascorbate with melatonin and vitamin E decreased the erythemal response to UV radiation (162,163).

Exogenous Antioxidants.

α-Hydroxy acids. α-Hydroxy acids possess a hydroxyl group on the adjacent carbon to a carboxyl group, a structure that enables them to act as chelators, especially for calcium ions. Thus they reduce epidermal calcium ions and cause a loss of calcium ions from the cadherins of the desmosomes and adherens junctions, resulting in disruption of cell adhesion and desquamation. This decrease of epidermal calcium ions also tends to promote cell growth and retard cell differentiation, giving rise to a younger-looking skin. This property of α-hydroxy acids, many of which are found in fruits, explains their use as topical rejuvenating agents. α-Hydroxy acids constitute the third class of topical agents widely used in the treatment of photoaging, besides topical retinoids and antioxidants (72,164,165). Some α-hydroxy acids are also antioxidants, such as gluconic, malic, tartaric, citric, and ascorbic acids (166), possibly owing to their direct reducing power or to their chelating properties toward transition metals able to initiate oxidative stress by Fenton and Haber-Weiss reactions. Glycolic acid was shown to increase type I collagen mRNA and hyaluronic acid content in human skin, thus indicating a potential benefit as a treatment for any condition leading to the loss of physical properties of the dermis, including photoaging (167). For more details on topical α-hydroxy acids in photoaging, the reader is invited to read the chapter devoted to this subject in this book.

Plant antioxidants. Plants are fascinating chemical factories and have to protect themselves from the sun. Thus plants synthesize many flavonoid and polyphenolic compounds that are powerful antioxidants (168). Many of these plant antioxidants are consumed in the diet and are believed to play an important role in human health (169). Recently, some of these compounds, including *Polypodium leucotomos* extracts, silymarin, soy isoflavones, and tea polyphenols, were shown to have photoprotective properties when applied to the skin (126).

Anapsos, a hydrophilic fraction of the tropical fern P. leucotomos, exerts antioxidant and immunomodulating properties in vitro (170,171). It was introduced 30 years ago to treat psoriasis (172), and then vitiligo (173). More recently, topical anapsos was shown to inhibit lipid peroxidation, ROS formation, phototoxicity, and acute sunburn in humans in vivo following acute UV exposure. (171,174). In a pilot study using hairless mice exposed to long-term UVB radiation, topical anapsos significantly decreased dermal elastosis, a typical photoaging parameter, and decreased the number of mice that developed skin tumors (175).

Silymarin is the name given to an extract of the thistle *Silybum marianum*, and consists of a mixture of three flavonoids: silybin, silydianin, and silychristine (176). It has been used for a long time in the treatment of liver diseases (177), and has powerful antioxidant properties (178). In mice, silymarin efficiently prevented tumor promotion (179), as well as UV-induced immunosuppression and oxidative stress (180,181). In human cultured keratinocytes, silymarin significantly inhibited UV-induced activation of the transcription factor NF-κB (182). According to these reported actions of silymarin on various in vitro and in vivo models, silymarin opposes to the direct actions of UV radiation on living cells, and thus could be a promising topical reagent in preventing and treating photodamage. New in vivo studies are needed to confirm this hypothesis in the case of photoaging.

Soybeans contain a variety of biologically active flavonoids. These compounds may be responsible for the lower risk of cardiovascular diseases and breast cancers in Asian populations who regularly consume soy derivatives. Indeed, soybean flavonoids have antioxidant (183), anticancer (184), and estrogen-like properties (185). The two major soy flavonoids are genistin and daidzin; both are glycosides and must be hydrolyzed in the gut in order to deliver their respective free aglycones: the isoflavones genistein and daidzein (186). Because of their biological properties, and because topical estrogens improve the skin condition of postmenopausal women (187,188), topical genistein and daidzein could be helpful in aging and photoaging conditions, but this has to be confirmed by in vivo studies.

Tea (*Camellia sinensis*) is a potential rich source of polyphenols, their precursors comprising up to 35% of the dry weight of tea leaves. These polyphenols are produced during tea leaf processing, and depending of the processing conditions, green, black, and other tea varieties can be obtained. Green tea contains predominantly monomeric polyphenol catechins, including epigallocatechin-3-gallate, whereas polymeric polyphenols are found in black tea (189,190). Green tea and black tea polyphenols have interesting properties in animal and human health when given orally or topically. Topical epigallocatechin-3-gallate (191,192) and oral green tea and black tea extracts (193) prevent photocarcinogenesis in mice, as well as UVB-induced infiltration of leukocytes, depletion of antigen-presenting cells, and oxidative stress (194). In humans, green tea polyphenols protects the skin against UV-induced erythema and inflammation (195). In mice and guinea pigs, epigallocatechin-3-gallate prevented UV-induced erythema and LPO, decreased collagen degradation, and inhibited activation of the transcription factors NF-κB and AP-1 (196). As for the plant antioxidants already described in this section, green tea and black tea polyphenols have interesting biological effects compatible with a possible preventive action on photoaging, but human studies are needed to ensure their potential actions in this context.

Besides the aforementioned plant antioxidant families, many other possibilities exist, such as *ginkgo biloba* and ginger extracts, resveratrol, and curcumin (197–200). These compounds are particularly promising in treating cutaneous diseases, since they usually combine several biological actions that interfere with oxidative stress, aging, photoaging, and cancer development.

SUMMARY AND DISCUSSION

Aging is a natural ineluctable process defining the progressive loss of the characteristics acquired during development, and finally leading to death. It has both genetic and metabolic bases that converge to a chronic oxidative stress in all tissues in general and in the skin in particular. Skin aging manifests clinically by fine and coarse wrinkling, roughness, dryness, a loss of dermal elasticity, and actinic keratosis. Photoaging or extrinsic aging is a similar process that superimposes to intrinsic aging, and is the consequence of long-term exposure to the UV radiation from the sun. Besides accelerating the biological processes involved in intrinsic aging, photoaging is more susceptible than intrinsic aging to give rise to skin cancers.

Since oxidative stress plays a pivotal role in the biological events leading to the clinical manifestations of aging and photoaging, any treatment that counteracts the effects of oxidative stress should have a therapeutical value in inhibiting the progression of aging and photoaging. However, UV radiation also interferes with the signal transduction pathways of extracellular messengers involved in cellular proliferation and differentiation. Two strategies are thus promising in the prophylaxis and treatment of photoaging: one should bring to the skin antioxidant molecules able to trap reactive oxidant intermediates and reduce the biomolecules that have been oxidized by these intermediates, and the other should bring to the skin messenger molecules that oppose the effects of UV radiation in signal transduction pathways. The best way to load the skin with high amounts of a compound is the direct application of this compound to the skin. Antioxidants can reduce both oxidant intermediates and oxidized biomolecules, and retinoids modulate the expression of genes involved in cellular proliferation and differentiation in an opposite direction to that induced by UV radiation. In this chapter, we described the molecular bases for the treatment of photoaging with topical retinoids or antioxidants, and then we reviewed the animal and human studies aimed at assessing the therapeutical value of these topical agents in preventing and treating photoaging.

Among topical retinoids, tretinoin (retinoic aid) has been extensively studied the last 15 years and has been shown to improve photoaging conditions when used every day for several months at 0.05% concentration. The main limitation of use comes from its potent irritating properties; for this reason, retinoic acid precursors, such as retinaldehyde, which are better tolerated and load the skin with sufficient amounts of retinoic acid to saturate its receptors, appear as an interesting alternative, although more controlled studies in humans have to be performed before this can be confirmed.

Topical antioxidants are another class of promising compounds used to treat photoaging because of their ability to protect the skin from oxidative stress. Since antioxidants have to be recycled in order to retain their efficiency and to avoid to become pro-oxidant, it is always better to combine various antioxidants acting in synergy than to apply one antioxidant at high concentrations. The predominant endogenous cutaneous antioxidants are vitamins C and E (ascorbate and tocopherols, respectively), which have been shown to slightly improve certain conditions of photoaging, although more human studies are needed to confirm the findings of these pilot studies. However, because of their various biological actions that counteract UV-induced direct effects on the skin, exogenous plant extracts from tea, ginger, ginkgo biloba, or grape are quite promising in the prevention and treatment of photoaging and nonmelanoma skin cancers. However, most of the studies performed to date have used in vitro or animal models, and more human studies are needed to confirm that these compounds are topical agents with therapeutical value in photoaging and photocarcinogenesis.

REFERENCES

1. Pereira-Smith OM. Genetic theories on aging. Aging (Milano) 1997; 9:429–430.
2. Martin GM. Genetics and the pathobiology of ageing. Philos Trans R Soc Lond B Biol Sci 1997; 52:1773–1780.
3. Cong YS, Wright WE, Shay JW. Human telomerase and its regulation. Microbiol Mol Biol Rev 2002; 66:407–425.
4. Neumann AA, Reddel RR. Telomere maintenance and cancer—look, no telomerase. Nat Rev Cancer 2002; 2:879–884.
5. Yaar M, Eller MS. Mechanisms of aging. Arch Dermatol 2002; 138:1429–1432.
6. Bodnar AG. Extension of life-span by introduction of telomerase into normal human cells. Science 1998; 279:349–352.
7. Cawthon RM. Association between telomere length in blood and mortality in people aged 60 years or older. Lancet 2003; 361:393–395.
8. Rothman DJ. Telomeres, telomerase, and cancer. New Engl J Med 2000; 342:1282–1286.
9. Campisi J. Replicative senescence: an old lives' tale. Cell 1996; 84:497–500.
10. Harman D. Aging : A theory based on free radical and radiation chemistry. J Gerontol 1956; 11:298–300.
11. Harman D. Free radical involvement in aging. Pathophysiology and therapeutic implications. Drugs Aging 1993; 3:60–80.
12. Halliwell B, Gutteridge JMC. Free Radicals in Biology and Medicine. 3rd ed.. Oxford: Oxford University Press, 1999.
13. Harman D. Aging: overview. Ann N Y Acad Sci 2001; 928:1–21.
14. Polla AS, Polla LL, Polla BS. Iron as the malignant spirit in successful ageing. Ageing Res Rev 2003; 2:25–37.
15. Biesalski HK. Free radical theory of aging. Curr Opin Clin Nutr Metab Care 2002; 5:5–10.
16. Sohal RS, Weindruch R. Oxidative stress, caloric restriction, and aging. Science 1996; 273: 59–63.
17. Hamilton ML. Does oxidative damage to DNA increase with age. Proc Natl Acad Sci U S A 2001; 98:10469–10474.
18. Mooradian AD, Thurman JE. Glucotoxicity: potential mechanisms. Clin Geriatr Med 1999; 15:255.
19. Rouse J, Jackson SP. Interfaces between the detection, signaling, and repair of DNA damage. Science 2002; 297:547–551.
20. Sander CS. Photoaging is associated with protein oxidation in human skin in vivo. J Invest Dermatol 2002; 118:618–625.
21. Tahara S, Matsuo M, Kaneko T. Age-related changes in oxidative damage to lipids and DNA in rat skin. Mech Ageing Dev 2001; 122:415–426.

22. Kuro-o M. Disease model: human aging. Trends Mol Med 2001; 7:179–181.
23. Hosokawa M. A higher oxidative status accelerates senescence and aggravates age-dependent disorders in SAMP strains of mice. Mech Ageing Dev 2002; 123:1553–1561.
24. Hekimi S, Guarente L. Genetics and the specificity of the aging process. Science 2003; 299: 1351–1354.
25. Kligman AM. Topical tretinoin for photoaged skin. J Am Acad Dermatol 1986; 15:836–859.
26. Green LJ, McCormick A, Weinstein GD. Photoaging and the skin. The effects of tretinoin. Dermatol Clin 1993; 11:97–105.
27. Montagna W, Carlisle K. Structural changes in ageing skin. Br J Dermatol 1990; 122(suppl 35):61–70.
28. Taylor CR. Photoaging/photodamage and photoprotection. J Am Acad Dermatol 1990; 22: 1–15.
29. Fisher GJ. Mechanisms of photoaging and chronological skin aging. Arch Dermatol 2002; 138:1462–1470.
30. Gilchrest BA. A review of skin ageing and its medical therapy. Br J Dermatol 1996; 135: 867–875.
31. Trautinger F. Mechanisms of photodamage of the skin and its functional consequences for skin ageing. Clin Exp Dermatol 2001; 26:573–577.
32. Yaar M, Gilchrest BA. Aging versus photoaging: postulated mechanisms and effectors. J Investig Dermatol Symp Proc 1998; 3:47–51.
33. Uitto J. Molecular aspects of photoaging. Eur J Dermatol 1997; 7:210–214.
34. Young AR. Chromophores in human skin. Phys Med Biol 1997; 42:789–802.
35. Halliwell B. Free radicals and antioxidants : a personal view. Nutr Rev 1994; 52:253–265.
36. Jacob RA, Burri BJ. Oxidative damage and defense. Am J Clin Nutr 1996; 63:985S–990S.
37. Kohen R, Gati I. Skin low molecular weight antioxidants and their role in aging and in oxidative stress. Toxicology 2000; 148:149–157.
38. Thiele JJ, Traber MG, Packer L. Depletion of human stratum corneum vitamin E : An early and sensitive In vivo marker of UV induced photo-oxidation. J Invest Dermatol 1998; 110: 756–761.
39. Wenk J. UV-induced oxidative stress and photoaging. Curr Probl Dermatol 2001; 29:83–94.
40. Mitchell DL, Nairn RS. The biology of the (6-4) photoproduct. Photochem Photobiol 1989; 49:805–819.
41. Rosenstein BS, Mitchell DL. Action spectra for the induction of pyrimidine(6-4)pyrimidone photoproducts and cyclobutane pyrimidine dimers in normal human skin fibroblasts. Photochem Photobiol 1987; 45:775–780.
42. Bykov VJ, Hemminki K. Assay of different photoproducts after UVA, B and C irradiation of DNA and human skin explants. Carcinogenesis 1996; 17:1949–1955.
43. Bykov VJ, Jansen CT, Hemminki K. High levels of dipyrimidine dimers are induced in human skin by solar- simulating UV radiation. Cancer Epidemiol Biomarkers Prev 1998; 7: 199–202.
44. Cadet J. Effects of UV and visible radiations on cellular DNA. Curr Probl Dermatol 2001; 29:62–73.
45. Ahmed NU. High levels of 8-hydroxy-2′-deoxyguanosine appear in normal human epidermis after a single dose of ultraviolet radiation. Br J Dermatol 1999; 140:226–231.
46. Toyokuni S. Reactive oxygen species-induced molecular damage and its application in pathology. Pathol Int 1999; 49:91–102.
47. Friedberg EC. DNA damage and repair. Nature 2003; 421:436–440.
48. Yarosh DB. Enhanced DNA repair of cyclobutane pyrimidine dimers changes the biological response to UV-B radiation. Mutat Res 2002; 509:221–226.
49. Vink AA, Roza L. Biological consequences of cyclobutane pyrimidine dimers. J Photochem Photobiol B 2001; 65:101–104.

50. Rittie L, Fisher GJ. UV-light-induced signal cascades and skin aging. Ageing Res Rev 2002; 1:705–720.
51. Seo M. Bi-directional regulation of UV-induced activation of p38 kinase and c-Jun N-terminal kinase by G protein beta gamma-subunits. J Biol Chem 2002; 277:24197–2203.
52. Miller CC, Hale P, Pentland AP. Ultraviolet B injury increases prostaglandin synthesis through a tyrosine kinase-dependent pathway. Evidence for UVB-induced epidermal growth factor receptor activation. J Biol Chem 1994; 269:3529–3533.
53. Marinissen MJ, Gutkind JS. G-protein-coupled receptors and signaling networks: emerging paradigms. Trends Pharmacol Sci 2001; 22:368–376.
54. Karin M, Liu Z, Zandi E. AP-1 function and regulation. Curr Opin Cell Biol 1997; 9:240–246.
55. Angel P, Szabowski A, Schorpp-Kistner M. Function and regulation of AP-1 subunits in skin physiology and pathology. Oncogene 2001; 20:2413–2423.
56. Fisher GJ. Molecular basis of sun-induced premature skin ageing and retinoid antagonism. Nature 1996; 379:335–339.
57. Fisher GJ. c-Jun-dependent inhibition of cutaneous procollagen transcription following ultraviolet irradiation is reversed by all-trans retinoic acid. J Clin Invest 2000; 106:663–670.
58. Kohler HB. Involvement of reactive oxygen species in TNF-alpha mediated activation of the transcription factor NF-kappaB in canine dermal fibroblasts. Vet Immunol Immunopathol 1999; 71:125–142.
59. Turpaev KT. Reactive oxygen species and regulation of gene expression. Biochemistry (Moscow) 2002; 67:281–292.
60. Kaminski KA. Oxidative stress and neutrophil activation: the two keystones of ischemia/reperfusion injury. Int J Cardiol 2002; 86:41–59.
61. Tyrrell RM. Ultraviolet radiation and free radical damage to skin. Biochem Soc Symp 1995; 61:47–53.
62. Sorg O. Oxidative stress-independent depletion of epidermal vitamin A by UVA. J Invest Dermatol 2002; 118:513–518.
63. Cooke MS. Induction and excretion of ultraviolet-induced 8-oxo-2′-deoxyguanosine and thymine dimers in vivo: implications for PUVA. J Invest Dermatol 2001; 116:281–285.
64. Petersen AB. Hydrogen peroxide is responsible for UVA-induced DNA damage measured by alkaline comet assay in HaCaT keratinocytes. J Photochem Photobiol B 2000; 59:123–131.
65. Halliday GM. UVA-induced immunosuppression. Mutation Res 1998; 422:139–145.
66. Grether-Beck S. Non-enzymatic triggering of the ceramide signaling cascade by solar UVA radiation. EMBO J 2000; 19:5793–5800.
67. Zhang Y. Requirement of ATM in UVA-induced signaling and apoptosis. J Biol Chem 2002; 277:3124–3131.
68. Krutmann J. Ultraviolet A radiation-induced biological effects in human skin: relevance for photoaging and photodermatosis. J Dermatol Sci 2000; 23(suppl 1):S22–S26.
69. de Laat A, van der Leun JC, de Gruijl FR. Carcinogenesis induced by UVA (365-nm) radiation: the dose-time dependence of tumor formation in hairless mice. Carcinogenesis 1997; 18:1013–1020.
70. de Gruijl FR. Photocarcinogenesis: UVA vs. UVB radiation. Skin Pharmacol Appl Skin Physiol 2002; 15:316–320.
71. Gasparro FP. Sunscreens, skin photobiology, and skin cancer: the need for UVA protection and evaluation of efficacy. Environ Health Perspect 2000; 108(suppl 1):71–78.
72. Griffiths CE. Drug treatment of photoaged skin. Drugs Aging 1999; 14:289–301.
73. Blomhoff R, Green MG, Norum KR. Vitamin A : Physiological and biochemical processing. Annu Rev Nutr 1992; 12:37–57.
74. Roos TC. Retinoid metabolism in the skin. Pharmacol Rev 1998; 50:315–333.
75. Fisher GJ, Voorhees JJ. Molecular mechanisms of retinoid actions in skin. FASEB J 1996; 10:1002–1013.
76. Napoli JL. Retinoic acid biosynthesis and metabolism. FASEB J 1996; 10:993–1001.

77. Pfahl M, Chytil F. Regulation of metabolism by retinoic acid and its nuclear receptors. Annu Rev Nutr 1996; 16:257–283.
78. Vahlquist A. Vitamin A in human skin: I. Detection and identification of retinoids in normal epidermis. J Invest Dermatol 1982; 79:89–93.
79. Vahlquist A. Vitamin A in human skin: II. Concentrations of carotene, retinol and dehydroretinol in various components of normal skin. J Invest Dermatol 1982; 79:94–97.
80. Duell EA. Extraction of human epidermis treated with retinol yields retro-retinoids in addition to free retinol and retinyl esters. J Invest Dermatol 1996; 107:178–182.
81. Sorg O. Retinol and retinyl ester epidermal pools are not identically sensitive to UVB irradiation and antioxidant protective effect. Dermatology 1999; 199:302–307.
82. Sorg O, Tran C, Saurat JH. Cutaneous vitamins A and E in the context of ultraviolet- or chemically-induced oxidative stress. Skin Pharmacol 2001; 14:363–372.
83. Randolph RK, Siegenthaler G. Vitamin A homeostasis in human epidermis: native retinoid composition and metabolism. In: Nau H, Blaner WS, Eds. The Biochemical and Molecular Basis of Vitamin A and Retinoid Action. Berlin: Springer-Verlag, 1999:491–520.
84. Siegenthaler G, Gumowski-Sunek D, Saurat JH. Metabolism of natural retinoids in psoriatic epidermis. J Invest Dermatol 1990; 95:47S–48S.
85. Saurat JH. How do retinoids work on human epidermis? A breakthrough and its implications. Clin Exp Dermatol 1988; 13:350–364.
86. Duell EA. Human skin levels of retinoic acid and cytochrome P-450-derived 4-hydroxyretinoic acid after topical application of retinoic acid in vivo compared to concentrations required to stimulate retinoic acid receptor-mediated transcription in vitro. J Clin Invest 1992; 90: 1269–1274.
87. Schaefer H, Zesch A. Penetration of vitamin A acid into human skin. Acta Derm Venereol Suppl 1975; 74:50–55.
88. Kang S. Application of retinol to human skin in vivo induces epidermal hyperplasia and cellular retinoid binding proteins characteristics of retinoic acid but without measurable retinoic acid levels or irritation. J Invest Dermatol 1995; 105:549–556.
89. Duell EA, Kang S, Voorhees JJ. Unoccluded retinol penetrates human skin in vivo more effectively than unoccluded retinyl palmitate or retinoic acid. J Invest Dermatol 1997; 109: 301–305.
90. Tran C. Topical delivery of retinoids counteracts the UVB-induced epidermal vitamin A depletion in hairless mouse. Photochem Photobiol 2001; 73:425–431.
91. Jensen BK. The negligible systemic availability of retinoids with multiple and excessive topical application of isotretinoin 0.05% gel (Isotrex) in patients with acne vulgaris. J Am Acad Dermatol 1991; 24:425–428.
92. Sass JO. Plasma retinoids after topical use of retinaldehyde on human skin. Skin Pharmacol 1996; 9:322–326.
93. Santana D. Plasma concentrations after three different doses of topical isotretinoin. Skin Pharmacol 1994; 7:140–144.
94. Nau H. Embryotoxicity and teratogenicity of topical retinoic acid. Skin Pharmacol 1993; 6(suppl.):35–44.
95. Chandraratna RA. Current research and future developments in retinoids: oral and topical agents. Cutis 1998; 61:40–45.
96. Ellis CN. Sustained improvement with prolonged topical tretinoin (retinoic acid) for photoaged skin. J Am Acad Dermatol , 1990; 23:629–637.
97. Lever L, Kumar P, Marks R. Topical retinoic acid for treatment of solar damage. Br J Dermatol 1990; 122:91–98.
98. Leyden JJ. Treatment of photodamaged facial skin with topical tretinoin. J Am Acad Dermatol 1989; 21:638–644.
99. Olsen EA. Tretinoin emollient cream for photodamaged skin: results of 48-week, multicenter, double-blind studies. J Am Acad Dermatol 1997; 37:217–226.

100. Weinstein GD. Topical tretinoin for treatment of photodamaged skin. A multicenter study. Arch Dermatol 1991; 127:659–665.
101. Weiss JS. Topical tretinoin improves photo aged skin. A double blind vehicle-controlled study. JAMA 1988; 259:527–532.
102. Sendagorta E, Lesiewicz J, Armstrong RB. Topical isotretinoin for photodamaged skin. J Am Acad Dermatol 1992; 27:S15–S18.
103. Kang S, Voorhees JJ. Photoaging therapy with topical tretinoin: an evidence-based analysis. J Am Acad Dermatol 1998; 39:S55–S61.
104. Prystowsky J. Comprehensive Dermatologic Drug Therapy. Philadelphia: Saunders, 2001.
105. Creidi P. Profilometric evaluation of photodamage after topical retinaldehyde and retinoic acid treatment. J Am Acad Dermatol 1998; 39:960–965.
106. Saurat JH. Topical retinaldehyde on human skin : biological effects and tolerance. J Invest Dermatol 1994; 103:770–774.
107. Didierjean L. Biological activities of topical natural retinaldehyde. Dermatology 1999; 199(suppl):19–24.
108. Sachsenberg-Studer EM. Tolerance of topical retinaldehyde in humans. Dermatology 1999; 199(suppl 1):61–63.
109. Saurat JH, Sorg O. Topical natural retinoids. The ''pro-ligand-non-ligand'' concept. Dermatology 1999; 199(suppl):1–2.
110. Saurat JH, Sorg O, Didierjean J. New concepts for delivery of topical retinoid activity to human skin, In: Nau H, Blaner WS, Eds. Retinoids The Biochemical and Molecular Basis of Vitamin A and Retinoid Action. Vol. 1999. Berlin: Springer-Verlag:521–538.
111. Phillips TJ. Efficacy of 0.1% tazarotene cream for the treatment of photodamage: a 12-month multicenter, randomized trial. Arch Dermatol 2002; 138:1486–1493.
112. Wang Z. Ultraviolet irradiation of human skin causes functional vitamin A deficiency, preventable by all-trans retinoic acid pre-treatment. Nat Med 1999; 5:418–422.
113. Xu XC. Progressive decreases in nuclear retinoid receptors during skin squamous carcinogenesis. Cancer Res 2001; 61:4306–4310.
114. Murata M, Kawanishi S. Oxidative DNA damage by vitamin A and its derivative via superoxide generation. J Biol Chem 2000; 275:2003–2008.
115. Halliday GM, Ho KKL, Barnetson RSC. Regulation of the skin immune system by retinoids during carcinogenesis. J Invest Dermatol 1992; 99:83S–86S.
116. Campanelli A, Naldi L. A retrospective study of the effect of long-term topical application of retinaldehyde (0.05%) on the development of actinic keratosis. Dermatology 2002; 205: 146–152.
117. Kligman LH. Retinoic acid and photocarcinogenesis. A controversy. Photodermatology 1987; 4:88–101.
118. Marks R. Retinoids in cutaneous malignancy. Frontiers in Pharmacology & Therapeutics. Vol. 619. Oxford: Blackwell Scientific, 1991:205.
119. Alirezai M. Clinical evaluation of topical isotretinoin in the treatment of actinic keratoses. J Am Acad Dermatol 1994; 30:447–451.
120. Misiewicz J. Topical treatment of multiple actinic keratoses of the face with arotinoid methyl sulfone (Ro 14-9706) cream versus tretinoin cream: a double-blind, comparative study. J Am Acad Dermatol 1991; 24:448–451.
121. Oikarinen A, Peltonen J, Kallioinen M. Ultraviolet radiation in skin ageing and carcinogenesis: the role of retinoids for treatment and prevention. Ann Med 1991; 23:497–505.
122. Moon TE. Retinoids in prevention of skin cancer. Cancer Lett 1997; 114:203–205.
123. Levine N. Role of retinoids in skin cancer treatment and prevention. J Am Acad Dermatol S62–S66; 39.
124. Vainio H, Rautalahti M. An international evaluation of the cancer preventive potential of vitamin A. Cancer Epidemiol Biomarkers Prev 1999; 8:107–109.

125. Stratton SP, Dorr RT, Alberts DS. The state-of-the-art in chemoprevention of skin cancer. Eur J Cancer 2000; 36:1292–1297.
126. Pinnell SR. Cutaneous photodamage, oxidative stress, and topical antioxidant protection. J Am Acad Dermatol 2003; 48:1–19; quiz 20–22.
127. Wulf HC, Stender IM, Lock-Andersen J. Sunscreens used at the beach do not protect against erythema: a new definition of SPF is proposed. Photodermatol Photoimmunol Photomed 1997; 13:129–132.
128. Autier P. Quantity of sunscreen used by European students. Br J Dermatol 2001; 144:288–291.
129. Cross SE. Can increasing the viscosity of formulations be used to reduce the human skin penetration of the sunscreen oxybenzone. J Invest Dermatol 2001; 117:147–150.
130. Xu C. Photosensitization of the sunscreen octyl p-dimethylaminobenzoate by UVA in human melanocytes but not in keratinocytes. Photochem Photobiol 2001; 73:600–604.
131. Dreher F, Maibach H. Protective effects of topical antioxidants in humans. Curr Probl Dermatol 2001; 29:157–164.
132. Stäb F. Topically applied antioxidants in skin protection. Meth Enzymol 2000; 319:465–478.
133. Tesoriere L. Synergistic interactions between vitamin A and vitamin E against lipid peroxidation in phosphatidylcholine liposomes. Arch Biochem Biophys 1996; 326:57–63.
134. Abreu RM, Santos DJ, Moreno AJ. Effects of carvedilol and its analog BM-910228 on mitochondrial function and oxidative stress. J Pharmacol Exp Ther 2000; 295:1022–1030.
135. Rao AV, Balachandran B. Role of oxidative stress and antioxidants in neurodegenerative diseases. Nutr Neurosci 2002; 5:291–309.
136. Cadenas E, Hochstein P, Ernster L. Pro- and antioxidant functions of quinones and quinone reductases in mammalian cells. Adv Enzymol Relat Areas Mol Biol 1992; 65:97–146.
137. Thiele JJ. The antioxidant network of the stratum corneum. Curr Probl Dermatol 2001; 29: 26–42.
138. Steenvoorden DP, van Henegouwen GM. The use of endogenous antioxidants to improve photoprotection. J Photochem Photobiol B 1997; 41:1–10.
139. Krol ES, Kramer-Stickland KA, Liebler DC. Photoprotective actions of topically applied vitamin E. Drug Metab Rev 2000; 32:413–420.
140. Jurkiewicz BA, Bissett DL, Buettner GR. Effect of topically applied tocopherol on ultraviolet radiation-mediated free radical damage in skin. J Invest Dermatol 1995; 104:484–488.
141. Lopez-Torres M. Topical application of a-tocopherol modulates the antioxidant network and diminishes ultraviolet-induced oxidative damage in murine skin. Br J Dermatol 1998; 138: 207–215.
142. Steenvoorden DPT, Beijersbergen van Henegouwen GMJ. Protection against UV-induced systemic immunosuppression in mice by a single topical application of the antioxidant vitamins C and E. Int J Radiat Biol 1999; 75:747–755.
143. Alberts DS. Disposition and metabolism of topically administered alpha-tocopherol acetate: a common ingredient of commercially available sunscreens and cosmetics. Nutr Cancer 1996; 26:193–201.
144. Gensler HL. Importance of the form of topical vitamin E for prevention of photocarcinogenesis. Nutr Cancer 1996; 26:183–191.
145. Bissett DL, Hillebrand GG, Hannon DP. The hairless mouse as a model of skin photoaging: its use to evaluate photoprotective materials. Photodermatology 1989; 6:228–233.
146. Bissett DL, Chatterjee R, Hannon DP. Photoprotective effect of superoxide scavenging antioxidants against ultraviolet-induced chronic skin damage in the hairless mice. Photodermatol Photoimmunol Photomed 1990; 7:56–62.
147. Fuchs J, Packer L. Vitamin E in dermatological therapy, in vitamin E in health and disease Packer L, Fuchs J, Eds, Marcel Dekker Inc.. 1992:739–763.
148. Pehr K, Forsey RR. Why don't we use vitamin E in dermatology. Can Med Assoc J 1993; 149:1247–1253.

149. Fuchs J. Potentials and limitations of the natural antioxidants RRR-alpha- tocopherol, L-ascorbic acid and beta-carotene in cutaneous photoprotection. Free Radic Biol Med 1998; 25:848–873.
150. Chan AC. Partners in defense, vitamin E and vitamin C. Can J Physiol Pharmacol 1993; 71: 725–731.
151. Englard S, Seifter S. The biochemical functions of ascorbic acid. Annu Rev Nutr 1986; 6: 365–406.
152. Levine M. A new recommended dietary allowance of vitamin C for healthy young women. Proc Natl Acad Sci U S A 2001; 98:9842–9846.
153. Pinnell SR. Topical L-ascorbic acid: percutaneous absorption studies. Dermatol Surg 2001; 27:137–142.
154. Darr D. Effectiveness of antioxidants (vitamin C and E) with and without sunscreens as topical photoprotectants. Acta Derm Venereol 1996; 76:264–268.
155. Darr D. Topical vitamin C protects porcine skin from ultraviolet radiation-induced damage. Br J Dermatol 1992; 127:247–253.
156. Podda M, Grundmann-Kollmann M. Low molecular weight antioxidants and their role in skin ageing. Clin Exp Dermatol 2001; 26:578–582.
157. Fitzpatrick RE, Rostan EF. Double-blind, half-face study comparing topical vitamin C and vehicle for rejuvenation of photodamage. Dermatol Surg 2002; 28:231–236.
158. Kobayashi S. Protective effect of magnesium-L-ascorbyl-2 phosphate against skin damage induced by UVB irradiation. Photochem Photobiol 1996; 64:224–228.
159. Kobayashi S. Postaministration protective effect of magnesium-L-Ascorbyl-2-phosphate on the development of UVB-induced cutaneous damage in mice. Photochem Photobiol 1998; 67:669–675.
160. Nayama S. Protective effects of sodium-L-ascorbyl-2 phosphate on the development of UVB-induced damage in cultured mouse skin (In Process Citation). Biol Pharm Bull 1999; 22: 1301–1305.
161. Muizzuddin N, Shakoori AR, Marenus KD. Effect of topical application of antioxidants and free radical scavengers on protection of hairless mouse skin exposed to chronic doses of ultraviolet B. Skin Res Technol 1998; 4:200–204.
162. Dreher F. Effect of topical antioxidants on UV-induced erythema formation when administered after exposure. Dermatology 1999; 198:52–55.
163. Dreher F. Topical melatonin in combination with vitamins E and C protects skin from ultraviolet-induced erythema: a human study in vivo. Br J Dermatol 1998; 139:332–339.
164. Wang X. A theory for the mechanism of action of the alpha-hydroxy acids applied to the skin. Med Hypotheses 1999; 53:380–382.
165. Clark CP III. New directions in skin care. Clin Plast Surg 2001; 28:745–750.
166. Van Scott EJ, Ditre CM, Yu RJ. Alpha-hydroxyacids in the treatment of signs of photoaging. Clin Dermatol 1996; 14:217–226.
167. Bernstein EF. Glycolic acid treatment increases type I collagen mRNA and hyaluronic acid content of human skin. Dermatol Surg 2001; 27:429–433.
168. Pietta PG. Flavonoids as antioxidants. J Nat Prod 2000; 63:1035–1042.
169. Nijveldt RJ. Flavonoids: a review of probable mechanisms of action and potential applications. Am J Clin Nutr 2001; 74:418–425.
170. Bernd A. In vitro studies on the immunomodulating effects of Polypodium leucotomos extract on human leukocyte fractions. Arzneimittelforschung 1995; 45:901–904.
171. Gonzalez S, Pathak MA. Inhibition of ultraviolet-induced formation of reactive oxygen species, lipid peroxidation, erythema and skin photosensitization by Polypodium leucotomos. Photodermatol Photoimmunol Photomed 1996; 12:45–56.
172. Padilla HC, Lainez H, Pacheco JA. A new agent (hydrophilic fraction of Polypodium leucotomos) for management of psoriasis. Int J Dermatol 1974; 13:276–82.

173. Mohammad A. Vitiligo repigmentation with Anapsos (Polypodium leucotomos). Int J Dermatol 1989; 28:479.
174. Gonzalez S. Topical or oral administration with an extract of Polypodium leucotomos prevents acute sunburn and psoralen-induced phototoxic reactions as well as depletion of Langerhans cells in human skin. Photodermatol Photoimmunol Photomed 1997; 13:50–60.
175. Alcaraz MV. An extract of Polypodium leucotomos appears to minimize certain photoaging changes in a hairless albino mouse animal model. A pilot study. Photodermatol Photoimmunol Photomed 1999; 15:120–126.
176. Pepping J. Milk thistle: Silybum marianum. Am J Health Syst Pharm 1999; 56:1195–1197.
177. Saller R, Meier R, Brignoli R. The use of silymarin in the treatment of liver diseases. Drugs 2001; 61:2035–2063.
178. Singh RP, Agarwal R. Flavonoid antioxidant silymarin and skin cancer. Antioxid Redox Signal 2002; 4:655–663.
179. Lahiri-Chatterjee M. A flavonoid antioxidant, silymarin, affords exceptionally high protection against tumor promotion in the SENCAR mouse skin tumorigenesis model. Cancer Res 1999; 59:622–632.
180. Katiyar SK. Treatment of silymarin, a plant flavonoid, prevents ultraviolet light-induced immune suppression and oxidative stress in mouse skin. Int J Oncol 2002; 21:1213–1222.
181. Katiyar SK. Protective effects of silymarin against photocarcinogenesis in a mouse skin model. J Natl Cancer Inst 1997; 89:556–566.
182. Saliou C. Antioxidants modulate acute solar ultraviolet radiation-induced NF- kappa-B activation in a human keratinocyte cell line. Free Radic Biol Med 1999; 26:174–183.
183. Arora A, Nair MG, Strasburg GM. Antioxidant activities of isoflavones and their biological metabolites in a liposomal system. Arch Biochem Biophys 1998; 356:133–141.
184. Yang CS. Inhibition of carcinogenesis by dietary polyphenolic compounds. Annu Rev Nutr 2001; 21:381–406.
185. Glazier MG, Bowman MA. A review of the evidence for the use of phytoestrogens as a replacement for traditional estrogen replacement therapy. Arch Intern Med 2001; 161: 1161–1172.
186. Setchell KD. Evidence for lack of absorption of soy isoflavone glycosides in humans, supporting the crucial role of intestinal metabolism for bioavailability. Am J Clin Nutr 2002; 76: 447–453.
187. Brincat M. Skin collagen changes in post-menopausal women receiving oestradiol gel. Maturitas 1987; 9:1–5.
188. Brincat MP. Hormone replacement therapy and the skin. Maturitas 2000; 35:107–117.
189. Balentine DA, Wiseman SA, Bouwens LC. The chemistry of tea flavonoids. Crit Rev Food Sci Nutr 1997; 37:693–704.
190. Harbowy ME, Balentine DA. Tea chemistry. Crit Rev Plant Sci 1997; 16:415–480.
191. Gensler HL. Prevention of photocarcinogenesis by topical administration of pure epigallocatechin gallate isolated from green tea. Nutr Cancer 1996; 26:325–335.
192. Lu YP. Topical applications of caffeine or (−)-epigallocatechin gallate (EGCG) inhibit carcinogenesis and selectively increase apoptosis in UVB-induced skin tumors in mice. Proc Natl Acad Sci U S A 2002; 99:12455–12460.
193. Record IR, Dreosti IE. Protection by black tea and green tea against UVB and UVA+B-induced skin cancer in hairless mice. Mutation Res 1998; 422:191–199.
194. Katiyar SK, Mukhtar H. Green tea polyphenol (−)-epigallocatechin-3-gallate treatment to mouse skin prevents UVB-induced infiltration of leukocytes, depletion of antigen-presenting cells, and oxidative stress. J Leukoc Biol 2001; 69:719–726.
195. Bickers DR, Athar M. Novel approaches to chemoprevention of skin cancer. J Dermatol 2000; 27:691–695.
196. Kim J. Protective effects of (−)-epigallocatechin-3-gallate on UVA- and UVB-induced skin damage. Skin Pharmacol Appl Skin Physiol 2001; 14:11–19.

197. Gupta S, Mukhtar H. Chemoprevention of skin cancer through natural agents. Skin Pharmacol Appl Skin Physiol 2001; 14:373–385.
198. Einspahr JG. Chemoprevention of human skin cancer. Crit Rev Oncol Hematol 2002; 41: 269–285.
199. Pietri S. Cardioprotective and anti-oxidant effects of the terpenoid constituents of Ginkgo biloba extract (EGb 761). J Mol Cell Cardiol 1997; 29:733–742.
200. Afzal M. Ginger: an ethnomedical, chemical and pharmacological review. Drug Metabol Drug Interact 2001; 18:159–190.
201. Babior BM, Lambeth JD, Nauseef W. The neutrophil NADPH oxidase. Arch Biochem Biophys 2002; 397:342–344.
202. Hruza LL, Pentland AP. Mechanisms of UV-induced inflammation. J Invest Dermatol 1993; 100:35S–41S.
203. Segal AW, Abo A. The biochemical basis of the NADPH oxidase of phagocytes. Trends Biochem Sci 1993; 18:43–47.
204. Ogura R. Mechanism of lipid radical formation following exposure of epidermal homogenate to ultraviolet light. J Invest Dermatol 1991; 97:1044–1047.
205. Antille C et al. J Invest Dermatol 2003; 121(5).

8

The Role of α-Hydroxy Acids in the Treatment of Photoaging

Alpesh Desai / Lawrence S. Moy *Manhattan Beach Skin and Laser Institute, Manhattan Beach, California, U.S.A.*

- α-Hydroxy acids (AHA), particularly glycolic acid, have been used extensively as peeling agents.
- Although used for a wide variety of dermatological conditions, glycolic acid improves photoaging by aiding with fine rhytides, lentigines, actinic damage, telangiectasia, dyspigmentation, laxity, and roughness.
- Glycolic acid may affect wrinkles because of its effects on glycosaminoglycans and other ground substances, unlike other peeling agents, such as trichloroacetic acid and phenol, which damage the skin and cause a thickened zone of papillary dermal collagen proportional to chemical damage.
- Glycolic acid can also be used in combination with other acids or as an ingredient in pharmaceutical or cosmetic products
- Possible side effects of glycolic acid peels include pigmentary problems, prolonged erythema, scarring, infection, and irregular surface texture.

The definition of a chemical peel is an application of a chemical agent that causes controlled destruction of the outer layers of the skin. The concept of treatment is to damage the skin that is deep enough to cause exfoliation of some of the layers of the skin but superficial enough to allow for regeneration from the appendage structures and papillary dermis (1). The damage to the outer layers of the skin induces superficial wound healing and is said to reduce scars, wrinkles, hyperpigmentation, actinic keratoses, and lentigines. These properties of chemical peels using glycolic acid have therefore been used in the treatment of photoaging.

The first documented use of chemicals to smooth and improve the skin was in first-century BC Egypt by Cleopatra, who bathed in sour milk (the cosmetic effect was probably due to lactic acid) (2). During the time of the French revolution, the ladies of the court would apply old wine (tartaric acid) to their faces. Gypsies in Europe applied various caustic chemicals to their skin, presumably for the same reasons. The first chemical peels in the United States were probably brought by dermatologists from Germany in the 1930s (1). It was during the early 1960s that phenol peels began to be used extensively. Other peeling agents were then used, including trichloroacetic acid (TCA), resorcinol, plant agents, pancreatic enzymes, salicylic acid, and α-hydroxy acids (AHAs) (3).

Three degrees of peels are performed by the dermatologist in the office, each entailing a different depth. Superficial peels penetrate through the epidermis and to the upper regions of the papillary dermis (e.g., glycolic acid) (1). Medium peels penetrate to the deeper areas of the papillary dermis and upper reticular dermis (e.g., 40% and 50% TCA). Deep peels penetrate to the depth of the midreticular dermis (e.g., phenol or pyruvic acid).

Superficial peels will cause less damage than other peels owing to their depth of penetration, and can be repeated within 4 weeks. More patients are candidates for superficial peels than for deeper peels. Medium-depth peels containing TCA or a combination of TCA (i.e., with dry ice, Jessner's solution, or AHAs) cannot be repeated as frequently (approximately once every 3 months) (4,5). It is known that medium-depth chemical peels do not cause systemic toxicity; however, higher Fitzpatrick skin types (III and IV) may have hyperpigmentation side effects from these peels. A small patch test may be indispensable for darker-skinned individuals who want a medium-depth chemical peel.

Because of the potential side effects, such as pigmentation changes, deeper chemical peels are usually not recommended for olive-skinned or dark-skinned patients (6). For example, many dermatologists do not recommend deeper chemical peels, such as the Bakers' phenol chemical peel, because of the pasty white complexion and hypopigmentation that occurs after the peel has been removed (7,8). Deeper peels can also cause systemic toxicity. A classic example is phenol peeling, which can induce cardiac arrhythmias (7). It is essential for the dermatologist to have cardiac monitoring and life support systems readily available when using these agents.

α-Hydroxy acid peels, among which glycolic acid is the most frequently used type, are therefore attractive peeling agents from a safety standpoint. The AHA peels are also efficacious in various dermatological defects and recently have been used to combat the deleterious effects of photoaging. New studies have clearly substantiated the effects of AHA on photoaging.

PHOTOAGING PROTECTION

The exact biological mechanism by which glycolic acid exerts it effects on photoaged skin is unknown. Rakic et al. (9) have studied the role of glycolic acid on human keratinocytes in vitro, and have shown that glycolic acid is not cytotoxic for keratinocytes at a neutral pH and will not alter fibroblast protein, collagen, or metalloproteinase production. These findings are in contrast to TCA peels, which are toxic to keratinocytes and fibroblastic activity. This makes glycolic acid a highly desirable peeling agent for rejuvenation purposes.

Much of the evidence that glycolic acid improves photodamaged skin comes from histological studies. Glycolic acid (15% glycolic acid for 10 weeks) showed a significant decrease in wrinkling, an increased thickness of dermal repair zone, and an increase in collagen synthesis when used to chronically ultraviolet (UV) B light-irradiated skin (10).

Many experts believe that topical glycolic acid acts as an antioxidant. To support this hypothesis, a study by Perricone et al. (11) showed that topically applied glycolic acid exerted a photoprotective effect of about 2.4 SPF (sun protection factor). Additional evidence indicates that topical glycolic acid accelerates the disappearance of erythema in irradiated skin (11).

The safety of glycolic acid-containing cosmetic products has been receiving increased public scrutiny owing to their increased use for skin rejuvenation and the treatment of the effects of photoaging. A study using guinea pigs treated with glycolic acid alone or in combination with UVB found that glycolic acid caused an increase in the level of skin damage in a dose- and time-dependent manner (12). Lower doses of glycolic acid caused primarily erythema and eschar. This progressed to edema and necrotic ulceration at higher doses. Interestingly, glycolic acid enhances UVB-induced skin damage; the magnitude of sun damage caused by combined UVB and glycolic acid treatment was much greater than that caused by glycolic acid or UVB alone. For these reasons, those individuals with photosensitive skin or those who use glycolic acid products on a regular basis should use glycolic acid with caution (12). Additionally, Tsai et al. (13) observed an increase in UVA and UVB tanning with a short-term topical regimen of glycolic acid and thus advised that patients who use AHA products should wear sunscreen.

To assess the safety of the topical application of α- and β-hydroxy acids in conjunction with UV light exposure, changes in the epidermal basal cell proliferation and edema response have been examined in SKH-1 mice using skin-thickness measurements (14). The findings indicated that a 6-week treatment with AHA changed the UV light sensitivity of mouse skin; however, treatment with these acids did not contribute to the UV light sensitivity of mice when only low doses of UV light were used (14). Additionally, increased epidermal cell proliferation was noted, thereby demonstrating a positive benefit from the use of glycolic acid (14).

EPIDERMAL/DERMAL EFFECTS

Numerous studies have validated the positive effects of AHA on the epidermis and dermis. Among these, histological studies have been done to analyze the effects of glycolic acid on different layers of the skin. The wound healing that occurs with glycolic acid is identical to that of dermabrasion, including cellular and connective tissue destruction in the papillary dermis (15–17).

Glycolic acid at lower concentrations decreases corneocyte cohesion, leading to a reduction of the stratum corneum. Histological effects of glycolic acid include decreased stratum corneum thickness, increased epidermal thickness, increased cellular differentiation, enhanced rete ridge pattern, and increased dispersal of melanin within the basal layer (18–20). Glycolic acid also affects the dermis by increasing the thickness of the papillary dermis, increasing collagen synthesis, increasing hyaluronic acid levels, and increasing the number and quality of elastic fibers (18–25). Data suggest that skin treated with glycolic acid (20% glycolic acid lotion) shows epidermal and dermal remodeling of the extracellular matrix. Longer treatments with glycolic acid may result in collagen deposition, as suggested by the measured increase in mRNA (26).

The epidermal proliferation is maximal 12 to 16 hours after treatment with glycolic acid-containing cream and is dose dependent (27). However, the proliferation is visibly seen just after 3 days of treatment with 10% glycolic acid-containing cream, but should be sustained for a 6.5-week time course (27). Data from fluorescence excitation spectroscopy also confirm that glycolic acid induces epidermal proliferation in a dose-dependent fashion (28). A unique connective tissue layer composed of fine collagen fibers beneath the epidermis was noted on UVB-irradiated hairless mice 28 days after a 20% glycolic acid peel was applied (29). Another study involving hairless mice investigated the contribution of glycolic acid in the formation and secretion of lamellar bodies, which are critical structures for epidermal barrier function. The findings suggest that glycolic acid in low concentrations (5%) may improve the skin barrier in hairless mice by inducing enhanced desquamation and by increasing the number and secretion of lamellar bodies without increased transepidermal water loss (30).

Many experts believe the quantitative and qualitative beneficial effects of AHA on photoaged skin are due to a combination of two effects: a reorganization in dermal structural elements and an increase in dermal volume (31).

EFFECTS ON UV-INDUCED TUMORS

Little is known about the functional role of glycolic acid in UV-induced skin tumorigenesis, but increasing evidence shows that glycolic acid reduces UV-induced skin tumor development. Glycolic acid has been shown to cause a 20% reduction of skin tumor incidence, a 55% reduction of tumor multiplicity, and a 47% decrease in the number of large tumors (> 2 mm in diameter) (32). Additionally, glycolic acid also delayed the first appearance of tumor formation by about 3 weeks (32).

Additionally, glycolic acid has been found to inhibit UV-induced skin tumor development in hairless mice. The antitumor effect of glycolic acid is related to its inhibitory effect on UVB-induced apoptosis and cytotoxicity. An inhibition of c-fos expression and activation of activator protein-1 as well as inhibitions of the p53–p21 response pathway are the proposed mechanisms (33).

GLYCOLIC ACID PEEL VARIATIONS

A multitude of glycolic acid variations exist in treating photoaging (Table 1). Key clinical aspects of photoaging include laxity, roughness, sallowness, irregular hyperpigmentation, and telangiectasia (34). Many studies have been conducted in order to determine which glycolic acid variation works the best. One study cites a 30% complete regression and a 60% partial regression of cutaneous hyperpigmentation treated with 50% glycolic acid and 10% kojic acid (35). A double-blind vehicle-controlled study tested the efficacy of glycolic acid (50%) on improving photoaged skin. Significant improvement was noted both histologically and clinically (36).

Table 1 Glycolic Acid Peel Variations in the Literature

1. 30% glycolic acid (39)
2. 50% glycolic acid (36,59)
3. 50% glycolic acid with 10% kojic acid (35)
4. 70% glycolic acid (short contact) (36,37,59)
5. 70% glycolic acid with 40% TCA (72,73)
6. 70% glycolic acid with 5% fluorouracil (56)

Another variation of the glycolic acid peel is contact time. A pilot study was undertaken to observe if there was any benefit with monthly, short-contact-time 70% glycolic acid peels. Although 90% of patients felt there was improvement in the visible effects produced by photoaging, there was no benefit associated with short-contact-time glycolic acid peels (37).

A novel application of 70% glycolic acid involves the concomitant use of 35% TCA. The 70% glycolic acid peel is applied for 2 min to the entire face and then diluted with water. The 35% TCA peel is then applied over the same areas. A dramatic improvement in photoaging was noted histologically and clinically (38). This GA-TCA combination affords the dermatologist a consistent approach when a medium depth peel is justified.

GLYCOLIC ACID PRODUCT VARIATIONS

Dermatologists are increasingly dispensing or formulating AHA-containing products through their offices (Table 2). The pharmaceutical and cosmetic industry has also contributed to this increasingly popular trend by adding AHA into various products (e.g., lotions, creams, gels, masks, sprays, and shampoos).

A study by Lim et al. (39) advocates the use of a cream containing 10% glycolic acid and 2% hydroquinone for improving fine facial wrinkling. Another study tested the efficacy of AHA in reversing photoaging and found a 25% increase in skin thickness, increased acid mucopolysaccharides, improved quality of elastic fibers, and increased collagen (40).

A double-blind study found either 8% glycolic acid or 8% lactic acid superior to placebo in the treatment of photoaging (41). Thus, patients can obtain a modest reduction in the signs of chronic cutaneous photodamage with over-the-counter products. The results of a double-blind clinical study demonstrated that daytime usage of 8% glycolic acid lotion along with nightly applications of Renova (tretinoin emollient cream 0.05%) is well tolerated as part of a comprehensive photoaging program (42). The addition of 2% kojic acid in a gel containing 10% glycolic acid and 2% hydroquinone achieves greater improvement for photodamage (43).

GLYCOLIC ACID

Glycolic acid is typically a superficial chemical peel that may have beneficial effects on photodamage (i.e., wrinkles, actinic keratoses, solar lentigines, and rough texture), acne, keratoses, and ichthyoses. Glycolic acid peels are used repetitively to achieve the best results. In addition to the additive effect, repeated peels also have fewer side effects than a single deeper chemical peel.

Table 2 Glycolic Acid Product Variations in the Literature

1. 8% glycolic acid + 8% L-lactic acid cream (41)
2. 8% glycolic acid + nightly use of tretinoin 0.05% emollient cream (42)
3. 10% glycolic acid + 2% kojic acid gel + 2% hydroquinone (43)
4. 20–30% glycolic acid + 4% hydroquinone (60)
5. 25% glycolic acid (40)

α-Hydroxy acids are a class of compounds derived from various fruits and other foods and are therefore sometimes called ''fruit acids.'' For instance, glycolic acid comes from sugar cane, lactic acid comes from sour milk, malic acid comes from apples, tartaric acid comes from grapes, and citric acid comes from citrus fruits. The principal structure of glycolic acid ($CH_2OHCOOH$) is composed of an α-hydroxy group, a carboxyl carbon, and two carboxyl oxygens lying in the same plane. Glycolic acid is the smallest molecule of all the AHAs (44). Other AHAs also have potential uses on the skin, although penetration of larger molecules may be more difficult.

The mechanism by which glycolic acid improves problems related to photoaging may relate to its similarity to ascorbic acid (45,46). Ascorbic acid, a derivative of AHA, has been shown to stimulate collagen production and possibly even decrease melanin production. As with ascorbic acid, glycolic acid may also have clinical relevance as an antioxidant, which protects against the effects of ultraviolet radiation. Glycolic acid may also affect wrinkles by its effects on glycosaminoglycans and other ground substances, and it may stimulate the production of collagen in fibroblasts. This is in contrast to other peeling agents, such as TCA and phenol, which damage the skin and cause a thickened zone of papillary dermal collagen proportional to damage (47,48). For glycolic acid, crusting, and tissue necrosis can be minimized while still improving the skin. In a mini pig study, 12% lactic acid was shown to deposit as much new papillary collagen as 25% TCA or 25% phenol after 21 days (48).

Glycolic acid can penetrate as efficiently as other chemical peels. When a 50–70% solution is left on the skin for 15 min, a depth of necrosis occurs that is comparable to 35% and 50% TCA. With shorter exposures, 50% and 70% glycolic acid will cause less depth of damage than 35% TCA.

Dr.Van Scott and Ruey Yu (44) have used glycolic acid for a variety of skin lesions. They originally used AHAs to treat conditions associated with excessive corneocyte cohesion, such as ichthyosis (49). It is thought that AHAs decrease corneocyte cohesion by interfering with ionic bonding. Dr. Van Scott began to successfully treat other epidermal lesions, including seborrheic keratoses, verrucae vulgaris, acne, and actinic keratoses (18,25). In addition, Dr. Van Scott found distinct resolution of wrinkles using glycolic acid (18,25).

SIDE EFFECTS OF GLYCOLIC ACID

Skin sensitivity to glycolic products can manifest itself in several different ways. Stinging on immediate application is common. With continual use, this reaction will usually last a few days and then subside. Higher therapeutic concentrations can be expected to cause stinging and patients should be forewarned. Daily-use home products with lower concentrations can cause erythema, dryness, and peeling. Patients with extreme sensitivity can occasionally develop acneiform papules soon after starting the products. When these reactions occur, it is suggested that the patient stop the product temporarily and use a milder glycolic acid lotion.

Complications of glycolic acid chemical peels are uncommon and can usually be avoided. Patients who may be more sensitive to chemical peeling agents should be identified so that the depth and type of peel can be tailored for each individual. The dermatologist's presence throughout the peel procedure is important so that any problems can be managed rapidly and efficiently. The dermatologist's presence will also give the patient a sense of security and comfort.

Possible side effects from glycolic peels include hyperpigmentation, post-peel erythema, and, rarely, irregular surface texture. Side effects will resolve after a short time and can be treated with specific topical agents. Hyperpigmentation may occur in darker skin types and in patients with melasma. Prolonged erythema is uncommon. A mild cortisone cream applied to the area very early will commonly clear the erythema. Irregular surface texture is defined as a ''step-off'' lesion that occurs when the peel is significantly uneven in a given area. The most common areas for this irregular healing are the upper cheek, upper nose, and perioral areas. Promoting rapid healing with an antibiotic ointment (Bacitracin ointment) is advantageous, and with time, the lesions will heal well. Additional superficial peels will also smooth these areas.

HISTOLOGICAL CHANGES AFTER CHEMICAL PEEL

Histological studies have analyzed the effects of glycolic acid peels on the different layers of the skin, and have shown that the initial reaction is epidermal coagulation, followed by the formation of a thin crust composed of keratin, necrotic keratinocytes, and a proteinaceous precipitate (16–20). Epidermal regeneration typically occurs after 2–7 days (16–20). After 2 weeks, the epidermis is completely healed with partially reformed rete ridges (16–21). In addition, dermal thickening with fibroblast proliferation and new collagen deposition is observed in the papillary dermis (22,23). This new dermal collagen deposition probably accounts for most of the cosmetic improvement and rejuvenation of the skin.

Biopsies show horizontally arranged new collagen with a predominance of fibroblasts 2 or 3 weeks after glycolic acid peels (22,23). The sun-induced elastotic changes with basophilic degeneration and homogenization of collagen disappear, and the zone of new collagen remains for up to 1 year (50). Finely wrinkled, actinically damaged skin is benefited most by treatment with glycolic acid peels. Subsequent biopsies performed after glycolic acid chemical peeling demonstrate both a reduction in the melanosis of the epidermis and fewer melanocytes at the dermal-epidermal junction (16–21).

The absorption of glycolic acid in human skin is pH, strength, and time dependent (51). A study by DiNardo et al. (20) demonstrated clinically and histologically that glycolic acid at all pH levels and concentrations showed significant improvement in skin condition, with data indicating that increasing the pH increases efficacy.

CLINICAL INDICATIONS

Glycolic acid chemical peels can be used for a variety of skin conditions. When used properly, glycolic acid can be comparable in effectiveness to other frequently used chemical peels. In addition, glycolic acid can be selectively used on a wider variety of skin types than other chemical peels. It is necessary to repeat the glycolic acid peels to achieve the desired clinical result. However, glycolic acid peels typically require less time to heal. Therefore, glycolic acid peels are ideal for patients that do not want extended healing times. Glycolic acid is especially desirable if the patient does not want it known that a specific treatment was performed since glycolic acid will cause gradual improvement and little postoperative disfigurement that has to be explained in social situations.

Recently, glycolic acid peels have been proposed as a primary treatment method for the treatment of photoaging. The following is a detailed review on the use of glycolic acid in improving the different aspects of photoaging.

Wrinkles

Wrinkled, sun-exposed skin shows accumulation of elastotic material. This elastotic deposition is thought to lack structural support quality leading to sagging, nonelastic, wrinkled skin. Some patients will have many fine wrinkles across the cheeks and around the eyes and mouth. On occasion, patients will have wrinkles that crosshatch. The reason for the elastotic deposition is not fully understood. One theory is that the fibroblasts are damaged by UV radiation and produce altered collagen and elastin (50).

The improvement of photoaged skin by glycolic acid involves new collagen deposition either on top of or in place of the upper papillary zone of elastotic damaged deposits (22,23,50). Medium and deep peels are thought to function histologically like dermabrasions by causing a similar scar formation in the upper papillary dermis (52–54). Superficial peels such as glycolic acid may achieve satisfactory results by repeatedly stimulating the skin and stimulating new collagen growth without causing the deeper wound healing of deep chemical peels.

Quantitative analysis on glycolic acid's ability to decrease wrinkling has been difficult and not generally examined. Funasaka et al. (55) assessed the efficacy of glycolic acid peeling on facial wrinkling in different age groups using computer-assisted analysis. Two parameters were measured: change in number of wrinkles and average wrinkle length. They found that erythema elicited by glycolic acid correlates with improvement of wrinkles. In addition, no significant differences in the aforementioned parameters were found when using 35%, 50%, or 70% concentrations.

Generally speaking, glycolic acid has not been uniformly accepted as an effective means for the removal of deep photodamage. Maximizing the concentration of the glycolic acid combined with a consistent pattern of repeated peels and a strong concentration of the daily glycolic acid lotions can give positive results for deep wrinkles (Fig. 1). These results are proportional to maximally applying high concentrations of glycolic acid. Deep wrinkles can be improved without causing necrosis. However, compared to other conditions, glycolic acid chemical peels must be applied longer and allowed to penetrate deeper when used for deep wrinkles (Fig. 2). It is also important to use the thick 70% glycolic acid gel when treating deep photodamage. A thin or water-based glycolic acid chemical peel will often penetrate unevenly and cause ''hot'' spots where the peel penetrates too deeply.

Glycolic acid chemical peels can be beneficial for lentigines and fine-crosshatched wrinkles caused by superficial cutaneous sun damage. These patients can be peeled with 70% glycolic acid, but caution must be taken not to peel too deeply. Some patients with superficial and minimal photodamage can react more than anticipated to the glycolic acid and, therefore, timing is very important. As photodamage becomes more significant, with deeper creases and prominent lentigines, the skin's tolerance to the 70% glycolic acid peel increases dramatically. The application time of the peel can be increased accordingly so the penetration may be enhanced.

Actinic Keratoses

Chemical peels can be used to treat actinic keratoses that are not excessively hyperkeratotic. Additionally, the blotchy appearance of the skin can be dramatically improved and made more uniform. There is a tendency to produce hypopigmentation scars when treating individual actinic keratoses lesions with spot liquid nitrogen or electrocautery. Repeated application of fluorouracil can effectively remove multiple lesions, but is very uncomforta-

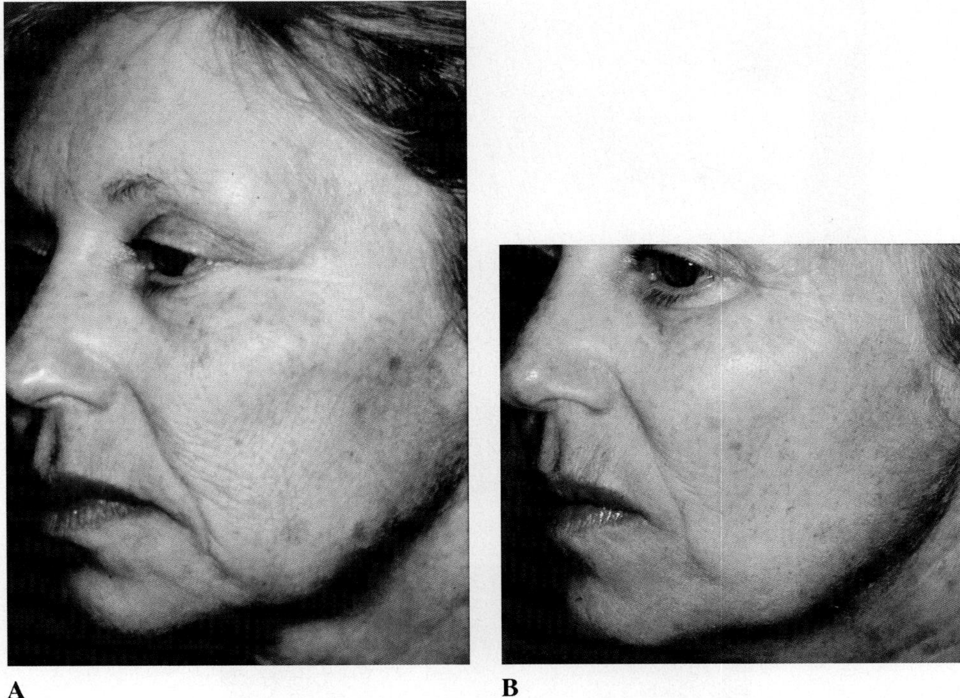

Figure 1 (A) This female patient had marked wrinkles. (B) Glycolic acid peels (50% concentration) applied for 4–6 min monthly for 4 months, combined with a daily regimen of 10% glycolic lotion, produced significant reduction in wrinkling.

ble and cosmetically noticeable for a longer period of time than a glycolic acid peel. It should also be noted that many patients will not be compliant with such a harsh therapeutic regimen. Topical retinoic acid has been reported to be only minimally effective as a solitary agent for actinic keratoses, although it can complement the penetration of fluorouracil for patients with thicker hyperkeratotic lesions.

Seventy percent glycolic acid causes increased epidermolysis and reduces cohesiveness of keratinocytes, thus thinning actinic keratoses (56). Patients will actually have resolution of most of their actinic keratoses. If some of the thicker actinic keratoses do not resolve, the lesions are always thinner, thus, making them easier to treat with fluorouracil or other modalities. The advantage of pretreating with glycolic acid before fluorouracil is the decreased discomfort and time required for application for the fluorouracil (56).

Actinic Damage

Actinic damage consists of hyperpigmentation, uneven texture, fine lines, dryness, and telangiectasias. A recent study by Gladstone et al. (57) evaluated the efficacy of LUSTRA® (4% hydroquinone and 2% glycolic acid) used alone or with salicylic acid peels in reducing actinic damage on the neck and upper chest areas. They found a 33–71% improvement in actinic damage, thereby reinforcing the concept of using AHA for photoaging.

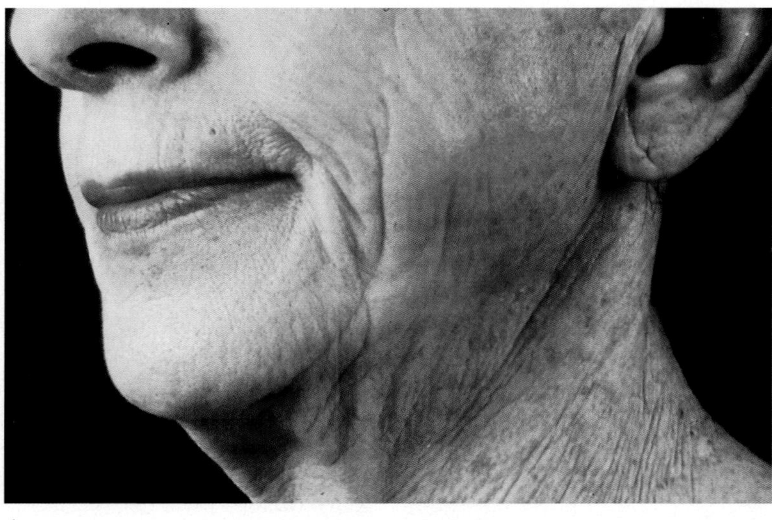

A

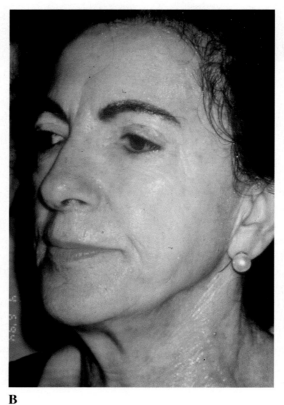

B

Figure 2 (A) Deep creases on the cheeks and around the mouth in an elderly woman. A series of more than twenty 70% glycolic acid peels applied for 6–8 min were performed in the course of a year. (B) The results observed 1 year after the series of glycolic acid peels are shown. The deep creases, which greatly improved, have remained improved.

Lentigines

Lentigines are enduring flat brown macules appearing on the sun-exposed areas of the skin such as temples and upper cheeks. Lentigines are due to an increase of melanocytes and melanocytic activity at the epidermal basal layer of the skin. Some dermatologists now believe that lentigines also have a keratotic component along with the hypermelanization component. These lesions have been called ''keratoses simplex.'' Much of the aging that occurs on the hands is a function of the number of these lesions.

The AHA peels can be very effective in the treatment of lentigines (Fig. 3). In our experience, the glycolic peel must penetrate the lentigo to the papillary dermal layer to be effective. On some patients, pretreatment with Jessner's (lactic acid, resorcinol and salicylic acid) formulation may allow the glycolic acid to penetrate deep enough to remove the lesions (58). It is recommended that the patient apply 10% glycolic acid or topical retinoic acid before and after the glycolic acid peel when treating lentigines.

Melasma

Melasma is a blotchy, irregular melanin hyperpigmentation that classically appears on areas of the face. Most notably, melasma appears on the forehead, upper cheeks, and upper lip; however, other areas of the face can also show the hyperpigmentation. Estrogens and progesterone are thought to be partially responsible for melasma, especially during pregnancy or with the use of oral contraceptives (Fig. 4).

Much of the difficulty in treating melasma is that patients prone to having melasma also have a tendency for postinflammatory hyperpigmentation. Dermabrasions and deeper peels have been used, but the results are not consistent and have a higher incidence of side effects than superficial chemical peels (52,54). The exact mechanism of glycolic acid on hyperpigmentation is not known. Some studies suggest that ascorbic acid has a direct melanocyte activity-inhibiting effect that may be similar to that produced by glycolic acid (45,46). Another possible effect of glycolic acid is to allow better penetration of the hydroquinone to the melanocytes in the epidermal basal layer and upper papillary dermis. In addition, glycolic acid may directly damage and decrease the number of melanocytes.

Patients can apply a mixture lotion of 10% glycolic acid and 2% hydroquinone or topical tretinoin, 4% hydroquinone, and a mild topical corticosteroid (59). The lotions are applied twice a day before and after a series of peels. Fifty percent glycolic acid chemical peels or 15–25% TCA peels are used, although TCA peels may cause more problems than glycolic peels. Crusting should be minimized because of the risk of hyperpigmentation on darker skin. A regimen of four or five peel treatments is recommended to the patients before obvious improvements are clinically made (Fig. 5). It is recommended to repeat the glycolic peel every 3 or 4 weeks. A sunscreen with maximum UVA and UVB protection coverage is strongly recommended to the patient to prevent further darkening.

A study by Hurley et al. (60) found a significant effect in reducing skin pigmentation (measured by the Melasma Area and Severity Index) by using 4% hydroquinone cream combined with 20–30% glycolic acid peels.

A study of Indian women with melasma found that a prepeel regimen of daily topical sunscreen (SPF 15) and 10% glycolic acid lotion at night for 2 weeks followed by a 50% glycolic acid peel monthly for 3 consecutive months proved to be an effective treatment modality (61). There were no significant side effects reported with this treatment program. Another study on Indian men demonstrated that serial glycolic acid peels provided an

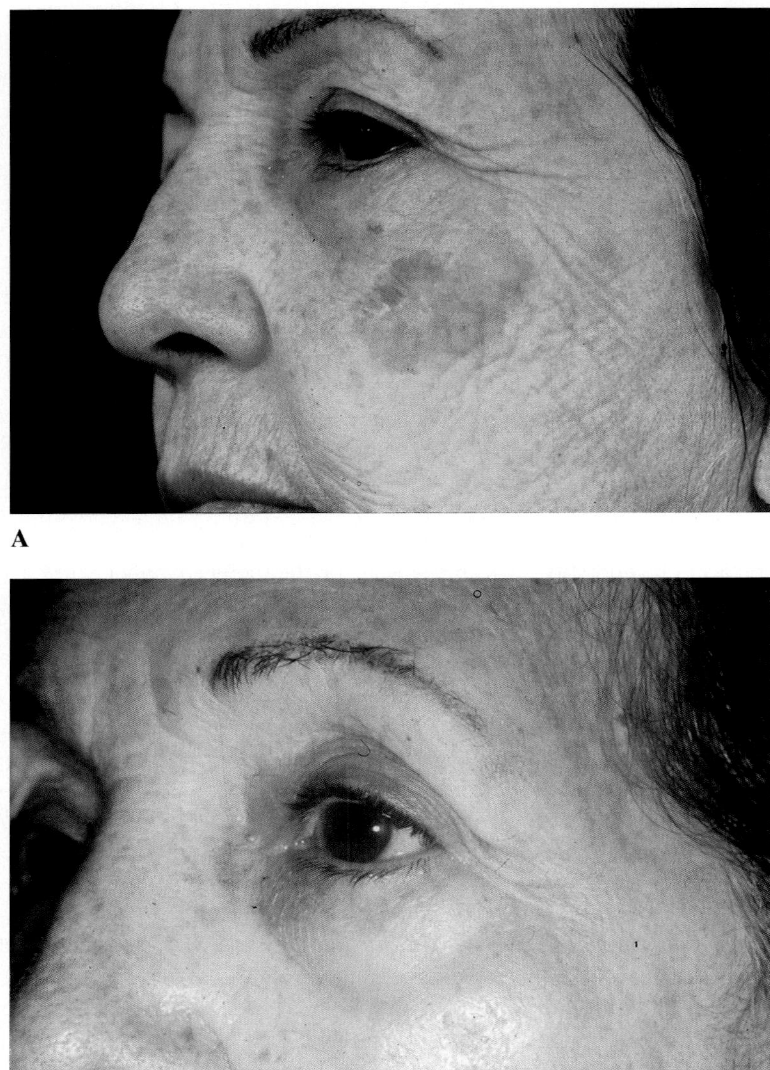

Figure 3 (A) A Latina patient with a solar lentigo on the left malar area resistant to various types of treatments. (B) Monthly repeated 70% glycolic acid peels were applied locally to the area, and lightened the lesion after 3 months.

additional benefit when combined with hydroquinone 5%, tretinoin 0.05%, and hydrocortisone acetate 1%, in a cream base (a modification of Kligman's formula) (62).

Cosmetic Benefits

A comparative study indicated that the cosmetic benefits from the use of AHA are due to the modification of the epidermis, especially of the basal and spinous layers (63). This

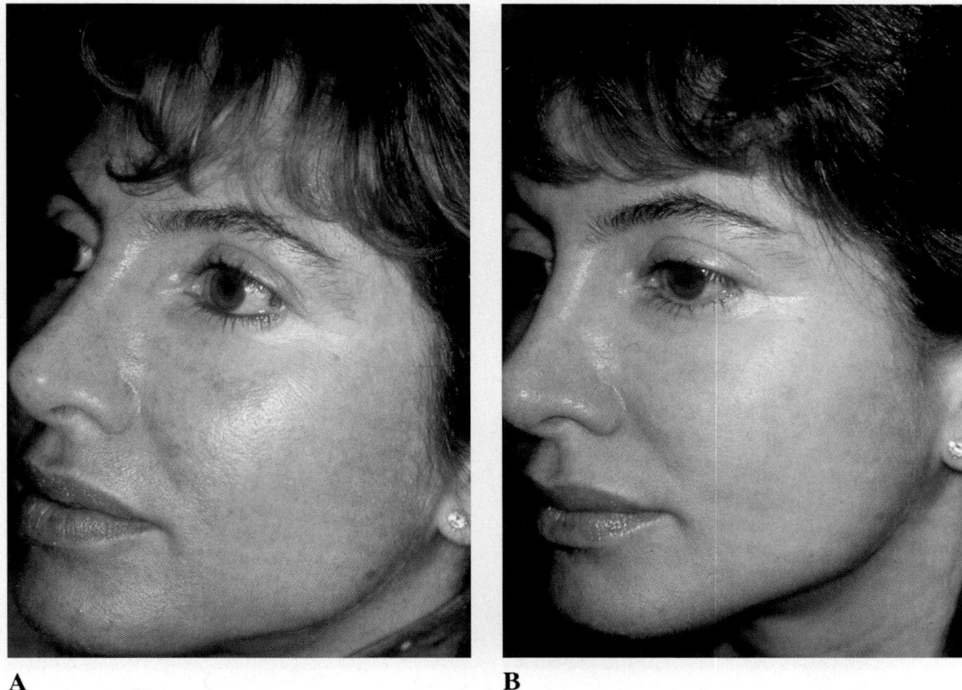

Figure 4 (A) A 42-year-old woman with melasma after long-term oral contraceptive use. Two 50% glycolic acid peels (6–8 min) were performed on this patient. (B) Note the dramatic improvement of hyperpigmentation, as well as improvement in overall skin texture and quality.

causes a decrease in laxity, roughness, sallowness, dyspigmentation, and telangiectasias (Fig. 6). A double-blind study by Newman et al. (36) showed significant improvement in mild to moderate photoaging with associated histological proof to support the clinical findings. Numerous other studies continue to validate these findings. It has been our experience that most patients prefer low-strength glycolic acid peels to low-intensity microdermabrasion for facial rejuvenation

TECHNIQUE

Planning the Peel: Considerations Before the Procedure

Before beginning a peel on a patient, it is important to assess possible risk factors or exposures that may affect the outcome of the peel. A history of topical retinoic acid, glycolic acid, or recently used topical fluorouracil may sensitize a patient's skin, as well as certain oral medications like 13-*CIS*-retinoic acid for acne. It is not clear if oral or systemic retinoids increase the risk of scarring after glycolic peels (64). Other medications such as photosensitizing drugs or oral contraceptives may increase the risk of pigmentary problems and scarring. Any underlying dermatological conditions, such as atopic dermatitis, may increase the complication rate.

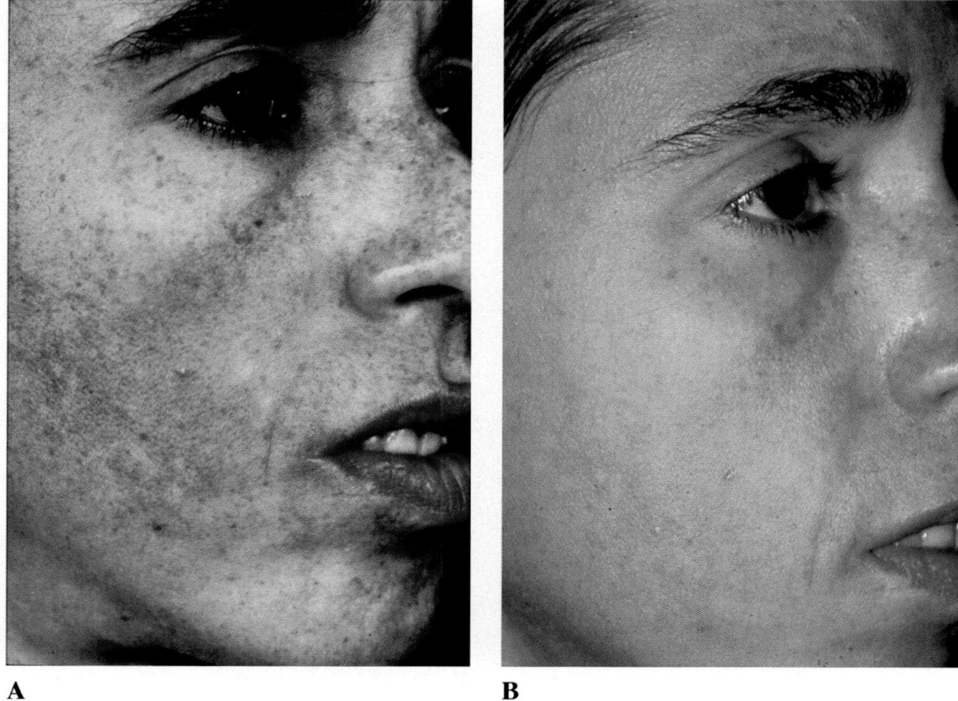

Figure 5 (A) A 32-year-old patient had a distinct area of melasma for several years. The use of prescription bleachers and retinoic acid did not improve this condition. Four 50% glycolic acid peels (6–8 min) and daily 10% glycolic acid lotion were used over a period of 8 weeks. (B) The treatment regimen totally cleared the melasma in 8 weeks.

Physical characteristics of skin are also very important. Those who tolerate stronger peeling agents tend to be older patients with more chronic sun exposure, solar lentigines, and deep wrinkles. A possible reason for this increased tolerance may be that the penetration of the peeling agent is partially blocked by the accumulation of solar elastosis in the upper papillary dermis. Ruddy, telangiectatic skin and/or skin with actinic keratoses can be less tolerant depending on how much erythema is associated with these lesions.

Thicker, more sebaceous skin quality may tolerate more stringent glycolic peels than thinner, less sebaceous skin. Part of the resistance to glycolic peels may be due to the quantity of sebaceous material on the surface. Skin preparation with alcohol and acetone need to be more vigorous and areas such as the nose may require more scrubbing to achieve an even, proper peel.

When considering deeper peels with glycolic acid, it is important to consider the Fitzpatrick skin type of the patient. The darker skin types will have a tendency to hyperpigment.

It is prudent to document the peeling process. Documentation is very important for procedures requiring consistency. Notes should include skin condition being treated and skin characteristics that may affect the peel. A record sheet helps keep track of variations

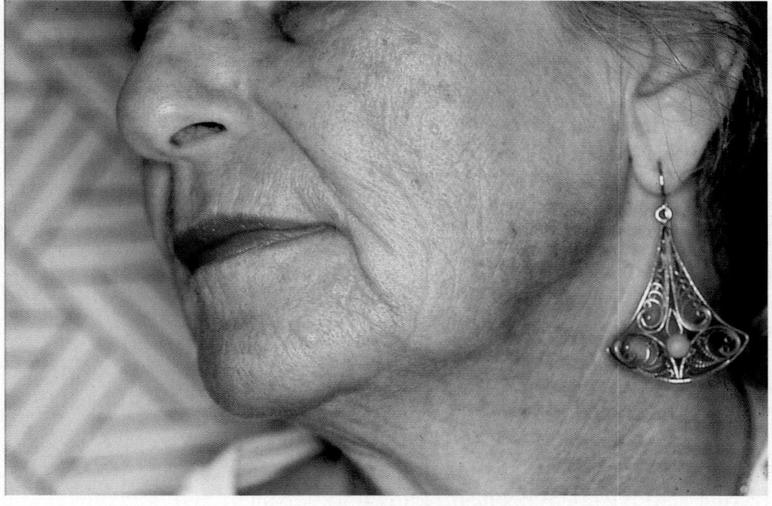

A

B

Figure 6 (A) This elderly patient had multiple features of photoaging consisting of solar lentigines, rhytides, and uneven texture. (B) The same patient was treated with 70% glycolic acid peels (6–8 min) for 6 months and daily glycolic lotions. A marked improvement in the signs of photoaging was noted after treatment.

in technique. Records should emphasize skin preparation method, duration of the peel, and the type and concentration of the agent. Photos can be difficult to take consistently from the same angle and same lighting, but can be very important for patient progress. Uniform pictures or digital images should be obtained. Taking a side angle view, one can always line the top of the ear horizontally with the lateral canthus of the eye and line the tip of the nose vertically with the edge of the contralateral cheek.

Pretreatment with daily topical retinoic acid or AHA may additively increase the efficacy of the peel (65). In our office, patients are given 10% glycolic acid to apply daily for 2 weeks prior to a peel.

Skin Preparation

Skin preparation is critical for consistent and successful peeling in the office. The skin-preparation steps will determine the depth and the control of the chemical peel. Improper preparation can give minimal, insufficient, or uneven results. Overzealous preparation can deepen the chemical peel below the penetration level needed for the specific patient. Even though glycolic acid chemical peels are known to be superficial, glycolic acid can cause deeper necrosis of dermal layers and unanticipated deeper peeling.

Cleansing the skin is typically performed with a gauze or cotton pad. The purpose of the preparation is to evenly remove debris and a variable amount of stratum corneum. Degreasing is important because even small amounts of oils from the skin will cause increased surface tension and cause less penetration of the peeling agent.

Alcohol is probably the easiest and most consistent skin-preparation cleanser and should be applied twice to properly prepare the skin. Other cleansing substances are acetone and chlorhexidine. If erythema occurs on sensitive skin after cleansing with any of the mentioned agents, lower-concentration peels or shorter application of the peels in these specific areas is recommended. Some dermatologists will gently scrub with alcohol and acetone until the dark film (probably keratin debris) appearing on the gauze disappears (1,4). Our experience shows that skin preparation with acetone causes a much deeper peel than gentle cleaning with a chlorhexidine solution.

Supplies and Application of the Glycolic Acid Peel

A simple tray is all that is required to perform the peel. The glycolic acid is applied using a fan-shaped brush. The fan brush ideally coats the skin surface with an even amount of glycolic acid gel while minimizing trauma to the skin. Additionally, the brush allows application of the peel with very close proximity to the eyes with no problems. The glycolic acid is carefully applied to one cosmetic unit at a time to ensure even coverage. The recommended method is to start on one cheek and completely cover the anatomical unit, and then apply around the forehead to the other cheek and down over the chin. The central face should be treated last. Glycolic acid peels do not cause frosting, thus, using this pattern ensures that the whole face is uniformly covered. Application over the face should take 15–20 seconds.

To ensure proper coverage of the area, one hand is used to stretch out furrows and creases while the other is used to apply the peel. Often, with a cotton applicator or the same brush, more of the glycolic acid will be firmly rubbed into furrows and fine crease areas, such as nasolabial folds or perioral creases, to enhance the effect in that area. Some keratotic areas will not respond as well and require firm rubbing to react properly. Because the 50% and 70% glycolic acid is a gel-like substance, some of the peeling agent may collect slightly more on certain areas; however, unlike TCA, glycolic acid does not react more in areas with more peeling agent on it. The area around the eyes has to be applied separately, using a semimoist cotton applicator, to ensure that the peeling agent does not get into the eyes. The patient is instructed to keep the eyes closed to minimize tearing. Tears are wiped away to avoid capillary movement of the chemical agent into the eye. The glycolic acid should be kept within 2 mm from the eyelid ciliary margin. This will likely cause mild stinging, but improves periocular photodamage. All types of peels should be feathered below the jaw and into the hairline to minimize a line of demarcation. The glycolic acid is left on the skin for a set amount of time using a stopwatch. The timer is set at the initial contact of the glycolic acid.

After glycolic acid has been applied for the specified time period, it must be neutralized. Complete neutralization is very important for glycolic acid. Unlike TCA, glycolic acid activity is not dissipated during the peeling action. Complete removal is required after the timed application. Caution should be taken using sodium bicarbonate for neutralization because the combination of glycolic acid and sodium bicarbonate creates an entropic reaction, which creates heat. This heat could intensify or damage the peeled skin. It is highly recommended to remove the peel in three steps, thereby stopping the reaction and improving patient comfort. First, with water-soaked gauze, excess glycolic acid should be removed from the skin. This will not absolutely stop the reaction, but will lift off a majority of the gel. Second, a buffered cleansing lotion should be applied. This acts as a neutralizer and the buffer will stop the reaction and inactivate glycolic acid on the skin. Additionally, the neutralizer cools the skin to give comfort from the mild stinging and heat caused by the glycolic acid chemical peel. The neutralizer ensures that the peel is stopped. Finally, the patient is asked to rinse off the excess glycolic acid and neutralizer from their skin. It is not sufficient to have the patient rinse off without the neutralizer, because it should not be the patient's responsibility to completely remove and inactivate the peel. Occasionally, a patient will complain of stinging of the eyes even if no glycolic acid has actually entered them, but this will resolve after the peel has been neutralized. A water-soaked gauze can be used to gently wipe the eyes or a squeeze bottle with water can be kept on hand to rinse the eyes if needed. Patients with moderate to severe erythema are given a mild corticosteroid cream to apply twice daily to affected areas for 2 days.

It is recommended that 50% and 70% solutions of glycolic acid gel be applied. Our experience has been that these concentrations are best and can be used for a large variety of skin conditions and disorders. Lower-concentration glycolic acid chemical peels are available but have not yet shown sufficient therapeutic benefits or undergone sufficient research. Unlike other chemical peels, glycolic acid is time dependent and contact time is therefore critical. The preparation should not have any runoff and should adhere to the skin surface during the peel time period. The peel should be carefully timed from the first contact of glycolic acid with the skin until it is washed off. Proportionally, the longer that the glycolic acid stays on the skin, the deeper the penetration and peeling of the skin. For deeper skin conditions, including actinic elastosis, actinic keratoses, and acne scars, 70% glycolic acid gel is left on for 4–8 min. For more superficial problems, such as acne and melasma, 2–5 min of 50% glycolic acid gel treatment is recommended. Again, sensitivity can vary significantly, so the length of time for a glycolic acid chemical peel must be individual.

Superficial glycolic acid chemical peels need to be repeated to have maximal benefit (4). The initial application is usually 50% solution and is left on for a carefully timed 3 min. If the patient has repeated peels every 2–4 weeks, the time is increased by 30 seconds or the concentration of the glycolic acid is increased to 70%. If the patient has very sensitive skin, the peel may be started at 2–2.5 min. Eventually, some patients will tolerate peels lasting up to 10 min, especially if they have severe chronic sun damage.

POST-PEEL CARE

Post-peel care includes preventing infection and minimizing inflammation. Various products are used to accomplish this including antibiotic ointments, Preparation H Ointment (mineral oil 14%, petrolatum 71.9%, phenylephrine HCl 0.25%, shark liver oil 3.0%, Wyeth home products, Philadelphia, PA), petroleum, and other agents. We recommend an antibiotic ointment (Bacitracin ointment) for the first 7 days to prevent any infection and promote wound healing. The patient is instructed to wash with cool water and a mild cleanser. Sunscreens are applied over the post-peel healing agent when the patient leaves the office and then reapplied regularly for 2 weeks. The patient is instructed not to apply their daily home glycolic acid products or topical retinoic acid for 2–4 days, depending on the depth and reaction of the glycolic acid peel. The application of glycolic acid-containing products immediately on the peel can cause deeper and unwanted peeling reactions and problems (66).

Patients are warned about crusting and erythema for 3–7 days after a peel procedure. Discomfort is usually only during the procedure and usually consists of stinging and pruritus. Normally, no oral analgesia or oral steroids are required after the peel procedure. A mild cortisone cream can be given if the inflammation and erythema are uncomfortable. Patients can apply makeup and other cosmetics 30–60 min after the peel. We find that providing patients with written post-peel instructions a valuable and important tool for patient education.

COMPLICATIONS

Hyperpigmentation is probably the most common side effect caused by AHA chemical peels. Usually, the deeper peels are more susceptible to postinflammatory hyperpigmentation. In fact, pigmentation problems occur in 67% of phenol peels (67). Many believe that color outcome cannot be fully predicted from peels. Medium-pigmented or olive-skinned patients (Asians, Hispanics, and Mediterranean skin types) can develop irregular pigmentation (1,4). If patients experience persistent hyperpigmentation 2 weeks after a peel, the patient can apply glycolic acid 10% with 2% hydroquinone lotion or 4% hydroquinone alone to lighten the effected areas. With TCA, hyperpigmentation can occur and be persistent even at concentrations of 10–35%. To this date, we have never seen any permanent hyperpigmentation problems from using glycolic acid.

Even deeper peels have caused very few complications (6). Theoretically, the skin of a darker person can result in a line of demarcation around certain anatomical areas. The most commonly affected areas include below the angle of the jaw, periorbital regions, periorally, and in the hairline. These areas, therefore, should be feathered when being treated. Post-peel factors that may enhance postinflammatory hyperpigmentation include pregnancy, prolonged sun exposure, and the use of oral contraceptives or photosensitizing drugs. One should restrict these factors as much as possible for 2–4 weeks following the procedure. Deeper peels need to be watched for 6 weeks to 6 months.

Persistent erythema occurs uncommonly with glycolic peels (67). Erythema should not last longer than 2 or 3 months, with the majority of cases fully resolving within 2 or

3 weeks. Mild hydrocortisone ointment is applied for 2 days after the peel for patients with severe erythema. Erythema may be due to sensitivity to the peel with a subsequent persistent inflammatory reaction. TCA tends to cause more erythema than glycolic acid.

Infections have not been a problem with superficial glycolic peels. The skin preparation agents and peeling agents themselves are bactericidal, although the crust that occurs after the peel may harbor and colonize organisms on the skin to cause infections. The crust produced in superficial peels is thinner and less adherent. It is recommended to patients to use triple-antibiotic ointment and to gently wash the face. The crust usually washes off in 2 or 3 days.

Herpes simplex infection has occurred after the use of glycolic acid peels. Hyperpigmentation and hypertrophic scarring are potential hazards of these viral infections. Patients should be questioned on history of herpetic outbreaks and incipient causes. Even if the patient has not had a herpetic outbreak for many years, he or she can develop postoperative scarring and herpetic flares due to the chemical peels (68). Susceptible patients are given acyclovir (400 mg twice daily by mouth) beginning 2 days prior to the peel and continuing 7 days after the peel (1,6). Candidiasis infection also can develop, for which a short course of ketoconazole can be used. Bacterial infections may also rarely occur and cultures should be taken. Based on sensitivity, appropriate antibiotics should be prescribed.

Hypertrophic scarring is very rare in AHA peels since this type of scarring may be a function of the depth of injury to the skin. Low-dose intralesional corticosteroid injections are recommended. The areas most often affected are the perioral areas and the jawline.

Some patients may develop acne 3–9 days after the peel, for which appropriate antibiotics (oral or topical) should be prescribed. Milia can also occur after a peel, usually 2 or 3 weeks after the peel, most likely due to the re-epithelialization process that occurs after the peel and occlusion of sebaceous glands due to ointment use.

No allergic reactions have been observed with AHA chemical peels

DAILY APPLICATION

Glycolic acid formulations are a useful adjunct to chemical peels. The use of lotions at 8–15% concentrations can help accelerate the effects of glycolic acid chemical peels. In addition, daily applications of glycolic lotions can maintain the beneficial effects noted with glycolic acid peels.

Efforts should be made to use an effective set of glycolic acid products. It is best to use a formulation line that is compatible with the therapeutic needs of the patient. The important qualities for such products include strength, specific intent (e.g., pigment, lentigines), and compatibility with glycolic acid chemical peels. There have been reported problems with glycolic peels and daily glycolic lotions not produced by experienced manufacturers. Experience in the production of glycolic acid is essential to ensure that irritation is minimized and the product will be effective. Many of the effectiveness claims of such products have not been substantiated.

To obtain the proper effect of the glycolic acid peeling agents, it is recommended to begin the daily-use home lotions 2 weeks before the first peel. This regimen is helpful for several reasons:

1. The patients' commitment is assessed for post-peel care. If the patient is not dedicated enough to use the daily products, then he or she may not be a proper peel candidate.

2. The 2 weeks of glycolic acid lotion use prepares the skin for a more even peel and increases the skin's tolerance for glycolic acid.
3. Any reaction or sensitivity to the daily-use lotions can help predict any adverse reactions that may occur from the glycolic acid peel.

COMBINATION PEELS

Combination peels have been used to some extent in different variations. The principles behind combining peels is that one agent can enhance the penetration of the other agent, while decreasing some of the toxic risk and morbidity of deeper peeling agents.

Retinoic acid has been used as a daily topical agent (64,69,70). Several studies have indicated the use of topical retinoic acid for the treatment of actinic keratoses, wrinkles, and pigmentation. Further investigations are still needed to evaluate the effectiveness of this modality. ''Retinizing'' the skin before procedures is thought to improve wound healing and speed epithelialization (69). Topical retinoic acid can be used in conjunction with a superficial peel such as glycolic acid peels to enhance the effects of the peel. Studies focusing on the use of these two modalities together have not been done, although it is commonly advocated. Extreme caution should be used when using retinoic acid in combination with glycolic acid peels because retinoic acid augments the effect of the peel possibly by thinning the upper portion of the epidermis (stratum corneum and upper malpighian layer).

An alternative to topical retinoic acids as a prepeel agent is 10% glycolic acid, which can be used for 2 weeks before any glycolic acid peel (71). Although further studies are warranted, prepeel 10% glycolic acid, like topical tretinoin, may enhance penetration of superficial peels.

Jessner's solution or 20% TCA can enhance 50% and 70% glycolic acid. These combinations allow for more accelerated peeling, while only producing mild erythema and only focal mild crusting. As with other superficial peels, these combinations can be repeated regularly in 2–4 weeks. Preliminary histological studies suggest that the depth of penetration will be enhanced when combinations with glycolic acid are used.

The procedure of applying a prepeel agent before glycolic acid is similar to the regular peel procedure for TCA. Jessner's solution is applied thinly and allowed to dry on the face for 2 min. Some clinicians will firmly rub the Jessner's solution or apply three even coats. Next, the glycolic acid is applied and subsequently neutralized as before (58). The skin is likely to have more erythema and on occasion more sloughing of epidermis with resulting crusting than with glycolic acid by itself.

A set of more than 3100 enrolled patients showed that 70% glycolic acid peels immediately augmented with 40% TCA produced excellent clinical outcomes, resulting in smoother skin texture, decreased wrinkling and striae, and fading of lentigines and other pigmentary abnormalities (72,73). Moreover, there was excellent blending into peeled facial skin and into adjacent areas of nonpeeled skin (72,73). Although this study was based on nonfacial skin, similar effects would be expected on the face.

CONCLUSION

The AHAs are a group of nontoxic organic acids that have been used throughout history for beautification purposes. More recently, AHA is thought to play an important role in reversing the effects of photoaging. The role of AHA in specific disorders (melasma, wrinkles, lentigines, etc.) has been reviewed, and recent experimental studies have substantiated its effects. It is critical to educate patients on the peeling process, expectations, and prevention of photoaging. This enhances patient compliance and leads to better results. As our understanding of AHA grows, it is evident that these peeling agents will be a forefront in the treatment of many different dermatological conditions.

REFERENCES

1. Stegman SJ, Tromovitch TA. Chemical peels in cosmetic dermatologic surgery. In: Stegman S, Tromovitch TA, Glogau RG, Eds. Cosmetic Dermatologic Surgery. Chicago: Year Book Publishing, 1984:27–46.
2. Collins PS. The chemical peel. Clin Dermatol 1987; 5:57–74.
3. Letessier SM. Chemical peel with resorcin. In:. Roenigk RK, Roenigk HH, Eds. New York: Marcel Dekker, 1989:1017–1024.
4. Rubin MG. Manual of Chemical Peels: Superficial and Medium Depth. Philadelphia: JB Lippincott Company, 1995.
5. Monheit GD. The Jessner's and TCA peel: a medium-depth chemical peel. J. Dermatol Surg Oncol 1989; 15:945–950.
6. Greenbaum SS, Lask GP. Facial peeling: a trichloroacetic acid. In: Parish LC, Lask GP, Eds. Aesthetic Dermatology. New York: McGraw-Hill Publishing, 1991:139–143.
7. Truppman ES, Ellenberg JD. Major electrocardiographic changes during chemical face peeling. Plast Reconstr Surg 1979; 64:44–48.
8. Baker TJ, Gordon HL. Chemical peel with phenol. In: Epstein E, Epstein E, Eds. Skin Surgery. 6th ed.. Philadelphia: WB Saunders, 1987:423–438.
9. Rakic L, Lapiere CM, Nusgens BV. Comparative caustic and biological activity of trichloroacetic and glycolic acids on keratinocytes and fibroblasts in vitro. Skin Pharmacol Appl Skin Physiol 2000; 13:52–59.
10. Moon SE, Park SB, Ahn HT, Youn JL. The effect of glycolic acid on photoaged albino hairless mouse skin. Dermatol Surg 1999; 25:179–182.
11. Perricone NV, DiNardo JC. Photoprotective and inflammatory effects of topical glycolic acid. Dermatol Surg 1996; 22:435–437.
12. Park KS, Kim HJ, Kim EJ, Nam KT, Oh JH, Song CW, Jung HK, Kim DJ, Yun YW, Kim HS, Chung SY, Cho DH, Kim BY, Hong JT. Effect of glycolic acid on UVB-induced skin damage and inflammation in guinea pigs. Skin Pharmacol Appl Skin Physiol 2002; 15: 236–245.
13. Tsai TF, Paul BH, Jee SH. Effects of glycolic acid on light-induced skin pigmentation in Asian and Caucasian subjects. J Am Acad Dermatol 2000; 43(2 Pt 1):238–243.
14. Sams RL, Couch LH, Miller BJ, Okerberg CV, Warbritton AR, Warner WG, Beer JZ, Howard PC. Effects of alpha- and beta-hydroxy acids on the edemal response induced n female SKH-1 mice by simulated solar light. Toxicol Appl Pharmacol 2002; 184:136–143.
15. Brody HJ, Hailey CW. Variations and comparisons in medium-depth chemical peeling. J Dermatol Surg Oncol 1989; 15:953–963.
16. Behin F, Feverstein SS, Marovitz WF. Comparative histological study of mini pig skin after chemical peel and dermabrasion. Arch Otolaryngol 1977; 103:271–277.
17. Baker TJ, Gordon H, Mosienko P, Seckinger DL. Long-term histological study of skin after chemical face peeling. Plast Reconstr Surg 1974; 53:522–525.
18. Van Scott EJ, Yu RJ. Alpha hydroxy acids: procedures for use in clinical practice. Cutis 1989; 43:222–228.
19. Clark CP. Alpha hydroxyl acids in skin care. Clin Plast Surg 1996; 23:49–56.
20. DiNardo JC, Grove GL, Moy LS. Clinical and histological effects of glycolic acid at different concentrations and pH levels. Dermatol Surg 1996; 22:421–424.

21. Maddin S. Current review of alpha hydroxyl acids. Skin Ther Lett 1998; 3:1–2.
22. Moy LS, Howe K, Moy RL. Glycolic acid modulation of collagen production in human skin fibroblast cultures in vitro. Dermatol Surg 1996; 22:439–441.
23. Kim SJ, Park JH, Kim DH, Won YH, Maibach HI. In creased in vivo collagen synthesis and in vitro cell collagen synthesis and in vitro cell proliferative effect of glycolic acid. Dermatol Surg 1998; 24:1054–1058.
24. Ayres S III. Dermal changes following application of chemical cauterants to aging skin. Arch Dermatol 1960; 82:578.
25. Van Scott EJ, Yu RJ. Substances that modify the stratum corneum by modulating its formation. In: Frost P, Horwitz SN, Eds. Principles of Cosmetics for the Dermatologist. St. Louis: CV Mosby, 1982:70–74.
26. Bernstein EF. Chemical peels. Semin Cutan Med Surg 2002; 21:27–45.
27. Sams RL, Couch LH, Miller BJ, Okerberg CV, Warbritton AR, Warner WG, Beer JZ, Howard PC. Basal cell proliferation in female SKH-1 mice treated with alpha- and beta-hydroxy acids. Toxicol Appl Pharmacol 2001; 175:76–82.
28. Doukas AG, Soukos NS, Babusis S, Appa Y, Kollias N. Fluorescence excitation spectroscopy for the measurement of epidermal proliferation. Photochem Photobiol 2001; 74:96–102.
29. Isoda M, Ueda S, Imayama S, Tsukahara K. New formulation of chemical peeling agent: histological evaluation in sun-damaged skin model in hairless mice. J Dermatol Sci 2001; suppl 1:60–67.
30. Kim TH, Choi EH, Kang YC, Lee SH, Ahn SK. The effects of topical alpha-hydroxyacids on the normal skin barrier of hairless mice. Br J Dermatol 2001; 144:267–273.
31. Butler PE, Gonzalez S, Randolph MA, Kim J, Kollias N, Yaremchik MJ. Quantitative and qualitative effects of chemical peeling on photodamaged skin: an experimental study. Plast Reconstr Surg 2001; 107:222–228.
32. Hong JT, Kim EJ, Ahn KS, Jung KM, Yun YP, Park YK, Lee SH. Inhibitory effect of glycolic acid on ultraviolet-induced skin tumorigenesis in SKH-1 hairless mice and its mechanism of action. Mol Carcinog 2001; 31:152–160.
33. Ahn KS, Park KS, Jung KM, Jung HK, Lee SH, Chung SY, Yang KH, Yum YP, Pyo HB, Park YK, Yun YW, Kim DJ, Park SM, Hong JT. Inhibitory effect of glycolic acid on ultraviolet B-induced c-fos expression, AP-1 activation and p53-p21 response in a human keratinocyte cell line. Cancer Lett 2002; 186:125–135.
34. Gilchrist BA. A review of skin aging and its medical therapy. Br J Dermatol 1996; 135: 867–875.
35. Cotellessa C, Peris K, Onorati MT, Fargnoli MC, Chimenti S. The use of chemical peels in the treatment of different cutaneous hyperpigmentations. Dermatol Surg 1999; 25:450–454.
36. Newman N, Newman A, Moy LS, Babapour R, Harris AG, Moy RL. Clinical improvement of photoaged skin with 50% glycolic acid. A double-blind vehicle-controlled study. Dermatol Surg 1996; 22:455–460.
37. Piacquadio D, Dobry M, Hunt S, Andree C, Grove G, Hollenbach KA. Sort contact 70% glycolic acid peels as a treatment for photodamaged skin. A pilot study. Dermatol Surg 1996; 22:449–452.
38. Coleman WP, Futrell JM. The glycolic acid trichloroacetic acid peel. J Dermatol Surg Oncol 1994; 20:76–80.
39. Lim JT, Tham SN. Glycolic acid peels in the treatment of melasma among Asian women. Dermatol Surg 1997; 23:177–179.
40. Ditre CM, Griffin TD, Murphy GF, Sucki H, Telegan B, Johnson WC, Yu RJ, Van Scott EJ. Improvement of photodamaged skin with alpha hydroxy acid (AHA): A clinical, histological and ultra-structural study. J Am Acad Dermatol 1996; 34(2 Pt 1):187–195.
41. Stiller MJ, Bartolone J, Stern S, Kolhas N, Gillies R, Drake LA. Topical 8% glycolic acid and 8% L-lactic acid creams for the treatment of photodamaged skin. A double-blind vehicle-controlled clinical trial. Arch Dermatol 1996; 132:631–636.

42. Appa Y. Retinoid therapy: compatible skin care. Skin Pharmacol Appl Skin Physiol 1999; 12: 111–119.
43. Lim JT. Treatment of melasma using kojic acid in a gel containing hydroquinone and glycolic acid. Dermatol Surg 1999; 25:282–284.
44. Van Scott EJ, Yu RJ. Alpha hydroxyl acids: therapeutic potentials. Can J Dermatol 1989; 1: 108–112.
45. Pinnell SR, Murad S, Darr D. Induction of collagen synthesis by ascorbic acid: a possible mechanism. Arch Dermatol 1987; 123:1684–1686.
46. Haas JE. The effect of ascorbic acid and potassium ferricyanide as melanogenesis inhibitors on the development of pigmentation in Mexican axolotols. Am Osteopath 1974; 73:674.
47. Brown AM, Kaplan LM, Brown ME. Phenol-induced histological skin changes: hazards, technique and uses. Br J Plast Surg 1960; 13:158.
48. Resnick SS. Chemical peeling with trichloroacetic acid. J Dermatol Surg Oncol 1984; 10: 549–550.
49. Van Scott EJ, Yu RJ. Hyperkeratinization, corneocyte cohesion, and alpha hydroxy acids. J Am Acad Dermatol 1984; 5:867–879.
50. Uitto J, Fazio MJ, Olsen DR. Cutaneous aging: molecular alterations in elastic fibers. J Cut Aging and Cosm Dermatol 1988; 1:13–26.
51. Jiang M, Qureshi SA. Assessment of in vitro percutaneous absorption of glycolic acid through human skin sections using a flow-through diffusion cell system. J Dermatol Sci 1998; 18: 181–188.
52. Stegman SJ. A comparative histologic study of the effects of three peeling agents and dermabrasion on normal and sun damaged skin. Aesthetic Plast Surg 1982; 6:123–135.
53. Baker TJ, Gordon HL. Chemical face peeling and dermabrasion. Surg Clin North Am 1971; 51:387–401.
54. Stegman SJ. A study of dermabrasion and chemical peels in an animal model. J Dermatol Surg Oncol 1980; 6:490–497.
55. Funasaka Y, Sato H, Usuki A, Ohashi A, Kotoya H, Miyamoto K, Hillebrand GG, Ichihashi M. The efficacy of glycolic acid for treating wrinkles: analysis using newly developed facial imaging systems equipped with fluorescent illumination. J Dermatol Sci 2001; 27(suppl 1): 53–59.
56. Marrero GM, Katz BE. The new fluor-hydroxy pulse peel. A combination of 5-fluorouracil and glycolic acid. Dermatol Surg 1998; 24:973–978.
57. Gladstone HB, Nguyen SL, Williams R, Ottomeyer T, Wortzman M, Jeffers M, Moy RL. Efficacy of hydroquinone cream (USP 4%) used alone or in combination with salicylic acid peels in improving photodamage on the neck and upper chest. Dermatol Surg 2000; 26: 333–337.
58. Tse Y, Ostad A, Lee HS, Levine VJ, Koenig K, Kamino H, Ashinoff R. A clinical and histologic evaluation of two medium-depth peels. Glycolic acid versus Jessner's trichloroacetic acid. Dermatol Surg 1996; 22:781–786.
59. Moy LS, Murad H, Moy RL. Glycolic acid peels for the treatment of wrinkles and photoaging. J Dermatol Surg Oncol 1993; 19:243–246.
60. Hurley ME, Guevara IL, Gonzales RM, Pandya AG. Efficacy of glycolic acid peels in the treatment of melasma. Arch Dermatol 2002; 138:1578–1582.
61. Javaheri SM, Handa S, Kaur I, Kumar B. Safety and efficacy of glycolic acid facial peel in Indian women with melasma. Int J Dermatol 2001; 40:354–357.
62. Sarkar R, Kaur C, Bhalla M, Kanwar AJ. The combination of glycolic acid peels with a topical regimen in the treatment of melasma in dark-skinned patients: a comparative study. Dermatol Surg 2002; 28:828–832.
63. Rodrigues LH, Maia Campos PM. Comparative study of the effects of cosmetic formulations with or without hydroxy acids on hairless mouse epidermis by histopathologic, morphometric, and stereologic evaluation. J Cosmet Sci 2002; 53:269–82.

64. Moy RL, Moy LS, Bennett RG, Zitelli JA, Uitto J. Systemic isotretinoin: effects on dermal wound healing in a rabbit ear model in vivo. J Dermatol Surg Oncol 1990; 16:1142–1146.
65. Hanke CW, Bullock SS. Tretinoin and glycolic acid treatment regimens. Facial Plast Surg 1995; 11:9–14.
66. Effendy I, Kwangsukstith C, Lee JY, Maibach HL. Functional changes in human stratum corneum induced by topical glycolic acid: comparison with all-trans retinoic acid. Acta Derm Venereol 1995; 75:455–458.
67. Brody HJ. Complications of chemical peeling. J Dermatol Surg Oncol 1989; 15:1010–1019.
68. Rappaport MJ, Kamer F. Exacerbation of facial herpes simplex after phenolic face peels. J Dermatol Surg Oncol 1984; 10:57–58.
69. Mandy SH. Tretinoin in preoperative and post operative management of dermabrasion. J Am Acad Dermatol 1986; 15:878–879.
70. Pierard GE, Kligman AM, Stoudernmayer T, veque JL. Comparative effects of retinoic acid, glycolic acid and a lipophilic derivative of salicylic acid on photodamaged epidermis. Dermatology 1999; 199:50–53.
71. Bergfeld W, Tung R, Vidimos A, Vellanki L, Remzi B, Stanton-Hicks U. Improving the cosmetic appearance of photoaged skin with glycolic acid. J Am Acad Dermatol 1997; 36(6 Pt 1):1011–1013.
72. Cook KK, Cook WR. Chemical peel of nonfacial skin using glycolic acid gel augmented with TCA and neutralized based on visual imaging. Dermatol Surg 2000; 25:994–999.
73. Cox S. Rapid development of keratoacanthomas after a body peel. Dermatol Surg 2003; 29: 201–203.

9

Laser and Light-Based Treatment of the Aging Skin

Jeffrey T. S. Hsu *SkinCare Physicians of Chestnut Hill, Chestnut Hill, Massachusetts, U.S.A.*

Murad Alam *Northwestern University, Chicago, Illinois, U.S.A.*

Jeffrey S. Dover *Yale University School of Medicine, New Haven, Connecticut; Dartmouth Medical School, Hanover, New Hampshire, U.S.A.*

- Since the 1980s, lasers have been indispensable in correcting signs of aging, complementing traditional modalities.
- Current lasers and light-based technologies are capable of treating signs of aging, such as lentigines, telangiectasias, and rhytides.
- Several emerging technologies hold tremendous promise in rejuvenating the photoaged skin with minimal recovery time.

INTRODUCTION

Aging of the skin can be attributed to both intrinsic physiological processes and external exposures in the form of ultraviolet light. This photoaging is characterized by rhytides, rough texture, dyspigmentation, and loss of elasticity. Histologically, epidermal thinning, disorganized collagen bundles, and clumping of elastic fibers are seen (1). Similar changes may induce formation of superficial capillaries that manifest as facial telangiectasia. Given rapidly advancing technology, the physician interested in treating these signs of cutaneous skin aging can select from among several different laser devices. Although different crystals, liquids, and gases can be used to produce laser light of various wavelengths, some have clinical efficacy limited to particular applications. This chapter reviews the most commonly used lasers and light-based treatments for targeting age-related skin changes.

Although the physiology of aging is similar among patients, the manifestations can vary widely among individuals; therefore, careful preoperative evaluation is critical for selecting the right combination of treatments. Understanding the patient's desires also should be a focus of this evaluation. Whereas one patient may not tolerate rhytides around her eyes but feels comfortable with lentigines on her forehead, the next patient may have the opposite set of concerns. A frank discussion should include physician assessment of the patient's tolerance of risk, recovery time, and financial expenditure.

HISTORY

The development of clinically applicable lasers began in 1960s with the work of Leon Goldman. His investigation of neodymium:yttrium-aluminum-garnet (Nd:YAG), ruby, and argon lasers for treatment of vascular and pigmented lesions initiated interest in the new treatment modality. In the early 1980s, Anderson and Parrish proposed the theory of selective photothermolysis, which clarified the biophysics underlying the treatment of specific targets with particular laser wavelengths and pulse durations. This theoretical advance led to the development of tunable dye lasers. Emitting 577-nm light, these lasers excite the absorption peak of oxyhemoglobin in the yellow region of the visible spectrum. Since the original dye lasers, which used microsecond pulses, technological advances have enabled the development of similar lasers with longer wavelengths and longer pulse durations (2,3). In recent years, a multitude of additional lasers and light-based devices have been perfected for cutaneous use. Lasers are now available for the selective treatment of various visible manifestations of photoaging, including vascular lesions, pigmented lesions, premalignant actinic damage, textural changes, and rhytides.

LASER AND LIGHT TISSUE INTERACTIONS

Modern cutaneous lasers operationalize the principles of selective photothermolysis (4). Structures in the skin serve as chromophores that preferentially absorb certain wavelengths of light, which are unique to a given laser. By limiting the exposure of the laser light to a time shorter than the target's thermal relaxation time, the energy is contained in the selected chromophores and collateral damage to the surrounding skin is limited. The energy level then can be modulated to achieve the desired effect. Chromophores that are targeted frequently include oxyhemoglobin in vascular lesions, melanin in pigmented lesions, and water in all cells.

The interaction of laser energy with tissue results in three types of biological effects: (1) photothermal reactions from the direct effect of heat; (2) photochemical reactions from the interaction between photosensitizers with light (e.g., porphyrin derivatives in photodynamic therapy [PDT]); and (3) photomechanical reactions from sudden thermal expansion, which leads to formation of shock waves. Traditionally, most therapeutic effects of lasers are related to photothermal reactions. As light energy is absorbed, it is transformed to heat. Between 50°C and 100°C, most biological tissues undergo denaturation or irreversible coagulation of proteins. The location and extent of the thermal injury depends on the intensity, duration, and wavelength of the laser light, but once the temperature surpasses 100°C, vaporization of the tissue occurs. Vaporized tissue is surrounded by a zone of coagulative necrosis, which in turn is surrounded by a zone of reversible thermal damage. Photomechanical damage is produced by laser pulses of short duration and high peak powers, such as those generated by Q-switched lasers. In the treatment of tattoos and pigmented lesions, Q-switched devices raise the tissue temperature by 300°C in nanoseconds, sufficiently fast to explode the pigment granules and the cells that contain them (5).

SKIN COOLING

Skin cooling is frequently an integral part of laser therapy both for cryoanesthesia and for protection. It is particularly crucial when treating darker-skinned individuals. Epidermal melanin can absorb light intended for the underlying targeted chromophores, such as oxyhemoglobin, leading to epidermal injury. One way to overcome this problem is to selectively cool the epidermis. Devices designed to cool the skin reduce epidermal damage and allow the use of higher fluences and treatment of darker skin types. All forms of cooling entail putting a cold medium, usually cold air, cryogen spray, cold gel, or cold sapphire window, in contact with the skin. To ensure adequate cooling, several parameters must be considered regardless of the medium: duration of contact, temperature of the cooling source, and quality of contact. There are three basic modes of cooling: precooling, parallel cooling, and postcooling (6). Precooling lowers the skin temperature prior to the laser pulse. Because of the possibility of freeze injury to the epidermis, there is a limit on the degree of safe precooling. Protective precooling is best for pulse widths shorter than 5 msec and best delivered by cryogen spray (7). Parallel cooling lowers the skin temperature concurrent with the laser pulse. With short pulse widths, the limited time of contact provided with parallel cooling tends to afford little epidermal protection. Parallel cooling becomes much more protective when it is coincident with pulses longer than 5 to 10 msec. A common parallel cooling medium is cold sapphire. Cryogen spray is less appropriate once the laser is firing because it may interfere with the laser beam. Postcooling is mainly used for minimizing pain and edema but has little effect on preventing thermal injury (8). The skin temperature also can be lowered with air chilled as low as −30°C. The cooling time for this medium can be longer than other methods, but this results in deeper penetration of the cooling effect. Consequently, the entire skin can be cooled (''bulk cooling'') with little selectivity for the epidermis (9). On the other hand, there are certain advantages to air cooling. This medium does not disturb the laser light, can be used regardless of skin topography, and requires no compression of the skin, which can be important when treating vascular lesions (10).

VASCULAR LASERS

Vascular lasers target oxyhemoglobin and deoxyhemoglobin in blood. As light energy is converted to heat in oxyhemoglobin, the temperature of blood rises enough to irreversibly damage the endothelial cells lining the vessel walls. Oxyhemoglobin has three absorption peaks: 418, 542, and 577 nm. Because melanin competes for absorption of light at these wavelengths, to treat vascular lesions selectively, it is important to select wavelengths that are preferentially absorbed by hemoglobin as opposed to melanin.

For selective treatment, pulse durations must be appropriately synchronized to the thermal relaxation time of oxyhemoglobin. Pulse durations also may be tailored to the size of the vessel being treated, as larger vessels require longer pulse duration than smaller ones. Additionally, longer pulse widths allow for less purpura. Purpura is the result of microvascular hemorrhage, thrombosis, and vasculitis, and pulse widths equal to or slightly longer than the thermal relaxation time of a given vessel can prevent purpura by selectively damaging this vessel without injuring the adjacent capillaries and smaller vessels (11). One may prevent purpura by using longer pulse widths that slowly and evenly heat the blood and cause endothelial damage without rupturing the vessel.

Given the absorption spectrum of oxyhemoglobin and depth of cutaneous vessels, lasers with wavelengths ranging from 532 to 1064 nm may be used to treat vascular lesions. Longer wavelengths may be desirable for treating deeper vascular anomalies because these wavelengths allow for deeper penetration into the dermis, whereas shorter wavelengths are more appropriate for superficial vessels. The most common vascular lasers include potassium titanyl phosphate (KTP) lasers, pulsed dye lasers (PDL), alexandrite lasers, diode lasers, and Nd:YAG lasers, as well as the intense pulsed light (IPL) devices. No single laser is ideal for all types of lesions. The caliber and depth from the skin surface of the target vessel must be considered when selecting the proper device and parameters.

Pulsed Dye Laser

The first PDL had an emission wavelength of 577 nm to coincide with one of the absorption peaks of hemoglobin. The more recent PDL lasers have wavelengths of 585 and 595 nm to enhance depth of penetration. Pulse duration may range from 350 μsec to the millisecond range, although rapid heating of the vessels at the shorter pulse widths can lead to purpura, a potentially significant cosmetic problem. Given overlapping absorption between hemoglobin and melanin, there is always a risk for epidermal damage. Light absorption by the melanin in the epidermis may lead to excessive heating of the epidermis, with subsequent injury and possible dyspigmentation. To prevent this, one should avoid treating tanned patients. Overall, the PDL has been used in successive iterations since 1986 when it was first approved by the U.S. Food and Drug Administration (FDA) for the treatment of port-wine stains. It has been proven to be safe and effective therapy for a variety of vascular lesions, including telangiectasia, hemangiomas, port-wine stains, and scars. Applications of PDL in aging skin include the treatment of photodistributed reticulated telangiectasias and erythema of the cheeks, as well as poikiloderma of Civatte of the neck and upper chest. Depending on the severity, these signs of aging can be effectively cleared with several treatments at fluences ranging from 6.5 to 7.5 J/cm^2 (Figs. 1 and 2).

Patients undergoing PDL treatment should be warned of mild discomfort, potential local tissue swelling, and possible immediate purpuric reaction, which may persist for as long as 7 to 10 days. Patients should be encouraged to avoid sun exposure prior to and after treatment to prevent dyspigmentation.

Diode Laser

At 810 nm, the diode laser offers more depth penetration than PDL. This wavelength is poorly absorbed by melanin, allowing less risk for epidermal damage. However, it also is relatively poorly absorbed by hemoglobin, requiring higher fluences to induce tissue heating. Studies have shown promising results in the treatment of facial lesions but less predictable outcome in the treatment of leg telangiectasias (12).

KTP and Nd:YAG Lasers

The long-pulse, frequency-doubled, 532-nm Nd:YAG laser has proven successful for treatment of superficial veins (13). The pulse duration of this laser, which ranges from 1 to 50 msec, allows for intravascular coagulation without vessel rupture, which prevents purpura.

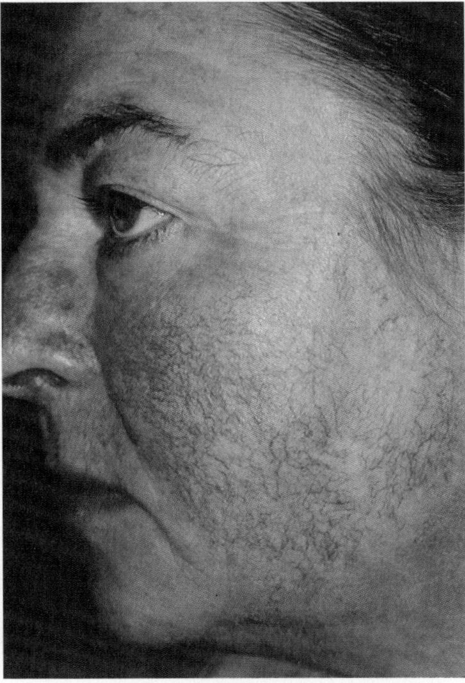

Figure 1 Severe telangiectasia before treatments with pulsed dye laser.

Using either a 1- or 2-mm spot size, individual vessels are treated without injuring the surrounding skin. Larger spot sizes and scanning hand pieces are available, but they usually are reserved for total face nonablative rejuvenation. Given the short wavelength and correspondingly shallower penetration, this laser is not effective at treating leg veins or deeper facial veins. High peak power, long pulse width Nd:YAG (1064 nm) has been used for deeper and larger caliber vessels more effectively (Figs. 3 and 4). Its longer wavelength allows for coagulation effect at a depth of 5 to 6 mm (14). Despite the incorporation of efficient, high-volume cooling mechanisms, the deep penetration and high energy of the Nd:YAG laser can lead to dermal necrosis and ulceration. It is important to cautiously monitor for signs of epidermal damage and to avoid overlapping laser spots.

Vascular Lasers

Vascular lesions are summarized in Table 1.

INTENSE PULSED LIGHT

In 1976, Muhlbauer et al. first described a polychromatic infrared light source for treatment of capillary hemangiomas and port-wine stains (15). In 1990, Goldman and Eckhouse developed a new high-intensity flashlamp to pave the way for the first commercial IPL system, introduced in 1994. Further refinement of this technology has made it one of the

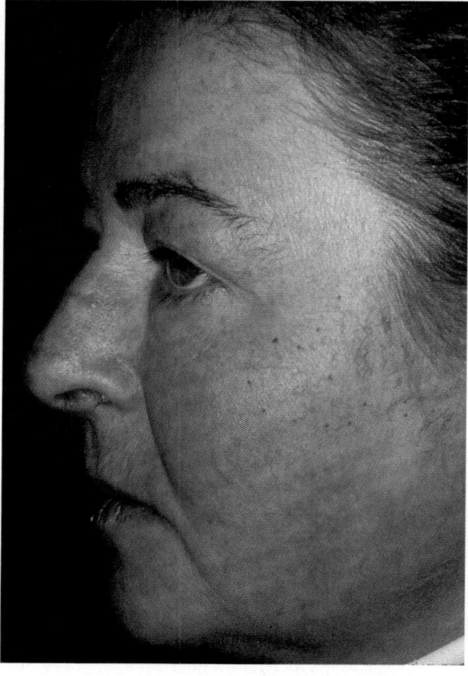

Figure 2 Severe telangiectasia after two treatments with pulsed dye laser.

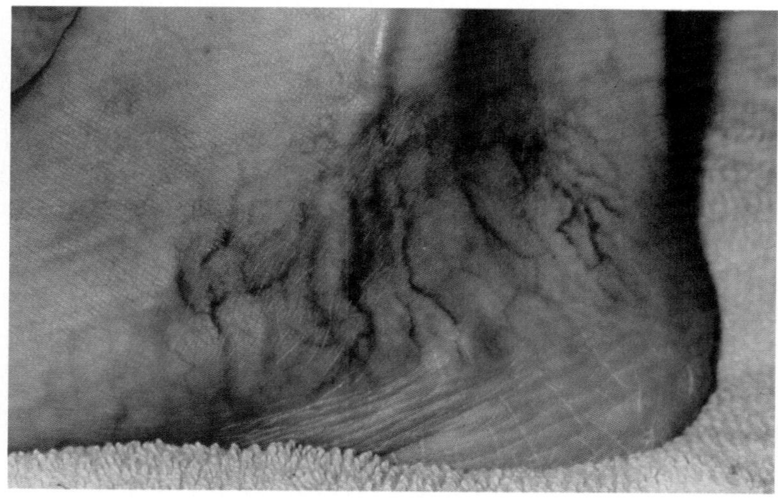

Figure 3 Spider veins on ankle before treatment.

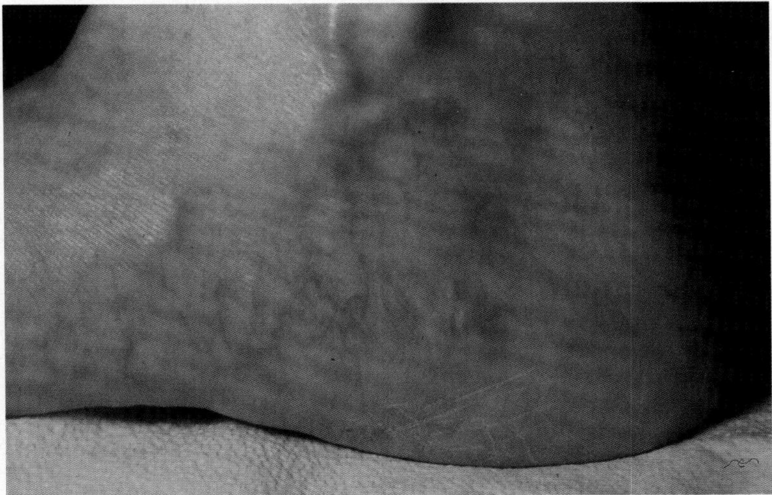

Figure 4 Spider veins on ankle improved with one treatment using 1064-nm long-pulse Nd:YAG laser.

most versatile tools for treating the aging skin. Unlike lasers, IPL is a noncollimated, noncoherent light source. It emits a continuous spectrum that ranges from 515 to 1200 nm. As with true lasers, the efficacy of IPL for treatment of vascular and pigmented lesions is based on selective destruction of target chromophores by particular wavelengths and pulse durations. Filters are used to eliminate the shorter than desired wavelengths from a particular treatment to focus the residual emissions on the feature to be treated. Pulse duration can range widely from 0.5 to over 20 msec. Pulses can be delivered singly, one after the other (double pulsing), or three in a row (triple pulsing), with variable delay between the pulses. The epidermis can be cooled by applying a thick layer of cold gel or, with newer models, by integrated cooling on the IPL crystal (16).

Studies have shown that IPL devices are effective for reduction of both lentigines and vascular lesions, such as telangiectasias, port-wine stains, and poikiloderma (17) (Figs. 5 and 6). IPL also has some efficacy as a nonablative resurfacing device and may improve fine rhytides through mild thermal denaturation of dermal collagen and subsequent repair

Table 1 Vascular Lasers

Lesions	KTP (532 nm)	PDL (595 nm)	Alexandrite (755 nm)	Diode (810 nm)	Long Pulse Nd:YAG (1064 nm)
Superficial facial vessels	+++	+++	+	+	+
Superficial leg veins	+	++	++	++	++
Deep reticular leg veins	–	–	++	+	++

KTP, potassium titanyl phosphate; Nd:YAG, neodymium: yttrium-aluminum-garnet; PDL, pulsed dye laser.

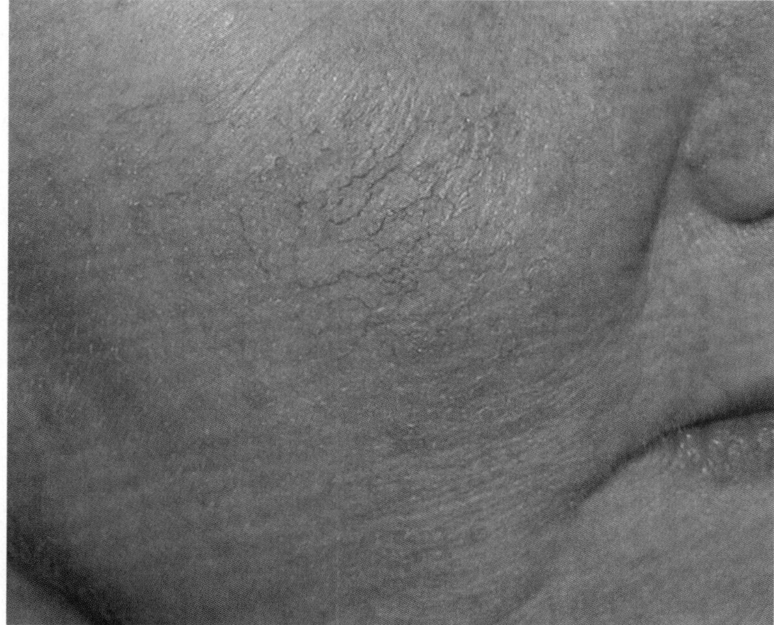

Figure 5 Cheek telangiectasias before treatment. (Courtesy of R. Weiss, M.D.)

(18). Along with improvement in red color tone, vessels, dyspigmentation, and lentigines, clinical studies have shown improvements in skin texture, pore size, and fine wrinkles (16). Histological studies have confirmed posttreatment epidermal regeneration and have suggested the production of collagen I, collagen III, elastin, procollagen, and hyaluronate receptors (19–21). Compared to other nonablative lasers, IPL technology allows for larger spot size and is well suited for treatment of nonfacial areas, such as the chest and extremities. For patients, the treatment is more comfortable than the deep penetrating infrared nonablative lasers.

Originally, due to the wide spectrum of potential combinations of wavelengths, pulse durations, delay times, and fluences, IPL technology was difficult to master. With improvements in software and the knowledge of effective settings, IPL treatments have become fairly standardized and much easier to master. The most common unwanted reaction is transient erythema, which lasts for 2 to 48 hours (15). Other side effects include temporary mild crusting, mild purpura, and facial edema. Rarely, hypopigmentation can be observed, but mostly in darker skinned patients and tanned skin. Other relative contraindications to consider are (1) patients with photosensitivity or who are taking photosensitizing medications, and (2) patients who took isotretinoin within the last 6 months (16). As with nonablative lasers, several treatments may be needed to produce visible results.

PIGMENTED LESION LASERS

Devices for Treating Lentigines

Devices for treating lentigines are summarized in Table 2.

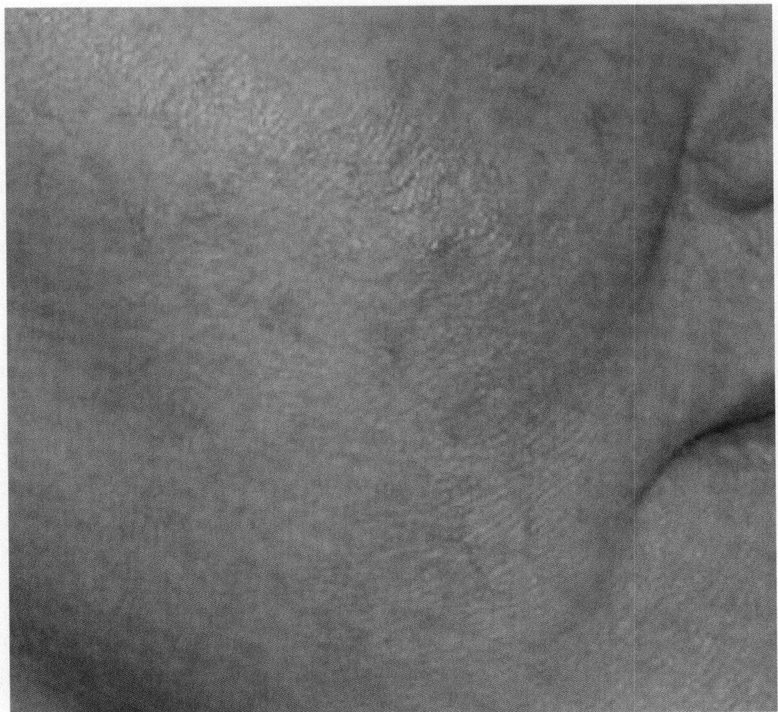

Figure 6 Improvement of cheek telangiectasias after only one treatment with intense pulsed light. (Courtesy of R. Weiss, M.D.)

Table 2 Devices for Treating Lentigines

Q-switched lasers	
Ruby	694 nm
Alexandrite	755 nm
Nd:YAG	1064 nm
Long-pulse laser	
KTP	532 nm
Others	
Intense pulsed light	515–1200 nm

KTP, potassium titanyl phosphate; Nd:YAG, neodymium: yttrium-aluminum-garnet.

The most common pigmented lesions in photoaged patient are lentigines. The target chromophore in lentigines is melanin, which competes with oxyhemoglobin for light absorption. However, unlike hemoglobin, which has several peaks and valleys in its absorption spectrum, the absorption of melanin is highest at approximately 200 nm and decreases steadily up to 2000 nm.

Lasers that target pigment are particularly successful in ameliorating superficial benign epidermal pigmented lesions, such as lentigines and ephelides. However, lesions with many active melanocytes, such as café-au-lait macules, nevi, and conditions such as melasma, are far less responsive to laser treatment (22).

The superficial nature of lentigines and the wide absorption spectrum of melanosomes make them accessible targets for lasers with a wide range of wavelengths. Given that the thermal relaxation time of melanosomes falls in the range from 250 to 1000 nsec (23), it was traditionally accepted that superficial pigmented lesions were most susceptible to similarly rapid firing Q-switched lasers, with wavelengths from 694 to 1064 nm (Q-switched ruby laser, 694 nm; Q-switched alexandrite laser, 755 nm; and Q-switched Nd:YAG laser, 1064 nm) and pulse durations in the nanosecond domain. More recent evidence indicates that longer pulse lasers, including the long-pulse alexandrite and the long-pulse KTP, also have substantial efficacy in the treatment of superficial pigment. Despite the elongated pulse duration, these devices are empirically successful in achieving clearing with minimal side effects, such as hyperpigmentation at the periphery, or persistent edema and erythema. This surprising efficacy and safety profile suggests that targets other than melanosomes also may mediate the laser-induced resolution of lentigines and similar lesions.

Patients must be warned of the likely transient darkening and possible week-long crusting resulting from the treatment of lentigines. Lightening occurs over the ensuing 3 to 6 weeks. Other side effects are erythema, hyperpigmentation, or hypopigmentation. Patients should take extra precautions to avoid any tanning prior to treatment.

Q-Switched Ruby Laser

The Q-switched ruby laser has a wavelength of 694 nm. With strong absorption by melanin and good depth of penetration, this laser is very effective in the treatment of cutaneous pigmented lesions. However, the intensity of its absorption by melanin increases the risk of hypopigmentation in darker skin types.

Alexandrite Laser

Alexandrite crystal lasers emit at 755 nm and can be Q-switched at 50- to 100-nsec pulse width or function in the normal mode at the millisecond domain. When Q-switched, the laser emissions are well absorbed by melanin, with little absorption by hemoglobin. This makes the Q-switched alexandrite laser ideal for treating epidermal and dermal pigmented lesions (Figs. 7 and 8). In the normal mode, this laser is effective for hair removal (24).

Nd:YAG Laser

This versatile laser may emit light at 1064 nm in the near-infrared spectrum or frequency-doubled as 532-nm green light. The 1064-nm wavelength is moderately well absorbed by melanin but has the deepest penetration of the pigment lasers; therefore, this laser is less efficacious for epidermal pigment but can be used to lighten deeper benign lesions such

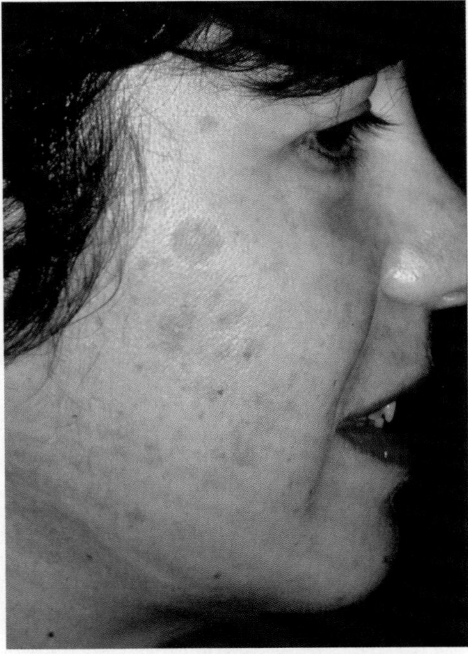

Figure 7 Facial lentigines before treatment using Q-switched alexandrite laser.

as nevus of Ota and dark tattoo ink. The shorter wavelength is useful for treating red colored tattoos, a topic outside the scope of this chapter. Its use for treatment of lentigines is limited by induced postinflammatory hyperpigmentation and hypopigmentation, especially in darker skinned patients, but recent results suggest that this problem is less significant than previously suspected (25).

Long-Pulse KTP

Unlike the Q-switched 532-nm laser, the long pulse width 532-nm laser has been found to be safe and efficacious for treatment of lentigines, even in darker skinned patients (25). Q-switched lasers produce intense energy that leads to rapid rise in temperature, damaging not only melanosome-containing cells but, at 532 nm, also damaging hemoglobin in superficial vessels and thus causing purpura. This leads to inflammation and possible hyperpigmentation. Longer pulse widths may help circumvent this problem. Whereas the clinical endpoint for Q-switched system is defined as immediate whitening, ashen-gray changes without purpura are the endpoint for the long-pulse system.

RESURFACING LASERS

Intrinsically and extrinsically aged skin is marked by rhytides. Rhytides can be classified in many ways, with one scheme separating them into solar rhytides, fine age-related rhytides, and rhytides caused by facial expression (26,27). Solar rhytides are characterized

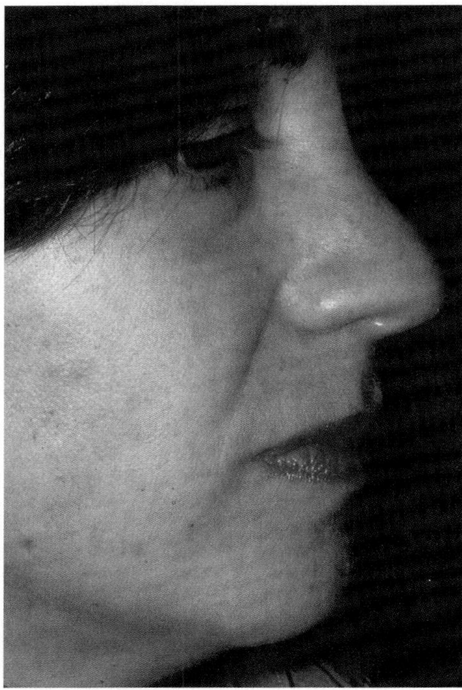

Figure 8 Facial lentigines improved 70% with one treatment using Q-switched alexandrite laser. Further improvement is likely with additional treatments, but the patient already is satisfied with the result.

by normal elastic fibers within the rhytide, which is encased in a zone of elastotic degeneration along the shoulders of the central depression (28). Fine age-related rhytides are caused by thinning of the elastic tissue and loss of subcutaneous fat. They disappear with stretching. Rhytides caused by facial expression come from chronic mechanical stress on the dermis from muscle contractions. Histology shows thickening and shortening of the hypodermal septa that connect the dermis to the superficial musculoaponeurotic system (29).

One way to produce smoother skin by modifying these markers of aging entails ablating superficial skin and allowing the generation of new dermal matrix proteins, as well as the formation of a new epidermal layer and new collagen synthesis at the dermal–epidermal junction. In the 1980s and early 1990s, continuous wave carbon dioxide lasers were used to resurface photoaged skin through this process of ablation and re-epithelialization. Although results were impressive in skilled hands, the difficulty in controlling dwell time occasionally led to excessive thermal damage and scarring. However, the subsequent development of short-pulse, high peak power, rapidly scanned focused beam CO_2 lasers and normal mode erbium:yttrium-aluminum-garnet (Er:YAG) lasers made precise, controlled skin ablation possible. The wavelengths of CO_2 (10,640 nm) and Er:YAG (2940 nm) lasers are absorbed by water. Because water is a major component of most cells, light from either laser will ablate any cell it strikes.

CO_2 Laser

The CO_2 laser (10,640-nm emission wavelength) can be used to both vaporize and cut tissue, while simultaneously sealing small blood vessels. Water is the chromophore, making CO_2 laser light highly absorbed in most biological tissues. Penetrating approximately 30 μm into the skin (30), CO_2 laser requires a fluence of 4 to 5 J/cm^2 to ablate to this level. As previously explained, until the mid 1990s, CO_2 lasers were available only in continuous wave mode. Unfortunately, when delivered with a continuous beam, CO_2 laser can induce a zone of thermal coagulation up to 1 mm thick because of heat diffusion. To control the depth of thermal damage, the laser beam needs to be scanned at a rate that results in tissue dwell time that is less than the thermal relaxation time. For a 30-μm slice of skin, the thermal relaxation time has been calculated to be less than 1 msec (31,32).

The first high-energy CO_2 was developed by Coherent, Inc. (ESC Medical Systems, Yokneam, Israel; now, Lumenis, Santa Clara, CA) and named the UltraPulse laser. It is capable of delivering more than 5 J/cm^2 to the target in less than 1 msec. The SilkLaser flashscanner (Sharplan SilkTouch, FeatherTouch, ESC Medical Systems, Yokneam, Israel; now, Lumenis, Santa Clara, CA) was among the early devices used to automatically scan the active laser across a target area of variable size and shape (33).

Several CO_2 lasers now are capable of achieving these parameters. Typically, the epidermis is removed with one pass, leaving a residual thermal necrosis zone of 20 to 70 μm (33). With each subsequent pass, less tissue is ablated, and a relatively greater zone of thermal damage is created. This likely is a consequence of tissue desiccation from the first pass, which leaves less water as target for later passes. Despite the potential for scarring, the nonselective thermal effect induced by the CO_2 laser on the dermis can be beneficial. The rejuvenation effect on the aged skin is not only through direct ablation of rhytides but also through heating of the collagen. Heating breaks the heat-labile intramolecular cross-links within collagen, and the protein undergoes a transition from a highly organized structure to a random, gel-like state. Collagen shrinkage occurs through the additive effect of the unwinding of the triple helix and the residual tension of the heat-stable intermolecular cross-links. This heat-induced denaturation typically occurs at approximately 65(C. New collagen deposition is observed, although the mechanism of this phenomenon is less well defined. Numerous studies have documented that thermally modified tissues undergo a remodeling process characterized by fibroplasia and increased collagen deposition (34). Collagen may contract by 20% to 30% from CO_2 laser resurfacing (35), and the dramatic effect is observable during the laser procedure (Figs. 9 and 10).

Er:YAG Laser

Water is also the main chromophore for Er:YAG lasers, which emit energy at 2940 nm. Compared to the wavelength of the CO_2 laser, the Er:YAG wavelength is absorbed 16 times better by water ands requires only 1.5 J/cm^2 to ablate 10 to 30 μm at a pulse duration of 250 to 350 μsec (36). This precise ablation leaves zones of thermal damage that are only 5 to 15 μm thick (37). Unlike the CO_2 laser, less desiccation occurs, and pulse stacking does not increase the depth of thermal damage. Because the absorption peak of collagen is 3030 nm, which is close to the 2940-nm wavelength of the Er:YAG, collagen is effectively targeted by the Er:YAG laser. With less nonselective heating of the dermis, contraction of the skin is much less dramatic, estimated to be 0% to 14% in most patients

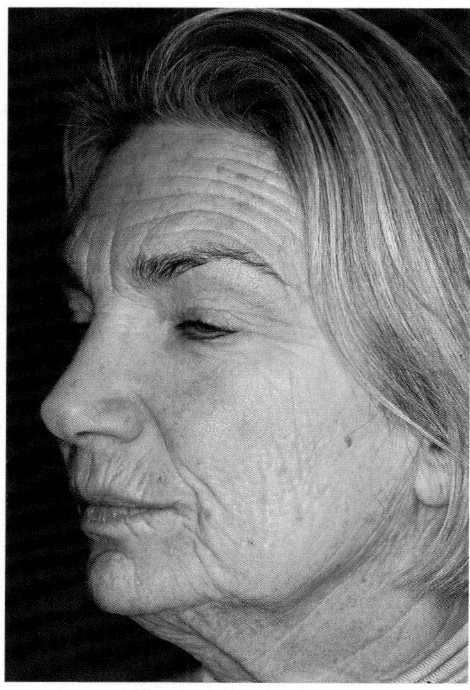

Figure 9 Before full-face resurfacing using CO_2 laser.

(38). The advantage of the smaller zone of thermal damage lies in the quicker healing time and reduced risk for scarring (39).

To achieve immediate tissue contraction, combinations of short ablative pulse and longer subablative pulse Er:YAG laser systems have been introduced to achieve both ablation and coagulation, much like CO_2 lasers (Sciton Contour, Palo Alto, CA). The longer pulse duration delivers the same energy over a longer exposure, resulting in increased thermal effects without vaporization. Additionally, immediate tissue contraction is achieved, and the overall healing rate is between that of CO_2 lasers and the short-pulse Er:YAG lasers (40). These hybrid lasers reduce erythema, swelling, and discomfort compared to CO_2 laser resurfacing alone, without compromising clinical results (41).

Combined CO_2 Laser and Er:YAG Laser

Using the CO_2 and Er:YAG lasers together for resurfacing is now the technique of choice of many laser surgeons for ablative resurfacing. The treatment begins with CO_2 laser to induce nonselective thermal heating of the dermis for tissue contraction. This is followed by Er:YAG to remove the layer of residual thermal damage. Such a two-step process achieves the impressive results seen with CO_2 laser alone but with shorter healing time (42). Several studies of the technique have found improvement in rhytides of 25% to 75%, depending on the laser used, the parameters selected, and the pretreatment wrinkle severity (43,44).

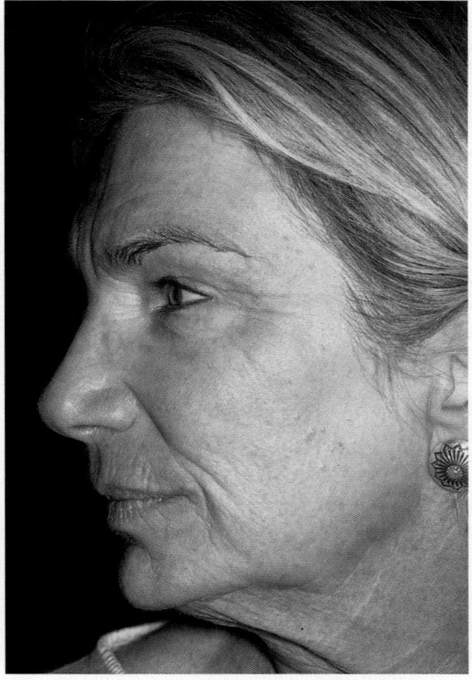

Figure 10 Six months after full-face resurfacing using CO_2 laser only.

Patient Selection

Several features of aging skin, including rhytides, actinic damage, and superficial pigmentation, can be treated by resurfacing lasers. Mild rhytides may be fully corrected with the CO_2 laser, the Er:YAG laser, or the combination laser. Moderate-to-severe rhytides respond better to either CO_2 or the combination treatment. Because of the superficial epidermal ablation achieved by all three systems, any of the lasers may improve superficial pigmentation, such as lentigines. However, if superficial pigmentation is the only target, the Er:YAG can more ablate more precisely and limit the zone of thermal damage, allowing for faster healing.

Perioral and periorbital regions should be evaluated in prospective patients. Redundancy of the skin of the upper eyelids often starts in the third decade. By the fourth decade, lateral canthal rhytides and lower eyelid folds are present, even at rest. Wrinkling in these areas may be unresponsive to facelift procedures, but laser resurfacing potentially could achieve excellent results (45). Even with laser ablation, lines of expression on the forehead, glabella, and nasolabial folds may only soften rather than resolve. These dynamic lines are best treated with additional modalities such as botulinum toxin to prevent contraction of the muscle and rewrinkling of the overlying skin during the skin remodeling that follows resurfacing.

Patient expectations must be managed prior to the procedure, during which the patient usually will require either oral or intravenous conscious sedation to tolerate. Specifically, patients must know that resurfacing can improve but not eliminate wrinkles. Patients should expect mild wrinkles to nearly resolve and moderate and severe wrinkles to improve significantly. The treated areas may continue to improve up to 18 months after the procedure because collagen remodeling persists for this period. Potential side effects, which range from prolonged erythema and dyspigmentation to scarring and ectropion, should be carefully and completed discussed with patients before any laser treatment is begun (46).

Patients of any age who are in reasonably good health can safely undergo laser resurfacing. Absolute contraindications include active infections, immunocompromise, use of isotretinoin within the past year, history of hypertrophic scar or keloid in the treatment area, and unrealistic expectations. Relative contraindications include history of dyspigmentation, skin types V and VI, koebnerizing diseases such as vitiligo or psoriasis, and history of recurrent infections (47).

NONABLATIVE LASER REJUVENATION

Nonablative Rejuvenation Devices

Nonablative rejuvenation devices are listed in Table 3.

Recently, several laser and light sources have been developed with the aim of stimulating new collagen growth and improving texture without the prolonged healing and side effects of the resurfacing lasers. So-called nonablative laser and light treatments are attractive to physicians and patients alike because of the associated minimal risk and inconvenience. A series of nonablative treatments are routinely required to yield a cosmetically significant benefit, and the cumulative aesthetic improvement is less than with traditional ablative resurfacing. Numerous laser and light devices, including the KTP laser (532 nm), PDL (585, 595 nm), Nd:YAG laser (1064, 1320 nm), diode laser (1450 nm), Er:glass laser (1540 nm), IPL (500–1200 nm), and light-emitting diodes (LEDs) have been used for this purpose. Most of these laser and light treatments are generally delivered in combination with epidermal precooling or postcooling that prevents injury to the epidermis while delivering thermal injury to the dermis. The thermal injury to the dermis initiates fibroblastic proliferation and upregulation of collagen expression. Weeks to months after a series of treatments, increased collagen may be observed histologically in the dermis

Table 3 Nonablative Rejuvenation Devices

Visible lasers	
KTP	532 nm
PDL	577, 585, 595 nm
Infrared lasers	
Nd:YAG	1064 nm
Nd:YAG	1320 nm
Diode	1450 nm
Er:glass	1540 nm
Intense pulsed light	
IPL	515–1200 nm
Low intensity light sources	
Light-emitting diode (LED)	

Er, erbium; IPL, intense pulsed light; KTP, potassium titanyl phosphate; Nd:YAG, neodymium: yttrium-aluminum-garnet; PDL, pulsed dye laser.

(20,48,49). Nonablative devices with shorter wavelengths (e.g., 532-nm KTP) or a wide-action spectrum including such wavelengths (e.g., IPL) may additionally improve epidermal, vascular, and pigmented lesions such as telangiectasias and lentigines. Although nonablative treatments are accomplished without significant downtime, the temporary discomfort induced by some lasers may warrant the use of topical anesthetic prior to treatment. Currently, many investigators disagree on the extent to which the positive histological findings seen after nonablative therapy correlate with objectively verifiable clinical improvement. The absence of a standardized means of evaluating improvement makes it difficult to draw conclusions.

Visible Lasers

The 532-nm KTP laser initially was developed to treat vascular lesions and superficial pigmented lesions, but also it serves as a skin-remodeling tool. After a series of treatments, it was found to not only improve redness and pigmentation, but also skin tone, texture, and fine rhytides (50,51). Histological studies have revealed new collagen and elastin formation.

The PDL has used for years to treat vascular lesions, such as port-wine stains. Keen observers have noted improvement in the texture of skin overlying port-wine stains after a series of treatments. This textural improvement has been demonstrated in photoaged skin in patients without vascular anomalies. Based on these findings, U.S. FDA approval of several PDLs for skin rejuvenation has been obtained. After treatment, histological markers such as type III procollagen, Grenz zone thickness, and hyuronidase are reported to be significantly increased, suggesting new dermal growth (52). It has been hypothesized that these vascular lasers induce nonablative remodeling by stimulating the release of inflammatory mediators from vascular endothelial cells, ultimately leading to the production of new dermal collagen by fibroblasts.

Infrared Lasers

Other than vascular lasers, mid-infrared lasers with deeply penetrating wavelengths also can stimulate new collagen production. The long-pulse 1064-nm Nd:YAG laser targets melanin, hemoglobin, and water, and can penetrate deep enough into the skin for selective dermal heating. However, a 6-month prospective study showed only mild improvement in skin texture, tone, and fine rhytides, and to a less degree than that resulting from the 532-KTP laser (51).

The 1540-nm Er:glass laser is one of three lasers in this class that targets water and penetrates to a depth of 0.4 to 2.0 mm (53). A prospective study showed slow, progressive clinical improvement of rhytides continuing throughout the 6-month follow-up period in all patients after treatment with 1540-nm laser. Side effects of treatment were limited to transient erythema and edema immediately following laser irradiation. Histological skin changes were not apparent until several months following treatment, when an increase in dermal collagen was noted (54). The 1320-nm Nd:YAG laser, another mid-infrared device, was the first commercially available system designed for nonablative skin remodeling. It is coupled with cryogen spray cooling to protect the epidermis. Several studies have shown that the 1320-nm laser can trigger new collagen formation and associated clinical improvement without epidermal ablation (55,56). The 1450-nm diode laser is similar in wavelength and penetration to the other two mid-infrared systems but differs in that it has a lower peak power, which leads to the need for longer exposure times. This protracted pulse, in turn, necessitates cooling that is delivered in a sequence of sprays before, during, and after the pulse (57). A controlled prospective study showed mild clinical improvement of facial rhytides after use of the 1450-nm diode laser (58). Based on these results, U.S. FDA clearance for treatment of periorbital wrinkles was obtained in 2002. All three infrared devices (1320, 1450, and 1540 nm) effectively improve textural changes found in photoaging and are effective for treatment of acne scarring.

Another emerging tool is LED devices. LEDs emit a band of light of wavelengths that are broader than typical laser sources but narrower than IPL sources. They can be assembled into large panels that treat the entire face at one time. At much lower energy than conventional laser or even IPL, LED devices effect positive changes in the skin through nonthermal subcellular signal pathways that are yet poorly understood. To date, preliminary data have shown their usefulness for rejuvenation of aging skin, acne treatment, and PDT when combined with photosensitizers (59). Some of the newest nonablative regiments incorporate several different laser procedures for overall facial rejuvenation. One popular technique advocates serial treatment with the 532-nm laser and the long-pulse 1064-nm Nd:YAG for maximal improvement of redness, pigmentation, skin texture, and rhytides (51).

Intense Pulsed Light

As discussed previously, IPL has been found effective in nonablative rejuvenation of the skin. Because they emit wide bandwidths, IPL devices are effective in treating red color tone, vessels, dyspigmentation, and lentigines, in addition to improving skin texture, pore size, and fine wrinkles. The large spot size facilitates treatment of large areas, such as the chest and extremities. For patients, the treatment is more comfortable than the deep penetrating infrared nonablative lasers.

Light-Emitting Diodes

LEDs are ubiquitous in our daily lives. They are commonly used as lecture pointers, but it is only recently that they have begun to make inroads into the practice of medicine as a result of newly manufactured higher-intensity diodes. For years we have known of the effects of what has been termed low-level energy lasers. These milliwatt devices have been demonstrated to have biological effects on tissue. The effects appear to be both wavelength and pulse duration sensitive. Early data suggest that if the correct wavelength and pulse characteristics are chosen, collagen stimulation can be induced with virtually no unwanted tissue effects. Further research is pending to better characterize these findings.

RADIOFREQUENCY DEVICES

A bipolar multielectrode device (Coblation System, ArthorCare Corp, Sunnyvale, CA) has been introduced as an alternative to laser skin resurfacing. Initially used for arthroscopic surgery, it has been adapted to induce controlled tissue injury that leads to cutaneous resurfacing (60). Coblation differs from traditional electrosurgery, which uses high-energy radiofrequency (RF), generating temperatures exceeding 400°C. In contrast, the multielectrode system used for skin resurfacing permits precise ablation of soft tissue while minimizing damage to surrounding epithelium. Electrical energy is delivered only to the skin, passing through a saline conductive medium and returning via the receptive electrode. Temperatures generated with this system are modest, ranging from 70°C to 100°C. Histologically, RF ablation causes epidermal separation and minor thermal damage in the upper dermis. A multicenter study found acceptable safety and efficacy for treatment of facial rhytides (61). However, the outcome appears technique dependent, and the potential for adverse outcomes, such as scarring, can be high in inexperienced hands.

A device combining both conducted RF and IPL for multiple applications was introduced recently (Syneron, Toronto, Canada). In this device, the addition of RF permits reduced delivery of light energy and a better safety profile. The IPL portion of the device appears to produce results similar to other IPL devices. Adding RF may increase the ability to rid blonde and white hairs and has been purported to improve the outcome after photorejuvenation. Further work is needed to confirm these findings (62).

Another device based on RF holds great promise for rejuvenation of the aging face via aggressive nonablative resurfacing and wrinkle reduction. Unlike noninvasive devices that require numerous treatments over many months to achieve modest cosmetic benefits, this technology of RF nonablative therapy (ThermaCool TC System, Thermage, Hayward, CA) purports to offer results in one or two treatments. Uniform heating is delivered at greater depths than possible with light-based technologies, and epidermal injury is avoided. Treatments can be performed in an outpatient setting with minimal recovery time. In November 2002, the U.S. FDA granted clearance to the ThermaCool TC System for noninvasive treatment of periorbital rhytides based on clinical data from a multicenter study showing that a single nonablative treatment with the device can safely improve the appearance of periorbital skin (63). Since then, this device has been applied to the lower face and neck to tighten the skin and produce significant improvement in facial contours (Figs. 11 and 12). Anecdotal reports indicate at least sporadic efficacy in lifting eyebrows and flattening nasolabial folds.

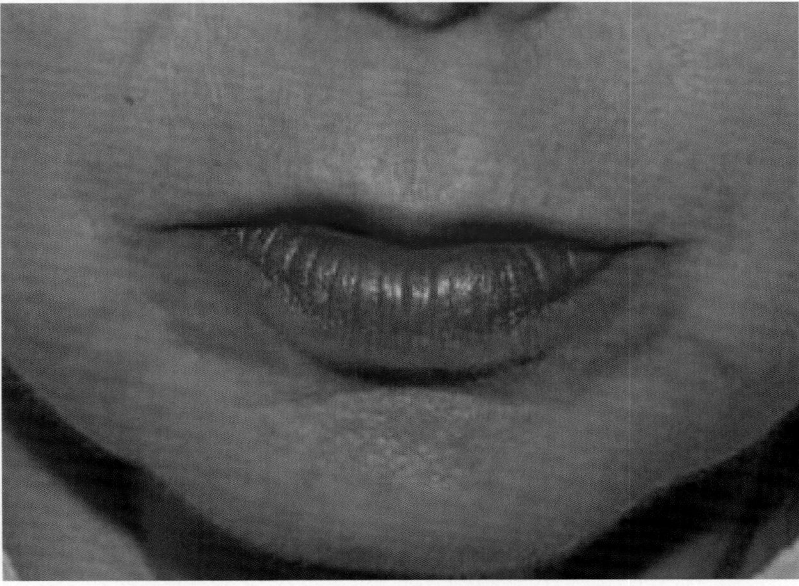

Figure 11 Before treatment with radiofrequency. (Courtesy of R. Weiss, M.D.)

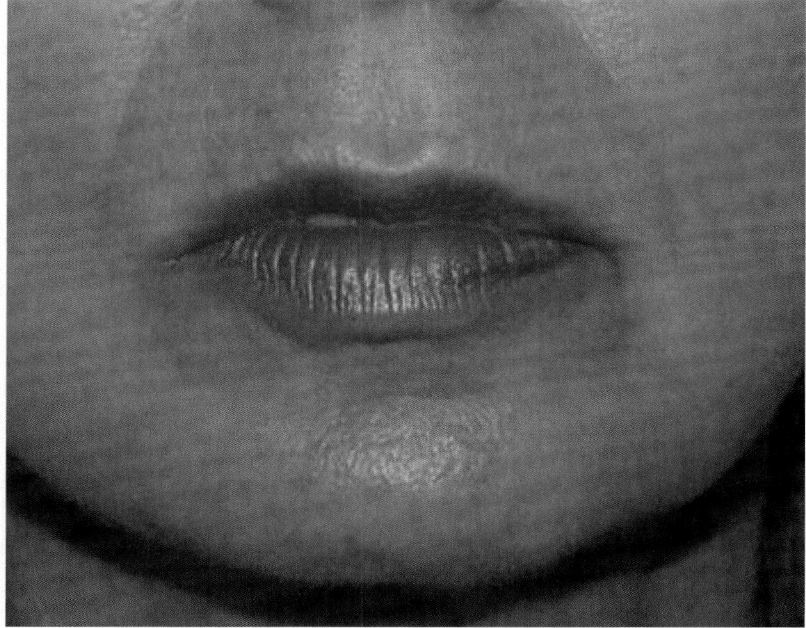

Figure 12 After one treatment with radiofrequency. Note tightening of the jaw line. (Courtesy of R. Weiss, M.D.)

Unlike lasers, which target specific chromophores using optically generated thermal energy, RF-related heat generation is derived from the tissue's natural resistance to the movement of electrons within an RF field. Once the energy reaches the skin, a dual effect is observed. First, primary collagen contraction, similar to that seen with ablative carbon dioxide laser (CO_2) resurfacing, is possibly the short-term mechanism of action. Secondary collagen synthesis in response to thermal injury may occur over a longer time period (64). Empirically, some patients see an immediate response, although the majority report improvement beginning at 4 to 8 weeks and continuing for as long as 6 months or more after a single treatment. With further study, nonablative RF treatment may become a primary tool for skin rejuvenation in the near future.

PHOTODYNAMIC THERAPY

Actinic keratoses (AK) are the most common incipient tumors in the aging skin. It has been estimated that 60% of predisposed persons older than 40 years have at least one AK (65). Left untreated, these lesions may progress to invasive squamous cell carcinomas. Cryotherapy is the most common method used to treat AK. It is a fast, effective, and inexpensive way to care for patients with only a few lesions. Aggressive treatment sometimes leads to hypopigmentation and scars, which are particularly disturbing to patients with multiple lesions. In these cases, topical treatments such as 5-fluorouracil or imiquimod, are indicated to achieve a treatment field effect over wide areas, but patient compliance becomes an issue because these treatments often lead to weeks of irritation and extreme erythema, which may be cosmetically unacceptable.

PDT is a promising alternative that couples the topical application of 5-aminolevulinate (ALA) to skin lesions with subsequent illumination by visible light. In vivo, preferential uptake of ALA by malignant cells is followed by enzymatic conversion to protoporphyrin IX (PpIX), a photosensitizer that promotes destruction of treated cells when exposed to light. The efficacy of this treatment is well documented (66). A single photodynamic treatment with topical ALA revealed a 71% to 91% response rate for lesions on the face and scalp (67). Cosmetic outcome has been excellent, due to the selectivity of the ALA for diseased cells.

Given that the absorption spectrum of PpIX peaks in the range from 350 to 450 nm, blue light was initially used to sensitize PpIX. This protocol called for overnight application of ALA followed by irradiation with a blue light source. However, significant pain, swelling, redness, and crusting ensued. It was later discovered that the absorption spectrum of PpIX is wide enough to allow the use of other light sources that may be less associated with inconvenient signs and symptoms. Recent data indicate efficacy with 1 to 3 hours of ALA application followed by either IPL or PDL, both of which induce less patient discomfort than blue light. The success of PDT treatment for AK has spurred trials for the treatment of Bowen's disease, basal cell carcinoma, and other tumors. Early results for various superficial tumors are promising. The use of PDT in acne, warts, port-wine stains, and alopecia areata is being investigated (68). It was discovered recently that the application of photosensitizers prior to IPL or PDL treatment may enhance rejuvenation of photoaged skin. This ''boost'' therapy may achieve the desired clinical endpoint with fewer treatments than conventional nonablative therapy.

CONTROVERSIES/NEW ON THE HORIZON

Although CO_2 and Er:YAG lasers remain the standard for rejuvenating photodamaged skin, nonablative lasers and IPL are able to effect modest collagen remodeling with much less downtime. As described earlier, one current challenge facing laser scientists is the further refinement of nonablative modalities to produce more consistent and noticeable results. IPL holds particular promise given its ability to harness multiple wavelengths to provide a balanced overall cosmetic benefit. Similarly, nonablative RF treatment is a nascent technology that likely will become increasingly effective as it is refined.

Presently, there is no evidence to suggest that nonablative laser treatments are harmful, but it is interesting that the histological description of horizontally distributed collagen in photodamaged skin resembles the findings observed after a series of nonablative laser treatment. Like skin treated with nonablative laser, photoaged dermis includes a broad band of eosinophilic material (Grenz zone) immediately under the epidermis (69). Better elucidation of the biochemical and biophysical mechanisms underlying nonablative therapy is likely to not only increase confidence in its safety but also permit magnification of its efficacy in a wide cross-section of photodamaged patients.

The availability of PDT to treat widespread AK, and possibly other superficial skin tumors, widens the applicability of lasers and light sources in the treatment of photoinjury. Now light can not only reduce the unattractive visible signs of photodamage but also potentially forestall the emergence of invasive nonmelanoma skin cancers.

REFERENCES

1. Bernstein EF, Andersen D, Zelickson BD. Laser resurfacing for dermal photoaging. Clin Plast Surg 2000; 27:221–240.
2. Anderson RR. Lasers in dermatology—a critical update. J Dermatol 2000; 27:700–705.
3. Dierickx CC, Casparian JM, Venugopalan V, Farinelli WA, Anderson RR. Thermal relaxation of port-wine stain vessels probed in vivo: the need for 1–10-millisecond laser pulse treatment. J Invest Dermatol 1995; 105:709–714.
4. Anderson RR, Parrish JA. Selective photothermolysis: precise microsurgery by selective absorption of pulsed radiation. Science 1983; 220:524–527.
5. Anderson RR. Laser tissue interactions in dermatology. In: Arndt KA, Dover JS, Eds. Lasers in Cutaneous and Aesthetic Surgery. Philadelphia: Lippincott-Raven, 1997:25.
6. Zenzie HH, Altshuler GB, Smirnov MZ, Anderson RR. Evaluation of cooling methods for laser dermatology. Lasers Surg Med 2000; 26:130–144.
7. Pfefer TJ, Smithies DJ, Milner TE, Gemert MJ, Nelson JS, Welch AJ. Bioheat transfer analysis of cryogen spray cooling during laser treatment of port wine stains. Lasers Surg Med 2000; 26:145–157.
8. Anderson RR. Lasers in dermatology—a critical update. J Dermatol 2000; 27:700–705.
9. Nelson JS, Majaron B, Kelly KM. Active skin cooling in conjunction with laser dermatologic surgery. Semin Cutan Med Surg 2000; 19:253–266.
10. Raulin C, Greve B, Hammes S. Cold air in laser therapy: first experiences with a new cooling system. Lasers Surg Med 2000; 27:404–310.
11. Polla LL, Margolis RJ, Dover JS, Whitaker D, Murphy GF, Jacques SL, Anderson RR. Melanosomes are a primary target of Q-switched ruby laser irradiation in guinea pig skin. J Invest Dermatol 1987; 89:281–286.
12. Eremia S, Li C, Umar SH. A side-by-side comparative study of 1064 nm Nd:YAG, 810 nm diode and 755 nm alexandrite lasers for treatment of 0.3–3 mm leg veins. Dermatol Surg 2002; 28:224–230.
13. Adrian RM, Tanghetti EA. Long pulse 532-nm laser treatment of facial telangiectasia. Dermatol Surg 1998; 24:71–74.
14. Groot D, Rao J, Johnston P, Nakatsui T. Algorithm for using a long-pulsed Nd:YAG laser in the treatment of deep cutaneous vascular lesions. Dermatol Surg 2003; 29:35–42.
15. Raulin C, Greve B, Grema H. IPL technology: a review. Lasers Surg Med 2003; 32:78–87.
16. Sadick NS, Weiss R. Intense pulsed-light photorejuvenation. Semin Cutan Med Surg 2002; 21:280–287.
17. Weiss RA, Weiss MA, Beasley KL. Rejuvenation of photoaged skin: 5 years results with intense pulsed light of the face, neck, and chest. Dermatol Surg 2002; 28:1115–1119.
18. Goldberg DJ, Cutler KB. Nonablative treatment of rhytids with intense pulsed light. Lasers Surg Med 2000; 26:196–200.
19. Zelickson KB, Kist KB. Effect of pulsed dye laser and intense pulsed light. Lasers Surg Med Suppl 2000; 12:68.
20. Goldberg DJ. Full-face nonablative dermal remodeling with a 1320 nm Nd:YAG laser. Dermatol Surg 2000; 26:915–918.
21. Goldberg DJ. New collagen formation after dermal remodeling with an intense pulsed light source. J Cutan Laser Ther 2000; 2:59–61.
22. Fitzpatrick RE, Goldman MP, Ruiz-Esparza J. Laser treatment of benign pigmented epidermal lesions using a 300 nsecond pulse and 510 nm wavelength. J Dermatol Surg Oncol 1993; 19: 341–347.
23. Murphy GF, Shepard RS, Paul BS, Menkes A, Anderson RR, Parrish JA. Organelle-specific injury to melanin-containing cells in human skin by pulsed laser irradiation. Lab Invest 1983; 49:680–685.
24. Stern RS, Dover JS, Levin JA, Arndt KA. Laser therapy versus cryotherapy of lentigines: a comparative trial. J Am Acad Dermatol 1994; 30:985–987.

25. Chan HH, Fung WK, Ying SY, Kono T. An in vivo trial comparing the use of different types of 532 nm Nd:YAG lasers in the treatment of facial lentigines in Oriental patients. Dermatol Surg 2000; 26:743–749.
26. Hardaway CA, Ross EV. Nonablative laser skin remodeling. Dermatol Clin 2002; 20:97–111, ix.
27. Glogau RG. Aesthetic and anatomic analysis of the aging skin. Semin Cutan Med Surg 1996; 15:134–138.
28. Tsuji T. Ultrastructure of deep wrinkles in the elderly. J Cutan Pathol 1987; 14:158–164.
29. Pierard GE, Lapiere CM. The microanatomical basis of facial frown lines. Arch Dermatol 1989; 125:1090–1092.
30. Green HA, Domankevitz Y, Nishioka NS. Pulsed carbon dioxide laser ablation of burned skin: in vitro and in vivo analysis. Lasers Surg Med 1990; 10:476–484.
31. Walsh JT, Flotte TJ, Anderson RR, Deutsch TF. Pulsed CO_2 laser tissue ablation: effect of tissue type and pulse duration on thermal damage. Lasers Surg Med 1988; 8:108–118.
32. Dover JS, Hruza GJ, Arndt KA. Lasers in skin resurfacing. Semin Cutan Med Surg 2000; 19: 207–220.
33. Chernoff KA, Schoenrock KA, Cramer KA. Cutaneous laser resurfacing. Int J Aesth Restor Surg 1995; 3:57–68.
34. Arnoczky SP, Aksan A. Thermal modification of connective tissues: basic science considerations and clinical implications. J Am Acad Orthop Surg 2000; 8:305–313.
35. Weinstein C, Roberts TL. Aesthetic skin resurfacing with the high-energy ultrapulsed CO2 laser. Clin Plast Surg 1997; 24:379–405.
36. Kaufmann R, Hibst R. Pulsed Erbium:YAG laser ablation in cutaneous surgery. Lasers Surg Med 1996; 19:324–330.
37. Hohenleutner U, Hohenleutner S, Baumler W, Landthaler M. Fast and effective skin ablation with an Er:YAG laser: determination of ablation rates and thermal damage zones. Lasers Surg Med 1997; 20:242–247.
38. Hughes PS. Skin contraction following erbium:YAG laser resurfacing. Dermatol Surg 1998; 24:109–111.
39. Khatri KA, Ross V, Grevelink JM, Magro CM, Anderson RR. Comparison of erbium:YAG and carbon dioxide lasers in resurfacing of facial rhytides. Arch Dermatol 1999; 135:391–397.
40. Adrian RM. Pulsed carbon dioxide and long pulse 10-ms erbium-YAG laser resurfacing: a comparative clinical and histologic study. J Cutan Laser Ther 1999; 1:197–202.
41. Rostan EF, Fitzpatrick RE, Goldman MP. Laser resurfacing with a long pulse erbium:YAG laser compared to the 950 ms pulsed CO(2) laser. Lasers Surg Med 2001; 29:136–141.
42. Goldman MP, Marchell N, Fitzpatrick RE. Laser skin resurfacing of the face with a combined CO_2/Er:YAG laser. Dermatol Surg 2000; 26:102–104.
43. Fitzpatrick RE, Tope WD, Goldman MP, Satur NM. Pulsed carbon dioxide laser, trichloroacetic acid, Baker-Gordon phenol, and dermabrasion: a comparative clinical and histologic study of cutaneous resurfacing in a porcine model. Arch Dermatol 1996; 132:469–471.
44. Rohrer TE. Lasers and cosmetic dermatologic surgery for aging skin. Clin Geriatr Med 2001; 17:769–794, vii.
45. Fitzpatrick RE, Goldman MP, Satur NM, Tope WD. Pulsed carbon dioxide laser resurfacing of photo-aged facial skin. Arch Dermatol 1996; 132:395–402.
46. Scarborough WD, Herron JB, Khan AJ, Bisaccia E. Periorbital rejuvenation for early signs of aging. Skin and Aging 2003; 11:45–52 .
47. Rohrer TE. Lasers and cosmetic dermatologic surgery for aging skin. Clin Geriatr Med 2001; 17:769–794, vii.
48. Goldberg DJ. New collagen formation after dermal remodeling with an intense pulsed light source. J Cutan Laser Ther 2000; 2:59–61.
49. Zelickson BD, Kilmer SL, Bernstein E, Chotzen VA, Dock J, Mehregan D, Coles C. Pulsed dye laser therapy for sun damaged skin. Lasers Surg Med 1999; 25:229–236.

50. Bernstein E. Nonablative skin rejuvenation. Controversies in Cutaneous Laser Surgery. Woodstock, Vt, 2000.
51. Lee MW. Combination visible and infrared lasers for skin rejuvenation. Semin Cutan Med Surg 2002; 21:288–300.
52. Zelickson BD, Kilmer SL, Bernstein E, Chotzen VA, Dock J, Mehregan D, Coles C. Pulsed dye laser therapy for sun damaged skin. Lasers Surg Med 1999; 25(3):229–236.
53. Ross EV, Sajben FP, Hsia J, Barnette D, Miller CH, McKinlay JR. Nonablative skin remodeling: selective dermal heating with a mid-infrared laser and contact cooling combination. Lasers Surg Med 2000; 26:186–195.
54. Lupton JR, Williams CM, Alster TS. Nonablative laser skin resurfacing using a 1540 nm erbium glass laser: a clinical and histologic analysis. Dermatol Surg 2002; 28:833–835.
55. Goldberg DJ. Non-ablative subsurface remodeling: clinical and histologic evaluation of a1320-nm Nd:YAG laser. J Cutan Laser Ther 1999; 1:153–157.
56. Trelles MA. Short and long-term follow-up of nonablative 1320 nm Nd:YAG laser facial rejuvenation. Dermatol Surg 2001; 27:781–782.
57. Hardaway CA, Ross EV. Nonablative laser skin remodeling. Dermatol Clin 2002; 20:97–111, ix.
58. Goldberg DJ, Rogachefsky AS, Silapunt S. Non-ablative laser treatment of facial rhytides: a comparison of 1450-nm diode laser treatment with dynamic cooling as opposed to treatment with dynamic cooling alone. Lasers Surg Med 2002; 30:79–81.
59. Weiss RA, McDaniel DH, Geronemus RG. Review of nonablative photorejuvenation: reversal of the aging effects of the sun and environmental damage using laser and light sources. Semin Cutan Med Surg 2003; 22:93–106.
60. Herne KB, Zachary CB. New facial rejuvenation techniques. Semin Cutan Med Surg 2000; 19:221–231.
61. Grekin RC, Tope WD, Yarborough JM, Olhoffer IH, Lee PK, Leffell DJ, Zachary CB. Electrosurgical facial resurfacing: a prospective multicenter study of efficacy and safety. Arch Dermatol 2000; 136:1309–1316.
62. Syneron company information. http://www.syneron.com/northamerica/
63. Fitzpatrick R, Geronemus R, Goldberg D, Kaminer M, Kilmer S, Ruiz-Esparza J. Vol. First Multi-Center Study of a New Non-Ablative Radiofrequency Device to Tighten Periorbital Tissue. Thermage, Inc., Hayward CA: 2002.
64. Kilmer SL. A New Nonablative Radiofrequency Device: Preliminary Results, Controversies and Conversations in Cutaneous Laser Surgery. Chicago: American Medical Association Press, 2002.
65. Drake LA, Ceilley RI, Cornelison RL, Dobes WL, Dorner W, Goltz RW, Graham GF, Lewis CW, Salasche SJ, Turner ML. Guidelines of care for actinic keratoses. Committee on Guidelines of Care. J Am Acad Dermatol 1995; 32:95–98.
66. Jeffes EW, McCullough JL, Weinstein GD, Fergin PE, Nelson JS, Shull TF, Simpson KR, Bukaty LM, Hoffman WL, Fong NL. Photodynamic therapy of actinic keratosis with topical 5-aminolevulinic acid. A pilot dose-ranging study. Arch Dermatol 1997; 133:727–732.
67. Szeimies RM, Karrer S, Sauerwald A, Landthaler M. Photodynamic therapy with topical application of 5-aminolevulinic acid in the treatment of actinic keratoses: an initial clinical study. Dermatology 1996; 192:246–251.
68. Fritsch C, Goerz G, Ruzicka T. Photodynamic therapy in dermatology. Arch Dermatol 1998; 134:207–214.
69. Chan HH. Photorejuvenation or photoaging: where does one draw the fine line. J Am Acad Dermatol 2002; 47:321–322.

10

Intense Pulsed Light and Nonablative Approaches to Photoaging

Mitchel P. Goldman *La Jolla Spa MD, La Jolla, California, U.S.A.*

Robert A. Weiss / Margaret A. Weiss *Johns Hopkins University School of Medicine, Baltimore, Maryland, U.S.A.*

- Indications for intense pulsed light (IPL) include facial telangiectasias and virtually all skin vascular conditions, scarring, pigmentation, poikiloderma of Civatte, and photorejuvenation for photoaging.
- The peak emission of IPL is the yellow 600-nm band, which most likely facilitates selective absorption by bright red superficial vessels.
- Use of a water-based coupling gel, along with allowing proper thermal relaxation time between synchronized pulses, prevents elevation of epidermal temperatures above 70°C and is an inherent advantage of "multiple sequential pulsing" of the programmable IPL device.
- Photorejuvenation has been described as a dynamic nonablative process involving the use of the IPL to reduce mottled pigmentation and telangiectasias and to smooth the textural surface of the skin.
- IPL treatment is generally administered in a series of three to six procedures in 3- to 4-week intervals with treatment of the entire face, and the patient can return to all activities immediately.

INTRODUCTION

One of the most controversial light-based technologies, first introduced for clinical studies in 1994 and cleared by the U.S. Food and Drug Administration (FDA) in late 1995 as the PhotoDerm™ (ESC/Sharplan, Norwood, MA, now Lumenis, Santa Clara, CA), is the noncoherent filtered flashlamp intense pulsed light (IPL) source. It initially was launched and promoted–as result of pressure from venture capital groups that funded its development in response to the perceived need for a new leg vein therapy–as a radical improvement over existing methods for elimination of leg telangiectasia. Another important feature that was recognized early on was the IPL's ability to be used as a specific modality to minimize the possibility of purpura common to pulsed dye lasers (PDLs). In reality, the device was found to be of far greater utility for indications other than leg telangiectasias. The road to usability, reproducibility, and good results was a long one. It is ironic that it now is considered the gold standard for treatment of many of the signs of photoaging.

The initial claims for use of IPL rather than a short pulsed PDL laser for less purpura were determined to be true and were confirmed by numerous investigators (1–9). Present-day indications have expanded far beyond the treatment of leg veins to include hair removal, facial telangiectasias, virtually all skin vascular conditions, scarring, pigmentation, and poikiloderma of Civatte. The most recent addition is the realm of nonablative treatment of photoaging known as facial rejuvenation or photorejuvenation (1,2,10,11).

The IPL device consists of a flashlamp housed in an optical treatment head with water-cooled reflecting mirrors. Some newer IPLs have water-cooled flashlamps for faster recycle times. An internal filter overlying the flashlamp prevents emission of wavelengths less than 500 nm. Optically coated quartz filters of various types (cutoff filters) are placed over the window of the optical treatment head to eliminate wavelengths lower than that of the filter. Available cutoff filters are 515, 550, 560, 570, 590, 615, 645, 690, and 755 nm. In order to allow optimal transmission of light by decreasing the index refraction of light to the skin, as well as promoting a ''heat sink'' effect, filter crystals are optically coupled to the skin with a water-based gel. The following discussion focuses on the Lumenis technology because our experience is primarily with this device. The IPL devices presently manufactured are listed in Table 1.

WAVELENGTH

The working premise for IPL is that noncoherent light, like many laser wavelengths, can be manipulated with filters to meet the requirements for selective photothermolysis. In this concept, for a broad range of wavelengths, the absorption coefficient of blood in the vessel is higher than that of the surrounding bloodless dermis. When filtered, the Lumenis IPL device is capable of emitting a broad bandwidth of light from 515 to approximately 1200 nm. (Other IPL devices have very different wavelength outputs.) This bandwidth is modified by application of filters that exclude the lower wavelengths. Although the output is not uniform across this spectrum, it has been shown that, during a 10-msec pulse, relatively high doses of yellow light at 600 nm are emitted, with far less red and infrared, although output has been demonstrated beyond 1000 nm (Fig. 1) (3). The peak emission of the optical treatment head in the 600-nm region and other yellow wavelengths most likely facilitates selective absorption by bright red superficial vessels.

Filters presently used for vascular lesions are 515, 550, 560, 570, and 590 nm. Longer filters of 615, 645, 695, and 755 nm, which cut off much more of the yellow wavelengths, are used most commonly for photoepilation and possibly fibroblast stimulation. Key factors in the successful use of IPL not only are filtering and eliminating the lowest wavelengths emitted by the flashlamp, but also the limitless capacity to manipulate pulse durations and to couple these pulse durations with precise resting or thermal relaxation times programmable in a Windows™ operating system environment using the C++

Table 1 Manufacturers and Brand Names of Intense Pulsed Light Devices

Manufacturer	Brand name	Output	Spot sizes	Fluence (max)
Lumenis, Santa Clara, CA www.lumenis.com	PhotoDerm VL/PL	515–1200 nm	4 × 8 mm	90 J/cm^2
	Epilight	590–1200 nm	8 × 35 mm	
	Multilight HR	515–1200 nm	10 × 45 mm	
	VascuLight HR	515–1200 and 1064 nm laser		
	Quantum SR	560–1200 nm		
	Quantum HR	560–1200 nm and 1064 nm laser		
	VascuLight–SR			
Energis Technology, Swansea, UK	Energis Elite IPL	600–950 nm	10 × 50 mm	19 J/cm^2
Danish Dermatologic Development A/S, Hørsholm, Denmark	Elipse	400–950 nm	10 × 48 mm	22 J/cm^2
Medical Bio Care	OmniLight FPL	515–920 nm		45 J
OptoGenesis	EpiCool–Platinum	525–1100 nm		60 J
Primary Tech	SpectralPulse	510–1200 nm		10–20 J
Syneron	Aurora DS	580–980 nm		10–30 J/cm^2
Palomar, Burlington, MA	EsteLux Y	525–1200 nm		15 J
	G	500–670/ 870–1400 nm		30 J
Alderm, Irvine, CA	Prolite	550–900 nm	10 × 20 mm 20 × 25 mm	10–50 J

programming language. This has been termed as multiple synchronized pulsing by the authors.

Selectivity is theoretically obtained for deoxy-hemoglobulin throughout the 600- to 750-nm range. Oxyhemoglobin is characterized by a very high absorption coefficient up to 630 nm; however, absorption drops at longer wavelengths but rises again to a broad peak in the near infrared in the 800- to 900-nm range. It has been shown that blue telangiectasias of the leg are only slightly more deoxygenated compared with red telangiectasias (12,13). In addition, by treating a vessel with multiple pulsing, oxygenated hemoglobin is converted to deoxygenated hemoglobin during the first portion of the sequential pulsing.

An additional advantage of working at higher wavelengths is that longer wavelengths are absorbed less by melanin. Melanin absorption is greatest in the ultraviolet range (240–360 nm) and decreases steadily as a function of increasing wavelength. Because absorption of light by skin is determined primarily by melanin, not only do longer wavelengths penetrate more deeply, reaching relatively deeper blood vessels, but more nonspecific melanin absorption with accompanying epidermal damage is avoided.

SPOT SIZE

When treating blood vessels of the legs, spot size plays a very important role because spot size, along with wavelength, affects penetration depth. A small spot size leads to

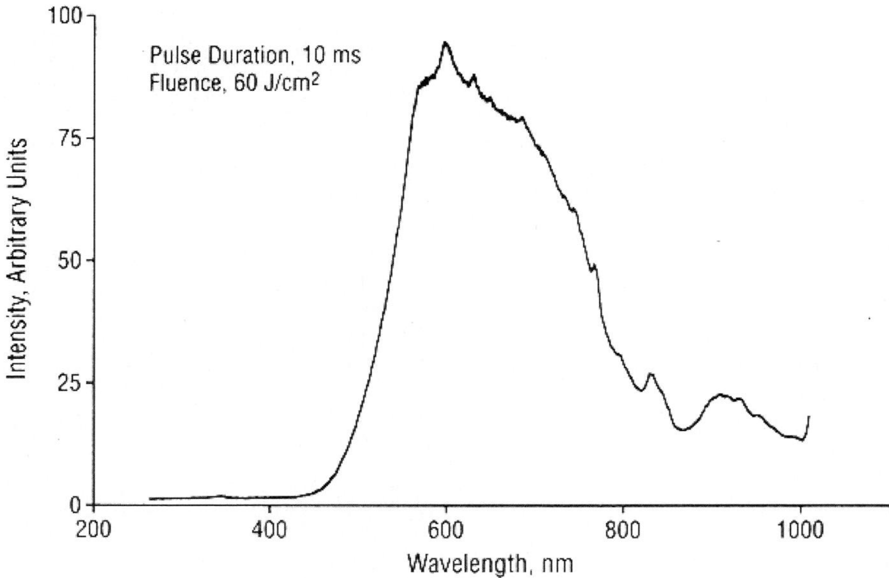

Figure 1 Emission spectrum of an intense pulsed light head with 515-nm filter at 10-msec pulse duration. Peak output at 600 nm is shown by the line. (Courtesy of H. Lubatschowski, Ph.D., Laser Zentrum, Hannover, Germany.)

rapid scatter with a rapid decay of fluence by depth (14); therefore, penetration is more efficient with a large spot size. A depth of 4 mm should be attainable with the 8-mm × 35-mm rectangular spot size of the IPL device considering an average wavelength of 800 nm.

With the large spot size, a tremendous amount of light energy is delivered to the skin. The large planar front of light emitted by the large-footprint IPL must be directed using a water-based interface between the crystal and skin. The water-based gel serves critical functions of enhancing optical coupling, minimizing reflections, and maintaining continuity of the index of refraction of the skin–air interface. Clinical experience has also emphasized the role of gel as a heat sink. Heat is generated by near infrared wavelengths in the epidermis during the programmed 2 to 8 msec of the flashlamp pulse. Water-based gel is efficient at absorbing heat from the epidermis; without use of water-based gel, the skin quickly overheats and protein denaturation of the epidermis occurs, causing subsequent blistering. The gel also may be necessary as a filter for higher wavelengths. Because water absorbs some wavelengths beyond 1000 nm, some of the ineffective or potentially tissue-damaging near infrared wavelengths may be removed prior to being absorbed by the target.

For treating deeper larger vessels requiring a much higher fluence, one may more safely increase fluence while protecting the overlying skin by chilling the gel. A general rule is that when working with the large footprint of IPL, a 1- to 2-mm layer of gel between the crystal and the skin is highly desirable (Fig. 2). This more recently has been termed *floating* the crystal on the gel and is the technique recommended when an integrated

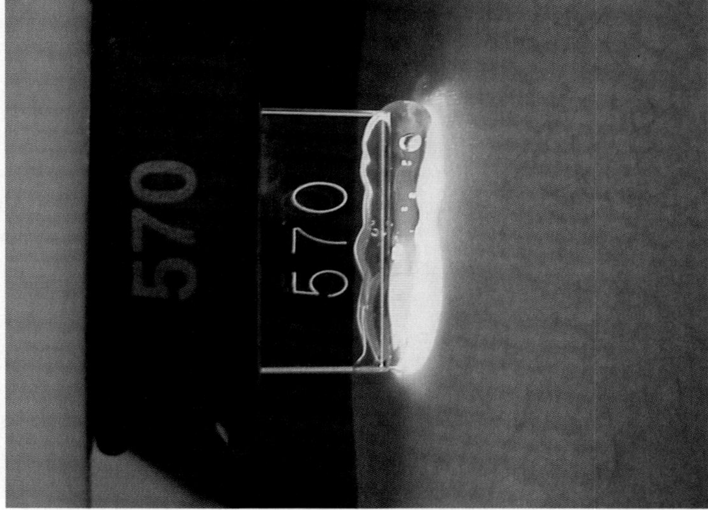

Figure 2 A: Proper spacing of the crystal from the skin with a 2-mm layer of gel or by floating the crystal in gel. If the crystal rests directly on the skin, the likelihood of epidermal injury is far greater. B: With a Peltier cooling device incorporated into the crystal, a smaller layer of gel is required.

chilled crystal is not being used. Use of a thermoelectric, ''refrigerated'' air cooling system with the topical gel provides even more comfort. The colder the gel, the more efficient it becomes as a heat sink. With a thermoelectrically chilled crystal, the ''direct contact'' method with 0.5 to 1 mm of gel is used.

PULSE DURATION

Allowing proper thermal relaxation time between pulses theoretically prevents elevation of epidermal temperatures above 70°C and is an inherent advantage of ''multiple sequential pulsing'' of the IPL device. Thermal relaxation time is the amount of time required for the temperature of a tissue to decrease by a factor $\varepsilon = 2.72$ as a result of heat conductivity. For a typical epidermis thickness of 100 μm, the thermal relaxation time is about 1 msec. For a typical vessel 100 μm (0.1 mm), the thermal relaxation time is approximately 4 msec; for a vessel of 300 μm (0.3 mm), the thermal relaxation time is approximately 10 msec. Therefore, vessels greater than 0.3 mm cool more slowly than the epidermis with a single pulse. For larger vessels, however, multiple pulses may be advantageous, with delay times of 10 msec or more between pulses for epidermal cooling. This delay time must be increased for larger vessels because thermal diffusion across a larger vessel elongates the thermal relaxation time. Multiple sequential pulsing with delay times permits successive heating of targeted vessel(s) with adequate cooling time for the epidermis and surrounding structures.

These theoretical considerations imply the following: (1) Vessels smaller than 0.3 mm should require only a single pulse, although a double pulse should have no adverse effect on treatment; (2) Double or triple pulses should be spaced 10 msec or longer to accommodate normal epidermal thermal relaxation times. A 15- to 20-msec thermal relaxation time might be even safer (and is recommended for patients with skin types that are highly reactive to thermal damage, such as Asian skin); (3) Bright red lesions (oxyhemoglobulin) are better treated with 515- to 590-nm filters; (4) Blue lesions (deoxyhemoglobulin) should be treated with 590 nm or higher filters; (5) Darker skin (melanin) should always be treated with the highest filter available and with double pulses, accompanied by increasing delay times between pulses (typically 20–40 msec) to allow for increased skin thermal relaxation times. For example, treatment of melasma in an individual with Asian skin would involve use of a 590- or 640-nm filter, double pulsed with 3- to 4-msec pulse durations, and fluence just enough to cause a slight pinkness of the treated areas.

Treatment of darker-skinned individuals (types IV–VI) and/or patients with hyperreactive melanocytes becomes of increasing concern when performing photoepilation. In these cases, the 755-nm filter is used primarily with delay times of 50 to 100 msec between pulses to allow sufficient time for the skin to cool down, thus preventing thermal damage.

CONCEPTS OF MULTIPLE PULSING

The newest concepts for IPL and what has contributed most to the success of the technique is the ability to elongate pulse durations for larger vessels, shorten pulse durations for smaller vessels, and use them in a variety of combinations of synchronized short and long pulse widths. For many laser devices used to treat leg veins, a longer pulse duration (up to 50 msec) has led to better clinical results (13,15). For a small vessel (0.3 mm), heat distribution is assumed to occur instantaneously. For a larger vessel, this cannot be assumed because more time is needed for heat to pass from just inside the superficial vessel wall through the vessel to the deeper wall. Additional cooling time is required to release the accumulated heat from the core to the vessel surface. These principles were demonstrated using double-pulse experiments with the 585-nm yellow dye laser in which larger vessels of port wine stain (>0.1 mm) absorbed greater energy fluences before reaching purpura after double pulses spaced 3 to 10 msec apart (16). In another study using pulsed laser irradiation at 585 nm, pulse durations were chosen between short pulse (0.45 msec) and long pulse (10 msec) (17). Results demonstrated that long-duration pulses caused coagulation of the larger-diameter vessels, whereas small-caliber vessels and capillaries showed resistance to photothermolysis at these parameters. This concept has been termed *photokinetic selectivity.*

Applying this to IPL, we have found that increasing pulse durations for IPL up to 12 msec causes larger vessels (≥0.5 mm) to undergo more effective clinical photothermal coagulation while sparing the epidermis (6). Obeying the principles of ''thermokinetic selectivity'' using IPL, we understand that the smaller overlying vessels in the papillary dermis do not absorb efficiently at longer pulse durations, causing less epidermal heating. Longer thermal diffusion times for larger vessels are best served with longer pulse durations for IPL.

The concept of double pulsing for larger telangiectasia is to allow preheating of vessels, with absorption by smaller vessels with the first pulse. This allows surrounding structures to cool. In addition, oxygenated hemoglobin turns to deoxygenated hemoglobin, which absorbs longer wavelengths, and the larger vessel starts to retain heat. The second coupled longer pulse then heats up the larger vessels further in the area under the crystal.

TREATMENT OF PHOTOAGING WITH IPL

Facial Telangiectasias

The treatment of facial telangiectasias is the foundation of treatment of photoaging by IPL. Suggested parameters are listed in Table 2. Clinical observations that skin texture became smoother following treatment of facial telangiectasias were made by authors when treating patients during the period from 1995 to 1997. The authors found it easier to treat facial telangiectasias than leg telangiectasias because facial telangiectasias are generally more uniform in size and depth and have a thinner overlying epidermis (18,19). Facial telangiectasia have thinner vessel walls than leg veins, making them more susceptible to endothelial thermal damage. Response is more predictable; our clinical results approach a 95% resolution rate of facial telangiectasias after one to three treatments. The parameters for IPL of facial telangiectasia include a double pulse of approximately 2.4- to 4-msec duration with a 550-nm filter for light skin and 570-nm filter for darker skin. Delay times are 10 to 20 msec between pulses, with 10-msec delay in light skin and 20 to 40 msec delay in dark and/or Asian skin. Fluences required are much less than for leg veins, typically between 28 and 35 J/cm^2. Higher fluences are used when the second pulse duration is greater than 4.0 msec so that a double pulse of 3.0 and 6.0 msec usually requires a fluence of 40 to 45 J/cm^2 to effectively treat a larger facial vessel (up to 1-mm diameter). The advantage of the IPL over the PDL is that, with the large spot size, an entire cheek of telangiectatic matting can be treated with fewer than a dozen pulses in less than 5 minutes (Fig. 3). In addition, there is little if any purpura. For the larger, more purple telangiectasias typically seen on the nasal alae or for venous lakes or adult port-wine stains, the same settings as for small vessels of leg can be used, i.e., a short pulse followed by a long pulse.

Table 2 Suggested Intense Pulsed Light Parameters for Common Facial Vascular Lesions and Photorejuvenation

Vascular Lesion	Filters (nm)	First pulse (msec)	Delay time (msec)	Second pulse (msec)	Fluence (J/cm^2)	No. of sequential pulses
Telangiectatic matting	550	2.4	10–15	4.0	22–30	Double
Nasal alae telangiectasia	570	2.4–3.0	10–15	5.0–7.0	32–44	Double
Hemangioma	570	2.4–3.0	10–20	6.0–8	32–42	Double
Poikiloderma	515, 550	1.5–2.4	10–20	2.4–4.0	22–36	Single or double
Photodamage, mild	550–570	2.4	10–20	4.0	25–38	Double
Photodamage, moderate (first treatment)	570–590	2.4	10–20	4.0–6.0	22–40	Double
Photodamage, severe	590 or higher	2.4–4.0	20–40	4.0–6.0	22–45	Double

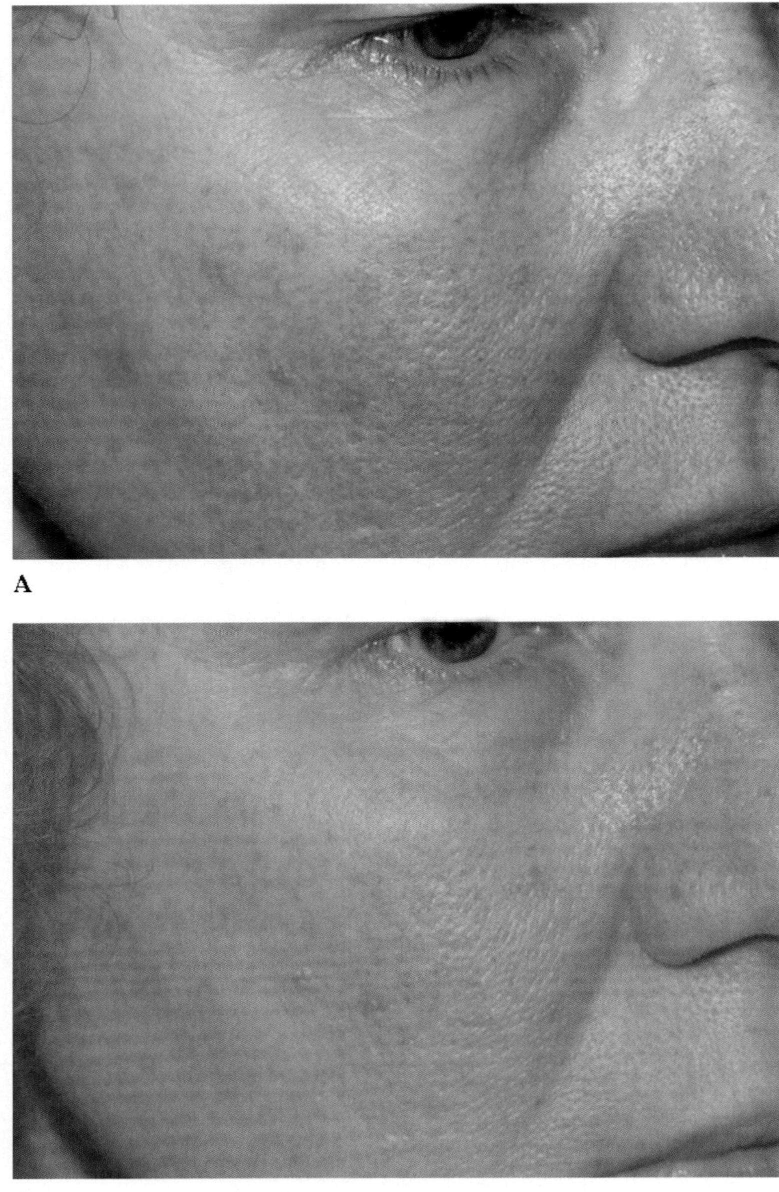

Figure 3 A: Patient with rosacea and the entire cheek is treated with 12 pulses. B: Results after two treatments spaced 1 month apart.

Poikiloderma

A frequently seen manifestation of photoaging is poikiloderma of Civatte. This photoaging process consists of an erythematous, pigmented, finely wrinkled appearance that occurs in sun-exposed areas, mostly the neck, forehead, and upper chest. For areas of poikiloderma consisting of pigmentation and capillary matting on the neck and lower cheeks, the IPL device is ideal with use of a 515-nm filter, which allows absorption simultaneously by melanin and hemoglobin (Fig. 4). For patients with more dyspigmentation, one begins with higher filters, such as 550 or 560 nm, to prevent excessive epidermal absorption that would result in crusting and swelling lasting for several days. Additional treatments with the IPL can be performed with a 550-, 560-, or 570-nm filter to treat the vascular component of poikiloderma. For patients with the most severe form of poikiloderma, one may need to begin with the 590-nm filter and use lower filters on subsequent treatments.

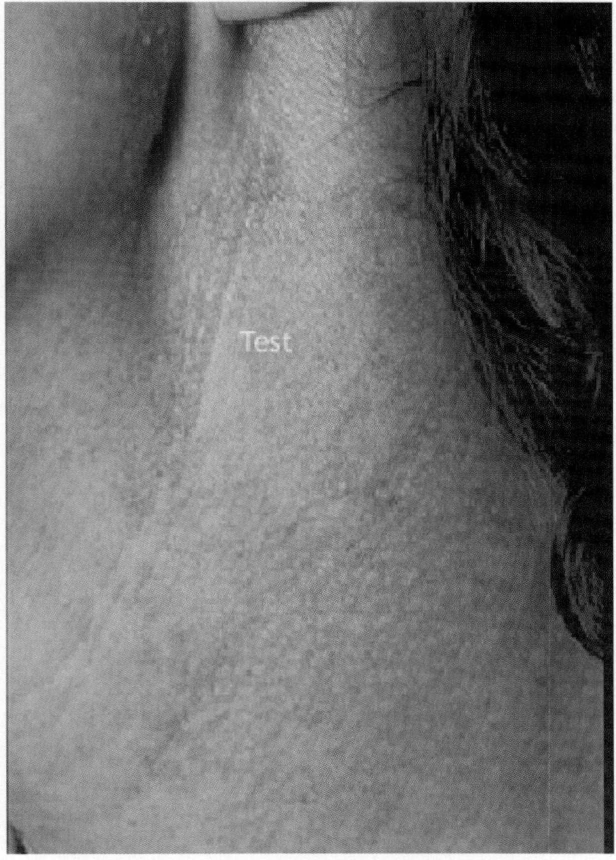

Figure 4 Treatment of poikiloderma of the neck. Initial treatment with single 3-msec pulse, 25 J/cm^2, 515-nm filter results in clearance in an area of two test pulses. Test area is outlined by arrows.

Treatment of poikiloderma is one of the most effective uses of IPL technology (1). In a previous study, 135 randomly selected patients with typical changes of poikiloderma of Civatte on the neck and/or upper chest underwent one to five IPL treatments (1). Parameters included the 515- and 550-nm filters with pulse durations of 2 to 4 msec, either single or double with a 10-msec delay. Fluences were between 20 and 40 J/cm^2. Clearance over 75% of both telangiectasia and hyperpigmentation was reported. The total incidence of side effects was 5%, including temporary hyperpigmentation and hypopigmentation. In many cases, improved skin texture as a result of treatment was noted by both the physician and the patient. Possibly due to either the near infrared component of IPL and/or an interaction of blood vessels with release of various endothelial and fibroblastic growth factors, there appears to be a collagen remodeling effect with improved skin texture reversing the cutaneous atrophy component of poikiloderma of Civatte.

PHOTOREJUVENATION

The overall appearance of aging skin is primarily related to the quantitative effects of sun exposure with resultant ultraviolet damage of structural components such as collagen and elastic fibers. However, appearance also is affected by genetic factors, intrinsic factors, disease processes such as rosacea, and overall loss of cutaneous elasticity associated with age. With excessive sun exposure in addition to depletion of the ozone layer, visible signs of aging have become more evident in younger individuals. Photorejuvenation has been described as a dynamic nonablative process involving use of the IPL to reduce mottled pigmentation and telangiectasias and to smooth the textural surface of the skin (2). The treatment is generally administered in a series of three to six procedures in 3- to 4-week intervals. The entire face is treated, rather than a limited affected area, and the patient can return to all activities immediately. Marketing has made the public and medical community aware of these changes through various unsuccessfully applied for service trademarks such as Photofacial, Fotofacial, Facialite, and others. An example of photorejuvenation of photoaging is shown in Fig. 5.

Zelickson et al. (20,21) demonstrated that IPL treatment results in an 18% increase in collagen type I transcripts, whereas pulse dye laser (PDL) treatment results in a 23% increase in collagen type I transcripts. This may explain the improvement in fine wrinkling with photorejuvenation. More details reveal that collagen I, collagen III, elastin, and collagenase increased in 85% to 100% of patients and procollagen increased in 50% to 70% of patients.

Hernandez-Perez et al. (22) evaluated the histological effects of five IPL treatments with 570 to 645 nm, 2.4 to 6.0 msec, delay 20 msec, and 25 to 42 J/cm^2. They showed epidermal thickening of 100 to 300 μm, better cellular polarity, a decrease in horny plugs, new rete ridge formation, decreased elastosis, and dermal neo-collagen formation.

However, in a histologic study in patients with rosacea, Prieto et al. (23) did not observe evidence of changes in collagen, elastic, or reticular fibers, but they did note coagulated Demodex that recurred after 3 months. They treated patients with the following parameters: 560 nm, 2.4 to 4.2 msec, 15-msec delay, and 28 to 36 J/cm^2, five times every month.

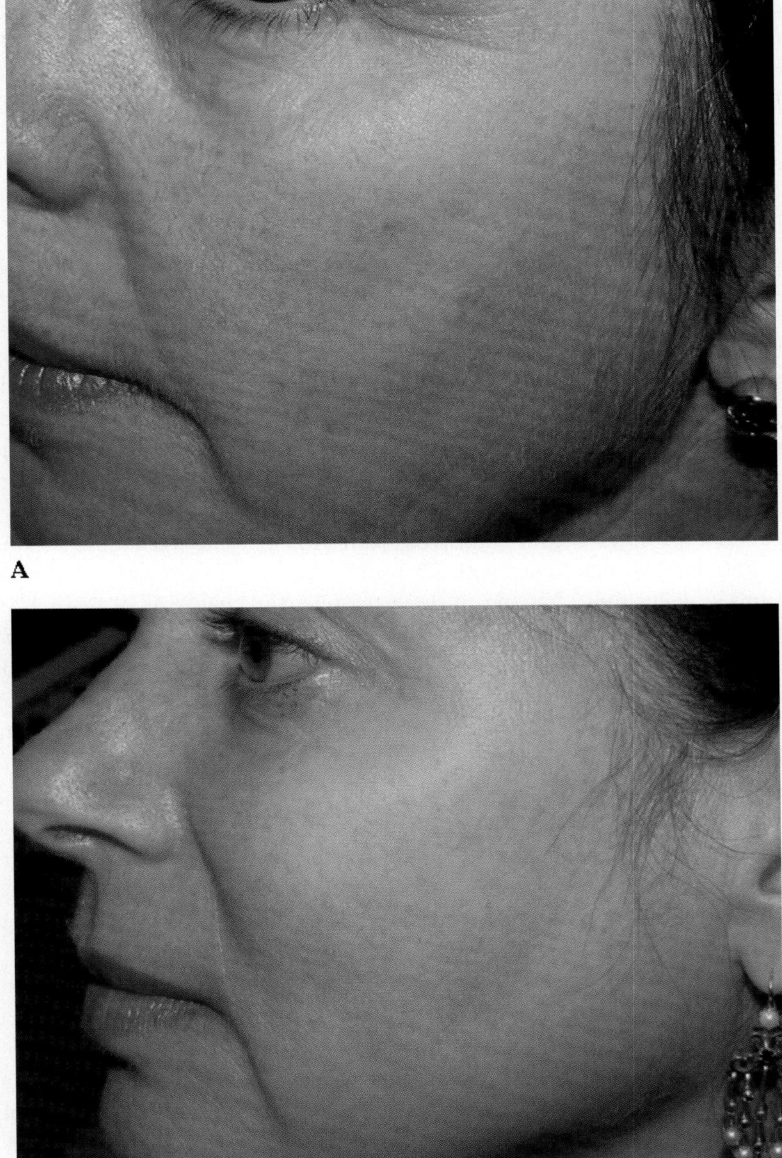

Figure 5 Photorejuvenation before (A) and after (B) three treatments. There is excellent reduction of the photoaging components of mottled pigmentation and telangiectasias, with smoothing of the textural surface of the skin.

Negishi et al. (24) treated 73 patients in five sessions with the Quantum IPL every 3 to 4 weeks at the following settings: 560 nm, 2.8 to 6.0 msec, 20- to 40-msec delay, and 23 to 27 J/cm^2. Eighty percent of their Japanese patients had greater than 60% improvement in pigmentation and erythema with smoother skin. The Quantum IPL has an integrated skin cooling crystal that cools the epidermis to 40°C during IPL versus 65°C without cooling.

With the original IPL, Negishi et al. (25) reported photorejuvenation in 97 Japanese patients using 550- to 570-nm cutoff filters (550 nm for pigment and 570 nm for telangiectasia). Patients were treated three to six times at 2- to 3-week intervals with IPL settings of 28 to 32 J/cm^2, 2.5 to 4.0/4.0 to 5.0 msec, 20- to 40-msec delay without topical anesthesia. They noted that 49% had greater than 75% improvement in pigmentation, 33% had greater than 75% improvement in telangiectasia, and 13% had greater than 75% improvement in skin texture. Approximately 50% of the other patients had greater than 50% improvement in these parameters as well. There were no episodes of hyperpigmentation, including four patients with melasma. Histological evidence of collagen and elastic fiber proliferation in the papillary and subpapillary layers was present in biopsies taken at the end of the study.

Treatment of freckling is improved with IPL photorejuvenation. Huang et al. (26) used 550- to 590-nm filters with 25 to 35 J/cm^2, 4-msec single or double pulse, 20- to 40-msec delay time, for one to three treatments (mean 1.4) at 4-week intervals. Their endpoint was graying or perilesional erythema. Of these patients, 91.7% were extremely/very satisfied with treatment. Kawada et al. (27) also treated freckling and lentigo in Asian skin. They used a Quantum IPL at the following parameters: 560 nm, 20 to 24 J/cm^2, 2.6 to 5.0 msec, 20-msec delay, for three to five treatments at 2- to 3-week intervals. No adverse effects were noted, and patients reported that small patches and ephelides responded best (48% of patients with >50% improvement; 20% of patients with >75% improvement).

Weiss et al. (28) evaluated 80 of their initial patients treated for vascular lesions to determine if ‘‘photorejuvenation’’ also occurred. Images from three subsequent visits including one follow-up at 4 years were graded. There was 80% improvement in pigmentation, telangiectasia, and skin texture. Hypopigmentation lasting for 1 year occurred in 2.5%, temporary mild crusting occurred in 19%, erythema lasting more than 4 hours in 15%, hypopigmentation or hyperpigmentation in 5%, and rectangular footprinting in 5%.

In a previous study, 49 subjects with varying degrees of photodamage were treated with a series of four or more full-face treatments at 3-week intervals using IPL (VascuLight™ IPL, Lumenis). Fluences varied from 30 to 50 J/cm^2, with typical settings of double or triple pulse trains of 2.4 to 4.7 msec and pulse delays of 10 to 60 msec. Cutoff filters of 550 or 570 nm were used for all treatments (2). Photodamage including wrinkling, skin coarseness, irregular pigmentation, pore size, and telangiectasias was improved in more than 90% of the patients. Treatments involved IPL of the entire facial skin, except in males who elected not to have treatment of the beard area because of potential for hair loss. In this study, 72% of subjects reported 50% or greater improvement in skin smoothness and 44% reported 75% or greater improvement. Minimal side effects were reported, with temporary discoloration consisting of a darkening of lentigines that resolved completely within 7 days. Two subjects reported a ‘‘downtime’’ of 1 and 3 days due to moderate-to-severe swelling.

The use of IPL with a thermoelectrically chilled crystal delivery system (Quantum SR) on 20 patients for photorejuvenation has been evaluated (29). These patients underwent three monthly IPL treatments on the face, neck, and/or anterior chest. A 560-nm cutoff filter was used with a double pulse of 2.4 and 6.0 msec, separated by a 15-msec delay time. Fluences ranged from 26 to 30 J/cm^2. Telangiectasia improved in 84% of patients, dyspigmentation in 78%, and skin texture in 78%. Side effects were minimal and consisted of localized edema in 50% for less than 8 hours and erythema lasting from 2 to 24 hours.

The dual-mode filtering IPL system Elipse Flex DDD for facial photorejuvenation was evaluated in 20 women (30). First, areas of telangiectasia were treated with a pulse duration of 14 to 30 msec. A second pass was made with a double pulse of 2.5 msec, with a 10-msec delay. Two types of filters were used: 530 to 750 nm at an energy of 11 to 17 J/cm^2, and 555 to 950 nm at a fluence of 13 to 19 J/cm^2. Both groups reported significant improvement in both telangiectasia and pigmentation without adverse sequelae.

Combination IPL and Photorejuvenation

Photorejuvenation may be enhanced with combination procedures, such as the use of IPL with 1064- and 1320-nm neodymium:yttrium-aluminum garnet (Nd:YAG) laser treatments (31,32), microdermabrasion (33), and botulinum toxin A (Botox®, Allergan, Irvine, CA) (34). Muscle relaxation with botulinum A allows for parallel collagen formation over a static dermis. The use of 1064-, 1320-, and 1450-nm wavelengths causes significant structural change in the dermis, which can enhance new collagen formation and further reducing wrinkling.

Miscellaneous Pigmentation

In addition to hyperpigmentation from photodamage as described in the preceding section, other forms of pigmentation have been treated successfully with IPL. Nineteen Chinese patients ranging in age from 8 to 51 years with postburn hyperpigmentation were treated in three to seven sessions with 550-, 570-, and 590-nm filters at the following parameters: 1.7 to 4 msec, 15- to 40-msec delay, and 28 to 46 J/cm^2 (35). Of these patients, 78% had greater than 50% improvement, 32% had greater than 5% improvement, and 2 of 19 had no improvement. There was no recurrence during follow-up of 11 to 32 months.

Photodynamic Skin Rejuvenation

The combination of IPL and photodynamic therapy sensitizers such as 5-aminolevulinic acid (ALA; Levulan, DUSA Pharmaceuticals, Wilmington, MA) allows for new options in the treatment of severely photodamaged skin (36) and may offer a significant cosmetically beneficial alternative to photodynamic treatments with blue light for conditions such as actinic keratoses (37), early skin cancers (38), and cystic acne (39).

We have termed this advanced technique photodynamic skin rejuvenation (PSR). The PSR application of PDT (photodynamic therapy) involves activation of a specific photosensitizing agent (ALA) by conventional IPL as provided by the VascuLight or Quantum system. This process produces activated oxygen species within cells, thus resulting in their elimination or destruction. The topically active agent ALA is the precursor in the heme biosynthesis pathway of protoporphyrin-9, which facilitates cellular destruction. Exogenous administration of ALA, along with 410-nm continuous blue light, has been cleared by the FDA for the treatment of actinic keratosis and appears to have significant long-term efficiency (40). In clinical practice, however, a variety of light sources has been used in photodynamic therapy in an effort to reduce time and discomfort for patients and to enhance the clinical and cosmetic outcome of the procedure. Alexiades-Armenakas et al. (41) were the first to describe the use of 595-nm pulsed light with ALA for treatment of actinic keratoses. Advantages over blue light therapy were decreased pain during treatment, as well as decreased posttreatment erythema and crusting.

Because 595 nm is not an optimal peak of absorption for ALA, a broader wavelength such as that found with the IPL should be even more efficacious in activating ALA. IPL treatments are being studied for such enhanced benefits of photodynamic therapy (42). Short-duration PDT using Levulan for 15 to 60 minutes coupled with a treatment of IPL has shown significant benefit in the treatment of precancerous conditions such as actinic keratoses, as well as actinically damaged skin. In addition, early evidence shows a significant degree of cosmetic enhancement (Fig. 6).

Other variations of the procedure being studied involve single IPL treatments with higher fluences and longer application times, resulting in dramatic decreases in actinic damage in a single treatment with a relatively short duration of healing. In addition, initial studies show promise in the application of topical ALA and IPL skin treatments using photorejuvenation for conditions such as moderate-to-severe acne and rosacea. The mechanism for improvement of acne and rosacea is enhanced absorption of ALA by sebaceous glands. This enhanced absorption, followed by photoactivation with IPL, damages the sebaceous gland, causing its involution. A decease in the size and/or activity of the sebaceous gland then leads to an improvement of acne.

Combination of the IPL procedure with pharmacologic treatments such as metronidazole topical cream (Metro Cream®, Galderma Laboratories, Ft. Worth, TX) has resulted in significant overall levels of success in the treatment of rosacea (43). The combination of IPL treatment with a variety of depigmenting agents also has resulted in greater resolution of melasma (44).

TREATMENT TECHNIQUE

Photorejuvenation

Floating Technique

For nonchilled crystals, a thick layer of gel must be placed onto the crystal and absolutely no pressure applied as the crystal is placed over the target area, floating the crystal in gel. Compressing this 2- to 3-mm layer of gel against the skin will result in crystal placement too close to the skin, which greatly increases the risks of epidermal injury. Plastic spacers are available to increase the uniformity of distance of crystal and thickness of gel, but most users simply float the crystal holding the weight of the IPL head in their hands.

To minimize rectangular footprinting, a 10% overlap of pulse placement is used. Alternatively, a second pass can be performed with a direction 90 degrees from the original direction.

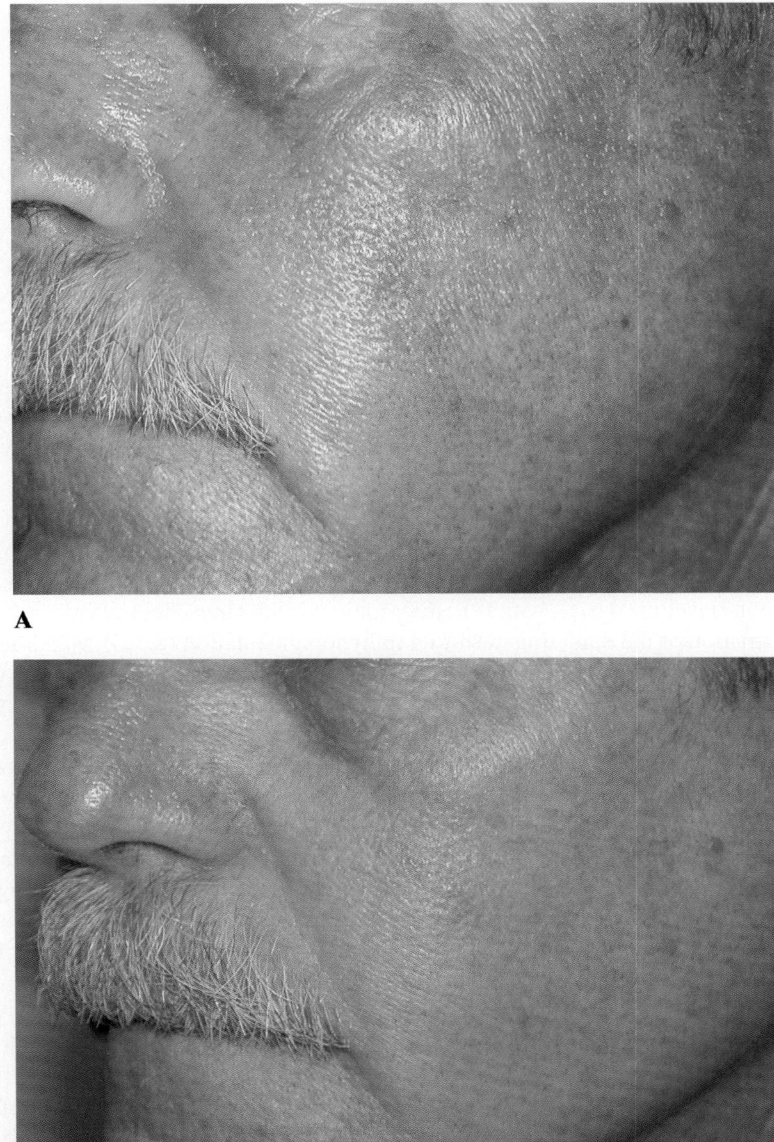

A

B

Figure 6 A: Extensive photodamage and actinic keratosis in a 55-year-old man. B: Six months after treatment with 5-aminolevulinic acid applied to the entire face.

Close Contact Technique

To minimize pain and facilitate uniform treatment among operators, contact cooling or epidermal anesthetic creams are used. Attaching a cooling device that surrounds the crystal has been shown to produce better results with fewer side effects (11). Cooling is maintained by circulating water at 1°C through the metal collar around the crystal. The newest devices incorporate a chilled crystal that is kept in close contact with the skin, while only a small layer of chilled water-based gel is placed between the crystal and the skin. Fluence must be lowered. With absolutely minimal pressure, the cooling device with the crystal is placed directly onto the skin overlying the targeted area. No pressure is applied because the target vessels may shut with compression. EMLA anesthetic cream is not used before treatment because there is a high incidence of vasoconstriction produced by the prilocaine component of EMLA. ELA-max 5% lidocaine (Ferndale Labs, Ferndale, MI) is a better choice and usually is requested by 50% of patients when lower fluences and the direct contact method of the chilled crystal are used.

ADVERSE REACTIONS

During our initial clinical trials with IPL, three patients with tanned legs developed immediate desquamation of the epidermis resulting in hypopigmentation (2.5%), which lasted for 4 to 6 months in two patients and 1 year in the third patient with no permanent pigment change. This occurred at 40 J/cm^2 with a single pulse of 3 msec. No such reaction has been observed on the face, and no long-term sequelae have been noted.

In our subsequent experience with thousands of treatment sessions, there has been an approximately 2% incidence of scattered crusting in areas of increased pigmentation. This typically heals by peeling off within 7 days. We accelerate this process by having the patients apply a moisturizer twice a day and/or undergo a microdermabrasion treatment 1 to 2 days after IPL treatment. When there is no underlying pigmentation, crusting occurs primarily on curved body areas such as the neck over the sternocleidomastoid muscle curvature. Purpura occurs in scattered isolated pulses in about 4% of treatments. Purpura is more likely to occur when the 515-nm filter is used or when the pulse durations are too short, as when a 2.4-msec pulse is coupled with another 2.4-msec pulse. The purpura from IPL is different than typical purpura from short-pulse PDL in that resolution from IPL occurs within 2 to 5 days versus 1 to 2 weeks with PDL.

Other adverse effects of IPL include a stinging pain described as a brief grease splatter, electric shock, or rubber band snapping on the skin during treatment. Typically patients tolerate more than 150 pulses per session. Treatment pain can be minimized by a number of topical anesthetic creams (except EMLA), such as ELA-max (lidocaine 4%; Ferndale Labs). Occasionally a thin nontreated stripe between reticular footprints can be seen. This is easily corrected with subsequent treatment applying the crystal over the nontreated sites or proceeding with treatment using the crystal rotated 90 degrees from the original direction. In the past 8 years, we have observed very few patients in whom small rectangular spots of hypopigmentation at the lateral neck margins persisted by the end of 2 years. This was preceded by epidermal desquamation.

With the newest progressive set of parameters, the incidence of acute side effects has been markedly reduced. Side effects include a mild burning sensation lasting less than 10 minutes noted in 45% and erythema typically lasting several hours to 3 days. Mild cheek swelling or edema occurs 25% of the time with full-face treatments, primarily after the initial treatment, and lasts from 24 to 72 hours. Short-term hyperpigmentation or hypopigmentation (<2 months) has been noted in approximately 8% to 15% of sites treated.

REFERENCES

1. Weiss RA, Goldman MP, Weiss MA. Treatment of poikiloderma of Civatte with an intense pulsed light source. Dermatol Surg 2000; 26:823–827.
2. Bitter PH. Noninvasive rejuvenation of photodamaged skin using serial, full-face intense pulsed light treatments. Dermatol Surg 2000; 26:835–842.
3. Goldberg DJ, Cutler KB. Nonablative treatment of rhytids with intense pulsed light. Lasers Surg Med 2000; 26:196–200.
4. Raulin C, Schroeter CA, Weiss RA, Keiner M, Werner S. Treatment of port-wine stains with a noncoherent pulsed light source: a retrospective study. Arch Dermatol 1999; 135:679–683.
5. Jay H, Borek C. Treatment of a venous-lake angioma with intense pulsed light [letter]. Lancet 1998; 351:112.
6. Weiss RA, Weiss MA, Marwaha S, Harrington AC. Hair removal with a non-coherent filtered flashlamp intense pulsed light source. Lasers Surg Med 1999; 24:128–132.
7. Raulin C, Schroeter C, Maushagen-Schnaas E. [Treatment possibilities with a high-energy pulsed light source (PhotoDerm VL)]. Hautarzt 1997; 48:886–893.
8. Raulin C, Weiss RA, Schonermark MP. Treatment of essential telangiectasias with an intense pulsed light source (PhotoDerm VL). Dermatol Surg 1997; 23:941–945.
9. Raulin C, Goldman MP, Weiss MA, Weiss RA. Treatment of adult port-wine stains using intense pulsed light therapy (PhotoDerm VL): brief initial clinical report [letter]. Dermatol Surg 1997; 23:594–597.
10. Schroeter C, Wilder D, Reineke T. Clinical significance of an intense, pulsed light source on leg telangiectasias of up to 1mm diameter. Eur J Dermatol 1997; 7:38–42.
11. Sadick NS, Weiss RA, Shea CR, Nagel H, Nicholson J, Prieto VG. Long-term photoepilation using a broad-spectrum intense pulsed light source. Arch Dermatol 2000; 136:1336–1340.
12. Weiss RA, Sadick NS. Epidermal cooling crystal collar device for improved results and reduced side effects on leg telangiectasias using intense pulsed light. Dermatol Surg 2000; 26: 1015–1018.
13. Sommer A, Van MP, Neumann HA, Kessels AG. Red and blue telangiectasias. Differences in oxygenation. Dermatol Surg 1997; 23:55–59.
14. Keijzer M, Jacques SL, Prahl SA, Welch AJ. Light distributions in artery tissue: Monte Carlo simulations for finite-diameter laser beams. Lasers Surg Med 1989; 9:148–154.
15. Adrian RM. Treatment of leg telangiectasias using a long-pulse frequency-doubled neodymium:YAG laser at 532 nm. Dermatol Surg 1998; 24:19–23.
16. Dierickx CC, Casparian JM, Venugopalan V, Farinelli WA, Anderson RR. Thermal relaxation of port-wine stain vessels probed in vivo: the need for 1-10 millisecond laser pulse treatment. J Invest Dermatol 1995; 105:709–714.
17. Kimel S, Svaasand LO, Hammer-Wilson M, Schell MJ, Milner TE, Nelson JS. Differential vascular response to laser photothermolysis. J Invest Dermatol 1994; 103:693–700.
18. Goldman MP, Eckhouse S. Photothermal sclerosis of leg veins. ESC Medical Systems, LTD Photoderm VL Cooperative Study Group. Dermatol Surg 1996; 22:323–330.
19. Green D. Photothermal sclerosis of leg veins [letter; comment]. Dermatol Surg 1997; 23: 303–305.
20. Zelickson B, Kist D. Pulsed dye laser and Photoderm treatment stimulates production of type-I collagen and collagenase transcripts in papillary dermis fibroblasts. Lasers Surg Med Abstract Suppl 2001; 3:33.

21. Zelickson B, Kist D. Effect of pulse dye laser and intense pulsed light source on the dermal extracellular matrix remodeling. Lasers Surg Med Abstract Suppl 2000; 12:17.
22. Hernandez-Perez E, Ibiett EV. Gross and microscopic findings in patients submitted to nonablative full face resurfacing using intense pulsed light. Dermatol Surg 2002; 28:651–655.
23. Prieto VG, Sadick NS, Lloreta J, Nicholson J, Shea CR. Effects of intense pulsed light on sun-damaged human skin, routine, and ultrastructural analysis. Lasers Med Surg 2002; 30: 82–85.
24. Negishi K, Wakamatsu S, Kushikata N, Tezuka Y, Kotani Y, Shiba K. Full-face photorejuvenation of photodamaged skin by intense pulsed light with integrated contact cooling. Lasers Surg Med 2002; 30:298–305.
25. Negishi K, Tezuka Y, Kushikata N, Wakamatsu S. Photorejuvenation for Asian skin by intense pulsed light. Dermatol Surg 2001; 27:627–632.
26. Huang YL, Liao YL, Lee SH, Hong HS. Intense pulsed light for the treatment of facial freckles in Asian skin. Dermatol Surg 2002; 28:1007.
27. Kawada A, Shiraishi H, Asai M, Kameyama H, Sangen Y, Aragane Y, Tezuka T. Clinical improvement of solar lentigines and ephelides with an intense pulsed light source. Dermatol Surg 2002; 28:504–508.
28. Weiss RA, Weiss MA, Beasley KL. Rejuvenation of photoaged skin: 5 yr results with IPL. Dermatol Surg 2002; 28:1115.
29. Beasley KL, Weiss RA, Weiss MA. New parameters for intense pulsed light rejuvenation with a thermoelectrically chilled crystal delivery system. Cosmetic Dermatol 2002; 15:14–16.
30. Troilius A, Bjerring P, Dierickx C, Christiansen K. Photorejuvenation with a double exposure procedure using a new IPL system. Laser Surg Med 2002; 14(suppl):29.
31. Goldberg DJ, Whitworth J. Laser skin resurfacing with the Q-switched Nd:YAG laser. Dermatol Surg 1997; 23:903–907.
32. Fatemi A, Weiss MA, Weiss RA. Short-term histologic effects of nonablative resurfacing: results with a dynamically cooled millisecond-domain 1320 nm Nd:YAG laser. Dermatol Surg 2002; 28:172–176.
33. Tan MH, Spencer JM, Pires LM, Ajmeri J, Skover G. The evaluation of aluminum oxide crystal microdermabrasion for photodamage. Dermatol Surg 2001; 27:943–949.
34. Fagien S, Brandt F. Primary and adjunctive use of botulinum toxin type A in facial aesthetic surgery. Clin Plast Surg 2001; 28:127–148.
35. Sun H, Nalim R, Yokota H. Prospective study on the treatment of postburn hyperpigmentation by IPL. Lasers Surg Med 2003; 32:42.
36. Ruiz-Rodriguez R, San-Sanchez T, Cordoba S. Photodynamic photorejuvenation. Dermatol Surg 2002; 28:742–744.
37. Fritsch C, Goerz G, Ruzicka T. Photodynamic therapy in dermatology. Arch Dermatol 1998; 134:207–214.
38. Kalla K, Merk H, Mukhtar H. Photodynamic therapy in dermatology. J Am Acad Dermatol 2000; 42:389–413.
39. Hongcharu W, Taylor CR, Chang Y, Aghassi D, Suthamjariya K, Anderson RR. Topical ALA-photodynamic therapy for the treatment of acne vulgaris. J Invest Dermatol 2000; 115:183–192.
40. Fowler JF, Zax RH. Aminolevulinic acid hydrochloride with photodynamic therapy: efficacy outcomes and recurrence 4 years after treatment. Cutis 2002; 69(6S):2–7.
41. Alexiades-Armenakas M, Kauvar ANB, Bernstein LJ. Laser-assisted photodynamic therapy of actinic keratoses. Lasers Surg Med Suppl 2002; 14:24.
42. Gold MH. The evolving role of aminolevulinic acid hydrochloride with photodynamic therapy in photoaging. Cutis 2002; 69(6S):8–13.
43. Dahl MV, Katz HI, Krueger GG, Millikan LE, Odom RB, Parker F, Wolf JE, Aly R, Bayles C, Reusser B, Weidner M, Coleman E, Patrignelli R, Tuley MR, Baker MO, Herndon JH, Czernielewski JM. Topical metronidazole maintains remission of rosacea. Arch Dermatol 1998; 143:679–683.

44. Taylor SC, Torok HM, Jones T, Lowe N, Rich P, Tschen E, Menter A, Baumann L, Wieder JJ, Jarratt MM, Pariser D, Martin D, Weiss J, Shavin J, Ramirez N. Efficacy and safety of a new triple combination agent for the treatment of facial melasma. Cutis 2003; 72:67–72.
45. Raulin C, Werner S, Hartschuh W, Schonermark MP. Effective treatment of hypertrichosis with pulsed light: a report of two cases. Ann Plast Surg 1997; 39:169–173.
46. Gold MH, Bell MW, Foster TD, Street S. Long-term epilation using the EpiLight broad band, intense pulsed light hair removal system. Dermatol Surg 1997; 23:909–913.
47. Schumults CD, Goldberg DJ. Blinded comparison of two intense pulsed light (IPL) systems for hair removal: clinical efficacy and complication rate. Lasers Surg Med 2003(Suppl 15): 31.

11

Chemical Peels

Gary D. Monheit *University of Alabama at Birmingham, Birmingham, Alabama, U.S.A.*

- Chemical peeling should be classified as superficial, medium, or deep based on the level of penetration and final results.
- Trichloroacetic acid remains the benchmark for all chemical peeling, and depth levels are determined by degree of frosting.
- Chemical peeling is technique sensitive, and complications can occur, which the dermatologist must learn how to handle.

BACKGROUND AND HISTORY OF PROCEDURE

The use of exfoliating agents to peel the epidermis and superficial dermis date back to ancient Egypt. Sour milk baths were used by ancient Egyptian women to soothe the skin. Alabaster, salt, brimstone, pumice stone, and various animal oils once were used to chemically exfoliate the skin and produce a more cosmetically elegant appearance. Fire was once used by the Turks to lightly singe the skin, causing exfoliation and an improved aesthetic glow (1).

In the early twentieth century, phenol was introduced as the premier peeling agent for postacne scarring (2). Paraprofessionals were the first to use phenol, resorcinol, and other acid emollients for exfoliation. Various formulations of phenol peels were tried, both with and without occlusion; however, its use became limited due to severe facial scarring and cardiac toxicity. Baker and Gordon first learned the safe use of thin phenol preparation from a Hungarian esthetician and promoted the present formula written in our literature today.

Between 1940 and 1970, a variety of exfoliating agents were introduced, some of which were combined to cause a deeper dermal injury. Examples include sulfur, resorcinol pastes, salicylic acid, and solid carbon dioxide. Resorcinol is commonly used today in combination with lactic acid, ethanol, and salicylic acid, a formulation known as Jessner's solution.

In the 1950s and 1960s, trichloroacetic acid (TCA) became the agent of choice for superficial, medium and deep peeling. However, use of 50% and greater TCA led to scarring and pigmentary complications that became common among patients treated by dermatologists and plastic surgeons. The need for safer media and deep peeling agents led to the search for combination products that would improve efficacy. Brody first combined solid CO_2 ice with 35% TCA, which produced a deeper resurfacing procedure. This was followed by Monheit's combination of Jessner's solution with 35% TCA. Other combinations were to follow.

The need for deeper dermal injury to improve contour deformities due to acne scarring led to the concept of chemabrasion (3). Chemabrasion, introduced in the 1970s, is the combined process of performing a full- or partial-face chemical peel followed by dermabrasion on the same day. Chemical peeling today often is combined with other mechanical resurfacing modalities, including laser resurfacing and dermasanding.

Over the past 20 years, a number of home treatment programs, cosmetic agents, and over-the-counter chemicals have entered the general market with the purpose of rejuvenating and erasing photodamage and marks of aging. Although most of these products do little more than abrasive chemexfoliation and moisturizing, the quest for youthful skin continues and the dermatologist remains at its forefront.

The explosion of interest in chemical peeling and laser resurfacing on the part of dermatologist has paralleled the general public's interest in acquiring a youthful appearance by rehabilitating the photoaged skin. Advertising has further heightened the public's interest in cosmetic agents, over-the-counter chemicals, and treatment programs that have entered the general market of products meant to rejuvenate skin and erase the marks of sun damage and age. It is the obligation of the physician to analyze the patient's skin type and degree of photoaging skin, and thus prescribe the correct facial rejuvenation procedure that will give the greatest benefit for the fewest risk factors and morbidity. The dermatologist should have available for the consumer the options of medical or cosmeceutical topical therapy, dermabrasion, chemical peeling, and lasers available for selective skin destruction and resurfacing. Each of these techniques maintains a place in the armamentarium of the cosmetic surgeon to provide the appropriate treatment for each individual patient and his or her specific problem.

The approach to photoaging skin has expanded beyond a one-stage procedure to now include preparatory medical therapy and posttreatment cosmeceutical topical therapy to maintain results and prevent further photodamage. Thus, the dermatologist's office has become not only a surgical treatment session but also an educational setting for skin protection and care and a marketplace for the patient to obtain the necessary topicals for skin protection. It is up to the dermatologist, cosmetic surgeon, and plastic surgeon to fully understand the nature of skin and sun damage, protective techniques available, and active agents that work as cosmeceutical preparations. Having multiple procedures available to solve these problems will make patients better candidates for the right procedure to restore and rehabilitate their skin.

ADVANTAGES AND DISADVANTAGES

Chemical peeling involves the application of a chemical exfoliant to wound the epidermis and dermis for the removal of superficial lesions and improve the texture of skin. Various acidic and basic chemical agents are been used to produce the varying effects of light to medium to deep chemical peels through differences in their ability to destroy skin. The level of penetration, destruction, and inflammation determines the level of peeling. Stimulation of epidermal growth through removal of the stratum corneum without necrosis consists of light superficial peel. Through exfoliation, it thickens the epidermis with qualitative regenerative changes. Destruction of the epidermis defines a full superficial chemical peel inducing regeneration of the epidermis. Further destruction of the epidermis and induction of inflammation within the papillary dermis constitutes a medium-depth peel (4). Further inflammatory response in the deep reticular dermis induces new collagen production and ground substances, which constitutes a deep chemical peel. These now have been well classified, and usage has been categorized for various degenerative conditions associated with photoaging skin based on levels of penetration. Thus, the physician has tools capable of solving problems that may be mild, moderate, or severe with agents that are very superficial, superficial, medium-depth, or deep peeling chemicals. The physician must choose the right agent for each patient and condition.

The advantages of chemical peeling include the following:

Low cost. The price of most chemicals is far more economical than lasers or light source tools on the market.

Simplicity. The procedures are fairly easy to learn yet may be technique sensitive.

Reliability. If performed properly on the correctly chosen patient, the procedure usually will produce what the physician predicts. Superficial peels are used for minimal damage with little downtime, whereas deep peels have significant downtime and morbidity to produce more dramatic and longer-lasting results.

Disadvantages of chemical peeling usually are related to the learning curve needed to choose the correct peel for each patient. Application of the peel is technique sensitive. Monitoring and caring for the healing patient requires experience in recognizing the normal appearance of the wound for each level of peel at different time intervals.

INDICATIONS AND PATIENT SELECTION

Analyzing the patient with photoaging skin must take into account skin color and skin type, as well as the degree of photoaging. Various classification systems have been available, and I would like to present a combination of three systems that would simplify and help the physician define the right program or therapeutic procedure for the patient. The Fitzpatrick skin type system classifies degrees of pigmentation and ability to tan using a graded I through VI. It prognosticates sun sensitivity, susceptibility to photodamage, and ability for facultative melanogenesis (one's intrinsic ability to tan) (5). In addition, this system classifies skin according to its risk factors for complications during chemical peeling. Fitzpatrick divides skin types I through VI, taking into account both color and reaction to the sun. Skin types I and II are pale white and freckled with a high degree of potential to burn with sun exposure. Types III and IV can burn but usually are an olive to brown coloration. Types V and VI are dark brown to black skins that rarely ever burn and usually do not need sunscreen protection (Table 1). The patient with type I or II skin with significant photodamage needs regular sunscreen protection prior to and after the procedure. This patient has little risk for hypopigmentation or reactive hyperpigmentation after a chemical peeling procedure. The patient with type III through VI skin has a greater risk for pigmentary dyschromia–hyperpigmentation or hypopigmentation–after a chemical

Table 1 Fitzpatrick Classification of Skin Types

Skin Type	Color	Reaction to sun
I	Very white or freckled	Always burns
II	White	Usually burns
III	White to olive	Sometimes burns
IV	Brown	Rarely burns
V	Dark brown	Very rarely burns
VI	Black	Never burns

peel and may need pretreatment and posttreatment with both sunscreen and bleaching to prevent these complications (6). Pigmentary risks are generally not a great problem with very superficial and superficial chemical peeling but may become a significant problem with medium and deep chemical peeling. It also can be a significant risk when regional areas such as lips and eyelids are peeled with deep peeling or pulsed CO_2 laser, creating a significant color change in these cosmetic units from the rest of the face. This has been classified as the ''alabaster look'' seen with taped deep chemical peels in regional areas. This is an objectionable side effect of deep taped phenol peeling and should be avoided now as patients demand a natural look. Although this was an acceptable look in the 1970s, it was not tolerated in the 1990s. The physician must inform the patient of this potential problem, especially if the patient is of skin type III through VI, justify the benefits of the procedure, outweigh these risks, and, in addition, plan for the appropriate techniques to prevent these unwanted changes in color.

The Glogau system classifies severity of photodamage, taking into account the degree of epidermal and dermal degenerative effects (7). Categorization is I through IV, ranging from mild, moderate, advanced, and severe photodamaged skin. These categories are devised for therapeutic intervention. Category I in young individuals or minimal degree photodamage should be treated with light chemical peeling and medial treatment. Categories II and III would entail medium-depth chemical peeling. Category IV would require the modalities listed plus cosmetic surgical intervention for gravitational changes (Table 2).

Monheit and Fulton have devised a system of quantitating photodamage and have developed numerical scores that would fit into corresponding rejuvenation programs (8). In analyzing photodamage, the major categories include epidermal color with skin lesions and dermal with textural changes. Dermal changes include wrinkles, cross-hatched lines, sallow color, leathery appearance, crinkly thin parchment skin, and the pebblish white nodules of milia. Each of these is classified, giving the patient a point score ranging from 1 to 4. In addition, the number and extent of lesions are categorized from freckles, lentigines, telangiectasias, actinic and seborrheic keratoses, skin cancers, and senile comedones. These are added in a classification system as 1 to 4 and the final score results are tabulated. A total score of 1 to 4 indicates very mild damage, and the patient would adequately respond to a five-step skin care program including sunscreen protection, retinoic acid, glycolic acid peels, and selective lesional removal. A score of 5 to 9 includes all of the above plus repetitive superficial peeling agents program such as glycolic acid, Jessner's solution, or lactic acid peels. A score of 10 to 14 includes medium-depth chemical peeling, and a score of 15 or more includes deep chemical peeling or laser resurfacing. With this system,

Table 2 Photoaging Group: Glogau's Classification

I. Mild (typically age 28–35)
   A. Little wrinkling or scarring
   B. No keratoses
   C. Requires little or no makeup
II. Moderate (age 35–50)
   A. Early wrinkling; mild scarring
   B. Sallow color with early actinic keratoses
   C. Little makeup
III. Advanced (age 50–65)
   A. Persistent wrinkling or moderate acne scarring
   B. Discoloration with telangiectasias and actinic keratoses
   C. Wears makeup always
IV. Severe (age 60–75)
   A. Wrinkling: photoaging, gravitational and dynamic
   B. Actinic keratoses with or without skin cancer or severe acne scars
   C. Wears makeup with poor coverage

during the consultation the patient can understand his or her degree of photodamage and the necessity for an individual peeling program (Table 3).

The peeling agent is a chemical escharotic that damages the skin in a therapeutic manner. It is important that the physician understand the patient's skin and its ability to withstand this damage. Certain skin types withstand the damage to a greater degree than others, and particular skin disorders have a greater tendency to produce side effects and complications from chemical peels. Patients with extensive photodamage may require stronger peeling agents and repeated applications of medium-depth peeling solutions to obtain therapeutic results. Patients with skin disorders such as atopic dermatitis, seborrheic dermatitis, psoriasis, or contact dermatitis may find their disease is exacerbated in the postoperative period, or they may develop problems with postoperative healing, such as prolonged healing, posterythema syndrome, or contact sensitivity, during the postoperative period. Rosacea is a disorder of vasomotor instability in the skin and may develop an exaggerated inflammatory response to the peeling agents. Other important factors include a history of radiation therapy to the proposed facial skin, as chronic radiation dermatitis decreases the body's ability to heal properly. A general rule of thumb is to examine the facial hair in the area treated by radiation. If the facial hair is intact, there are enough pilosebaceous units to heal the skin properly after medium or even deep chemical peeling; however, this rule is not absolute. One should find in the patient's history the dates of radiation treatment and how many rads were used for each individual treatment. Some of our patients with the greatest amount of radiation dermatitis underwent treatments for acne in the mid 1950s, and over the years the skin developed the resultant degenerative changes (9).

Herpes simplex fascial can be a postoperative problem with significant morbidity. Susceptible patients should be pretreated with antiherpetic agents such as acyclovir or valacyclovir to prevent herpetic activation. These patients can be identified in the preoperative consultation and placed on appropriate therapy at the time of the chemical peel. All antiherpetic agents act by inhibiting viral replication in the intact epidermal cell. The

Table 3 Monheit Dermatology Associates
2100 16th Avenue South, Suite 202, Birmingham, AL 35205 (205) 933-0987 Fax (205) 930-1750

Index of photoaging

Texture changes	Points				Score
Wrinkles	1	2	3	4	
(% of potential lines)	<25%	<50%	<75%	<100%	
Cross-latched line	1	2	3	4	
(% of potential lines)	<10%	<20%	<40%	<60%	
Sallow color	1	2	3	4	
	Dull	Yellow	Brown	Black	
Leathery appearance	1	2	3	4	
Crinkley (thin and parchment)	1	2	3	4	
Pebbly (deep whitish nodules)	2	4	6	8	
(% of face)	<25%	<50%	<75%	<100%	
Lesions	**Points**				**Score**
Freckles, mottled skin	1	2	3	4	
(# present)	<10	<25	<50	>100	
Lentigenes (dark and irregular) and SKs	2	4	6	8	
(size in mm)	<5	<10	<15	>20	
Telangiectasias erythema flush	1	2	3	4	
(no. present)	<5	<10	<15	>15	
AKs and SKs	2	4	6	8	
(no. present)	<5	<10	<15	>15	
Skin cancers	2	4	6	8	
(no. present, now or by history)	1ca	2ca	3ca	>4ca	
Senile comedones	1	2	3	4	
(in cheek bone area)	<5	<10	<20	>20	

Total Score____________

Corresponding rejuvenation program

Score	Needs
1–4	Skin care program with tretinoin, glycolic acid peels
5–9	Same plus Jessner peels; pigmented lesion laser and/or vascular laser
10–14	Same plus medium peels – Jessner/TCA peel; skin fillers and/or Botox
15 or more	Above plus laser resurfacing

Staff Signature ______ Date ______ Patient Signature ______ Date ______

AK, ; SK, .

significance of this in chemical peeling is that the skin must be re-epithelialized before the agent has its full effect. Thus, the antiviral agent must be continued for the entire 2 weeks in deep chemical peeling or for at least 10 days in medium-depth peeling (10). I rarely use antiviral agents in light or superficial chemical peeling because the injury pattern usually is not enough to activate the herpes simplex virus.

The chief indications for chemical peeling are associated with reversal of actinic changes such as photodamage, rhytides, actinic growths, pigmentary dyschromias, and acne scars (11). The physician thus can use the various systems to quantitatively and qualitatively classify the level of photodamage and prescribe the appropriate chemical peeling combination (12–14).

TECHNIQUE, PROCEDURE, AND RESULTS OF PEELING AGENTS

Superficial Chemical Peeling

Superficial chemical peeling is truly an exfoliation of the stratum corneum or the entire epidermis to encourage regrowth with less photodamage and a more youthful appearance. It usually takes repetitive peeling sessions to obtain maximal results. These agents have been broken down into very superficial chemical peels, which will remove the stratum corneum only, and superficial chemical peels, which will remove stratum corneum and damage the epidermis. It is to be noted that the effects of superficial peeling on photoaging skin is subtle and will not produce a prolonged or very noticeable effect on dermal lesions such as wrinkles and furrows. Agents used include TCA 10% to 25%, Jessner's solution, glycolic acid 40% to 70%, and salicylic acid-beta-hydroxy acid (15) (Table 4). Each of these agents has its own characteristics and methodology, and a physician must be thoroughly familiar with the chemicals, methods of application, and nature of healing. The usual time for healing is ranges from 1 to 4 days, depending on the chemical and its strength.

Very light peeling agents include low concentrations of glycolic acid, 10% TCA, and 20% salicylic acid, a beta-hydroxy acid.

TCA is the most versatile of all peeling agents; its concentration correlates directly with the depth of penetration and thus the degree of destruction within the skin. The concentration usually is compounded in a weight per volume measurement. It is important to distinguish this from the volume per volume formulation because the concentrations do not correlate. Most of the medical literature on TCA peeling uses a weight per volume measurement. TCA usually is standardized as an aqueous solution, although it has been formulated as a cream and a paste. I believe there is no distinct advantage to these formulations.

TCA destroys epidermis and partial dermis through keratocoagulation and protein precipitation, producing a white coating referred to as frosting. The degree of whitening or frosting can be correlated to penetration of the TCA within the epidermis and related

Table 4 Agents for Medium-Depth Chemical Peel

Agent	Comment
1. TCA 50%	Not recommended because of risk of scarring
2. Combination 35% TCA and solid CO_2 (Brody)	Most potent combination
3. Combination 35% TCA and Jessners (Monheit)	Most popular combination
4. Combination 35% TCA and 70% glycolic acid (Coleman)	Effective combination
5. 89% Phenol	Rarely used

TCA, trichloroacetic acid.

to the depth of the peel. Level I frosting has the appearance of erythema with a streaky white frosting, which indicates superficial penetration. Level II frosting is a white enamel color with no erythema. Level III indicates the deepest penetration and usually is found with full medium-depth peels through the epidermis with superficial dermal destruction (9).

It is important to note that TCA applications are cumulative, increasing penetration and peel depth with more quantity applied, even in low concentrations. Overcoating will always produce a deeper peel so that once the desired level of frosting is obtained, no further acid should be applied. Trichloroacetic acid 10% to 20% will produce a light whitening or frosting effect on the skin, with resultant sloughing of the upper third of the epidermis. Before this peel, the skin is prepared by washing the face thoroughly and using acetone, which removes surface oils and excessive stratum corneum. The TCA is applied evenly with either saturated 2 × 2 gauze or a sable brush, and it usually takes 15 to 45 seconds for the frosting to become evident. This would be categorized as a level I frosting with the appearance of erythema and streaky whitening on the surface. Level II and III frosting is seen in medium-depth and deeper peels (Fig. 1). The patient experiences stinging and some burning during the procedure, but these sensations subside rapidly and the patient then can resume normal activities. There is erythema and resulting desquamation that can last anywhere from 1 to 3 days. Sunscreens and light moisturizers are permitted and care is minimal in this superficial chemical peel.

Repetitive superficial TCA peels are useful for treatment of dyschromias and superficial skin lesions such as lentigines, ephelides, and thin seborrheic keratoses, as well as fine surface texture.

Jessner's solution is a combination acid–escharotic that has been used for more than 100 years for treatment of hyperkeratotic skin disorders (Table 5). It has been used as part of acne treatment for removal of comedones and inflammatory acne activity. Its performance as a superficial peeling agent is as an intense keratolytic agent. The application is similar to superficial TCA application with wet gauze, sponges, or a sable brush, producing an erythema with blotchy frosting. Tentative applications are done on an every-other-week basis, and the levels of Jessner's solution coatings can be increased with repetitive applications. The visual endpoint produces a predictable outcome with epidermal exfoliation and regrowth. The superficial Jessner's peel is a relatively inflammatory peel and is useful for mild photoaging textural changes. It can, however, produce postinflammatory hyperpigmentation, which limits its usefulness for melasma and dyschromias. This usually occurs within 2 to 4 days and is treated with mild cleansers, moisturizing lotion, and sunscreen protection.

Alpha-Hydroxy Acids

Alpha-hydroxy acids, specifically glycolic acid, became the wonder drug of the early 1990s, with promises of skin rejuvenation with home use and topical therapy. Hydroxy acids are found in various foods, e.g., as glycolic acid naturally present in sugar cane, lactic acid in sour milk, malic acid in apples, citric acid in fruits, and tartaric acid in grapes. Lactic acid and glycolic acid are widely available and can be purchased for physician use. Glycolic acid is found in unbuffered concentrations of 20% to 70% for use as a superficial chemical peel. Weekly or biweekly applications of 20% to 70% unbuffered glycolic acid treatments have been used for wrinkles by applying the solution to the face with a cotton swab, sable brush, or saturated 2 × 2 gauze. The time of application is critical for glycolic

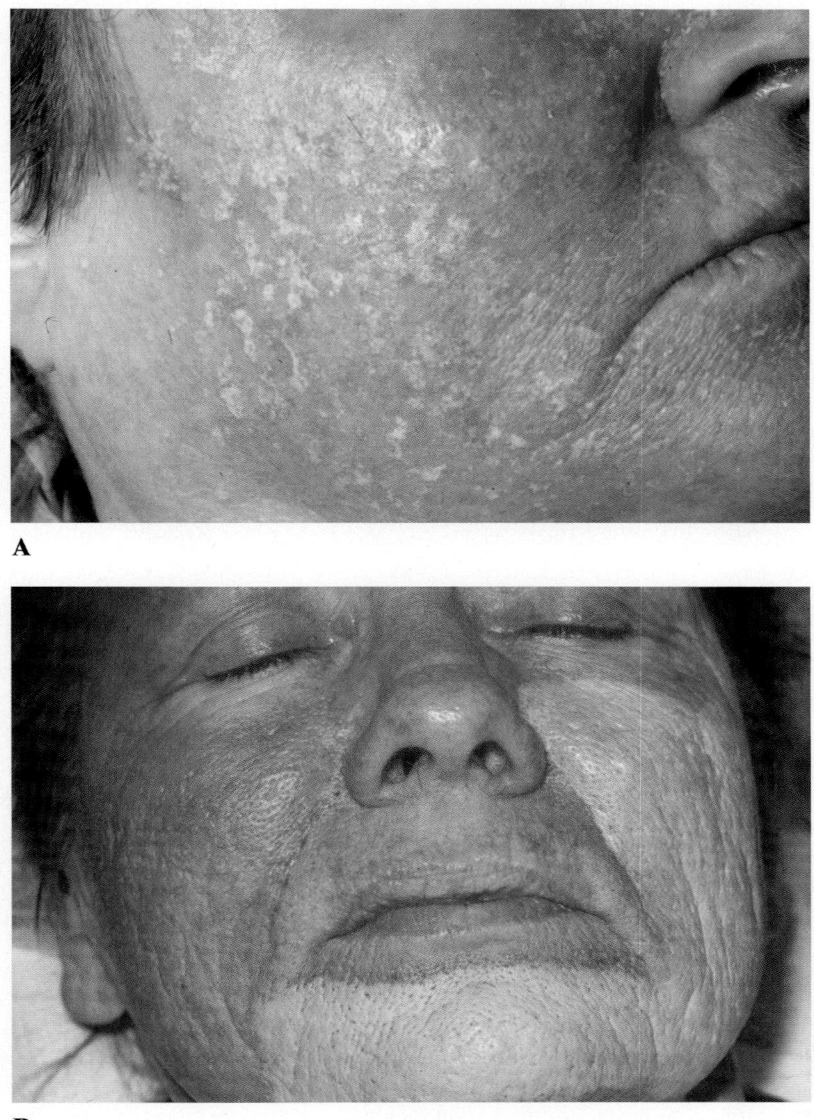

Figure 1 A: Level I frosting as found with light chemical peeling–erythema with streaky frosting. B: Level II–erythema with diffuse white frosting. C: Level III–solid white enamel frosting.

acid; it must be rinsed off with water or neutralized with 5% sodium bicarbonate after 2 to 4 minutes. Mild erythema may occur for 1 hour, with slight stinging and minimal result in scaling. Superficial wrinkle reduction and removal of benign keratoses have been reported from repeated applications of these peeling solutions (16).

Many proprietary forms of glycolic acid with novel approaches to limit the burning and stinging, such as buffering the acid and altering the pH and pKa, have emerged on

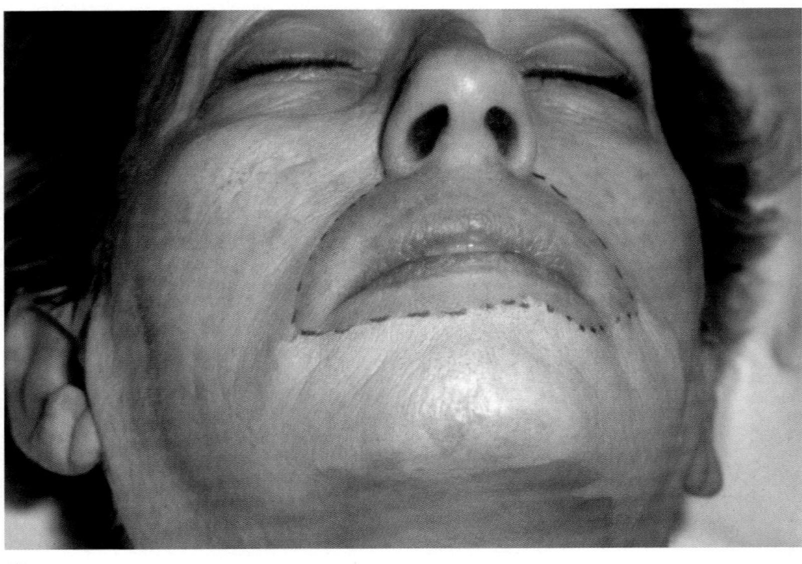

C

Figure 1 Continued.

the marketplace. Although many of these prepackaged treatments are elegant and simple to use, the physician should be concerned about the efficacy because the peel is pH dependent. The strength of the product is dependent on available free acid, which is limited with buffers and higher pHs. I find it most practical to use concentration as the parameter for patient comfort and begin with 20% glycolic acid peels and gradually work up to the more potent concentrations of 50% and 70% as the patient tolerates the procedure.

Salicylic Acid

Salicylic acid peeling or, as commonly called, the beta-hydroxy acid peel, is unique in that it is a lipophilic agent formulated in ethanol. It is a noninflammatory superficial peeling agent that creates keratolysis of the epidermal cells and sebaceous glands. Used as a 20% to 30% solution, it produces a white color, which is not a true frosting but rather a precipitation of salicylic acid crystals (Fig. 2).

This peel is especially useful for treatment of active acne, comedones, and pores. Its lipophilic character targets sebaceous glands, pores, and comedones, with active crystals

Table 5 Jessner's Solution Formula

Resorcinol	14 g
Salicylic acid	14 g
Lactic acid	14 mL
Ethanol (qs)	100 mL

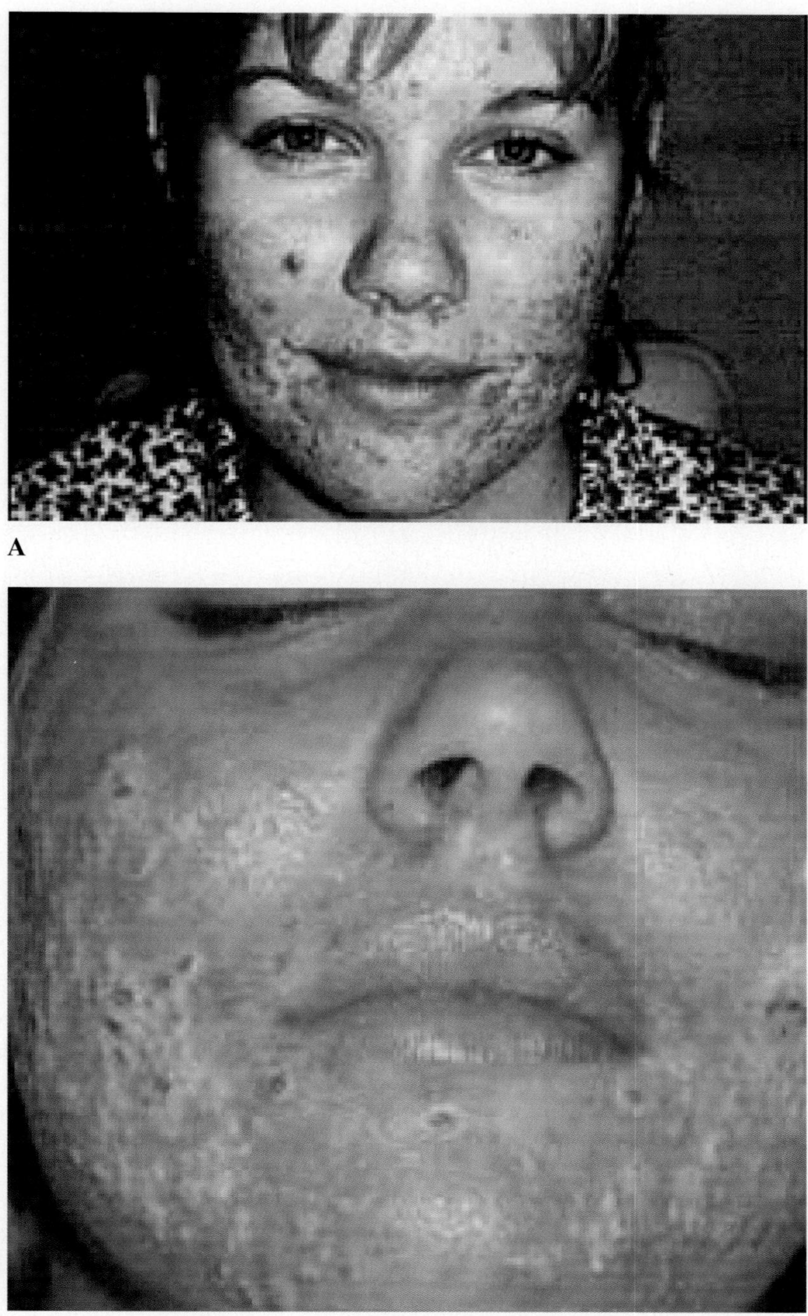

Figure 2 Salicylic acid peels are effective for treatment of acne and comedones. Repetitive treatment over 6 weeks with acne treatment will hasten resolution of the condition. A: Before treatment, active acne. B: Perifollicular frosting seen with salicylic acid, a lipophilic chemical. C: Six weeks after treatment.

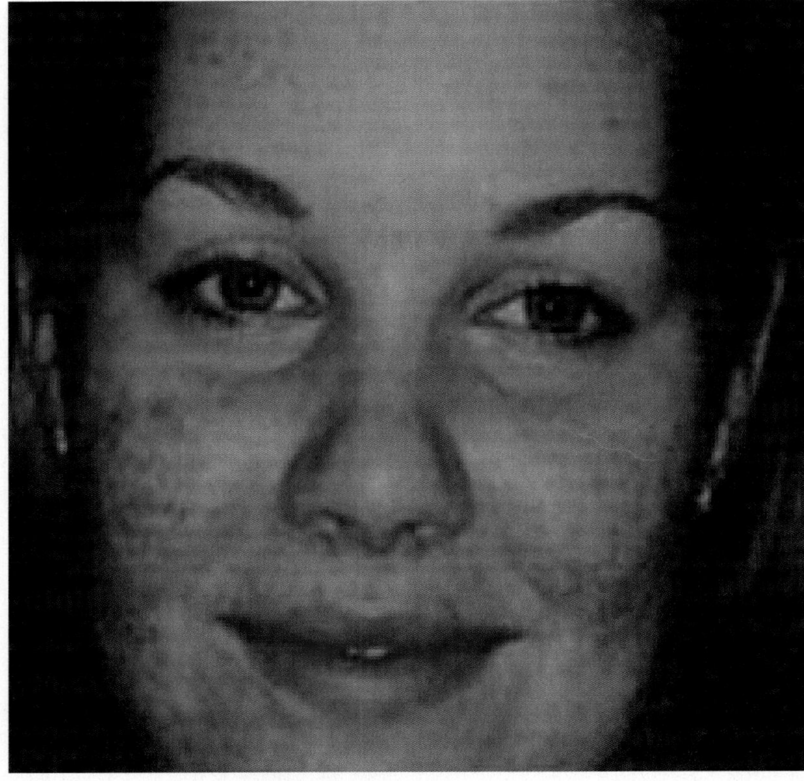

C

Figure 2 Continued.

penetrating the skin surface. The peel produces mild desquamation with little erythema and healing within 1 to 3 days. The effect in pores may continue for 5 to 7 days, as penetrant crystals remain active with the pilosebaceous units. This superficial peel is the least inflammatory and thus can be used safely on patients with darker skin. It also is an effective adjunct agent used for melasma because there is little risk of postinflammatory hyperpigmentation.

Preparation for the peel includes daily use of retinoic acid up to 6 weeks prior to the peeling event (17). Various strengths of retinoic acid are available on the market, and one must use a weaker formulation for sensitive skin and a stronger formulation for significant photodamaged skin. A retinoid dermatitis may ensue 1 or two weeks after initiation of the agent. One should not perform a peeling procedure when retinoid dermatitis is present because the inflamed skin may develop problems with healing or even postoperative complications. The dermatitis should subside by decreasing treatment so that the skin does not appear inflamed when the chemical peel is performed (11). Use of tretinoin prior to a chemical peel will enhance peel solution absorption and promote an even and uniform peel (13).

Superficial chemical peels can be used for treatment of comedonal acne and postinflammatory erythema or pigmentation from acne, mild photoaging skin (Glogau I and II), and melasma.

To treat melasma effectively, the skin must be pretreated and posttreated with sunscreen, hydroquinone 4% to 8%, and retinoic acid. Hydroquinone is a pharmacological agent that blocks the enzyme tyrosinase from developing melanin precursors for the production of new pigment. Its use essentially blocks new pigment as the new epidermis is healing after a chemical peel. Thus, its use is necessary when peeling for the treatment of pigmentary dyschromias and when using chemical peels on Fitzpatrick type III to VI skin, the skin type most prone to developing pigmentary problems (14).

When using superficial chemical peels, the physician must understand that repetitive peeling will not summate into medium-depth or deep peels. A peel that does not affect the dermis will have very little effect on textural changes that originate from dermal damage. The patient must understand this preoperatively so that he or she will not be disappointed with the results. On the other hand, repetitive peeling procedures are necessary to obtain maximal benefits with superficial chemical peeling. These procedures are timed every week or every other week for a total of six to eight chemical peels and enhanced by the appropriate cosmeceutical agents. The ease of the procedure with little downtime makes these ''lunch time'' chemical peels a favorite with the baby boomers who will not take time off.

Medium-Depth Chemical Peeling

Medium-depth chemical peeling is defined as controlled damage from a chemical agent to the papillary dermis resulting in specific changes that can be performed in a single setting. Agents currently used include combination products: (1) Jessner's solution with 35% TCA, (2) 70% glycolic acid with 35% TCA , and (3) solid carbon dioxide with 35% TCA. The hallmark for this level peel was 50% TCA, which traditionally achieved acceptable results in ameliorating fine wrinkles, actinic changes, and preneoplasia. However, because TCA in higher concentrations itself is an agent more likely to be fraught with complications, especially scarring, at strengths of 50% or higher, it has fallen out of favor as a single-agent chemical peel (18). It is for this reason that the combination products along with a 35% TCA formula have been found equally effective in producing this level of control damage without the risk of side effects or complications.

Brody (19) first developed the use of solid CO_2 applied with acetone to the skin as a freezing technique prior to the application of 35% TCA. This appears to break the epidermal barrier for more even and complete penetration of the 35% TCA (19).

Monheit (20) then demonstrated the use of Jessner's solution prior to the application of 35% TCA. Jessner's solution was found effective in destroying the epidermal barrier by breaking up individual epidermal cells. This allowed deeper and more even penetration of the 35% TCA with homogenous application of the peeling solution (20). Similarly, Coleman demonstrated the use of 70% glycolic acid prior to the application of 35% TCA, a similar effect to that of the Jessner's solution (21).

All three combinations have been proven equally effective and safer than the use of 50% TCA. The application and frosting can be controlled with the combination, so the ''hot spots'' with higher concentrations of TCA that can produce dyschromias and scarring are not a significant problem with lowered concentration TCA as used in this combination medium-depth peel. The Monheit version of the Jessner's solution–35% TCA peel is a relatively simple and safe combination. The technique is used for mild-to-moderate photoaging, including pigmentary changes, lentigines, and epidermal growths including actinic keratoses, seborrheic keratoses, sebaceous hyperplasia, dyschromias, and fine rhytides. It is a single procedure with a healing time of 7 to 10 days. It also is useful for removing diffuse actinic keratoses as an alternative to chemical exfoliation with topical 5-fluorouracil chemotherapy. It reduces the morbidity significantly and gives the cosmetic benefits of improved photoaging skin (22).

The procedure usually is performed with mild preoperative sedation and nonsteroidal anti-inflammatory agents. The patient is told that the peeling agent will sting and burn temporarily. Gr-X (grains 10) aspirin is given before the peel and continued through the first 24 hours if the patient can tolerate the medication. Its anti-inflammatory effect is especially helpful in reducing swelling and relieving pain. If given before surgery, it may be all the patient requires during the postoperative phase. For full-face peels, however, it is useful to give preoperative sedation (diazepam 5–10 mg orally) and mild analgesia, meperidine 50 mg (Demerol-Sanofi-Synthelabo, Inc., New York, NY), and hydroxyzine hydrochloride 25 mg intramuscularly (Vistaril-Pfizer Laboratories, New York, NY). The discomfort from this peel is not long lasting, so short-acting anxiolytics and analgesics are all that is necessary (23).

Vigorous cleaning and degreasing are necessary for even penetration of the solution. The face is scrubbed gently with Ingasam (Septisol, Vestal Laboratories, St. Louis, MO) applied with 4-inch × 4-inch gauze pads and water, then rinsed and dried. Next, an acetone preparation is applied to remove residual oils and debris. The skin is essentially debrided of stratum corneum and excessive scale. The necessity for thorough degreasing for an even, fully penetrating peel cannot be overemphasized. The physician should feel the dry clean skin to check the thoroughness of degreasing. If oil or scale is felt, degreasing should be repeated, especially in areas of the hairline and nose. A splotchy peel usually is the result of uneven penetration of peel solution because of residual oil or stratum corneum from inadequate degreasing.

The Jessner's solution is applied with either cotton-tipped applicators or 2-inch × 2-inch gauze. The Jessner's solution is applied evenly, usually with one coat to achieve a light but even frosting with a background of erythema. The frosting achieved with Jessner's solution is much lighter than that produced by TCA, and the patient usually is not uncomfortable. Even strokes are used to apply the solution to the unit area covering the forehead to the cheeks to the nose and chin. The eyelids are treated last, creating the same erythema with blotchy frosting (Fig. 3). The Jessner's solution will open the epidermal barrier for a more even and penetrant TCA peel.

The TCA is applied evenly with one to four cotton-tipped applicators that are rolled over different areas with light or heavier doses of the acid. Four cotton-tipped applicators are applied in broad strokes over the forehead and on the medial cheeks. Two mildly soaked cotton-tipped applicators can be used across the lips and chin, and one damp cotton-tipped applicator on the eyelids. Thus, the dosage of application is dependent on the amount of acid used and the number of cotton-tipped applicators applied. The cotton-tipped applicator is useful for quantitating the amount of peel solution to be applied.

The white frost from the TCA application appears on the treated area within 30 seconds to 2 minutes. Even application should eliminate the need to go over areas a second or a third time, but if frosting is incomplete or uneven, the solution should be reapplied. TCA takes longer to frost than Baker's formula or straight phenol, but a shorter period of time than the superficial peeling agents. The surgeon should wait at least 3 to 4 minutes

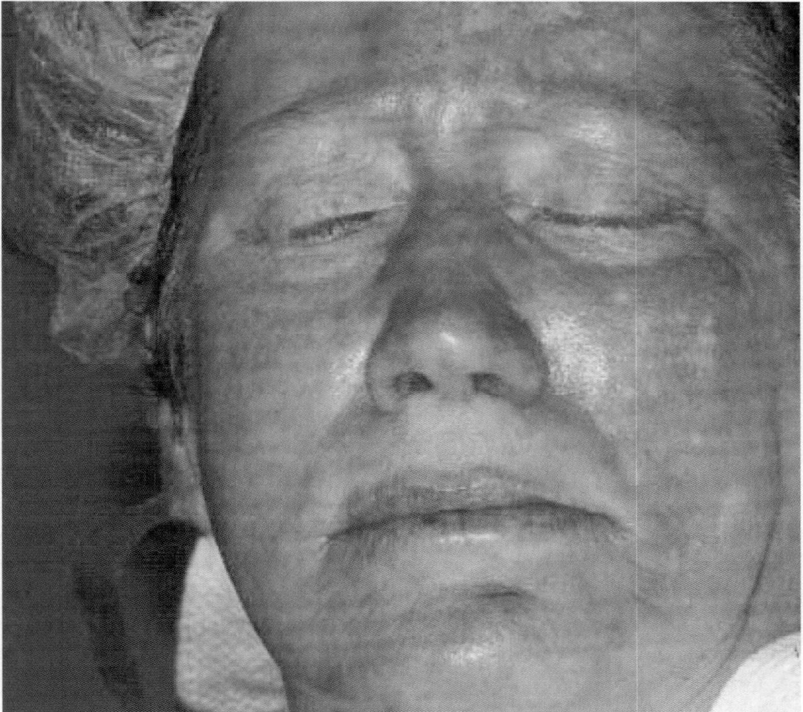

Figure 3 A: Jessner's solution technique: one or two applications to produce a level I frosting.

after TCA application to ensure the frosting has reached its peak. The surgeon can analyze the completeness of a frosted cosmetic unit and touch up the area as needed. Areas of poor frosting should be re-treated carefully with a thin application of TCA. The physician should achieve a level II to III frosting. Level II frosting is defined as white-coated frosting with a background of erythema (24). Level III frosting, which is associated with penetration to the reticular dermis, is a solid white enamel frosting with no background of erythema. A deeper level III frosting should be restricted only to areas of heavy actinic damage and thicker skin. Most medium-depth chemical peels use a level II frosting, and this is especially true over eyelids and areas of sensitive skin. Areas with a greater tendency to scar formation, such as the zygomatic arch, the bony prominences of the jaw line, and chin, should receive only up to a level II frosting. Overcoating TCA will increase its penetration so that a second or third application will dry the acid further, creating further damage. One must be careful in overcoating only areas in which the take-up was not adequate or the skin is much thicker.

Anatomical areas of the face are peeled sequentially from forehead to temple to cheeks and finally to the lips and eyelids. The white frosting indicates keratocoagulation, and at that point the reaction is complete. Careful feathering of the solution into the hairline and around the rim of the jaw and brow conceals the line demarcation between peeled and nonpeeled areas. The perioral area has rhytides that require a complete and even application of solution over the lip skin to the vermilion. This is accomplished best with the help of an assistant who stretches and fixates the upper and lower lips when the peel solution is applied.

Certain areas and skin lesions require special attention. Thicker keratoses do not frost evenly and thus do not pick up peel solution. Additional applications rubbed vigorously into the lesion may be needed for peel solution penetration. Wrinkled skin should be stretched to allow an even coating of solution into the folds and troughs. Oral rhytides require peel solution to be applied with the wood portion of a cotton-tipped applicator and extended into the vermilion of the lip. Deeper furrows such as expression lines will not be eradicated by peel solution and thus should be treated like the remaining skin.

Eyelid skin must be treated delicately and carefully. A semidry applicator should be used to carry the solution within 2 to 3 mm of the lid margin. The patient should be positioned with the head elevated at 30 degrees and the eyelids closed. Excess peel solution on the cotton tip should be drained gently on the bottom before application. The applicator then is rolled gently on the lids and periorbital skin. Never leave excess peel solution on the lids because the solution can roll into the eyes. Dry away tears with a cotton-tipped applicator during peeling because the tears may pull the peel solution into the puncta and eye by capillary attraction (Fig. 4). The solution is neutralized immediately with cool saline compresses at the conclusion of the peel. The Jessner's–TCA peel procedure is as follows:

1. The skin is cleaned thoroughly with Septisol to remove oils.
2. Acetone or acetone alcohol is used to further debride oil and scale from the surface of the skin.
3. Jessner's solution is applied.
4. Thirty-five percent TCA is applied until a light frost appears.
5. Cool saline compresses are applied to neutralize the solution.
6. The peel will heal with 0.25% acetic acid soaks and a mild emollient cream.

There is an immediate burning sensation as the peel solution is applied, but this subsides as frosting is completed. Cool saline compresses offer symptomatic relief for a peeled area as the solution is applied to other areas. The compresses are placed over the face for 5 to 6 minutes after the peel until the patient is comfortable. The burning subsides fully by the time the patient is ready to be discharged. At that time, most of the frosting has faded and a brawny desquamation is evident.

Edema, erythema, and desquamation are expected postoperatively. With periorbital peels and even forehead peels, eyelid edema can be severe enough to close the lids. For the first 24 hours, the patient is instructed to soak with a 0.25% acetic acid compress made of 1 tablespoon of white vinegar in 1 pint of warm water four times a day. A bland emollient is applied to the desquamating areas after soaks. After 24 hours, the patient can shower and clean gently with a mild nondetergent cleanser. The erythema intensifies as desquamation becomes complete within 4 to 5 days. Healing is completed within 7 to 10 days. At the end of 1 week, the bright red color has faded to pink and has the appearance of a sunburn. This can be covered by cosmetics and will fade fully within 2 to 3 weeks.

The medium-depth peel is dependent on three components for therapeutic effect: (1) degreasing, (2) Jessner's solution, and (3) 35% TCA. The amount of each agent applied creates the intensity and thus the effectiveness of this peel. The variables can be adjusted according to the patient's skin type and the areas of the face being treated. It is the workhorse of peeling and resurfacing in my practice because it can be individualized for most patients we see.

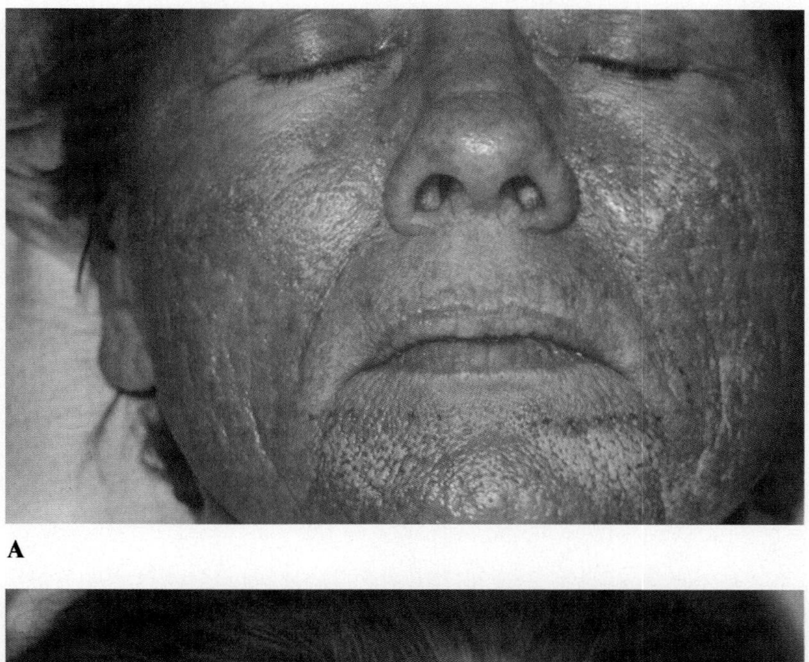

A

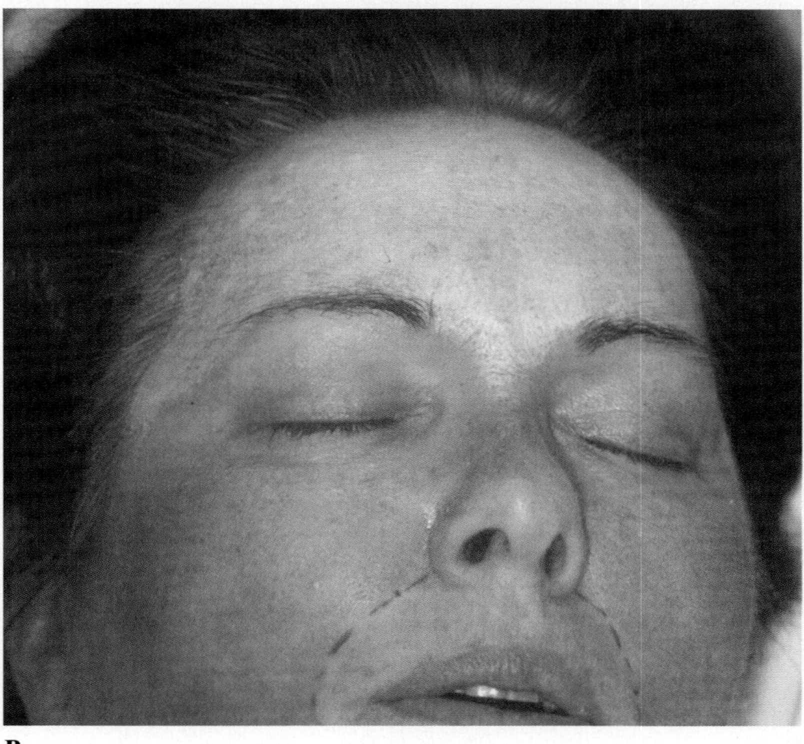

B

Figure 4 Technical aspects of the Jessner's solution + 35% trichloroacetic acid (TCA) peel. A: Appearance of level I frosting after application of Jessner's solution–erythema with blotchy frosting. B: The 35% TCA applied after Jessner's solution dries with an even application using one to four cotton-tipped applicators. A level III or white enamel frosting is obtained.

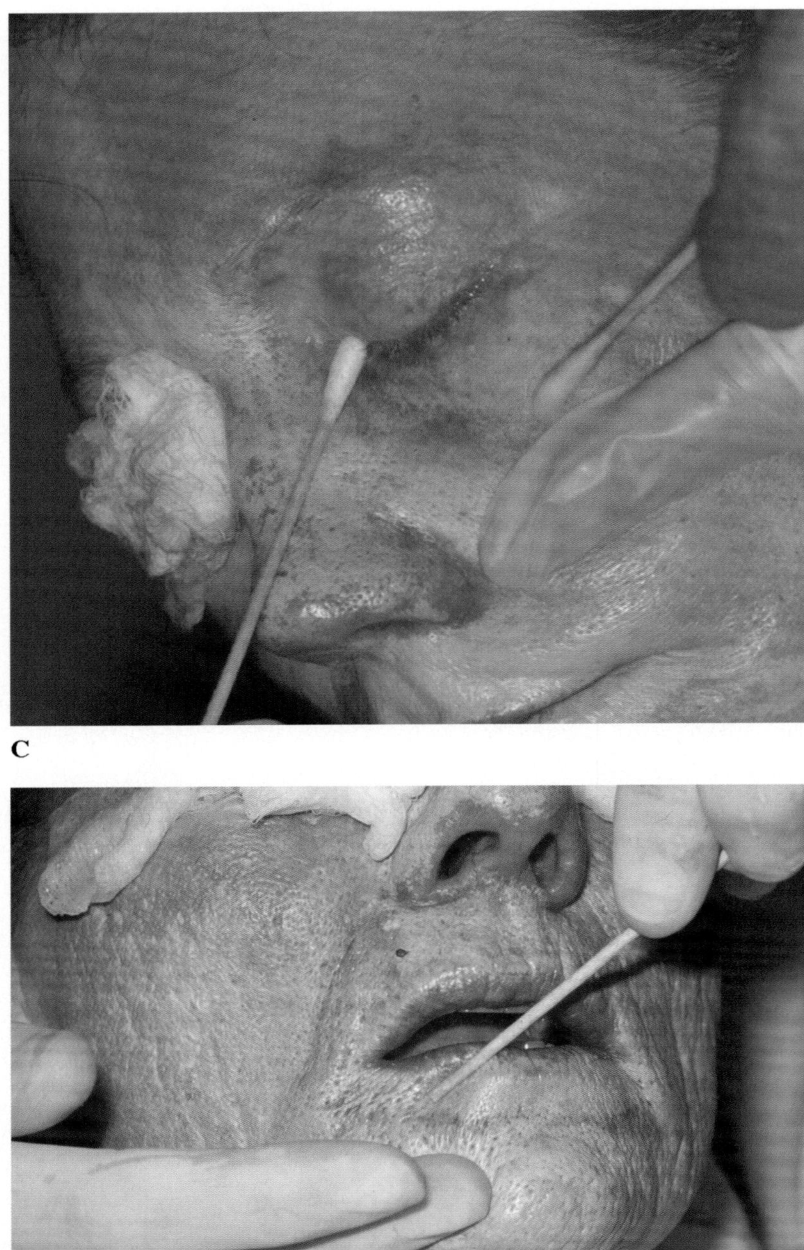

Figure 4 Continued. C: Eyelids are treated with one cotton-tipped applicator moistened with 35% TCA. A dry applicator is used to absorb tears during eyelid peeling. D: Lip rhytides are peeled with saturated cotton-tipped applicators. The wooden shaft is used to rub peel solution further into the lip rhytides.

The medium-depth chemical peel has five major indications: (1) destruction of epidermal lesions, e.g., actinic keratoses, (2) resurfacing level II moderate photoaging skin, (3) pigmentary dyschromias, (4) mild acne scars, and (5) blending photoaging skin with laser resurfacing and deep chemical peeling.

Actinic Keratoses

This procedure is well suited for males with epidermal lesions, such as actinic keratoses, which has required repeated removal with either cryosurgery or chemoexfoliation (5-fluorouracil). The entire face can be treated as a unit. A subfacial cosmetic unit, such as the forehead, temples, and cheeks, can be treated independently. Active lesions can be removed, and incipient growths, as yet undetected, will be removed as the epidermis is sloughed. Advantages for the male patient include a short recovery period of 7 to 10 days, with little postoperative erythema after healing. There is little risk of pigmentary changes (either hypopigmentation or hyperpigmentation); thus, the patient can return to work after the skin has healed (Fig. 5).

Moderate Photoaging skin

Glogau level II damage responds well to this peeling combination, with removal of the epidermal lesions and dermal changes that will freshen sallow atrophic skin and soften other rhytides. This also is an excellent peel for the male patient because it will heal in 10 days with minimal risk of textural or color complications (Fig. 6).

Pigmentary Dyschromias

Although color change can be treated with repetitive superficial chemical peeling, the medium-depth peel is a single treatment preceded and followed by the use of bleaching agents and retinoic acid. In most cases, the pigmentary problems are resolved with this single-treatment program (Fig. 7).

Blending Other Resurfacing Procedures

In a patient in whom there is advanced photoaging changes, such as crow's feet and rhytides in the periorbital area with medium-depth changes on the remaining face, a medium-depth peel can be used to integrate these procedures, that is, laser resurfacing or deep chemical peeling can be performed over the periorbital and perioral areas, which may have more advanced photoaging changes, while the medium-depth chemical peel is used for the rest of the face (25). Patients who require laser resurfacing in a localized cosmetic unit will have the remaining areas of the face blended with this medium-depth chemical peel. Patients who undergo laser resurfacing or deep peeling to the perioral or periorbital areas alone develop a pseudo-hypopigmentation that is a noticeable deformity. The patient who requires laser resurfacing at a localized cosmetic unit will have the remaining areas of the face blended with this medium-depth peel. The alternative–a full-face deep peel or laser resurfacing–has increased morbidity, longer healing, and risk of scarring over areas such as the lateral jaw line, malar eminences, and forehead. If deep resurfacing is needed only over localized areas such as perioral or periorbital face, a blending medium-depth peel does reduce morbidity and healing time. I find that almost all of my patients who require laser resurfacing in a localized cosmetic unit have the remaining areas of the face blended with this medium-depth chemical peel (26) (Fig. 8).

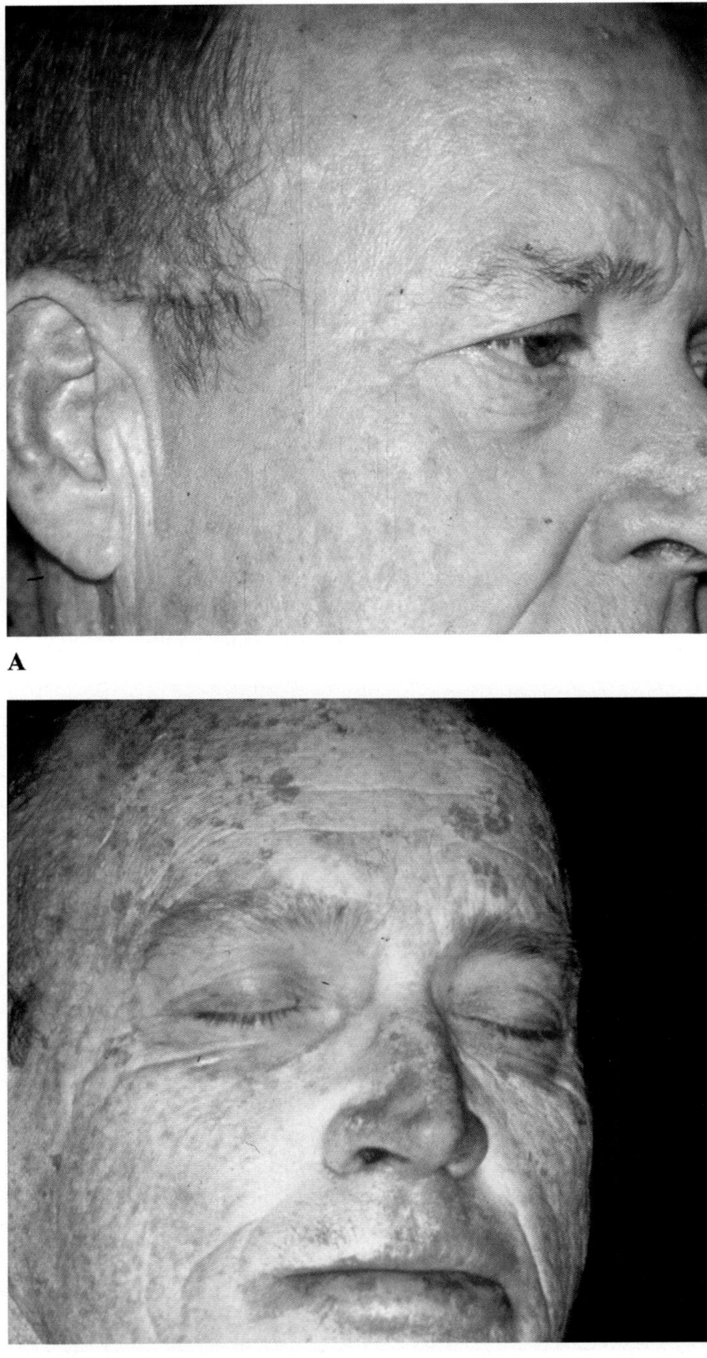

Figure 5 Medium-depth chemical peel for treatment of diffuse actinic keratoses and photoaging. Jessner's solution + 35% trichloroacetic acid (TCA) was used as a single treatment, with healing in 8 days. A: Preoperative. B: Frosting after TCA. C: One month postoperative.

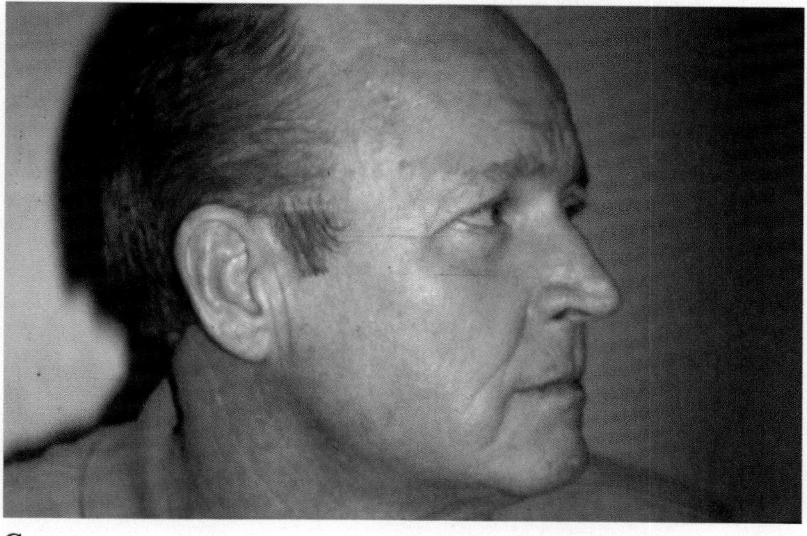

C

Figure 5 Continued.

Deep Chemical Peeling

Level III photodamage requires deep chemical peeling or laser resurfacing to correct the deeper dermal damage. This entails the use of either TCA above 50% or the Gordon-Baker phenol peel. Laser resurfacing also can be used to reliably reach this level of damage. TCA above 45% has been found to be unreliable, with a high incidence of scarring and postoperative complications. For this reason, it is not included as a standard treatment for deep chemical peeling. The Baker-Gordon phenol peel has been used successfully for more than 40 years for deep chemical peeling and produces reliable results. It is a labor-intensive procedure that must be taken seriously, as all major surgical procedures are. The patient requires preoperative sedation with an intravenous line and preoperative intravenous hydration. Usually 1 L of fluid is given preoperatively, and 1 L of fluid is given during the procedure. Phenol is both a cardiotoxin and a hepatotoxin, and it has nephrotoxicity. For this reason, one must be concerned with the serum concentration of phenol as a result of cutaneous absorption. Methods to limit this include the following:

1. Intravenous hydration prior to and during the procedure to flush the phenolic products through the serum.
2. Extend the time of application for a full-face peel to over 1 hour. Cosmetic units are applied in 15-minute periods, that is, the forehead, cheeks, chin, lips, and eyelids each is given a 15-minute application period for a total of 1 to 1.5 hours for the entire procedure.
3. All patients are monitored and if there is any electrocardiographic abnormality, i.e., premature ventricular contractions or premature atrial contractions, the procedure is stopped and the patient is watched carefully for other signs of toxicity.
4. Many physicians believe that administration of O_2 during the procedure can be helpful in preventing arrhythmic complications.

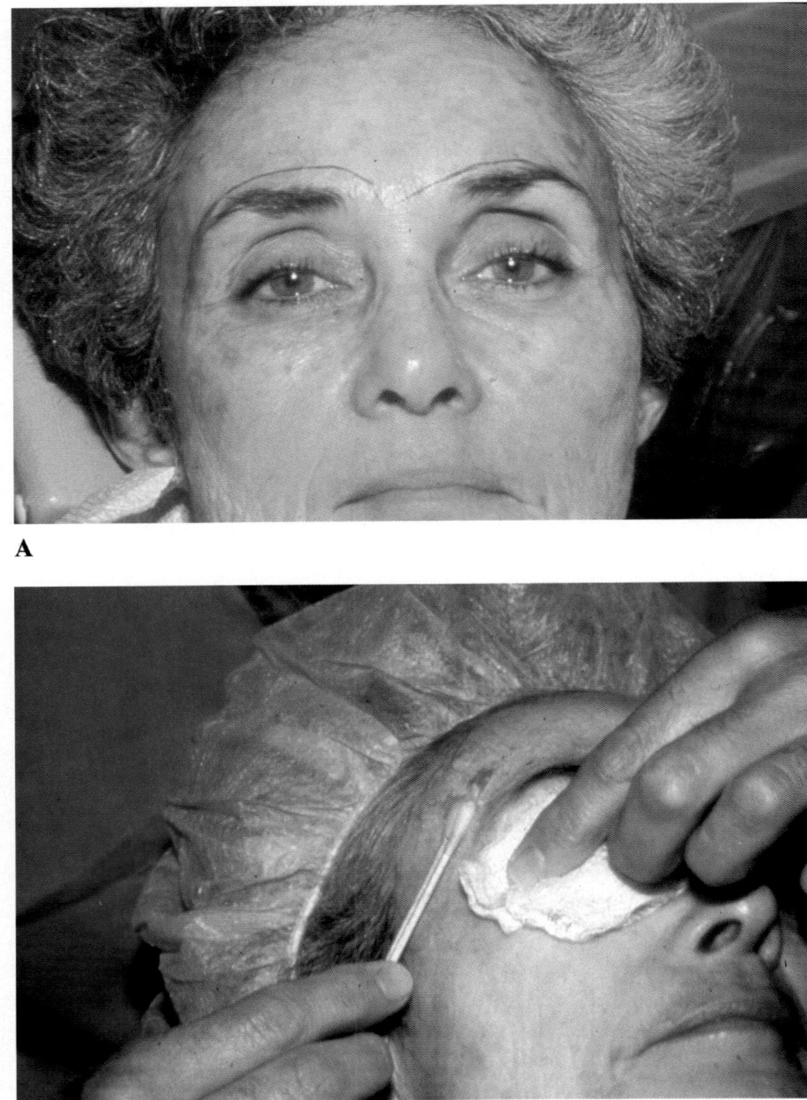

Figure 6 Medium-depth chemical peel used to treat moderate photoaging skin. A: Preoperative. Epidermal growths with aging textural changes. B: Application of 35% trichloroacetic acid (TCA) directly after Jessner's solution. C: White enamel frosting (level III) from 35% TCA. D: Desquamation and inflammation 4 days after peel. E: Final results 6 months later.

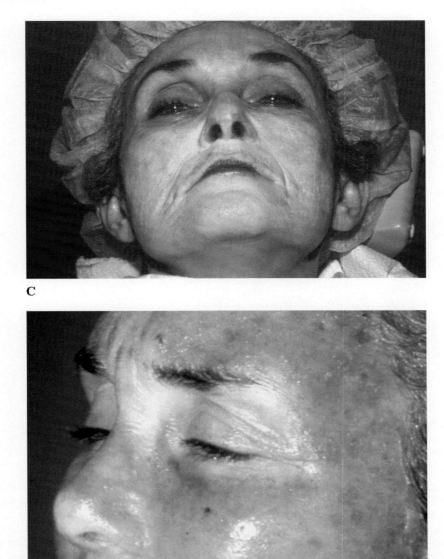

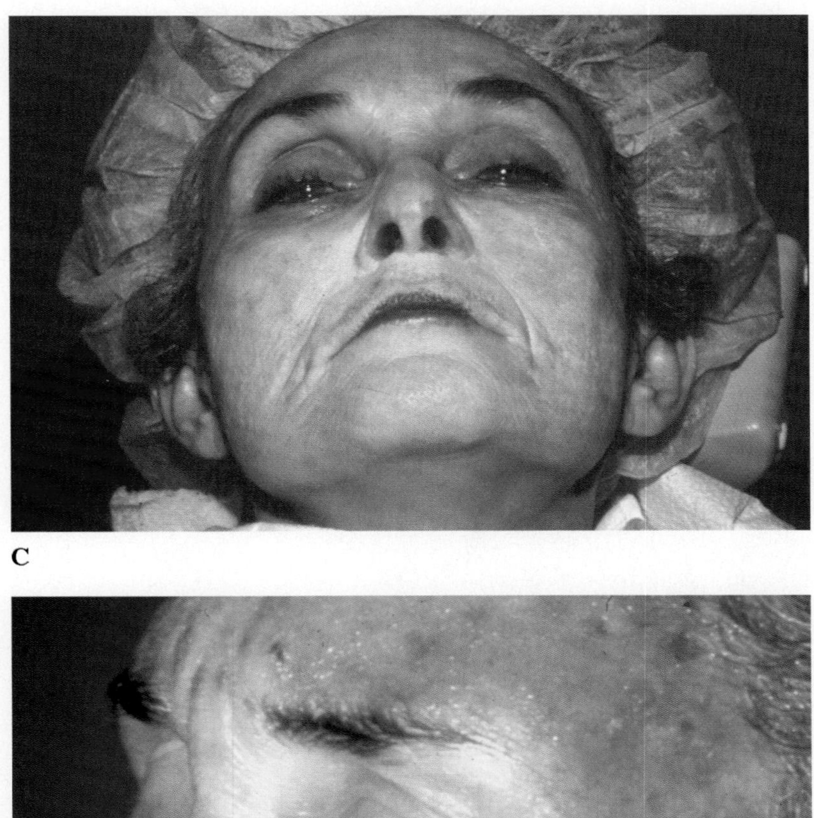

C

D

Figure 6 Continued.

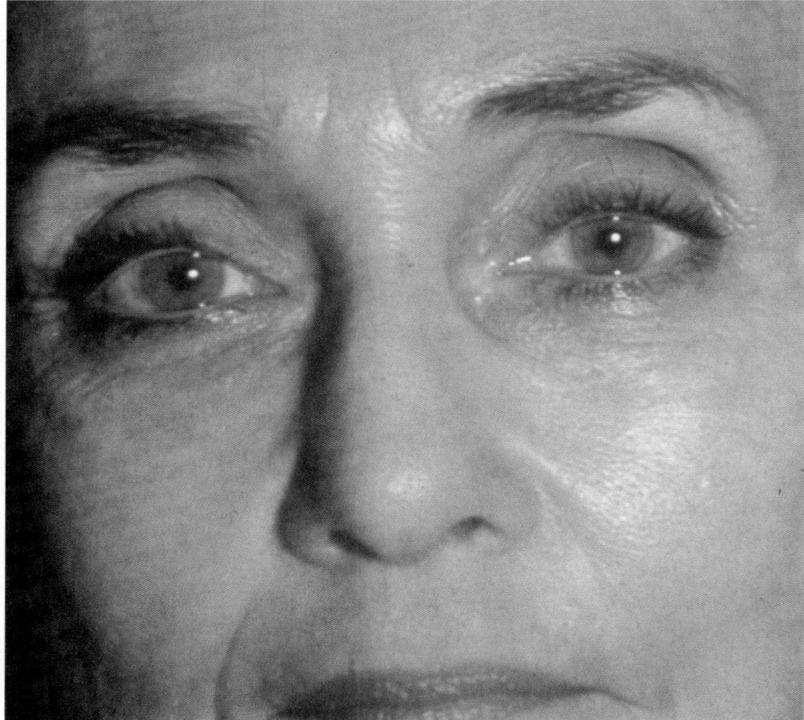

E

Figure 6 Continued.

5. Any patient with a history of cardiac arrhythmia or hepatic or renal compromise, or is taking medication with a propensity for arrhythmias, should not undergo the Baker-Gordon phenol peel (27).

The patient undergoing deep chemical peeling must recognize the significant risk factors, increased morbidity, and possible complications associated with this procedure so that the benefits can be weighed positively against these particular factors. In the hands of those that perform this technique regularly, it is a reliable and safe method of rejuvenating advanced-to-severe photoaged skin including deeper perioral rhytides, periorbital rhytides and crow's feet, forehead lines and wrinkles, and other textural and lesional changes associated with the more severe photoaging process.

There are two modalities for deep chemical peeling: (1) Baker's formula phenol unoccluded and (2) Baker's formula phenol occluded. Occlusion is accomplished with the application of waterproof zinc oxide tape such as 0.5-inch Curity tape. The tape is placed directly after the phenol is applied to each individual cosmetic unit. Tape occlusion increases the penetration of the Baker's phenol solution and is particularly helpful for deeply lined ''weather-beaten'' faces. A taped Baker's formula phenol peel creates the deepest damage in midreticular dermis, and this form of chemical peeling should be performed only by the most knowledgeable and experienced cosmetic surgeons who understand the

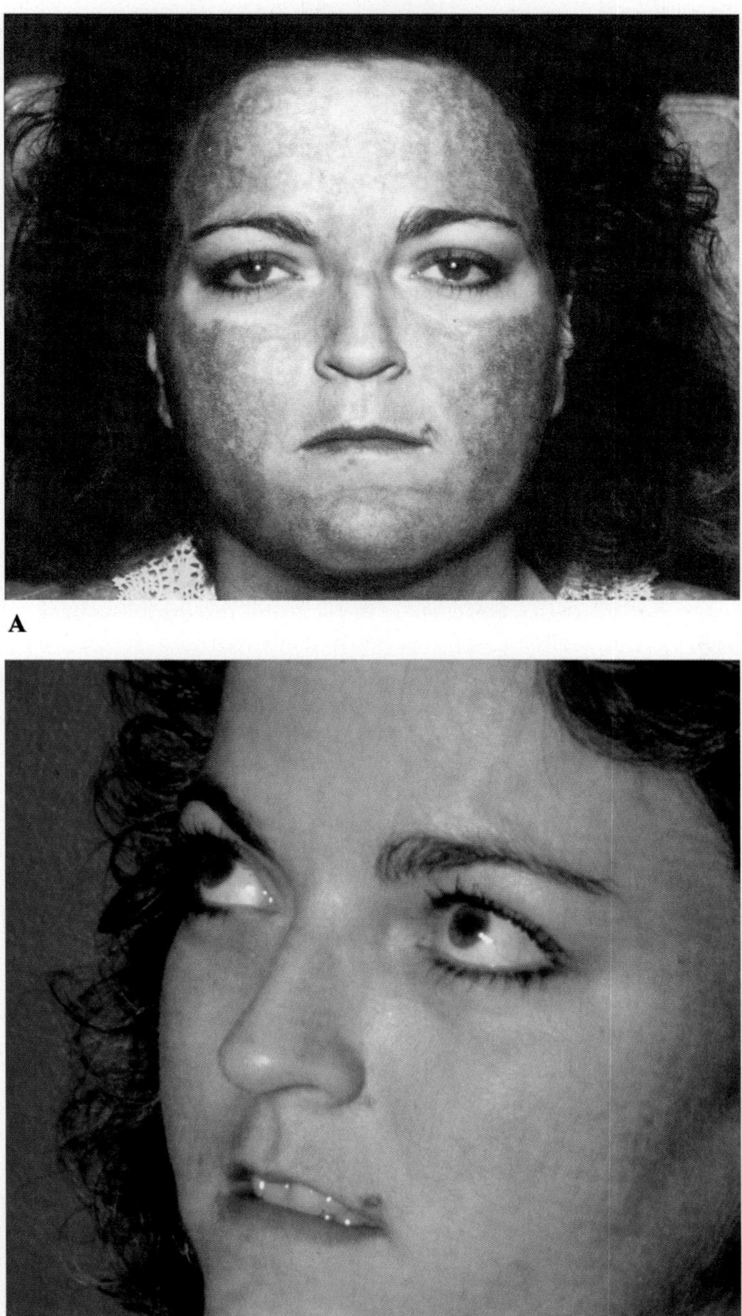

A

B

Figure 7 Postinflammatory hyperpigmentation unresponsive to topical agents (hydroquinone and tretinoin) and superficial chemical peeling. Full response to medium-depth chemical peel and topical agents. A: Preoperative. B: Six weeks postoperative.

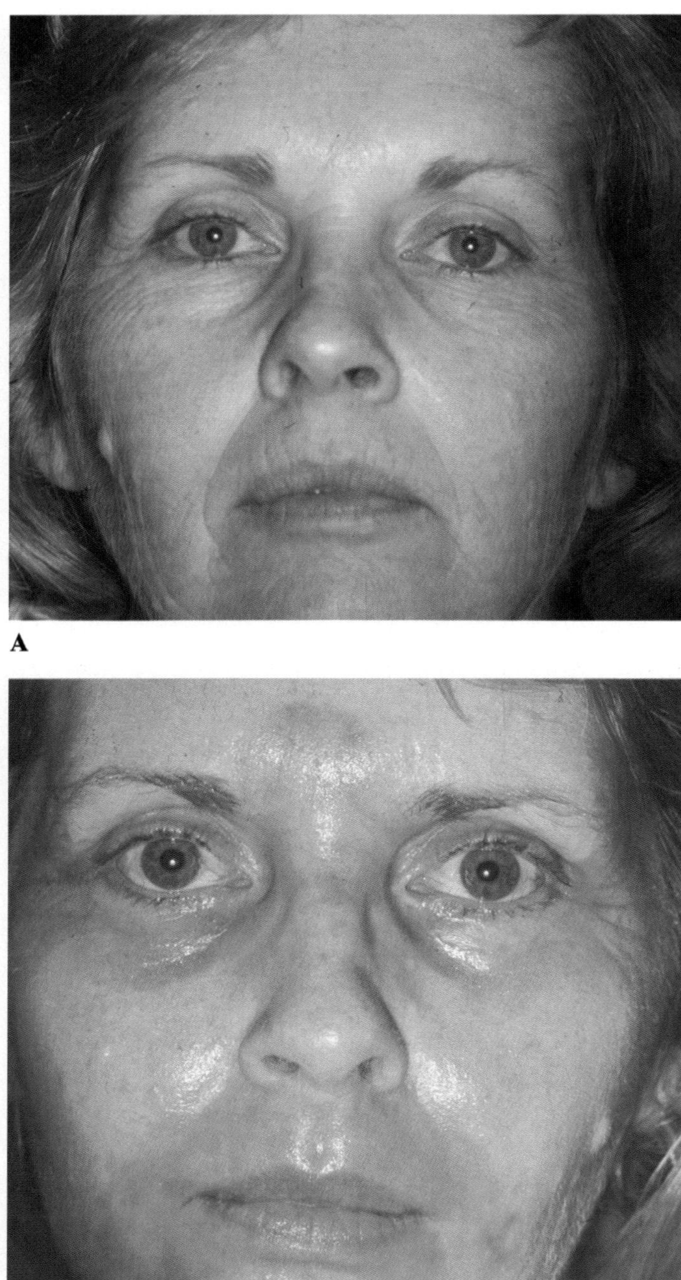

Figure 8 Combination procedure utilizing perioral–periorbital CO_2 laser resurfacing with Jessner's solution + 35% trichloroacetic acid (TCA) peel over the remaining face. The peel will blend color and texture of the laser treated areas. A: Preoperative. The eyelids and lips need deeper resurfacing than the cheeks, which require only medium-depth injury. B: Four days postoperative. Note difference in rate of healing between laser- and peel-treated areas. C: One year postoperative.

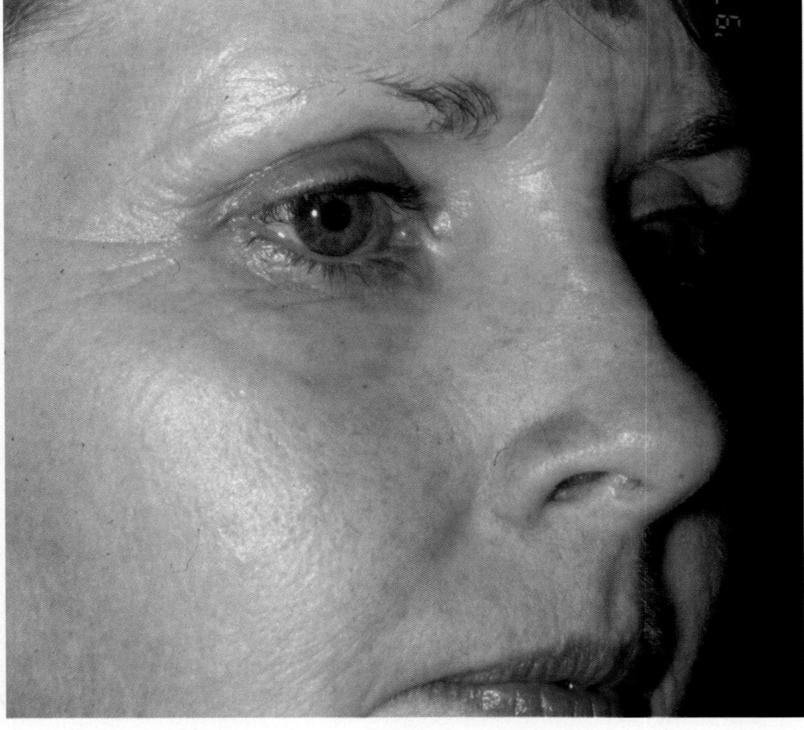

C

Figure 8 Continued.

risks of overpenetration and deep damage to the reticular dermis (28). These complications include hyperpigmentation and hypopigmentation, textural changes such as the ''alabaster skin,'' and the potential for scarring. The unoccluded technique as modified by McCollough involves more skin cleansing and application of more peel solution. On the whole, this technique does not produce as deep a peel as the occluded method (29).

The Baker-Gordon formula for this peel was first described in 1961 and since then has been used successfully for more than 25 years. The Baker-Gordon formula (Table 6) penetrated further into the dermis than full-strength undiluted phenol because full-strength phenol allegedly causes an immediate coagulation of epidermal keratin proteins and ''self-blocks'' further penetration. Dilution to approximately 50% to 55% in the Baker-Gordon formula causes keratolysis and keratocoagulation resulting in greater penetration. The liquid soap Septisol is a surfactant that reduces skin tension, allowing more even penetration. Croton oil is a vesicant that enhances phenol absorption. Only recently has the importance of croton oil been rediscussed. Hetter (33) investigated the reaction of phenol to croton oil in the Baker formula. He altered both ingredients in an elegant controlled study and discovered that croton oil plays a much greater role than previously assumed in the penetration and thus destruction of skin in the peel. By reducing the phenol/croton oil concentrations from 50% phenol/2.1% croton oil to 33% phenol/0.35% croton oil,

Table 6 Formula for Baker–Gordon Phenol Peel

3 mL USP liquid phenol 88%
2 mL tap water
8 drops liquid soap (Septisol)
3 drops croton oil

he demonstrated that the resultant peel was less aggressive and thus had less risk of complications.

Techniques

Before administration of anesthesia, the patient's face is marked while the patient is in the seated position. Landmarks such as the mandibular angle, the chin, the preauricular sulcus, the orbital rim, and the forehead are noted. This is done to extend the peel thoroughly throughout the limits of the face and slightly over the mandibular rim to blend any color change. This peel requires sedation. An intravenous combination such as fentanyl citrate (Sublimaze) and midazolam (Versed) can be administered intravenously by an anesthetist while the patient is being monitored and given intravenous sedation. It is helpful to use local nerve blocks, e.g., bupivacaine (Marcaine), along the supraorbital nerve, infraorbital nerve, and mental nerve, which should provide some local anesthesia for up to 4 hours.

The patients should arrive NPO (nothing by mouth) and have shaved and cleansed their face the morning of surgery. The face then is cleansed and degreased with a keratolytic agent such as hexachlorophene with alcohol (Septisol) over the entire face, with emphasis on oily areas such as the nose, hairline, and midfacial cheeks. A thorough and evenly distributed cleansing or degreasing of the face will ensure a more uniform peel without skipped areas. The chemical agent then is applied sequentially to six aesthetic units: forehead, perioral, right and left cheeks, nose, and periorbital areas. Each cosmetic area takes 15 minutes for application, allowing 60 to 90 minutes for the entire procedure. Cotton-tipped applicators are used with a similar technique as discussed for the medium-depth Jessner–35% TCA peel. Less of the agent is used because frosting occurs very rapidly. The last area for the peel is the periorbital skin on which the chemical is applied with only damp cotton-tipped applicators, taking care to keep the drops away from the eye and keep tears off the skin. Tearing may allow the peel solution to reach the eye by capillary attraction. It is important to remember that water dilution of this chemical may increase the absorption; therefore, if the chemical does get into the eye, it should be flushed with mineral oil rather than water. An immediate burning sensation is present for 15 to 20 seconds but then subsides. The pain returns in 20 minutes and persists for 6 to 8 hours.

Following the full application of peel solution, the frosting becomes evident and the tape can be applied for an occluded peel. Ice packs can be applied at the conclusion of the peel for comfort; if this is an untaped peel, petrolatum is used. A biosynthetic dressing such as Vigilon or Flexzan can be used for the first 24 hours (30). The patient usually is seen in 24 hours to remove the tape or the biosynthetic dressing and to monitor the healing. It is at this time the patient is again reinstructed on methods of compresses and occlusive ointments or dressings. It is important to keep the skin crust-free.

The four stages of wound healing are apparent after a deep chemical peel. They consist of (1) inflammation, (2) coagulation, (3) re-epithelializaiton, and (4) fibroplasia (31). At the conclusion of the chemical peel, the inflammatory phase has already begun, with a brawny, dusky erythema that will progress over the first 12 hours. There is an accentuation of pigmented lesions on the skin as the coagulation phase separates the epidermis, producing serum exudation, crusting, and pyoderma. During this phase it is important to use debridant soaks and compresses, as well as occlusive salves, which will remove the sloughed necrotic epidermis and prevent the serum exudate from hardening as crust and scab. I prefer to use of 0.25% acetic acid soaks found in the vinegar/water preparation (1 teaspoon of white vinegar, 1 pint of warm water), as it is antibacterial, especially against *Pseudomonas* and gram-negative bacteria. In addition, the mildly acidic nature of the solution is physiological for the healing granulation tissue and it is mildly debridant, as it dissolves and cleanses the necrotic material and serum. I prefer to use bland emollients and salves such as Vaseline petrolatum, Eucerin, or Aquaphor, as the skin can be monitored carefully day by day for potential complications.

Re-epithelializtaion begins on day 3 and continues until day 10 to 14. Occlusive salves promote faster re-epithelialization and less tendency for delayed healing. The final stages of fibroplasia continue well beyond the initial closure of the peeled wound and continues with neoangiogenesis and new collagen formation for 3 or 4 months. Prolonged erythema may last 2 to 4 months in unusual cases of sensitive skin or with contact dermatitis. New collagen formation can continue to improve texture and rhytides for a period up to 4 months during this last phase of fibroplasia.

RISKS AND COMMONLY ASSOCIATED PROBLEMS

Many of the complications seen in peeling can be recognized early during the healing stages. The dermatological surgeon should be well acquainted with the normal appearance of a healing wound and its time frame for both medium and deep peeling. Prolongation of the granulation tissue phase beyond 7 to 10 days may indicate delayed wound healing. This could be the result of viral, bacterial, or fungal infections, contact dermatitis interfering with wound healing, or other systemic factors. A red flag should alert the physician to careful investigation, and prompt treatment should be instituted to forestall potential irrepairable damage that may result in scarring.

Complications can be caused either intraoperatively or postoperatively. The two inherent errors that lead to intraoperative complications are (1) incorrect peel pharmacology and (2) accidental solution misplacement. It is the physician's responsibility to know that the solution and its concentration are correct. Trichloroacetic acid concentrations should be measured weight by volume because this is the standard for measuring depth of peel. Glycolic acid and lactic acid solutions, as well as Jessner's solution, must be checked for expiration date because their potency decreases with time. Alcohol or water absorption may inappropriately increase the potency, so one must assure the shelf life is appropriate. The peel solution should be applied with cotton-tipped applicators. In medium and deep peels, it is best to pour the peel solution in a secondary container rather than apply the solution spun around the neck of the bottle. Intact crystals may give the solution a higher concentration of solution as it is taken directly from its container. One should be careful to apply the solution to the appropriate location and not pass the wet cotton-tipped applicator directly over the central face, where a drop may inadvertently reach sensitive areas such as the eyes. Saline and bicarbonate of soda should be available to dilute TCA or neutralize glycolic acid if it is inappropriately placed in the wrong area. Likewise, mineral oil should be present for Baker's phenol peels. Postoperative complications most commonly result from local infection or contact dermatitis. The best deterrent for local infection is the continuous use of soaks to debride crusting and necrotic material. Streptococcal and staphylococcal infections can occur under biosynthetic membranes or thick occlusive ointments. Use of 0.25% acetic acid soaks seems to deter this, as does judicious removal of the ointment with each soak. *Staphylococcus, Escherichia coli,* and even *Pseudomonas* may result from improper care during healing and should be treated promptly with the appropriate oral antibiotic.

Frequent postoperative visits are necessary so that early onset of bacterial infection can be noted. Infection may present itself as delayed wound healing, ulcerations, and buildup of necrotic material with excessive scabbing, crusting, purulent drainage, and odor. Early recognition and treatment will prevent the spread of infection and scarring.

Herpes simplex infection is the result of reactivation of the herpes simplex virus (HSV) on the face and most commonly on the perioral area. A history of previous HSV infection should necessitate the use of prophylactic oral antiviral medications. Patients with a positive history can be treated with acyclovir 400 mg three times per day or 500 mg valcyclovir twice a day beginning on the day of the peel and continuing for 7 to 14 days, depending on whether it is a medium-depth or deep chemical peel. The mechanism of action is to inhibit viral replication in the intact epidermal cell. This means that the drug would not have an inhibitory effect until the skin is re-epithelialized, which is 7 to 10 days in medium and deep peels. In the past, these agents were discontinued at 5 days and clinical infection became apparent in 7 to 10 days (32).

Active herpetic infections can be treated easily with antiviral. When caught early, they usually do not cause scar.

Delayed wound healing and persistent erythema are signs that the peel is not healing normally. The dermatologist must know the normal time table for each of the healing events so that he or she can recognize when time healing is delayed or the erythema is not fading adequately. Delayed wound healing may respond to physical debridement if an infection is present, corticosteroids if the delay is due to contact allergic or contact irritant dermatitis along with the change of the offending contact agent, or protection with a biosynthetic membrane such as Flexzan or Vigilon. When this diagnosis is made, these patients must be followed daily with dressing changes and a close watch on the healing skin.

Persistent erythema is a syndrome where the skin remains pink to red beyond what is normal for the individual peel. A superficial peel loses its erythema in 2 to 4 days, a medium-depth peel within 60 days, and a deep chemical peel within 90 days. Erythema and/or pruritus beyond this period of time are considered abnormal and fit this syndrome. It may be contact dermatitis, contact sensitization, re-exacerbation of prior skin disease, or a genetic susceptibility to erythema, but it also may indicate potential scarring. Erythema is the result of the angiogenic factors stimulating vasodilation, which also indicates that the phase of fibroplasia is being stimulated for a prolonged period of time. For this reason, it can be accompanied by skin thickening and scarring. It should be treated promptly and appropriately with topical steroids, systemic steroids, intralesional steroids if thickening is occurring, and skin protection, which would eliminate the factors of irritancy and allergy. If thickening or scarring becomes evident, other measures that be helpful include the daily use of silicone sheeting and the pulsed dye laser to treat the vascular factors. With prompt intervention, scarring in many cases can be averted.

OTHER TECHNIQUES ARE COMBINED WITH PEELING

Correcting photoaging skin includes more than chemical peeling alone. Peeling helps resurfacing for epidermal and dermal aging and atrophic defects, as well as pigmentary growths; however, it will not solve problems of facial volume depletion, granulation changes, dynamic wrinkles, telangiectasias and vascular growths, or special conditions such poikiloderma.

Combining other procedures will solve problems and add benefits not obtained with peeling alone, including the following:

1. Cosmeceutical agents: Retinoids, glycolic acid lotions, bleaching agents, and home care exfoliants will enhance the results from a solitary peel and maintain the results. An appropriate sunscreen is very important.
2. Skin fillers will augment deeper rhytides and atrophic tissue so that peels can then refine the surface. Using collagen, cosmoplast, or hyaluronic acid products will smooth deeply wrinkled skin that peels cannot change.
3. Botox is used for the relaxation of dynamic wrinkles, especially in the glabella, forehead, and crow's feet. Injection prior to medium or deep peeling procedures will enhance the final results. Immobilizing the dynamic wrinkle will further lighten the dermal collagen remodeling in these areas, producing a better peeling result.
4. Peeling will not correct granulation changes or problems with excessive skin. If a patient needs rhytidectomy or blepharoplasty, these procedures should precede the peel procedure.

Chemical peeling thus does not stand alone as a solitary aesthetic procedure but should be combined with other tools to gain the best results.

CONCLUSION

The physician has the responsibility of choosing the correct modality to treat skin conditions such as photoaging skin, scars, dyschromias, and for the removal of skin growths. Many agents are available, including the three levels of chemical peels reviewed. It is the responsibility of the physician to have a thorough knowledge of all of these tools to give each patient the correct treatment his or her condition warrants.

REFERENCES

1. Brody HJ, Monheit GD, Resnick SS, Alt TH. A history of chemical peeling. Dermatol Surg 2000; 26:405–409.
2. Mackee GM, Karp FL. The treatment of post-acne scars with phenol. Br J Dermatol 1952; 64:456.
3. Stagnone JJ. Chemoabrasion. A combined technique of chemical peeling and dermabrasion. J Dermatol Surg Oncol 1977; 3:217.
4. Stegman SJ. A comparative histologic study of the effects of three peeling agents and dermabrasion on normal and sun-damaged skin. Aesthetic Plast Surg 1982; 6:123–125.
5. Fitzpatrick TB. The validity and practicality of sun-reactive skin types I through VI. Arch Dermatol 1988; 124:869–871.
6. Monheit GD. Chemical peeling for pigmentary dyschromias. Cosmetic Dermatol 1995; 8: 10–15.

7. Glogau RG. Chemical peeling and aging skin. J Geriatr Dermatol 1994; 2:30–35.
8. Monheit GD. Consultation for Photoaging Skin. Presentation at the American Academy of Dermatology at the New Orleans Hilton, March 25, 1999.
9. Wolfe SA. Chemical face peeling following therapeutic irradiation. Plast Reconstr Surg 1982; 69:859.
10. Monheit GD. Facial resurfacing may trigger the herpes simplex virus. Cosmetic Dermatol 1995; 8:9–16.
11. Glogau RG. Chemical peeling and aging skin. J Geriatr Dermatol 1994; 2:30–35.
12. Rubin M. Manual of Chemical Peels. Philadelphia: Lippincott, 1995:50–67.
13. Moy LS, Murad H, Moy RL. Glycolic acid peels for the treatment of wrinkles and photoaging. J Dermatol Surg Oncol 1933; 19:243–246.
14. Monheit GD. Skin preparation: an essential step before chemical peeling or laser resurfacing. Cosmetic Dermatol 1996; 9:13–14.
15. Mandy SH. Tretinoin in the preoperative and postoperative management of dermabrasion. J Am Acad Dermatol 1986; 15:879–879.
16. Monheit GD. Skin preparation: an essential step before chemical peeling or laser resurfacing. Cosmetic Dermatol 1996; 9:13–14.
17. Monheit GD. Chemical peeling for pigmentary dyschromias. Cosmetic Dermatol 1995; 8: 10–15.
18. Brody HJ. Trichloracetic acid application in chemical peeling, operative techniques. Plast Reconstr Surg 1995; 2:127–128.
19. Brody HJ. Variations and comparisons in medium depth chemical peeling. J Dermatol Surg Oncol 1989; 15:953–963.
20. Monheit GD. The Jessner's + TCA peel: a medium depth chemical peel. J Dermatol Surg Oncol 1989; 15:945–950.
21. Lawrence N, Brody H, Alt T. Chemical Peeling. In: Coleman WP III, Hanke W, eds. Cosmetic Surgery of the Skin. St. Louis, MO: Mosby, 1997:86–112.
22. Marrero GM, Katz BE. The new fluor-hydroxy pulse peel. Dermatol Surg 1998; 24:973–978.
23. Monheit GD. The Jessner's-trichloracetic acid peel. Dermatol Clin 1995; 13:277–283.
24. Rubin M. Manual of Chemical Peels, Lippincott. 1995:120–121.
25. Monheit GD. The Jessner's-TCA peel. Facial Plast Surg Clin North Am 1994; 2:21–22.
26. Monheit GD, Zeitouni NC. Skin resurfacing for photoaging: laser resurfacing versus chemical peeling. Cosmetic Dermatol 1997; 10:11–22.
27. Baker TJ, Gordon HL. Chemical Face Peeling. Surgical Rejuvenation of the Face. St. Louis: Mosby, 1986.
28. Alt T. Occluded Baker/Gordon chemical peel. Review and update. J Dermatol Surg Oncol 1989; 15:998.
29. McCollough EG, Langsdon PR. Chemical peeling with phenol. In: Roenigk H, Roenigk R, Eds. Dermatologic Surgery: Principles and Practice. New York: Marcel Dekker, 1989:997–1016.
30. Falanga V. Occlusive wound dressings. Arch Dermatol 1988; 124:877.
31. Goslen JB. Wound healing after cosmetic surgery. In: Coleman WP, Hanke CW, Alt TH, Eds. Cosmetic Surgery of the Skin. Philadelphia: BC Decker, 1991:47–63.
32. Monheit GD. Facial resurfacing may trigger the herpes simplex virus. Cosmetic Dermatol 1995; 8:9–16.
33. Hetter GP. An examination of the phenol-croton oil peel: Part I. Dissecting the formula. Plast Reconstr Surg 2000; 105:227–239, discussion 249–251.

12

Microdermabrasion for Treatment of Photoaging

Walter K. Nahm *University of California, San Diego School of Medicine, San Diego, and Dermatologic Surgery, West Los Angeles VA Medical Center, Los Angeles, California, U.S.A.*

Adam M. Rotunda *Dermatologic Surgery, West Los Angeles VA Medical Center, Los Angeles, California, U.S.A.*

Karen F. Han *Palo Alto Medical Foundation, Palo Alto, California, U.S.A.*

Adriana N. Schmidt / Ronald L. Moy *Dermatologic Surgery, West Los Angeles VA Medical Center, Los Angeles, California, U.S.A.*

- Microdermabrasion offers patients a simple, relatively inexpensive treatment for photoaging with rapid recovery time.
- One of the most popular cosmetic procedures.
- Requires no anesthesia, can be used on all Fitzpatrick skin types, and has minimal risk for dyschromia, infection, or scarring.
- Can be used in conjunction with other approaches to improve treatment results.

Cutaneous resurfacing methods using lasers, chemical peels, and physical agents have conventionally been used to improve wrinkles, texture, and pigmentation alteration. In this chapter, we discuss a subset of mechanical peeling called microdermabrasion and evaluate its utility for these signs of photoaging.

Microdermabrasion offers patients a simple, relatively inexpensive treatment for photoaging, with rapid recovery time. Since its introduction in the United States in 1996, microdermabrasion has become one of the most popular cosmetic procedures, with more than one million patients receiving treatment in 2002 (1). Although other resurfacing techniques offer potentially more effective results, microdermabrasion requires no anesthesia, can be used on all Fitzpatrick skin types, and has minimal risk for dyschromia, infection, or scarring (2). Microdermabrasion is used to treat the fine lines (and textual, and pigmentary) irregularities common in photoaged skin, as well as comedonal acne, lentigines, striae, and scars (due to acne, surgery, and trauma). It recently was demonstrated to help with palmoplantar keratoderma, Darier's disease, and actinic keratoses (2–8). The face, dorsal hands, anterior neck, and chest are most commonly treated.

Microdermabrasion was invented in Italy in 1985 when Molimed Engineering developed the first closed-circuit, negative pressure system (9). In 1988, Monteleone further investigated its clinical usefulness for treatment of scars (10). In the mid-1990s, Mattioli Engineering partnered with Aesthetic Lasers to submit an Italian-designed machine to the U.S. Food and Drug Administration (FDA). The microdermabrasion instrument was approved and granted exempt status, which meant that American manufacturers did not require clearance from the FDA. This subsequently led to a vast explosion in the number of manufacturers (more than two dozen) and machines that currently are available for use in the United States. However, with its unrestricted status, there is little incentive for manufacturers of microdermabrasion units to conduct controlled clinical trials evaluating clinical efficacy and the mechanism of action on photoaged skin. Reported clinical and histological effects of microdermabrasion derive from a limited number of peer-reviewed clinical trials, case series, physician and patient surveys, and comparison with other similar superficial rejuvenating techniques, such as chemical peels.

REGULATORY STATUS

Of particular concern in the health care system is the increasing number of complications resulting from nonphysicians performing cosmetic procedures. At the time of this writing, there is considerable variability in the types of professional status of individuals permitted by state medical boards to perform microdermabrasion. As of May 2002, 13 states permitted only physicians to perform microdermabrasion, and 21 states allowed physicians or other licensed health professionals (physician assistant, registered nurse, nurse practitioner, licensed cosmetologist, or aesthetician) supervised directly by a physician to treat patients (11). With such variation, physicians should be advised to check with their state medical board before having other licensed health and cosmetic professionals perform microdermabrasion. It is unclear at this time whether there will be subsequent national standardization and regulatory guidelines on the type of professional status of individuals who are allowed to perform microdermabrasion.

EQUIPMENT

Despite the vast array of machines available, all microdermabrasion units deliver an adjustable high-pressure stream of aluminum oxide, sodium bicarbonate, or sodium chloride crystals through a handpiece and use a self-contained vacuum to remove spent particles and debris (dirt and shed skin). Some machines provide the option of using positive pressure, which boosts the density of crystal abrasives that are projected to the skin, and provide greater flexibility in treating problem areas, such as scars. Handpieces are disposable or reusable; the latter must be sterilized before use on another patient. Most manufacturers sell aesthetician and physician models, which deliver a greater force of crystal flow and generally allow for greater suction, potentially introducing greater risk to the patient. Such devices cost between $8,000 and $20,000, depending upon the model, manufacturer, and often who provides on-site training and video instruction.

TECHNIQUE

The depth of treatment, and therefore the degree of injury produced during microdermabrasion, is dependent upon several variables, including crystal type, particle flow rate, vacuum (or negative) pressure, skin thickness, rate of movement across the skin surface, and number of passes (2,12). The crystals used are medical-grade aluminum oxide (commonly 100 μm in size), sodium chloride, or sodium bicarbonate. The sodium salts provide a smoother and less abrasive treatment than aluminum oxide crystals, which are very angular and second only to diamond in hardness (Fig. 1) (13). However, aluminum oxide and sodium chloride produce comparable histological changes and effects on epidermal barrier function (including decreased transepidermal water loss and increased stratum corneum hydration) (14,15). Crystal flow rate can be adjusted in some models by increasing positive pressure. The strength of its vacuum, or negative pressure, is operator dependent, as are the number of passes and contact time with the skin surface. Accordingly, more negative pressure, a greater number of passes, and longer time spent in contact at any one location all produce a deeper abrasion and inflammatory reaction.

The technique of microdermabrasion is relatively straightforward, and its application to the face is described here. First the treatment site is wiped thoroughly with an astringent cleansing solution (i.e., 70% alcohol) to remove dirt, makeup, and oil, and then air dried. Jewelry and contact lenses are removed, and the patient wears a cap or ties any loose hair away from the treatment field. The patient lies in a supine, partially reclined position and covers the eyes with goggles, pads, or moistened gauze. There is considerable variability in microdermabrasion negative-pressure settings reported in the literature, ranging from less than 10 mm Hg to greater than 380 mm Hg (4,5,13,16,17). Such discrepancies may be due to calibration differences between microdermabrasion vacuum units. After confirm-

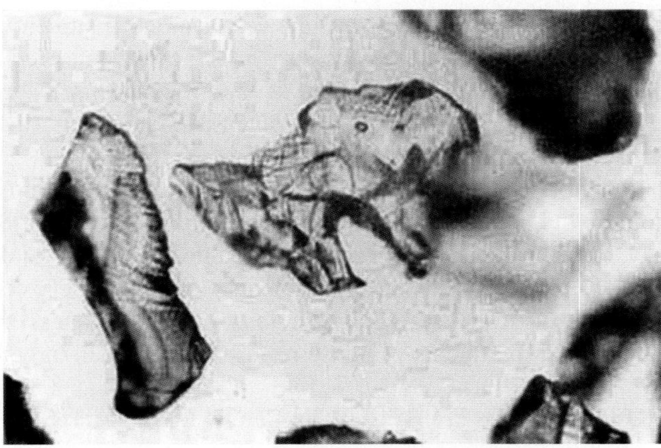

Figure 1 Microcrystals of aluminum oxide. (From Ref. 13.)

ing the recommended vacuum settings from the manufacturer, it is advisable to apply the handpiece to the medial forearm or other appropriate body part so that the vacuum settings can be adjusted to leave the treated area mildly pink. Using the dominant hand, the operator maintains constant contact with the skin as the nondominant hand stretches the area being treated. The handpiece usually is moved quickly along the surface in one direction (usually medial to lateral) for the duration of the stroke, whose length should stay consistent within the treatment site. Movement may be slower over the nose, chin, and forehead skin, which generally is more sebaceous and thicker. After a single pass, the motion is repeated in the opposite direction over the same site and then moved onto untreated skin. The negative vacuum pressure should be reduced on the thinner and sensitive infraorbital and malar skin. After treatment is completed, crystal remaining on the skin can be wiped away with a soft brush. A second pass may be made in a perpendicular direction to prevent streaking. Additional passes may be performed directed obliquely from the previous pass, although it is recommended to start with fewer passes and add another at subsequent sessions. Similarly, negative pressures may be increased at future visits.

Certain areas, including scars or hyperpigmented skin, may require more aggressive treatment with additional passes, increased crystal flow, or greater vacuum. Discomfort usually is minimal to none during the procedure. Depending upon the site, most treatments take between 15 and 30 minutes. After the procedure, patients should wash the skin with a nonabrasive moisturizing soap, dry, and apply a moisturizer with at least an SPF 15 sunscreen. Patients are advised to decrease sun exposure and apply a moisturizer with a broad-spectrum sunscreen at least once daily between treatment sessions. Most patients choose to return to work immediately and report no disruption in daily activity.

Although the face is the most commonly treated area, photodamage to the dorsal hands, chest, and neck make these sites particularly suitable for microdermabrasion. Some suggestions while treating these areas are as follows. The neck should be comfortably hyperextended before treatment, and only vertical strokes should be used. The patient should make a fist prior to hand treatments, and handpiece movement should be directed parallel to the long axis of the forearm. The chest is treated in a fashion similar to that of the face, where two perpendicular passes are initially performed.

TREATMENT REGIMENS

Although patients may notice a textural difference after one treatment, they should be aware that multiple sessions usually are necessary to achieve the desired effects. As with any cosmetic procedures, patients' expectation of the procedure must be addressed, and patients must be educated about the indications, potential side effects, and long-term outcome of microdermabrasion treatments.

Most manufacturers and clinicians recommend between four and eight treatments, spaced weekly to monthly, although up to 15 treatments have been reported for acne scars (13). Alternatively, some physicians recommend more intensive therapy initially (biweekly for 6 weeks) with subsequent maintenance treatments performed every couple of months. Moreover, there is a statistically significant increase in effectiveness between patients receiving fewer than three treatments vs. those receiving more than three treatments (18).

ADJUNCTIVE USE OF OTHER REJUVENATION MODALITIES

Patients seeking softening of skin lines, actinic damage, and pigment irregularities may benefit from other adjunctive skin care regimens during microdermabrasion treatment.

Many physicians in practice have observed that a combination of microdermabrasion with glycolic or trichloroacetic acid peels is a more effective treatment for photoaging than microdermabrasion alone. Moreover, 15% trichloroacetic acid used immediately after microdermabrasion was shown to be slightly more effective than microdermabrasion alone for the treatment of cutaneous facial hyperpigmentation (8). A combination of hydroquinone, topical retinoids, azelaic or kojic acid, and a short 2-month course of a low-potency topical steroid is effective for treating pigment irregularities (19–22).

Use of topical retinoids such as tretinoin and tazarotene are effective in diminishing the tactile roughness, coarse wrinkling, pore size, and irregular depigmentation associated with actinic damage. These products are discontinued at least 2 days prior to treatment because their associated inflammation may make subsequent microdermabrasion uncomfortable (23). Topical retinoids and over-the-counter antioxidants (vitamin A or C) or alpha-hydroxy acid (AHA) products (glycolic and lactic acid) may be resumed 3 days postprocedure.

Many speculate that microdermabrasion alters the skin barrier, resulting in improved penetration and efficacy of topical agents that make them more effective (4,24). On the subject of improved topical delivery, sonophoresis (low-intensity ultrasound focused to deliver energy into the skin) has been used to enhance the transport of topical agents such as AHAs and retinoids into the dermis after the skin's barrier has been disrupted by microdermabrasion. Although use of this process is well documented, its effectiveness has yet to be determined (25).

Others have used microdermabrasion as a means of eliciting erythema immediately before performing vascular targeted laser therapy. Microdermabrasion may aid the effectiveness of pulsed dye laser and intense pulsed light therapy for the treatment of background erythema and poikiloderma.

HISTOLOGICAL EFFECTS

Depth of Abrasion and Changes in the Epidermis

The depth of abrasion varies presumably with how aggressive the abrasion was performed. Tan et al. (13) demonstrated that even at a high level of vacuum at 65 mm Hg, there was only a slight thinning of the stratum corneum noted on histology after four passes, underscoring the very superficial nature of microdermabrasion (Fig. 2). However, another study showed that the stratum granulosum was penetrated from a different microdermabrasion unit at 30 mm Hg (26). Nonetheless, many authors have demonstrated a reduction and compaction of the stratum corneum in the acute posttreatment phase and epidermal thickening with flattening of the rete ridges in the chronic posttreatment phase, with decreased loss of polarity, typically seen in actinically aged skin (Fig. 3) (4,15,17,27,28).

Dermal Effects

In addition to the superficial effects of microdermabrasion, vascular dilation, perivascular mononuclear cell infiltrate, and edema in the dermis are consistently noted in histological studies (13). These changes may be responsible for the erythema and the perceived smoothening sensation of skin posttreatment. After a series of six microdermabrasion treatments, Freedman et al. (27) demonstrated with posttreatment histology a statistically significant increase in papillary dermal thickness, an increase perivascular infiltrate, and conspicuous fibroblasts, especially around the ectatic blood vessels (Fig. 4).

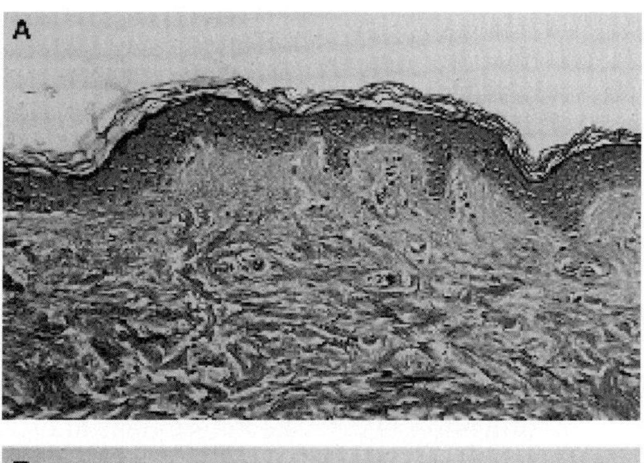

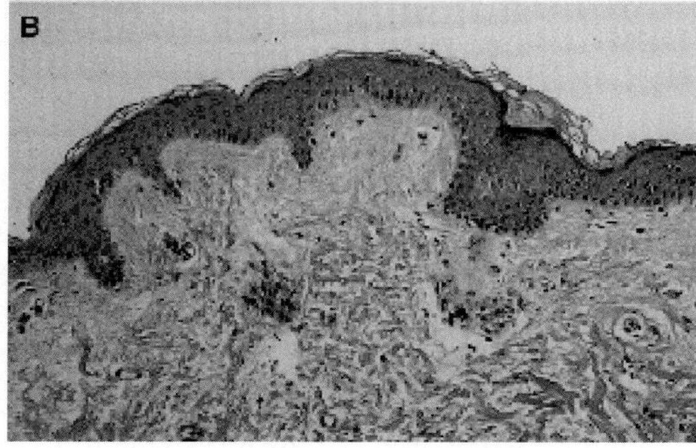

Figure 2 Histologic appearance of the volar forearm skin (A) pretreatment and (B) posttreatment with slight thinning of the stratum corneum and slight dermal edema (hematoxylin and eosin). (From Ref. 13.)

Changes in the concentration and quality of elastin and collagen have been recognized. Shim et al. (4) noted an increase in elastin in two of three patients who underwent biopsies, and Tsai et al. (6) noted slight upper dermal fibrotic changes in the only biopsy performed on 26 treated patients. Rubin and Greenbaum (26) noted an increase in fibroblast activity with new collagen deposition in the superficial papillary dermis. Hernandez-Perez and Ibiett (17) noted an increase in fibrillar collagen bundles, decreased elastosis, and new rete ridge formation.

As noted by several authors, in addition to direct abrasion of the epidermis, the dermal effects noted earlier perhaps can be attributed to the negative-pressure suction of this technique (4,13,29). Whether the dermal effects described earlier can be reproduced by suction alone, without superficial abrasion, is an area of study to be addressed.

CLINICAL EFFECTS

Biophysical Characteristics

Patients often feel a dry but much softer skin texture immediately after treatment. Posttreatment erythema may last from several hours to 1 week, depending upon the treatment parameters. Patients may experience mild painless exfoliation after several days. Rajan and Grimes (15) investigated skin barrier function at 24 hours and 7 days after microderma-

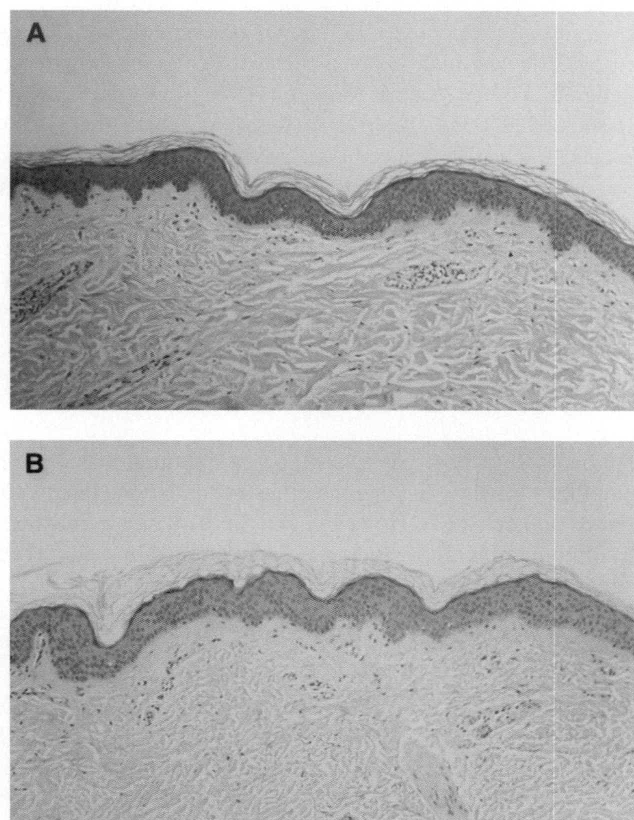

Figure 3 Biopsy specimen of the dorsal forearm (A) before and (B) after treatment series, 12 weeks later. Note the increased epidermal thickness. (From Ref. 4.)

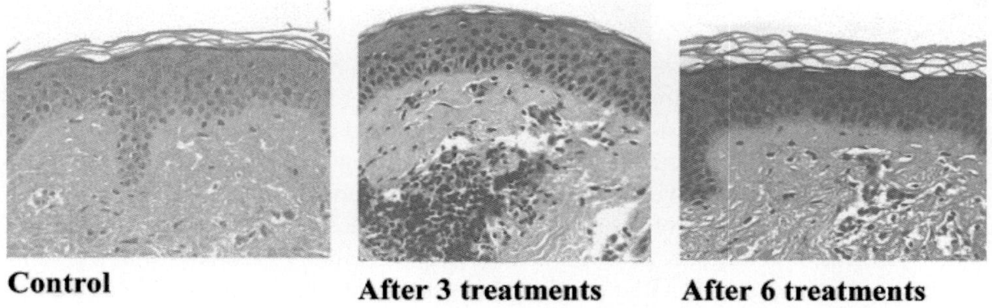

Figure 4 Histologic changes prior to and during a microdermabrasion series. Basal cell hyperplasia, increased fibroblasts, and inflammatory changes are seen after three and six treatments. (From Ref. 27.)

brasion. They reported that transepidermal water loss was highest 24 hours posttreatment and renormalized by 7 days, which is consistent with an acute abrasive injury followed by successful regeneration of the stratum corneum. A very slight decrease in transepidermal water loss was observed at day 7 relative to baseline, which the authors attributed to improved lipid barrier function. Enhanced lipid barrier function, and thus enhanced hydration in the stratum corneum, was demonstrated by a statistically increased capacitance 7 days posttreatment. Furthermore, Tan et al. (13) found a statistically significant decrease in skin stiffness between the first and sixth treatment (using 30 mm Hg weekly), with associated increase in skin compliance. These physical findings are consistent with the improved quality and quantity of dermal elastin and collagen demonstrated on histological findings discussed earlier.

Texture

Immediately after treatment, most patients report a smoother skin texture. This is felt even though a temporary increase in roughness has been demonstrated using skin surface topography in treated subjects (13). However, roughness disappeared 1 week after treatment. Immediate softening of wrinkles has been demonstrated immediately after treatment, but transient hydration and edema may account for these effects (13,15).

Pigmentation

Changes in mottled pigmentation seen in photoaging are difficult to measure objectively, although most patient and clinician surveys report favorable results (2). Shim et al. (4) found that there was comparatively more regular distribution of melanosomes and less melanization of the epidermis after six treatments (using 8–15 mm Hg every 2 weeks). Conservative microdermabrasion may be less effective than more aggressive treatment given the superficial histological component of lentigines. Reports using microdermabrasion for melasma are lacking, but they addressed melasma in the context of facial cutaneous hyperpigmentation with good results (complete remission in 40% and partial remission in 50% of 20 patients using up to eight treatments every 2 weeks) (8). It would be thought that without concomitant bleaching agents, effects would be minimal given the dermal pigment common to melasma (30).

Rhytides

Regardless of the intervention chosen, wrinkles are one of the most difficult signs of aging to treat. The most dramatic improvements result from aggressive procedures such as CO_2 laser resurfacing, dermabrasion, and deep chemical peels (e.g., trichloroacetic acid or phenol). However, the associated downtime makes patients less enthusiastic about these procedures. More conservative techniques, such as microdermabrasion or superficial chemical peels, are not as effective for rhytides and thus are deemed a ''rejuvenation'' rather than a resurfacing technique. In fact, the temporary flattening of wrinkles following microdermabrasion is thought to be due to the underlying dermal edema (13,15). One can speculate that if the dermal collagen remodeling described earlier is significant, then perhaps some wrinkle reduction should be clinically apparent and measurable. To our knowledge, there is no report to date that objectively demonstrates chronic improvement in rhytides resulting from microdermabrasion.

Scars

Tsai et al. (6) conducted the most extensive investigation of the use of microdermabrasion for superficial scars. Over a 2-year period they treated 41 patients with acne, traumatic, chicken pox, and burn scars. A mean of nine treatments, with a setting of 1 to 4 bar (19–76 mm Hg), was needed to achieve the endpoint of ''sufficient clinical improvement'' as appreciated by the patient or the operator. Good-to-excellent improvement was seen in the 18 patients with traumatic scars after a mean of four treatments. Three patients with surgical scars also had good-to-excellent improvement after a mean of four treatments (Fig. 5). However, a mean of 15 treatments was required to obtain good results in the 16 patients treated for acne scars, and some patients required up to 40 treatments for response. It was suggested that patients with acne scars must undergo more treatments than those with traumatic or surgical scars because acne scars are more depressed whereas traumatic ones are more elevated (6).

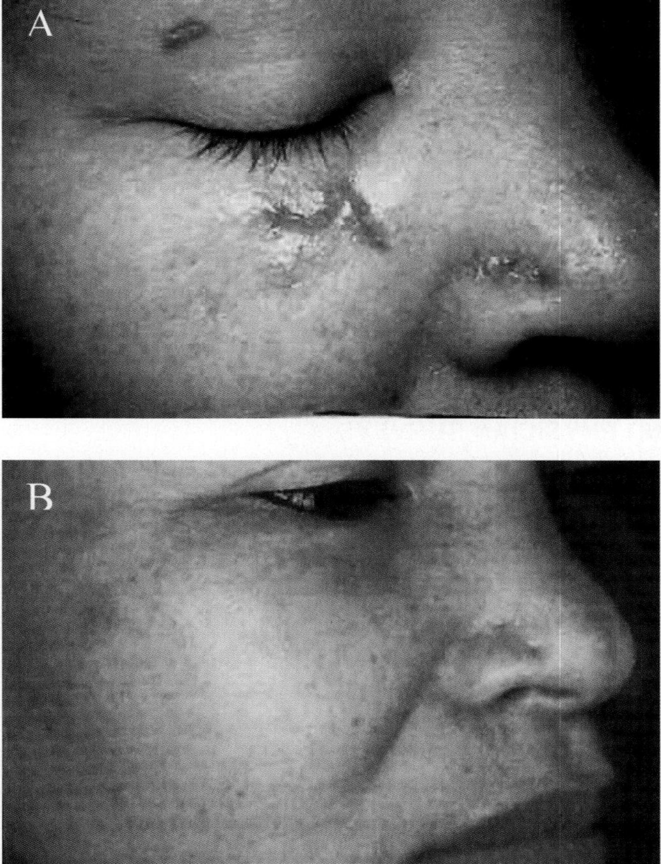

Figure 5 A: Surgical scar over the right eyelid. B: Appearance 2 months after four sessions of microdermabrasion. (From Ref. 6.)

In a study by Shim et al. (4), one patient with moderate acne scarring of ice pick-type scars had good improvement, and one of two patients with severe acne scarring consisting of shallow depressed scars had fair improvement. The authors state that good response requires aggressive treatment resulting in pinpoint bleeding. This raises the question whether medium-strength chemical peels, rather than microdermabrasion, is a more efficacious approach to acne scar treatment.

For treatment of abdominal striae, the MACROdermabrasion/Derma Phoresis Topical Kit (IntegreMed, LLC, Scottsdale, AZ), designed specifically for use with positive-pressure salt microdermabrasion, was shown in a 12-week study of 29 women to have 44% improvement when combined with microdermabrasion. A 39% improvement in striae was seen with positive-pressure salt microdermabrasion alone (25). The underlying mechanism by which microdermabrasion works on striae is unclear and again is speculated to be due to its dermal effects described earlier.

Acne

In a pilot study, Lloyd (5) evaluated microdermabrasion for the treatment of grade II to III acne and demonstrated promising results. Seventy-one percent of patients noted greater than 50% improvement in their condition based on four-graded pretreatment and posttreatment photographic evaluation. However, these patients were still using their oral (except for isotretinoin) and topical regimens originally prescribed (5). The author concluded that the benefits of microdermabrasion are greatest against postinflammatory acne lesions. A controlled trial is necessary to assess whether microdermabrasion alone can improve acne. In another study, Shim et al. (4) found that microdermabrasion did not statistically improve comedonal acne. Although Rajan and Grimes (15) did not demonstrate a statistically significant change in sebum production, Tan et al. (13) found as much as a four-fold decrease in sebum secretion after treatment. This decrease in sebum may be one of the reasons why microdermabrasion seems to improve noninflammatory acne conditions.

PATIENT AND PHYSICIAN SURVEYS

It can be argued that patient satisfaction with the simplicity and immediate effects of microdermabrasion, rather than dramatic clinical improvement, led to the extraordinary popularity of microdermabrasion. Moreover, some authors believe that patient satisfaction may dictate the success of the procedure and is the most valid measure of effectiveness (16,31). However, only a few studies reporting patient satisfaction with microdermabrasion appear in the literature (4,16,18).

A report by Bridges (18) surveyed 43 patients, 91% women, who had a mean of 4.51 microdermabrasion treatments for treatment of fine lines and skin texture. Overall short-term (<30 days) effectiveness was rated 2.91 (on a five-point scale of increasing effectiveness) and 2.5 for long-term effectiveness (>30 days). Shim et al. (4) reported significant improvement in patient self-graded signs of photoaging, including textural irregularities, mottle pigmentation, and overall complexion, but no improvement in acne/milia and fine wrinkling after six to seven treatments. A similar patient self-assessment 1 week after six microdermabrasion sessions in 10 patients revealed, on average, slight improvement in erythema, brown pigmentation, and skin softness, but no change in wrinkles and slight worsening in skin smoothness (16). In this study, these patients underwent six weekly, paired treatments of microdermabrasion on one side of the face and 20%

glycolic acid peels on the other side. Based on self-assessment survey between the two techniques, patients feel glycolic acid peels are associated with a greater overall improvement in smoothness and softness, but slight worsening in redness. Although the differences of each of the skin features assessed were not statistically significant, overall 7 of 10 preferred glycolic acid peels over microdermabrasion. To our knowledge, this was the only study in which the authors addressed a head-to-head comparison of microdermabrasion and glycolic acid peels. Because the results were not statistically significant, it is difficult to conclusively say that glycolic acid peels are a preferred technique. A larger comparative study with microdermabrasion vs. other superficial exfoliation modalities using objective measurements of biophysical characteristics of the skin are necessary. Nevertheless, it is now common practice to combine both modalities to synergistically treat mottled pigmentation and fine lines.

ADVERSE EVENTS

Despite is availability in nonmedical settings, microdermabrasion should be viewed as a medical procedure. Posttreatment erythema and possibly mild desquamation are to be expected after treatment and last hours to a couple of days (6,18). However infrequent, complications may arise and most often result from using too strong a vacuum suction, multiple passes, and/or moving too slowly on sensitive skin such as the periorbital region or areas of significant actinic damage. Additional caution is advised when using adjuvant skin rejuvenation therapy such as chemical peels and topical retinoids, which may make the skin susceptible to deeper ablation by microdermabrasion.

Potential adverse effects include patient discomfort, significant postprocedure xerosis and erythema, irritation, linear purpuric streaking, telangiectases, acneiform pustules, corneal abrasion, and scarring (although never reported) (2,6,13,16,18). Petechiae and pinpoint bleeding are more likely to arise on severely sun damaged skin or in patients using aspirin or nonsteroidal anti-inflammatory agents (4). Aggressive treatment is cautioned in Fitzpatrick skin types III and IV and should be avoided in darker skin to prevent postinflammatory hyperpigmentation. Depending upon their nature and extent, adverse effects may take several days (for streaking and petechiae) to several weeks (for hyperpigmentation) to resolve (4,13).

Ocular irritation can occur with microdermabrasion and can manifest as pain, photophobia, tearing, chemosis (swelling of the bulbar conjunctiva), and injection (13). In rare cases, the crystals can be adherent to the corneal epithelium, producing a punctate keratitis (13). Patients who wear contact lenses should remove them prior to treatment, and an eyewash should be kept available. Some physicians advocate the use of protective eyewear for both patients and operators.

There has been one reported case of an acute urticarial response after dermabrasion in a patient with latex allergy and dermatographism (32). The authors affirm that such complications are rare but require immediate medical intervention. This case emphasizes the importance of obtaining a detailed patient history and maintaining physician supervision over an office staff that may be performing the procedure. Clinicians should require from the microdermabrasion unit manufacturers a warning that latex exposure may occur at any time during a microdermabrasion procedure.

There has been considerable discussion about the acute and chronic effects of aerosolized aluminum exposure on the patient and operator. Aluminum oxide has been reported to cause laryngeal and tracheal papillomas, respiratory complications such as pulmonary fibrosis and decreased pulmonary function tests, and chest radiographic abnormalities in workers exposed to occupational aluminum (33–37). However, these findings are rare and inconsistent (35). Aluminum oxide microdermabrasion crystals are larger (100 μm) relative to industrial crystals (5 μm); therefore, they do not reach the alveoli (38–40). Furthermore, aluminum oxide has not been demonstrated to be a significant particulate after dental air abrasion (41). Aluminum salts inoculated into experimental animals have been found to produce neurofilamentous lesions that are similar, but not identical, to the neurofilamentous tangles of Alzheimer's disease (42–44). Nonetheless, although a few reports suggest that increased amounts of aluminum are found in the brains of patients with Alzheimer's disease, ongoing research still cannot ascribe a causative link (17,45).

The World Health Organization considers aluminum oxide a ''nuisance dust,'' such that it does not cause a biological response (40). Despite their size and unlikelihood of reaching the alveoli, some clinicians suggest having a high-efficacy particulate resistance (HEPA) filter nearby, avoiding positive-pressure foot pedal microdermabrasion units, and having the operator, who may be subject to prolonged exposure to the dust, use a filtration mask (4). Concerned operators may feel more comfortable choosing sodium chloride or bicarbonate crystals rather than aluminum oxide. Furthermore, a recent advance in microdermabrasion technology includes particle-free ''wands'' that have diamond chips directly attached to the probe, eliminating the environmental and health concerns of aluminum oxide (DiamondTome, Altair Instruments, Inc., Camarillo, CA).

CONTRAINDICATIONS

Contraindications to microdermabrasion include concurrent use of isotretinoin (patients should wait at least 1 year), impetigo or evidence of other infection (including verruca and herpes simplex), active dermatoses (e.g., inflammatory acne, rosacea, seborrheic dermatitis), significant dermatographism, pressure urticaria, latex allergy, untreated malignant skin tumors, and autoimmune disorders (4,32,46). Patients with a history of recurrent oral herpes simplex should be started on antiviral prophylaxis 2 days before and continued up to 1 week after treatment.

CONCLUSION

Microdermabrasion has gained widespread popularity in recent years because of its ability to improve the appearance of mild-to-moderate skin abnormalities. Aggressive marketing of the procedure can account for some of its popularity, which may have created unrealistic patient expectations. Although its effect on reversing the process of photoaging is modest, it appears that microdermabrasion is a useful adjunct to other skin care regimens. Furthermore, the increased epidermal thickness after multiple treatments may serve as a protective barrier against environmental damage, most notably from the sun. Finally, although the beneficial effects of microdermabrasion at the level of fibroblast activity, collagen synthesis, and elastic fibers remain to be further studied, microdermabrasion remains a quick painless procedure that can be performed easily in many settings.

REFERENCES

1. Cosmetic Surgery National Data Bank 2003. American Society for Aesthetic Plastic Surgery, 2002:5.

2. Bernard RW, Beran SJ, Rusin L. Microdermabrasion in clinical practice. Clin Plast Surg 2000; 27:571–577.
3. Glaser DA, Shah P, Nahass G, Schnoring H. The use of microdermabrasion in the treatment of striae distensae-a clinical open uncontrolled study of twelve patients. American Academy of Dermatology 61st Annual Meeting. San Francisco. California, 2003:628.
4. Shim EK, Barnette D, Hughes K, Greenway HT. Microdermabrasion: a clinical and histopathologic study. Dermatol Surg 2001; 27:524–530.
5. Lloyd JR. The use of microdermabrasion for acne: a pilot study. Dermatol Surg 2001; 27: 329–331.
6. Tsai RY, Wang CN, Chan HL. Aluminum oxide crystal microdermabrasion. A new technique for treating facial scarring. Dermatol Surg 1995; 21:539–542.
7. Imperio W. Tips on performing ablative rejuvenation procedures. Skin Allergy News 2001; 32(4):7.
8. Cotellessa C, Peris K, Fargnoli MC, Mordenti C, Giacomello RS, Chimenti S. Microabrasion versus microabrasion followed by 15% trichloroacetic acid for treatment of cutaneous hyperpigmentations in adult females. Dermatol Surg 2003; 29:352–356.
9. Clark CP 3rd. New directions in skin care. Clin Plast Surg 2001; 28:745–750.
10. McLachlan DR. Aluminum and Alzheimer's disease. Neurobiol Aging 1986; 7:525–532.
11. State board's position on microdermabrasion. PCI J 2002; 10:31–35.
12. Worcester S. Microdermabrasion is not limited to superficial use. Skin Allergy News 2001; 32(7):46.
13. Tan MH, Spencer JM, Pires LM, Ajmeri J, Skover G. The evaluation of aluminum oxide crystal microdermabrasion for photodamage. Dermatol Surg 2001; 27:943–949.
14. Boschert S. Histology data dribble in on microdermabrasion. Skin Allergy News 2001; 32(2): 7.
15. Rajan P, Grimes PE. Skin barrier changes induced by aluminum oxide and sodium chloride microdermabrasion. Dermatol Surg 2001; 28:390–393.
16. Alam M, Omura NE, Dover JS, Arndt KA. Glycolic acid peels compared to microdermabrasion: a right-left controlled trial of efficacy and patient satisfaction. Dermatol Surg 2001; 28: 475–479.
17. Hernandez-Perez E, Ibiett EV. Gross and microscopic findings in patients undergoing microdermabrasion for facial rejuvenation. Dermatol Surg 2001; 27:637–640.
18. Bridges MA. The efficacy of facial microdermabrasion. Cosmet Dermatol 2003; 16:19–20.
19. Grimes PE. Melasma. Etiologic and therapeutic considerations. Arch Dermatol 1995; 131: 1453–1457.
20. Pathak MA, Fitzpatrick TB, Kraus EW. Usefulness of retinoic acid in the treatment of melasma. J Am Acad Dermatol 1986; 15:894–899.
21. Breathnach AS. Melanin hyperpigmentation of skin: melasma, topical treatment with azelaic acid, and other therapies. Cutis 1996; 57:36–45.
22. Kligman AM, Willis I. A new formula for depigmenting human skin. Arch Dermatol 1975; 111:40–48.
23. Griffiths CE. The role of retinoids in the prevention and repair of aged and photoaged skin. Clin Exp Dermatol 2001; 26:613–618.
24. Fields KA. Skin breakthroughs in the year 2000. Int J Fertil Womens Med 2000; 45:175–181.
25. McDaniel DH. Laser therapy of stretch marks. Dermatol Clin 2002; 20:67–76.
26. Rubin MG, Greenbaum SS. Histologic effects of aluminum oxide microdermabrasion on facial skin. J Aesthet Derm Cosmet Surg 2000; 1:237–239.
27. Freedman BM, Rueda-Pedraza E, Waddell SP. The epidermal and dermal changes associated with microdermabrasion. Dermatol Surg 2001; 27:1031–1033.
28. Szachowicz EH. Microepidermabrasion: an adjunct to medical skin care. Otolaryngol Clin North Am 2002; 35:135–151.

29. Brunk D. Abrasion secondary? Suction could be the key to microdermabrasion. Skin Allergy News 2001; 32(4):36.
30. Sanchez NP, Pathak MA, Sato S, Fitzpatrick TB, Sanchez JL, Mihm MC. Melasma: a clinical, light microscopic, ultrastructural, and immunofluorescence study. J Am Acad Dermatol 1981; 4:698–710.
31. Ching S, Thoma A, McCabe RE, Antony MM. Measuring outcomes in aesthetic surgery: a comprehensive review of the literature. Plast Reconstr Surg 2003; 111:469–480.
32. Farris PK, Rietschel RL. An unusual acute urticarial response following microdermabrasion. Dermatol Surg 2002; 28:606–608.
33. Townsend MC, Enterline PE, Sussman NB, Bonney TB, Rippey LL. Pulmonary function in relation to total dust exposure at a bauxite refinery and alumina-based chemical products plant. Am Rev Respir Dis 1985; 132:1174–1180.
34. Townsend MC, Sussman NB, Enterline PE, Morgan WK, Belk HD, Dinman BD. Radiographic abnormalities in relation to total dust exposure at a bauxite refinery and alumina-based chemical products plant. Am Rev Respir Dis 1988; 138:90–95.
35. Schwarz Y, Kivity S, Fischbein A, Abraham JL, Fireman E, Moshe S, Dannon Y, Topilsky M, Greif J. Evaluation of workers exposed to dust containing hard metals and aluminum oxide. Am J Ind Med 1998; 34:177–182.
36. Jederlinic PJ, Abraham JL, Churg A, Himmelstein JS, Epler GR, Gaensler EA. Pulmonary fibrosis in aluminum oxide workers. Investigation of nine workers, with pathologic examination and microanalysis in three of them. Am Rev Respir Dis 1990; 142:1179–1184.
37. Berman E. Toxic Metals and Their Analysis. London: Heydon & Son, 1980.
38. Ess SM, Steinegger AF, Ess HJ. Experimental study on the fibrogenic properties of different types of alumina. Am Ind Hyg Assoc J 1993; 54:360–370.
39. Wentzell JM, Robinson JK, Wentzell JM, Schwartz DE, Carlson SE. Physical properties of aerosols produced by dermabrasion. Arch Dermatol 1989; 125:1637–1643.
40. Evaluation of exposure to airborne particles in the work environment. WHO Offset Publ 1984; 80:1–75.
41. Wright GZ, Hatibovic-Kofman S, Millenaar DW, Braverman I. The safety and efficacy of treatment with air abrasion technology. Int J Paediatr Dent 1999; 9:133–140.
42. Kowall NW, Pendlebury WW, Kessler JB, Perl DP, Beal MF. Aluminum-induced neurofibrillary degeneration affects a subset of neurons in rabbit cerebral cortex, basal forebrain and upper brainstem. Neuroscience 1989; 29:329–337.
43. Perl DP, Brody AR. Alzheimer's disease: X-ray spectrometric evidence of aluminum accumulation in neurofibrillary tangle-bearing neurons. Science 1980; 208:297–299.
44. Perl DP, Good PF. The association of aluminum, Alzheimer's disease, and neurofibrillary tangles. J Neural Transm Suppl 1987; 24:205–211.
45. Exley C. A molecular mechanism of aluminium-induced Alzheimer's disease? J Inorg Biochem 1999; 76:133–140.
46. Morgenstern KE, Foster JA. Advances in cosmetic oculoplastic surgery. Curr Opin Ophthalmol 2002; 13:324–330.

13

Ablative Laser Resurfacing

Mark Steven Nestor *Center for Cosmetic Enhancement, Aventura, and University of Miami School of Medicine, Miami, Florida, U.S.A.*

- Ablative laser resurfacing using carbon dioxide and erbium:yttrium-aluminum-garnet resurfacing lasers can be safe and effective in treating photodamaged and wrinkled skin.
- Careful consideration must be given to proper patient selection, preoperative and postoperative care, and proper technique.
- Significant complications may occur but can be minimized when they are recognized and treated quickly.
- Ablative resurfacing procedures can be used alone or in combination with a variety of nonablative procedures to maximize patient outcome.

INTRODUCTION

The use of lasers in clinical dermatology dates back more than 30 years with the initial use of continuous wave argon lasers and continuous wave CO_2 lasers (1). The mid- to late 1980s and early 1990s produced an influx of lasers for dermatology, such as neodymium:yttrium-aluminum-garnet (Nd:YAG), pulsed dye, and Q-switched lasers, which had significant efficacy (with certain side effects profiles) but were used by a more limited number of physicians (2–4). Clearly, the great wave of interest in lasers for both patients and physicians came during the mid 1990s with the advent of the ultrapulsed and scanned CO_2 lasers (5).

Carbon dioxide laser resurfacing provided physicians with the tools to significantly improve a patient's facial texture and mild-to-moderate wrinkling in a nonsurgical manner and opened the door to the widespread use of lasers by dermatologic and facial plastic surgeons. This advent of ''ablative laser resurfacing'' paved the way for future ablative and nonablative technologies, which now are in widespread use. Ablative laser resurfacing, first using CO_2 and then erbium:YAG (Er:YAG) lasers, had for many replaced traditional resurfacing techniques such as dermabrasion and deep chemical peels. The early promise of laser resurfacing was improvement in the results over the classic technologies, with a decrease in the relative incidence of side effects such as scarring, hyperpigmentation, and hypopigmentation (6). In retrospect, after hundreds of thousands of procedures were performed, it is clear that laser resurfacing has some significant benefits and advantages, but also some disadvantages. Laser resurfacing, whether CO_2 or erbium, has clearly shown side effects in both the short and long term. Recently, many physicians have virtually abandoned ablative procedures and replaced them with a variety of nonablative technologies. For many, however, ablative resurfacing with either CO_2 or newer combination long and short pulsed erbium lasers provides a significant tool for enhancement in carefully selected patients (7,8).

ABLATION

The end result of ablative laser resurfacing is the removal and heating of the epidermis and portions of the dermis, followed by associated biological and physiological reactions resulting in collagen shrinkage, remodeling, and thus an ultimate improvement in the appearance and texture of the skin (5). The classic targets for improvement of the skin using ablative laser resurfacing includes photoaging, color and textural changes, rhytides, benign lesions, and acne scarring (5,9). As ablative lasers remove the epidermis and at least a portion of the dermis, one can expect improvement of benign lesions such as lentigines and superficial nevi, seborrheic keratosis, and other benign neoplasms. Studies have shown that both CO_2 and erbium laser resurfacing can lead to significant changes in the topography of the skin (10).

Ablative laser resurfacing can be performed alone as a single treatment or in combination with a variety of treatment modalities, including surgical rhytidectomies, face lifts, blepharoplasties (11), punch excision or grafting (in the case of acne scarring), and even nonablative techniques such as pulsed dye laser and radiofrequency (Thermage, Hayward, CA) dermal remodeling.

THE LASERS

CO_2 Laser

The standard is the high-energy, short pulsed, carbon dioxide laser. It is the workhorse of ablative resurfacing because of the extremely rapid pulsing or computer-controlled scanning, which allows reproducible levels of ablative damage in the skin. Two classic examples of these technologies are the UltraPulse pulsed CO_2 laser (Lumenis, Santa Clara, CA) and the Silk and FeatherTouch scanned lasers (Lumenis) (12,13). Both of these devices reproducibly remove or ablate a layer of epidermis and dermis, and cause additional thermal injury to the remainder of the dermal tissue. The UltraPulse CO_2 laser and other pulsed lasers reproducibly ablate by using a pulse technology. This allows energy pulsing on a specific part of the skin for an exact amount of time. This pulse then is multiplied rapidly using computerized pattern generators to cover large areas of treated skin. The scanned units achieved similar results by using computer-controlled mirrors to scan a continuous beam across the skin and thereby achieve similar precise ablative tasks.

Although the results of CO_2 laser resurfacing certainly are impressive, the widespread use of these lasers showed that they were not without side effects and complications.

Virtually all patients treated with CO_2 laser have at least 1 week with an open wound, followed by at least 8 to 12 weeks of erythema. A significant potential for permanent hypopigmentation now is known to exist, and many patients have complained of a glassy-like appearance to their skin (6). There were a number of iterations of the CO_2 laser that sought to address these issues, including extremely short pulsed CO_2 lasers and rapidly scanned CO_2 lasers. In some physicians' hands these lasers did result in fewer side effects (14), but some patients still experienced the typical side effects of the CO_2 laser.

Er:YAG Laser

In the late 1990s, the Er:YAG laser was introduced with tremendous fanfare as an alternative to CO_2 laser resurfacing. The promise was that the Er:YAG laser would achieve similar results without long healing times, prolonged erythema, and side effects (15). The Er:YAG proved to have a shorter duration of healing and erythema and a slightly smaller incidence of complications, including scarring. There were significant limitations associated with the Er:YAG laser, including lack of significant tightening in many patients and lack of hemostasis (16). Erbium ablative resurfacing was not without complications and produced a certain number of scars, as well as hypopigmentation (16,17).

In the late 1990s, a number of companies introduced combination of short and long pulsed Er:YAG lasers, which were designed to take advantage of the benefits of microsecond pulsed erbium while offering offer additional benefits of millisecond pulsed erbium for improved hemostasis and thermally induced tightening. The goal was to achieve controlled effects of heat production that were somewhere between those of the CO_2 and traditional short pulsed Er:YAG lasers. These systems included the Contour (Sciton, Palo Alto, CA), variable pulse, Er:YAG, the Cynosure CO_3, long pulsed Er:YAG, and the DermaK CO_2 Er:YAG hybrid. These laser systems offered significant improvement and coagulation by either combining short and long pulsed erbium pulses or combining CO_2 with erbium (16–18).

Newer Er:YAG devices such as the Sciton Contour also allow for extremely superficial treatments; therefore, the concept of a ''weekend laser peel'' emerged. Patients could be treated using a low-fluence superficial erbium laser and heal within 2 to 3 days, with some improvement in skin texture and signs of photoaging (17).

PATIENT SELECTION

Patient selection prior to ablative resurfacing procedures is critical to a successful outcome. Not only will selection of the appropriate patient yield the best results from an ablative procedure, but it also will minimize side effects and complications. Depending upon the type of ablative laser used, patients with mild-to-moderate rhytides or signs of photoaging plus scarring associated with acne are the usual candidates for laser ablative therapy. Although patients can achieve significant improvement in tone and apparent tightening with CO_2 laser and some of the long pulsed erbium lasers, ablative laser resurfacing is clearly not a substitute for surgical intervention in patients with extremely lax skin. In addition, although ablative laser certainly can improve coloration and textural changes associated with sun damage, there is a limit to improvement of the vascular component of photoaging.

Acne scarring can improve significantly with ablative laser resurfacing; however, deeper scars of all types and ice-pick scars do not fair as well (9,19). Other options include excision or punch grafting of ice pick scars immediately prior to laser resurfacing.

Fitzpatrick skin type is also a significant criterion in patient selection. Many have incorrectly assumed that the lighter type skin types I and II fair best with laser resurfacing. Whereas patients with these skin types might not have problems with hyperpigmentation, lighter-skinned individuals tend to have more problems with long-term, if not permanent, hypopigmentation. Fitzpatrick type I and II patients also may suffer more complications associated with delayed healing (20). Darker-skinned individuals, specifically Fitzpatrick types IV, V, and VI, often have significant pigmentary abnormalities and generally are not good candidates for deeper laser procedures. In some physicians' hands, however, type IV and even type V patients may benefit from superficial erbium resurfacing (21). Although type V and type VI skin has been known to be more prone to hypertrophic and keloidal scars, it is clear that all skin types can be subject to hypertrophic scars (22). Thus, patients with all skin types must be informed of the long-term risks, and patients must be judged on an individual basis.

There are other contraindications to laser resurfacing (16). Patients who smoke are known to have a relatively increased risk of complications from any surgical procedure. This is due to reduced oxygenation of the skin as well as vascular contraction. Although the exact risk of an increased incidence of side effects of laser resurfacing is not clear, most laser surgeons suggest that patients stop smoking during the healing process for at least 2 weeks; many recommend that patients stop smoking up to 1 month prior to the procedure. Patients in poor health, with autoimmune conditions, undergoing radiation treatment, or with immunosuppression may have increased risk of complications because of increased susceptibility to infection and poor healing attributes. These certainly are contraindications, albeit not absolute. Most physicians believe that the use of isotretinoin within the preceding 6 months is an absolute contraindication (23,24). It is our practice to wait 1 year after a patient has completed a course of isotretinoin before proceeding with laser resurfacing. There is an increased risk of hypertrophic scar development in patients who received isotretinoin within 6 months prior to laser resurfacing. We even have seen cases of hypertrophic scar formation in patients who were placed on isotretinoin therapy as late as 3 to 4 months after laser resurfacing was performed. These patients appear to have healed satisfactorily but develop hypertrophic scars once placed on isotretinoin after laser resurfacing.

Patient selection also involves assessing the psychological needs and expectations of a patient (25). Patients must be informed about what to expect during the procedure and the potential final outcome. Ablative procedures can be significantly distressing because of the presence of either bandages or an open wound for at least 1 week or more. Patients also have significant erythema for a number of weeks. Despite the significant improvement that can be achieved with ablative laser resurfacing, no technique is perfect. Patients may not achieve their desired goals even with the best outcome.

Patient selection therefore involves the specific needs of the patient as well as their psychological willingness to undertake the risks. All patients need to understand all the choices that are available, including nonlaser resurfacing procedures such as dermabrasion and chemical peels. The numerous nonablative resurfacing and rejuvenation procedures also must be explained. With the guidance of the physician, a patient will weigh the pros and cons of all procedures and make an informed decision.

PREPARATION FOR ABLATIVE RESURFACING

Patients need to prepare for the recovery time of ablative procedures. Preparations include planning time off from work or other responsibilities and having time away from social interaction. They need to understand that, in the best of circumstances, it will take a number of days to heal and that they will need to start wearing makeup anywhere from 7 to 14 days after the procedure (25). Although some controversy exists about preoperative medications, most physicians choose prophylaxis with both oral antibiotics and oral antiviral agents for their patients. In addition, some believe that pretreatment with tretinoin for several weeks improves healing and enhancement of results (26).

The choice of oral antibiotics includes broad-spectrum antibiotics effective for gram-positive bacteria such as *Staphylococcus* and *Streptococcus*, and efficacy for gram-negative bacteria including *Pseudomonas* (27). We start patients on azithromycin (Zithromax Z-Pak, Pfizer, New York, NY) 1 day prior to the resurfacing procedure and in most cases switch them over to ciprofloxacin 500 mg twice a day for 7 days when they finish the initial course of the azithromycin. The combination tends to be very well tolerated by most individuals. Others choose to use more traditional cephalosporins or penicillin derivatives.

Most physicians feel the need for prophylaxis with antivirals (28). Our choice is to use famciclovir 250 mg twice a day starting approximately 2 days prior to the procedure and continuing for approximately 10 days until full re-epithelialization has occurred. In patients who are highly susceptible and with a significant history of herpes simplex, the dose is increased to 500 mg twice a day. Additional preparation often is necessary for patients who are undergoing level II or level III anesthesia, which involves a preoperative workup for the anesthesiologist and in most cases restriction to fluids after midnight of the day of surgery. Normally our patients shower the evening prior to the procedure, although some physicians tend to have a more significant ritual of antimicrobial washes both immediately and 1 day prior to the procedure.

ANESTHESIA

Anesthesia for resurfacing procedures varies considerably, depending upon the procedure that is being performed. For a variety of erbium laser procedures, patients often can tolerate the procedure with just the use of topical ELA-Max (Ferndale Laboratories, Ferndale, MI) or other topical anesthetics based on lidocaine or tetracaine. Somewhat deeper erbium resurfacing may also necessitate the use of infraorbital, supraorbital, and submental blocks using 2% lidocaine (Xylocaine) with epinephrine and/or intralesional Xylocaine with epinephrine in the periorbital region. For deeper laser procedures, many physicians tend to use either intravenous sedation with midazolam (Versed), Propofol, and/or other level II anesthetics or full level III intubation procedures using paralyzing agents as well as inhaled anesthetics. Whenever flammable anesthetics and/or oxygen are used, a major concern is shielding the patient well. The combination of oxygen and resurfacing lasers increases the risks of flame burning or an explosion (29). The use of level II or level III sedation requires adequate training in resuscitation techniques by operating room personnel, appropriate postanesthesia care, and, in most states, a specific certification or licensure.

ABLATIVE RESURFACING PROCEDURES

Articles too numerous to mention have been written about the specific technique for CO_2 laser resurfacing, but generally physicians perform either one or multiple passes using the laser, making sure that there is little if any overlap of the pulses or scans and that the char is removed completely prior to additional passes. The technique is split into two schools of thought. In the first, the initial pass is made over the deeper wrinkles and damaged skin only, followed by removal of the char and then a complete pass over the entire face. The second technique involves a straightforward one or two passes performed over the entire face (6,30). There is significant controversy about use of the CO_2 laser to resurface areas other than the face. Although some physicians choose to use the CO_2 laser on areas such as the neck and the chest, most believe that the risk of scarring increases dramatically when the CO_2 laser is used on areas other than the face (31).

The erbium laser is generally utilized to accomplish superficial laser resurfacing and generally requires some overlap of the resurfacing beam. Unless significant coagulation is caused by the long pulsed erbium laser, removal of material between passes is not required. Newly designed long pulsed erbium lasers, such as the Sciton Contour, allow specific depths to be programmed for consistent and reproducible results. This laser even allows for extremely superficial depths of approximately 10 to 20 μm, which allows for a ''micro laser peel'' in which healing can occur in 2 to 3 days (16–18).

POSTOPERATIVE MANAGEMENT

To minimize the risks of infection and to enhance healing, there are two methods of postoperative care. These can be divided into open techniques, which use topical emollients such as Aquaphor or Vaseline, and closed techniques, which use a variety of artificial dressing materials. Both of these techniques have their advantages and disadvantages. In the open technique, the patient is much more actively involved in the recuperative phase because the patient is kept busy applying topical emollient multiple times a day. The open technique tends to be a little more uncomfortable but allows the physician better visibility of healing. The closed technique can speed healing and may be more comfortable for the patient, but it is thought to be associated with a higher risk of infection. This risk of infection when using the closed technique seems to be minimized when closed bandages are left on for no more than 24 to 48 hours (32,33).

We prefer the open technique. The patient is seen in the office once or twice over the 7 to 10 days immediately postoperatively. Instructions are to soak with sterile saline and reapply Aquaphor frequently. Some physicians have patients soak with diluted acetic acid or utilize a variety of topical agents including topical antibiotics. Systemic antibiotics and antivirals are continued during the initial postoperative course until full re-epithelialization occurs. Although some utilize systemic prednisone to decrease swelling, most believe that oral steroids are not beneficial and could increase the risk of postoperative infection.

Depending upon the type of laser used, initial re-epithelialization occurs anywhere from the first 3 to 4 days up to 7 to 14 days after deep erbium or deeper CO_2 laser treatment. Patients continue to use open and/or closed dressing systems until complete re-epithelialization occurs, and most are placed on topical moisturizers, emollients, and/or sun blocks after re-epithelialization occurs. Early in the re-epithelialization process, patients have a tendency to bruise easily and may even desquamate easily upon moderate tension on the skin (25,34). The edema associated with ablative resurfacing abates slowly. Initially there is a significant swelling, but the swelling diminishes as re-epithelialization occurs. Some swelling may remain for up to 4 to 8 weeks. Patients may see immediate significant reduction of wrinkles because of the presence of edema, but they become disillusioned in 4 to 8 weeks because many of the wrinkles recur once the edema subsides.

Erythema or bright redness can remain for up to 2 to 3 months, depending on the depth of resurfacing. Erythema gradually fades and is easily covered with makeup. Many physicians believe that it is easier to camouflage full-face resurfacing than to hide regional resurfacing erythema and pigmentation changes.

Patients begin observing improvement approximately 2 to 3 months after the procedure, with continued improvement at least 6 to 8 months postprocedure (10). Most physicians wait at least 6 months before considering a second procedure or touching up areas. Patients who undergo regional resurfacing in the perioral or periorbital regions have more problems during the early stages of erythema because of the marked contrast with adjacent untreated areas.

The results are clear and consistent improvement in superficial and moderately significant rhytides and damage. CO_2 laser resurfacing can yield dramatic and significant improvement in patients with moderate-to-severe wrinkling and can result in significant toning and tightening of lax skin (Figs. 1 through 4). Significant improvement in patients with pigmentary abnormalities and fine lines can be obtained using the erbium laser (Fig. 5).

SIDE EFFECTS AND COMPLICATIONS

Side effects occur to some degree in virtually all patients, are expected, and tend to be self- limited. As mentioned, erythema or redness occurs in virtually all patients

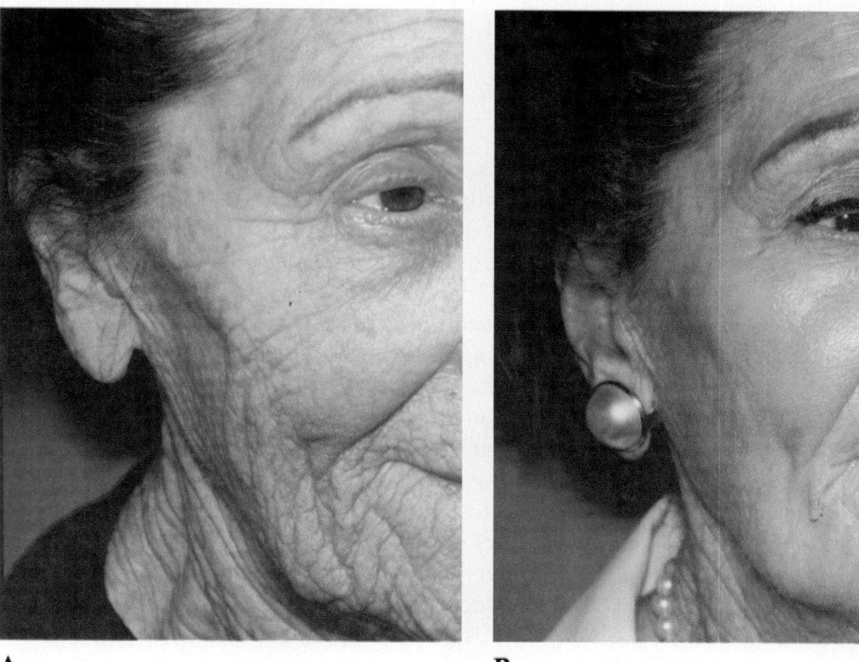

A B

Figure 1 CO_2 laser resurfacing using the FeatherTouch scanned resurfacing laser preoperatively (A) and at 1-year follow up (B).

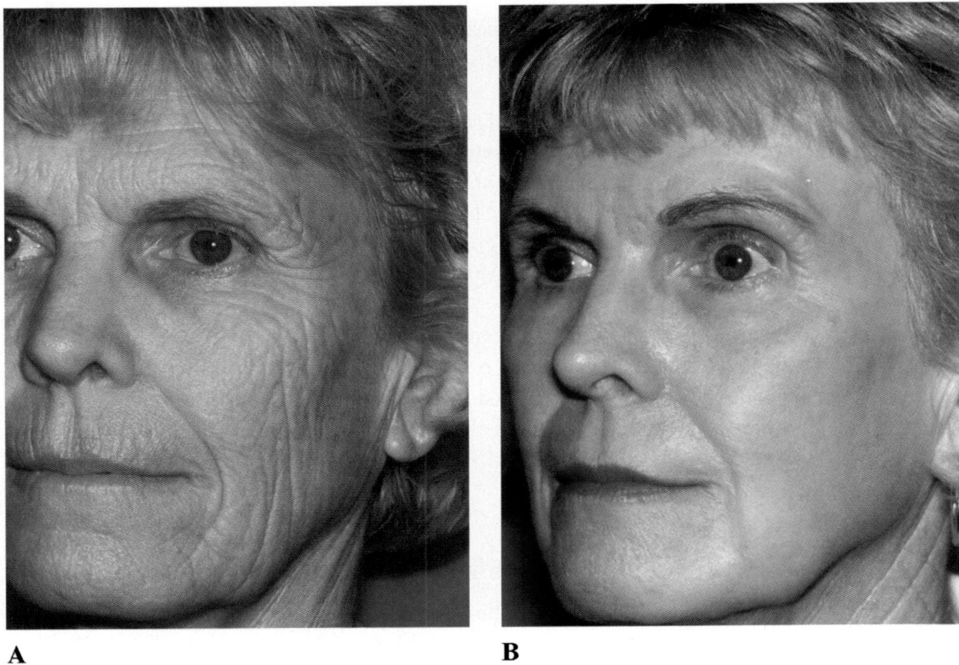

A B

Figure 2 CO_2 laser resurfacing using the FeatherTouch scanned resurfacing laser preoperatively (A) and at 1-year follow up (B).

and generally lasts anywhere from 2 weeks to 3 or 4 months. Milium or acne occur in the majority of patients and usually resolves on its own (6,25). Some patients benefit from the use of topical tretinoin for a period of time. A few patients experience intense burning pain, but the majority of patients have only minor discomfort associated with the procedure.

Edema occurs in almost 100% of patients and generally abates over time. Although hypopigmentation can be considered a complication when significant alabaster nontanning hypopigmentation occurs, most patients experience some relative hypopigmentation because of removal of hyperpigmented sun-damaged skin.

Complications of laser resurfacing include hyperpigmentation, hypopigmentation, infection, scarring, and, in a small minority of patients, nonhealing or delayed healing. Healing difficulties eventually may lead to permanent scarring after approximately 8 to 10 months (35–37). Hyperpigmentation occurs in many patients with type III and IV skin. Hyperpigmentation is much rarer in patients with type I and II skin. Some believed that hyperpigmentation could be decreased by the use of preoperative bleaching agents such as hydroquinone. Studies have shown that postoperative hyperpigmentation incidence is not changed (37). Patients who develop postoperative hyperpigmentation are treated with a combination of broad-spectrum sun blocks, hydroquinones, or combination treatments such as Triluma (Galderma Laboratories, LP, Fort Worth, TX). The vast majority of laser hyperpigmentation occurring after the procedure resolves in 4 to 8

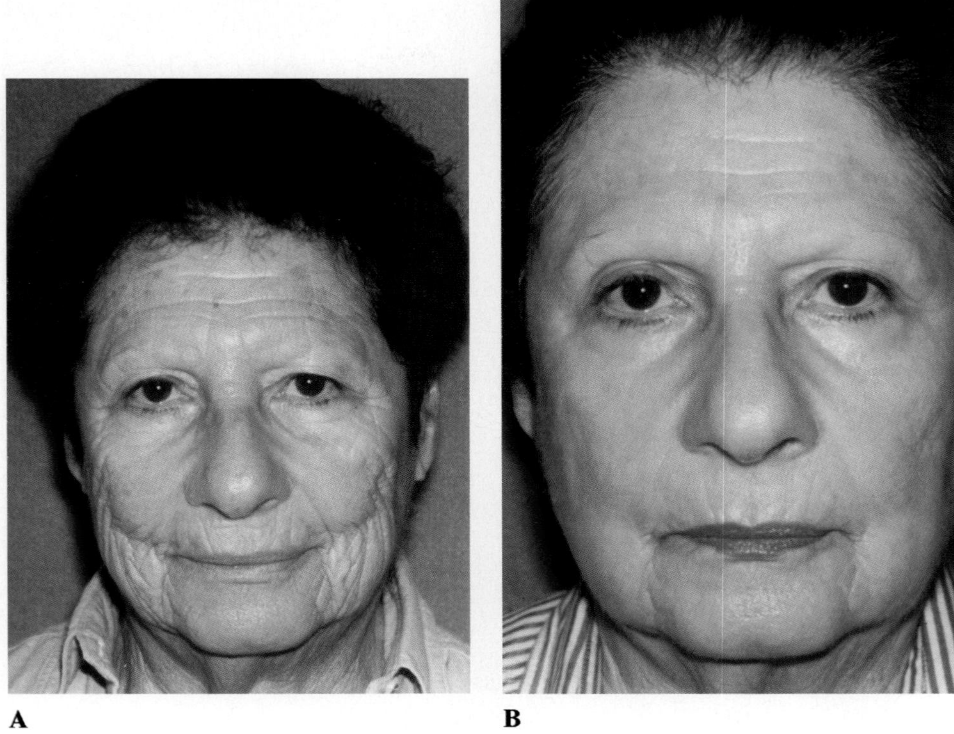

A B

Figure 3 CO_2 laser resurfacing using the FeatherTouch scanned resurfacing laser preoperatively (A) and at 1-year follow up (B).

weeks. In some patients, additional treatment such as microdermabrasion may be helpful.

Hypopigmentation can be a side effect of the procedure or a significant complication. Most patients experience relative hypopigmentation because of removal of tanned and dyspigmented sun-damaged skin. Significant permanent loss of pigmentation occurs in a subset of patients who undergo deeper CO_2 resurfacing and some deep erbium resurfacing procedures. This hypopigmentation is the alabaster type, similar to that seen with deep chemical peels (36). This complication occurs over the first 6 to 8 months but may appear even years later. Recently the excimer laser (Xtrac, PhotoMedex, PA) and the Relume narrow-band UVB device (Lumenis) have given hope for repigmentation, but the results are preliminary.

Infection is a risk and has been reported as bacterial, viral, or fungal (22,31,38–40). Covered wounds are more prone to infection. Signs include increasing redness, increasing pain, and new formation of ulcerations (20). A clue to atypical infections, including herpes simplex virus, fungal infection, and atypical bacteria, is the lack of response to broad-spectrum antibiotics and chronic unrelenting course (40). Cultures and specific antibiotics often are necessary for diagnosis and treatment. Untreated infection can lead to scarring.

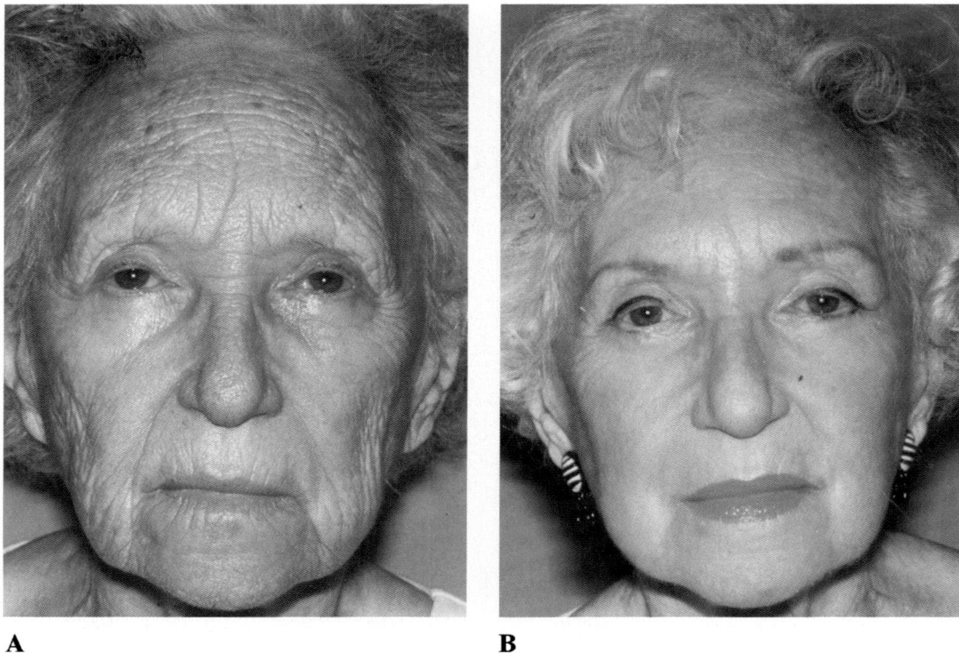

Figure 4 CO_2 laser resurfacing using the FeatherTouch scanned resurfacing laser preoperatively (A) and at 1-year follow up (B).

Scarring certainly is not common, but it can occur after any ablative procedure (35). The thought that scarring only occurs in deeper laser procedures is not true, although depth is related to a higher incidence of scarring. Scarring most often occurs on the upper lip and angle of the jaw and is much less frequent in regions of high sebaceous gland concentration. Hypertrophic scars often start with an area of discreet erythema appearing 3 to 4 weeks after the procedure and become dusky or darker hued over time. The hypertrophic scar itself may not appear until 6 to 10 weeks after the laser procedure. Hypertrophic scars need to be treated aggressively using combinations of intralesional triamcinolone, topical gels, and pulsed dye laser relatively early (41) (Fig. 6). Scars become more difficult to manage with time, but even mature scars can respond to pulsed dye laser, intense pulsed laser, and/or intralesional triamcinolone.

A small minority of patients have reported difficulties with healing after laser resurfacing (42). These patients generally have type I or II skin type and often are treated using closed dressing type procedures. Although the etiology of this complication is not clear, it is believed that a combination of infection and some sort of autoimmune phenomenon causes delayed re-epithelialization. The ''nonhealing'' or ''delayed healing'' syndrome can be associated with deeper laser procedures but has been reported in patients who underwent just single-pass or two-pass procedures. Although management is difficult, we have had the most success using combinations of oral antibiotics, antivirals, open wound care with gentle topical treatment, and judicious use of topical cortisones such as betamethasone dipropionate ointment. When patients finally heal,

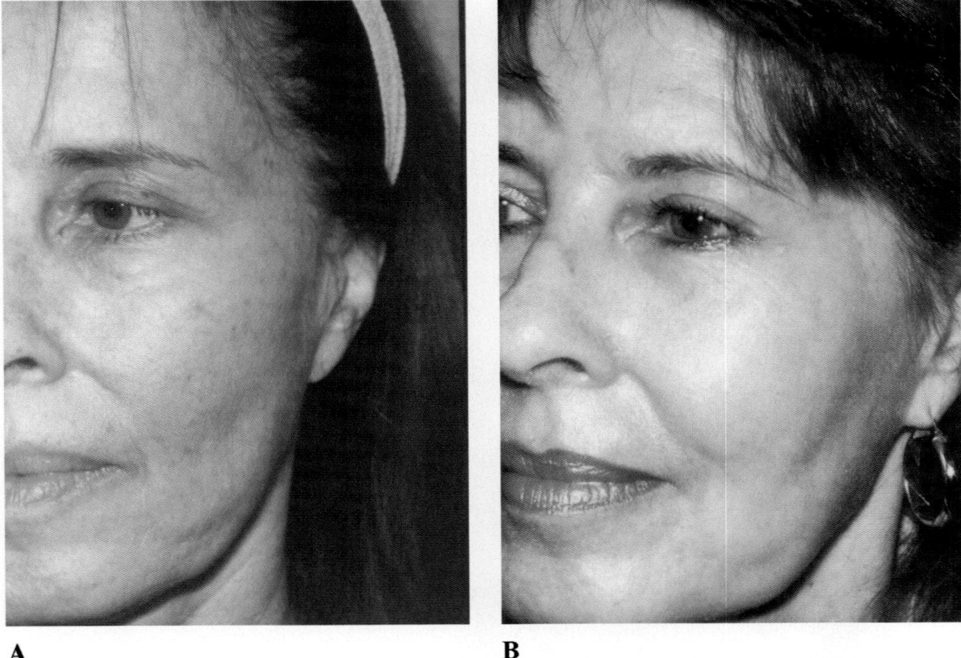

Figure 5 Erbium laser resurfacing preoperatively (A) and at 1-year follow-up (B). Multiple passes with short pulse erbium laser.

which may take 8 to 10 months, they heal with significant scarring, which then must be addressed (Fig. 7).

FUTURE OF ABLATIVE RESURFACING

As more physicians embrace nonablative treatments, some question the future of ablative laser resurfacing procedures. A significant number of patients now can see adequate and significant improvement with use of a variety of nonablative procedures. These procedures include photorejuvenation using intense pulsed light (43), as well as nonablative wrinkle improvement procedures such as the 1320-nm Nd:YAG laser (44) and the 1450-nm diode laser (45). Tightening and toning procedures may use radiofrequency (46). A novel combination treatment called photodynamic skin rejuvenation (47), which utilizes a combination of microdermabrasion, amino levulinic acid, and either intense pulsed light or pulsed dye laser, can be an option, especially for patients with significant actinic keratoses and other signs of photoaging previously amenable only to ablative procedures. A combination of ablative laser procedures including superficial and deeper erbium laser resurfacing with intense pulsed light for the vascular component and skin tightening with radiofrequency (ThermaCool TC, Thermage) may turn out to be the ultimate and ideal method for treatment of photoaging. We may find that use of the combination of nonablative procedures with superficial ablative procedures offers pa-

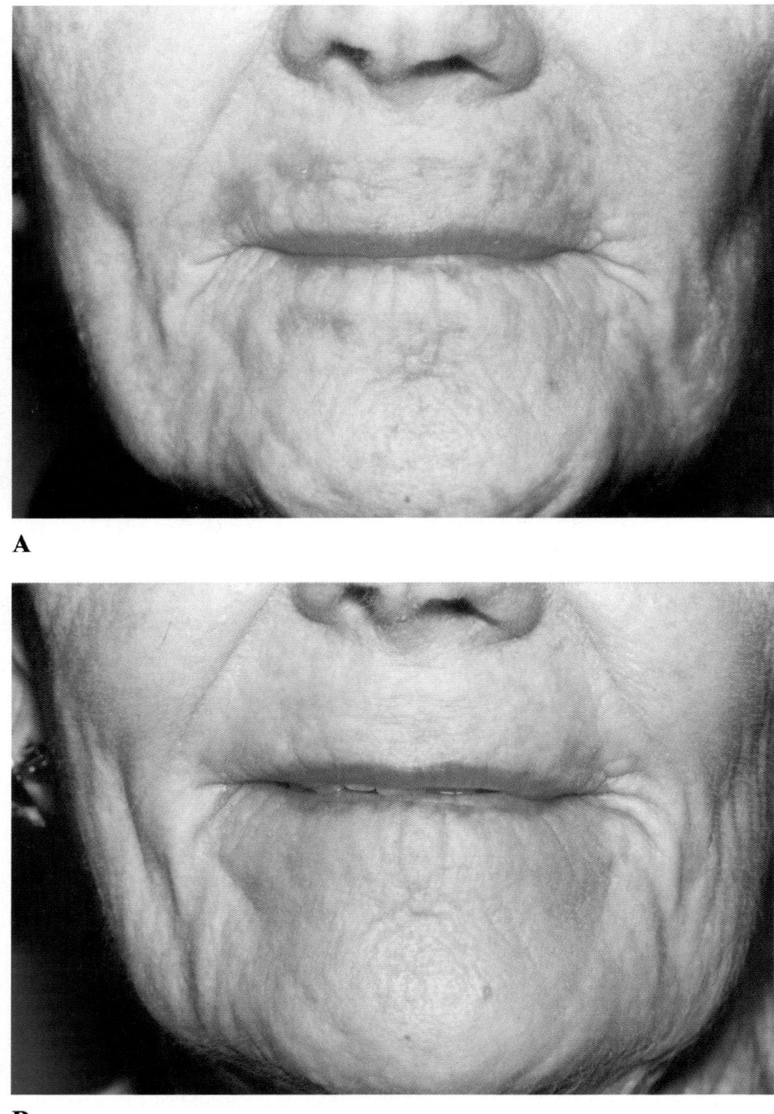

Figure 6 Hypertrophic scarring caused by CO_2 laser resurfacing before (A) and after (B) five treatments with 585-nm pulsed dye laser.

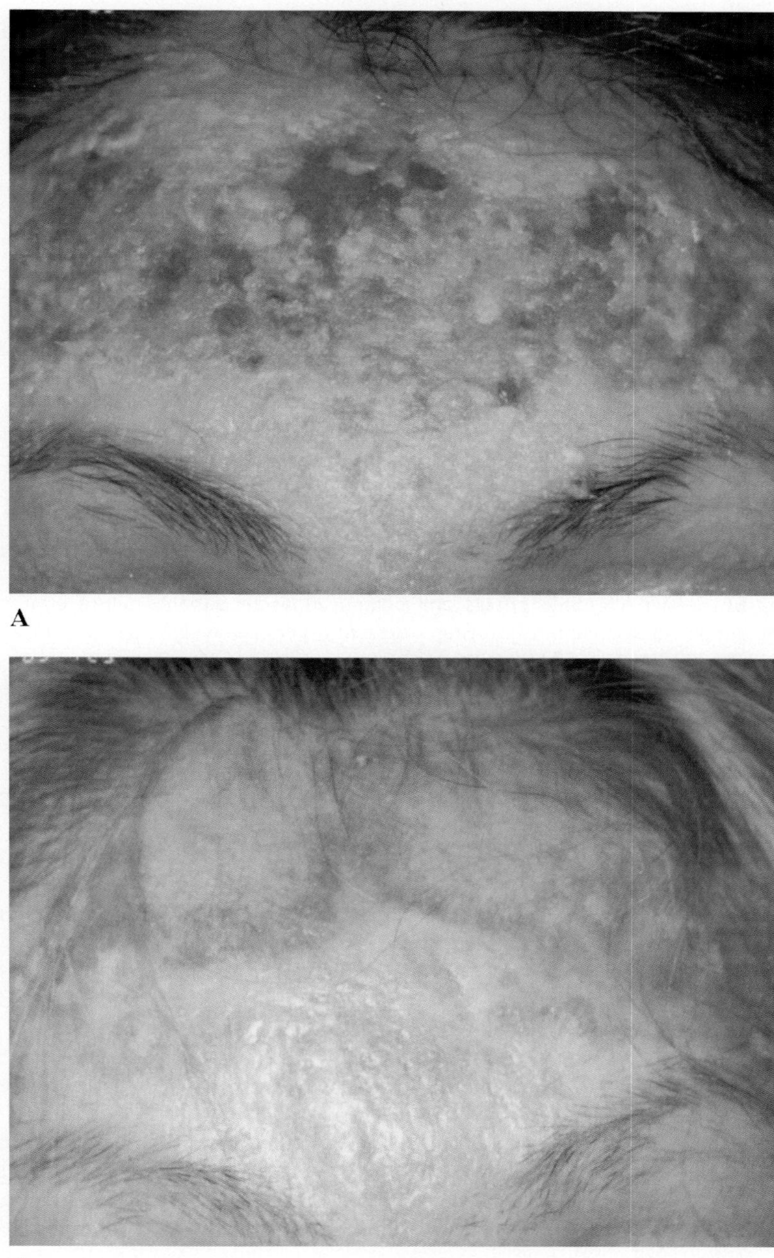

Figure 7 Delayed healing syndrome. A: Eight months post-laser resurfacing. B: Ten months post-laser resurfacing after treatment with antibiotics and topical cortisones.

tients the best results. Although it is clear that the use of ablative, CO_2, and erbium technology has been significantly supplanted by newer nonablative procedures, the older technology is extremely flexible and certainly will continue to have a place in the overall scheme of rejuvenation and resurfacing for photoaging.

REFERENCES

1. Goldman L. Pathology of the effect of the laser beam on the skin. Nature 1963; 197:912.
2. Anderson R. Selective photothermolysis of cutaneous pigmentation by Q-switched Nd:YAG laser pulses at 1964, 532, and 355 nm. J Invest Dermatol 1989; 93:28.
3. Tan O. Treatment of children with port-wine stains using the flashlamp-pulsed tunable dye laser. N Engl J Med 1989; 320:416.
4. Nehal K. The treatment of benign pigmented lesions with the Q-switched ruby laser: a comparative study using the 5.0 and 6.5 nm spot size. Dermatol Surg 1996; 22:683.
5. Fitzpatrick R. Laser resurfacing of rhytides. Dermatol Clin 1997; 15:431.
6. Bernstein L. The short- and long-term side effects of carbon dioxide laser resurfacing. Dermatol Surg 1997; 23:519.
7. Fitzpatrick RE. Maximizing benefits and minimizing risk with CO_2 laser resurfacing. Dermatol Clin 2002; 20:77–86.
8. Tanzi EL, Alster TS. Side effects and complications of variable-pulsed erbium:yttrium-aluminum-garnet laser skin resurfacing: extended experience with 50 patients. Plast Reconstr Surg 2003; 111:1524–1529.
9. Alster TS, West TB. Resurfacing of atrophic facial acne scars with a high energy, pulsed carbon dioxide laser. Dermatol Surg 1996; 22:151–155.
10. Fitzpatrick RE, Rostan EF, Marchell N. Collagen tightening induced by carbon dioxide laser versus erbium:YAG laser. Lasers Surg Med 2000; 27:395–403.
11. Roberts TL III, Pozner JN. Lasers, facelifting, and the future. Clin Plast Surg 2000; 27: 293–298.
12. Weinstein C, Roberts TL. Aesthetic skin resurfacing with the high-energy ultrapulsed CO2 laser. Clin Plast Surg 1997; 24:379–405.
13. Chernoff G, Slatkine M, Zair E. SilkTouch: a new technology for skin resurfacing in aesthetic surgery. J Clin Laser Med Surg 1995; 13:97–100.
14. Alster TS, Nanni CA, Williams CM. Comparison of four carbon dioxide resurfacing lasers: a clinical and histologic evaluation. Dermatol Surg 1999; 25:153–159.
15. Goldman MP. Techniques for erbium:YAG laser skin resurfacing: initial pearls from the first 100 patients. Dermatol Surg 1997; 23:1219–1221.
16. Alster TS. Clinical and histologic evaluation of six erbium:YAG lasers for cutaneous resurfacing. Lasers Surg Med 1999; 24:87–92.
17. Pozner JN, TL III. Variable-pulse width Er:YAG laser resurfacing. Clin Plast Surg 2000; 27:263–270.
18. Zachary CB, Grekin RC. Dual mode Er:YAG laser systems for skin resurfacing.
19. Kye YC. Resurfacing of pitted facial scars with a pulsed Er:YAG laser. Dermatol Surg 1997; 23:880–883.
20. Christian MM, Behroozan DS, Moy RL. Delayed infections following full-face CO_2 laser resurfacing and occlusive dressing use. Dermatol Surg 2000; 26:32–36.
21. Alster TS. Clinical and histologic evaluation of six erbium:YAG lasers for cutaneous resurfacing. Lasers Surg Med 1999; 24:87–92.
22. Nanni CA, Alster TS. Complications of cutaneous laser surgery: a review. Dermatol Surg 1998; 24:209–219.
23. Katz BE, MacFarlane DF. Atypical facial scarring after isotretinoin therapy in a patient with previous dermabrasion. J Am Acad Dermatol 1994; 30:852–853.

24. Bernestein LJ, Geronemus RG. Keloid formation with the 585-nm pulsed dye laser during isotretinoin treatment. Arch Dermatol 1997; 133:111–112.
25. Horton S, Alster TS. Preoperative and postoperative considerations for carbon dioxide laser resurfacing. Cutis 1999; 64:399–406.
26. McDonald WS, Beasley D, Jones C. Retinoic acid and CO_2 laser resurfacing. Plast Reconstr Surg 1999; 104:2229–2235.
27. Manuskiatti W, Fitzpatrick RE, Goldman MP. Prophylactic antibiotics in patients undergoing laser resurfacing of the skin. J Am Acad Dermatol 1999; 40:77–84.
28. Wall SH, Ramey SJ, Wall F. Famciclovir as antiviral prophylaxis in laser resurfacing procedures. Plast Reconstr Surg 1999; 104:1103–1108.
29. Wald D, Michelow BJ, Guyuron B. Fire hazards and CO_2 laser resurfacing. Plast Reconstr Surg 1998; 101:185–188.
30. Alster TS, Garg S. Treatment of facial rhytides with a high-energy pulsed carbon dioxide laser. Plast Reconstr Surg 1996; 98:791–794.
31. Fitzpatrick RE, Goldman MP, Sriprachya-Anunt S. Resurfacing of photodamaged skin on the neck with an UltraPulse(R) carbon dioxide laser. Lasers Surg Med 2001; 28:145–149.
32. Weiss RA, Goldman MP. Interpenetrating polymer network wound dressing versus petrolatum following facial CO_2 laser resurfacing: a bilateral comparison. Dermatol Surg 2001; 27:449–451.
33. Christian MM, Behroozan DS, Moy RL. Delayed infections following full-face CO_2 laser resurfacing and occlusive dressing use. Dermatol Surg 2000; 26:32–36.
34. Alster TS. cutaneous resurfacing with Er:YAG lasers. Dermatol Surg 2000; 26:73–75.
35. Ragland HP, McBurney E. Complications of resurfacing. Semin Cutan Med Surg 1996; 15:200–207.
36. Laws RA, Finley EM, McCollough ML. Alabaster skin after carbon dioxide laser resurfacing with histologic correlation. Dermatol Surg 1998; 24:633–636.
37. West TB, Alster TS. Effect of pretreatment on the incidence of hyperpigmentation following cutaneous CO_2 laser resurfacing. Dermatol Surg 1999; 25:15–17.
38. Bellman B, Brandt FS, Holtmann M. Infection with methicillin-resistant Staphylococcus aureus after carbon dioxide resurfacing of the face. Successful treatment with minocycline, rifampin, and mupirocin ointment. Dermatol Surg 1998; 24:279–282.
39. Monheit GD. Facial resurfacing may trigger the herpes simplex virus. Cosmetic Dermatol 1995; 8:9–16.
40. Rao J, Golden TA, Fitzpatrick RE. Atypical mycobacterial infection following blepharoplasty and full-face skin resurfacing with CO_2 laser. Dermatol Surg 2002; 28:768–771.
41. Alster TS, Lupton JR. Treatment of complications of laser skin resurfacing. Arch Facial Plast Surg 2000; 2:279–284.
42. Rendon-Pellerano MI, Lentini J, Eaglstein WE. Laser resurfacing: usual and unusual complications. Dermatol Surg 1999; 25:360–366.
43. Nestor MS, Goldberg DJ, Goldman MP. Photorejuvenation: non-ablative skin rejuvenation using intense pulsed light. Skin Aging 1999; 7:3.
44. Goldberg DJ. Non-ablative subsurface remodeling: clinical and histologic evaluation of a 1320-nm Nd:YAG laser. J Cutan Laser Ther 1999; 1:153–157.
45. Goldberg DJ, Rogachefsky AS, Silapunt S. Non-ablative laser treatment of facial rhytides: a comparison of 1450-nm diode laser treatment with dynamic cooling as opposed to treatment with dynamic cooling alone. Lasers Surg Med 2002; 30:79–81.
46. Hsu TS, Kaminer MS. The use of nonablative radiofrequency technology to tighten the lower face and neck. Semin Cutan Med Surg 2003; 22:115–123.
47. Nestor MS, Goldberg DJ, Goldman MP. New prospectives on photorejuvenation. Skin Aging 2003; 11:68–74.

14

Botulinum Toxin A in Photoaging

Alastair Carruthers / Jean Carruthers *University of British Columbia, Vancouver, British Columbia, Canada*

- Botulinum toxin can be used for treatment of rhytides and other signs of photoaging.
- Careful technique is required for optimizing cosmetic results.
- Proper dilution and handling of material are important.
- Appropriate patient selection and setting of expectations are critical for maximizing patient satisfaction.

INTRODUCTION

The face is the center of human communication, social interaction, and the perception of attractiveness. For some, the appearance of static facial lines—a natural occurrence in the aging process–adversely affects communication, attractiveness, and potentially even self-esteem (1). Botulinum toxin type A (BTX-A) has been used extensively over the last few years to treat hyperfunctional facial lines and now is one of the most frequently performed nonsurgical procedures on the face and neck. Effective in the treatment of dynamic facial lines, BTX-A relaxes the underlying muscular activity responsible for the formation of wrinkles. However, BTX-A alone cannot address nondynamic rhytides and other signs of photodamage. This chapter reviews the history and basic principles of BTX-A therapy, alone and as adjunctive therapy, for the treatment of facial aging.

BACKGROUND AND HISTORY

The anaerobic bacterium *Clostridium botulinum*—identified more than 100 years ago as the cause of muscle paralysis secondary to food poisoning (2)—produces seven distinct serotypes of BTX, each with varying potencies, mechanism of action, and clinical effects (3,4).

Pharmacology and Mechanism of Action

The commercially available subtypes, BTX-A and botulinum toxin type B (BTX-B), both are 150-kDa di-chain polypeptides composed of heavy and light chains linked by disulfide bonds (5). During biosynthesis, BTX-A and BTX-B form neurotoxin—protein complexes of 900 and 700 kDa, respectively (6). Following successful binding of the heavy chain to the motor nerve terminal, the toxin is internalized via receptor-mediated endocytosis, a process in which the plasma membrane of the nerve cell invaginates around the toxin receptor complex, forming a toxin-containing vesicle inside the nerve terminal. The neurotoxin molecule is released into the cytoplasm and cleaved into the heavy and light chains. The light chain of BTX-A cleaves a 25-kDa synaptosomal associated protein (SNAP-25), integral to the successful docking and release of acetylcholine from vesicles situated within nerve endings. The light chain of BTX-B cleaves vesicle-associated membrane protein (VAMP or synaptobrevin). Initial recovery of muscle contraction after BTX-A and BTX-B is accompanied by collateral sprouting of active, but transitory, terminal buds near the parent terminal. These new sprouts eventually disappear, and neurotransmission is restored at the original nerve ending (4).

History of Cosmetic Use

Pure BTX-A was first isolated in its crystalline form in 1946 (7). In the late 1970s, Alan Scott (Smith-Kettlewell Eye Research Foundation, San Francisco, CA) began to study BTX-A for strabismus in both monkeys and humans and first described its safety and efficacy in humans in 1980 (8). Scott's prediction that botulinum neurotoxins could be useful in a number of conditions caused by muscle spasms or hyperactivity proved correct: the U.S. Food and Drug Administration (FDA) approved BTX-A for the treatment of strabismus and blepharospasm in 1989, followed by approval for the use of both BTX-A and BTX-B for cervical dystonia in 2000.

Convinced of its safety and efficacy, we began using BTX-A in 1983, noted improvement in the appearance of glabellar lines in patients treated for blepharospasm in 1987, and published the first report of its cosmetic use in 1992 (9). Around that time, other physicians began reporting aesthetic benefits in patients treated for facial dystonias (10,11). The FDA approved BTX-A for the treatment of glabellar lines in 1992. Now, virtually all dynamic facial rhytides in the face and neck are treated routinely with BTX-A.

Sources

BTX-A (BOTOX®, BOTOX Cosmetic™) and BTX-B (MYOBLOC®) currently are the only botulinum neurotoxins commercially available in North America, while Dysport® (BTX-A) is available in Europe.

Each vial of BOTOX contains 100 mouse units of vacuum-dried *C. botulinum* type A neurotoxin complex. The vacuum-dried product must be stored in a freezer at or below −5°C or in a refrigerator between 2°C and 8°C. Before its use, BOTOX must be reconstituted with physiological saline (5).

MYOBLOC is available in a liquid formulation containing BTX-B 5000 U/mL and is available in 0.5-, 1.0-, and 2.0-mL vials containing BTX-B, saline, human serum albumin, and sodium succinate, with a pH of approximately 5.6 (which accounts for the stinging sensation reported on injection). Reconstitution is not required and is hampered by "overfill" of the vials. Clinicians who wish to add saline are advised to do so in the syringe.

The unopened vial is stable for months or years; once opened, the labeling is similar to BTX-A (12).

Dysport is available as a lyophilized vial containing 500 U of BTX-A, as well as sodium chloride, lactose, and human serum albumin. The smaller amount of albumin in Dysport compared to BOTOX may account for some of the difference in efficacy between the two products' units. In Europe, Dysport is labeled for transport at ambient temperature and storage at 2°C to 8°C, and the guidelines for reconstitution and use are similar to those for BOTOX (13).

Potency and Clinical Efficacy

There is a wide range of potency among the different serotypes in humans. BTX-A is the most potent in producing muscular paralysis in humans, followed by types B and F (3). The ''gold standard'' of assessing potency of BTX is the mouse lethality assay (MLA), in which 1 U is defined as the murine LD_{50} of intraperitoneal-injected BTX. For reasons that are not clear, the potencies in humans of 1 U of BOTOX, Dysport, and MYOBLOC are vastly different. The literature describes a BOTOX to Dysport potency ratio of 1:2 to 1:6 (14,15) and a BOTOX to MYOBLOC potency ratio of 1:50 to 1:100 (16,17). Doses of one formulation cannot be substituted for another formulation, and precise dosage conversion factors have not been established.

The clinical efficacy and safety of BTX-A have been well documented (9,18) and reported beneficial for a wide range of cosmetic indications (3,19); fewer data assessing the efficacy of BTX-B are available. In cosmetic clinical trials, BTX-B has demonstrated a more rapid onset of action, a wider diffusion, and a shorter duration of action, and is associated with greater pain upon injection and other side effects compared to BTX-A (20–25).

ADVANTAGES AND DISADVANTAGES

The use of BTX-A in facial rejuvenation has become increasingly popular due to its impressive safety and efficacy profile. Rather than simply treating the appearance of facial rhytides, BTX-A addresses the underlying muscular activity responsible for the development of wrinkles and folds. The procedure is quick and relatively painless; can be performed during lunch so that the patient can return to work immediately; and results in few skin blemishes, in contrast to the extensive skin wounding that occurs with chemical peels and laser skin rejuvenation. The clinical effects appear in 1 to 2 days, peak at 1 to 4 weeks, and gradually decline within 3 to 4 months. As the number of treatment sessions increases, the duration of clinical effect may lengthen. Patients who have undergone a series of treatments over a period of 1 year or more may experience clinical effects for as long as 6 to 12 months.

Although the temporary duration of action may be considered a disadvantage, the absence of a permanent effect produces a self-correcting situation and allows fine adjustments to the effect over time. In fact, some patients use BTX-A injections as ''rehearsals'' for more invasive surgical procedures. Side effects that occur with BTX-A are minimal and transient. More serious complications, such as ptosis, are due to both poor injection technique and lack of proper patient education (see Patient Selection and Side Effects and Complications).

PATIENT SELECTION

Appropriate patient selection is critical in ensuring satisfaction with clinical outcomes in facial rejuvenation.

Contraindications and Precautions

BTX-A is contraindicated in the presence of any neuromuscular disorder that could amplify the effect of the drug, such as myasthenia gravis, Eaton-Lambert syndrome, myopathies, or amyotrophic lateral sclerosis. Other contraindications include pregnancy, the presence of infection at the injection site, or a known hypersensitivity to any of the product contents. Caution should be used in patients with disorders that produce a depletion of acetylcholine (5).

BTX-A works best in younger patients, aged 20 to 45 years, and is most effective in reducing facial lines due to underlying muscle pull rather than to age-induced loss of dermal elasticity. A number of patients do not achieve a satisfactory aesthetic response to BTX-A alone (26). These patients have a marked display of facial lentigines, telangiectasia, and telangiectatic matting with fine rhytides and diminished skin texture, leading to an overall appearance of fatigue, frustration, and age that persists after treatment with BTX-A (27).

Patient Education

Assessment and education of the patient seeking facial aesthetic neuromodulation is critical, because some patients may have unrealistic expectations and may be unsatisfied irrespective of the outcome. Clinicians should inquire about the basis for the request and the areas of concern to the patient, because the face the patient views in the mirror may not always match the face in his or her imagination. A history of previous cosmetic interventions (and the patient's satisfaction with each outcome) may yield important background information.

In preparing patients for treatment, it is important to address their safety concerns. Ensure that they understand the procedures, what to expect before and after treatment, potential side effects (including ptosis or bruising), the typical time course of the clinical effects, and the need for re-treatment after 3 to 6 months. Patients must be instructed to remain upright and not to press or manipulate the injected areas in the immediate postinjection period.

Documentation

Document each patient's current anatomy with careful photographs that provide ''before'' and ''after'' comparisons and note any atypical features. Digital photography is an optimal method of documenting preoperative, intraoperative, and postoperative results in the clinical setting. A digital camera is a wise investment for cosmetic practitioners, not only for its cost savings and ability to capture both still and moving images of facial disorders or areas of concern, but also for its superior archiving capabilities (on office network, disks, or CD-ROM), documentation, and reproduction.

GENERAL TECHNIQUE

There currently are two commercially available sources of BTX-A: BOTOX and Dysport. The majority of our clinical experience is with BOTOX, and all references in this chapter are to the BOTOX or BOTOX Cosmetic formulations, unless otherwise specified. However, the clinician should be aware of the significant clinical differences between the two sources of BTX-A and adjust dosages accordingly.

Reconstitution and Dilution

Although manufacturers' guidelines recommend reconstitution with sterile, nonpreserved 0.9% saline solution and discarding the vial after 4 hours (5), other physicians have reported efficacy up to 6 weeks following reconstitution. (28,29). In addition, reconstitution with preserved saline has proved considerably less painful upon injection (30) and does not impair the stability of BTX-A (28,31).

The appropriate diluent volume must be selected based on the desired concentration of the injection solution, although higher doses of BTX-A delivered in smaller volumes (50 or 100 U/mL) keep the effects more localized and allow for the precise placement of the toxin with little diffusion (3,32).

General Procedures

Immediately prior to treatment, standardized, same-magnification color photographs or images of the glabellar region are recorded both when muscles are at rest and during maximal frowning. This aids in determining individual characteristics of the patient's muscular structure. Performing preinjection markings with the patient sitting upright will produce the most accurate representation of the natural movement of the muscles and corresponding facial rhytides. Draw up the appropriate dose of BTX-A into the syringe and express the air. In our clinic, we use the Becton-Dickinson Ultra-Fine II short needle 0.3 insulin syringe, which has an integrated 30-gauge, silicon-coated needle, which minimizes both patient discomfort and drug waste compared to traditional syringes having a needle hub (33). The needle dulls after approximately six injections and should then be discarded. We use a bottle opener to gently remove the rubber stopper so that the injecting needle remains sharp. Wear gloves and follow the usual precautions of sterility and skin preparation. In general, infusing slowly with a 30-gauge needle, injecting small volumes of relatively concentrated solutions, and reconstituting with preserved saline will minimize the pain associated with injections (34).

TREATMENT SITES AND TECHNIQUES

When discussing the technique used for individual injection sites, it is important to remember that all facial muscles vary in size and location, and what works for one patient may not work for another. The sites and techniques described in this section are those that we use in our clinic and are areas in which we have found BTX-A useful for the treatment of photoaged skin.

Glabellar Rhytides

Approved by Health Canada in 2001 and by the FDA in 2002, BTX-A for the treatment of glabellar rhytides leads to clinical benefits that generally last 3 to 4 months, with some patients continuing to benefit for as long as 6 to 8 months. Doses and sites are largely dependent on the type of brow arch, brow asymmetry, whether the brow is ptotic or crosses the orbital rim, and the amount of regional muscle mass (Fig. 14-1). In general, the male brow, which is associated with greater muscle bulk, requires larger doses of 60 or 80 U to produce paresis, whereas women achieve the greatest reduction in glabellar lines with 30 and 40 U BTX-A (35,36). Halving the volume of saline used to reconstitute the vial when treating males is a simple technique to reduce the injected volume while doubling the dose. We initially begin with 30 and 60 U for women and men, respectively, diluted to 1 U per 0.01 mL. If the initial dose fails to provide a sufficient response, we then titrate doses to 40 and 80 U in women and men, respectively.

We always inject above the bony supraorbital ridge at a point where it is safe to apply postinjection pressure. After injecting 4 to 6 units, the needle is slowly withdrawn (with its tip kept superficially beneath the skin), repositioned, and advanced superiorly and superficially to at least 1 cm above the previous injection site in the orbicularis oculi, where an additional 4 to 5 units of toxin is injected. The procedure is repeated on the opposite side of the brow to obtain a balanced appearance. We inject another 5 to 10 units into the procerus in the midline, at a point below a line joining the brows and above the crossing point of the ''X'' formed by joining the medial eyebrow to the contralateral inner canthus. Finally, we inject an additional 4 to 5 units into a point 1 cm above the supraorbital rim in the midpupillary line in those with horizontal brows.

Following treatment, patients must remain vertical and frown as much as possible within the next 2 to 3 hours (while the toxin is binding) but not manipulate the treated area. We perform ''touchups'' no earlier than 2 to 3 weeks postinjection, when the patients return for a follow-up examination. For patients who still have deep furrows at 2 weeks, one may consider adding a filler (see Adjunctive Therapy). Most patients experience clinical benefit for a period of 3 to 4 months following injection (Fig. 14-2). In patients with deep glabellar frown lines, we recommend further injections at 3- to 4-month intervals over a period of 1 year, which keeps the musculature paralyzed and allows the glabellar furrows to drop out (37).

Horizontal Forehead Lines

BTX-A injected into the forehead lessens undesirable horizontal forehead lines for a period of 4 to 6 months (38). Because the frontalis muscle is responsible for eyebrow elevation, excessive weakening of the frontalis without weakening of the depressors will result in unopposed action of the depressors, producing a lowering of the brow and an angry expression. BTX-A injections must therefore be conservative, allowing some function to remain intact. Softening the horizontal forehead rhytides can be accomplished by keeping injection sites well above the brow to prevent ptosis or a complete lack of expressiveness. Treatments are individualized for each patient: those with a narrow brow receive fewer injections (four sites, compared to five) and lower doses than patients with broader brows.

We have found that a total of 48 U injected in the procerus, frontalis, lateral orbicularis oculi, and depressor muscles gives the greatest improvement in horizontal rhytides and a longer duration of response (Fig. 14-3), although clinicians must be aware that adverse effects are dose related (38).

Crow's Feet

BTX-A diminishes the appearances of crow's feet rhytides, even in severely photoaged skin, by relaxing or weakening (rather than paralyzing) the orbicularis oculi. In general, two to three injection sites lateral to the lateral orbital rim are used (11,19,39,40), and equal doses of toxin are injected into each site (approximately 4–7 U/site; 12–20 U/side).

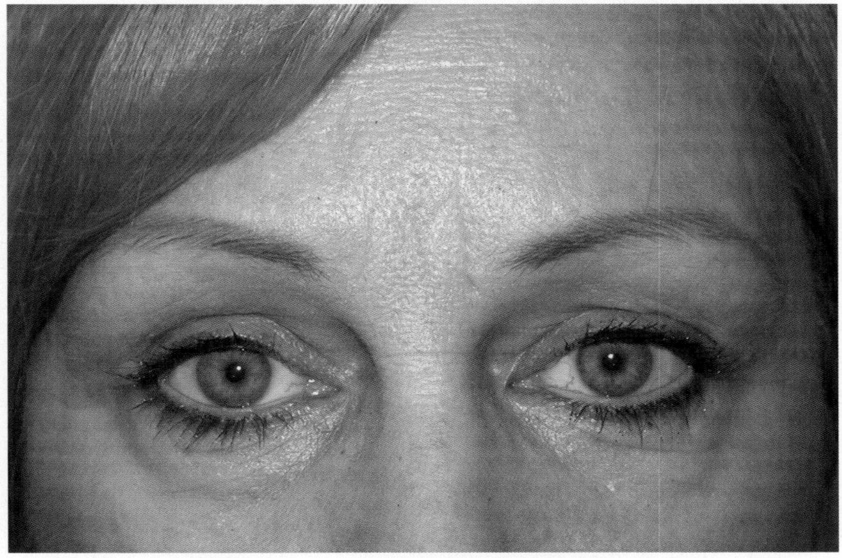

A

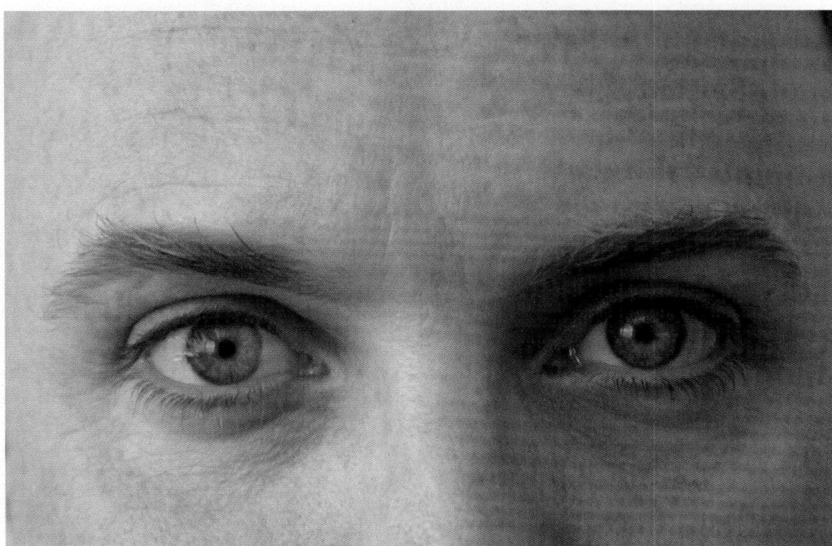

B

Figure 1 Botulinum toxin type A doses and sites are largely dependent on type and size of the brow. A: Typical female brow. B: Typical male brow.

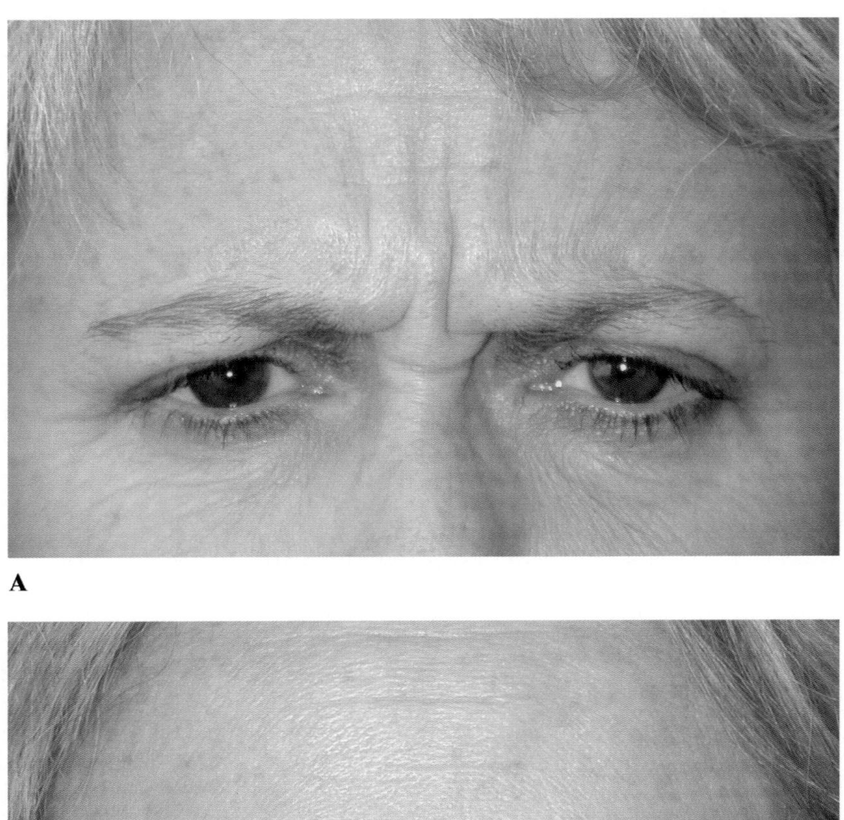

A

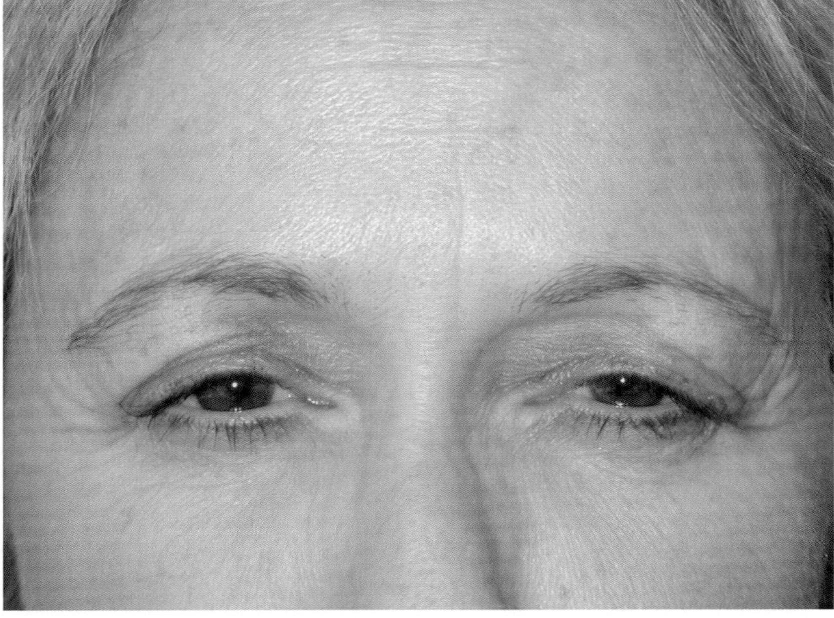

B

Figure 2 Glabellar rhytides before (A) and after (B) treatment with botulinum toxin type A.

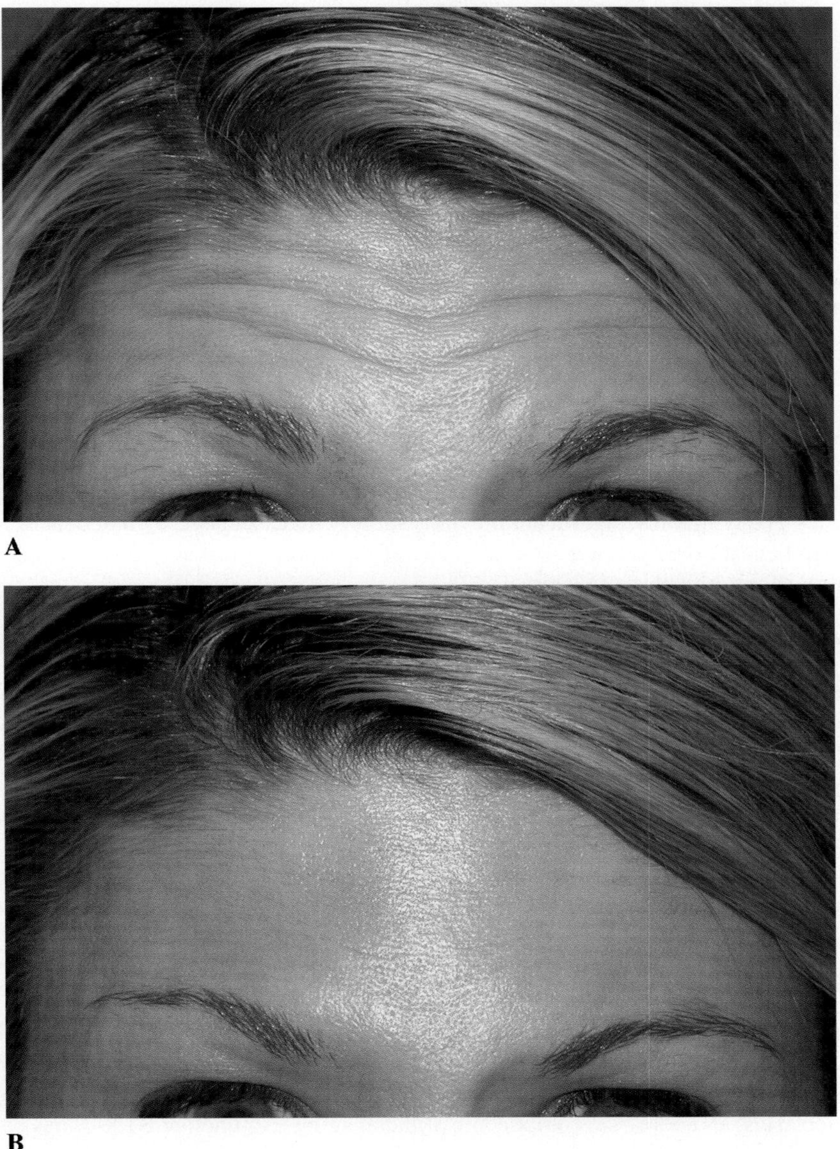

Figure 3 Horizontal forehead rhytides before (A) and after (B) botulinum toxin type A.

The dosage used in the lateral orbital region can vary. A recent dose-ranging study found no significant difference in efficacy between 6 and 18 U/side (40). Total dose ranges used by others include 5 to 15 U (41) and 4 to 5 U per eye over two or three injections sites (39). We use 12 to 15 U per side, distributed in equal parts over two to four injection sites, and recommend using as few and as superficial injections as possible to minimize bruising (19).

To identify the injection sites, ask the patient to smile maximally and note the center of the crow's feet. The first injection site is in the center of the area of maximal wrinkling, approximately 1 cm lateral to the lateral orbital rim. The second and third injection sites are approximately 1 to 1.5 cm above and below the first injection site, respectively. In some cases, crow's feet are distributed equally above and below the lateral canthus; in others, crow's feet are primarily below the lateral canthus. In these individuals, the injection sites may be in a line that angles from anteroinferior to superoposterior. In any case, the most anterior injection should be lateral to a line drawn vertically from the lateral canthus. The injection should not be made while the subject is still smiling, as the BTX-A then may affect the ipsilateral zygomaticus complex, causing upper lip ptosis. Results from the first injection session last approximately 3 months, although a duration of greater than 4 months has been noted following subsequent treatments (Fig. 14-4). (40).

Injection of the lateral orbital area will produce mild weakening of the infraorbital orbicularis, which can widen the palpebral aperture in some individuals. To accentuate this effect, the muscle immediately below the lash margin can be injected with 2 to 4 U in one or two injection sites (51). Patients with a significant degree of scleral show pretreatment, dry eye symptoms, significant previous surgery under the eye, a great deal of redundant skin beneath the eye, or a slow snap test of the lower eyelid are not good candidates for infraorbital orbicularis injections (42).

Perioral Rhytides

Overactive orbicularis oris causes vertical perioral rhytides radiating outward from the vermilion border (Fig. 14-5). Small doses of BTX-A (1–2 U per lip quadrant) usually are sufficient to weaken the orbicularis oris without causing a paresis that could interfere with elocution and suction, especially when used in combination with a soft-tissue augmenting agent. We increase the dilution and inject a total of 6 U in eight injection sites (0.75 U in 0.03 mL per injection), carefully measuring the sites to balance on either side of the columella or the lateral nasal ala. Appropriate patients must be chosen carefully; those who play wind instruments or are professional singers and speakers are not ideal candidates.

ADJUNCTIVE THERAPY

The use of BTX-A appeals to clinicians because it permits the underlying musculature causing wrinkles to be deactivated. However, BTX-A alone is not useful for nondynamic rhytides, and most physicians believe that another agent is necessary to treat lentigines, telangiectasias, and pore-size components of facial aging. Adjunctive BTX-A has become an integral aspect of facial rejuvenation.

Surgery

The constant action of facial muscles can interfere with or reverse the results of cosmetic surgery; therefore weakening the muscles with preoperative BTX-A may make it easier to manipulate tissues, allowing for greater surgical correction or better concealment of the incisions. In addition, some experts report that BTX-A administered during or after the procedure prevents or slows the return of the wrinkles by reducing the action of the responsible muscles (3). A variety of BTX-A surgical applications have been reported in the literature. Preoperative relaxation of the muscular brow depressor complex with BTX-A 1 week prior to brow lift surgery may allow for a greater brow elevation, whereas

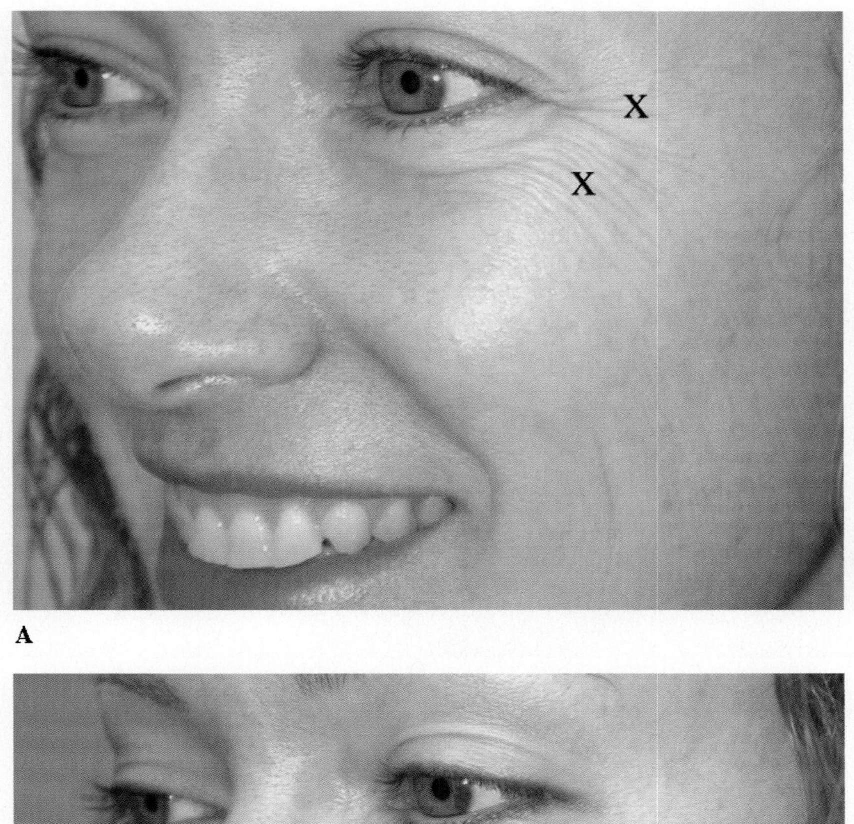

A

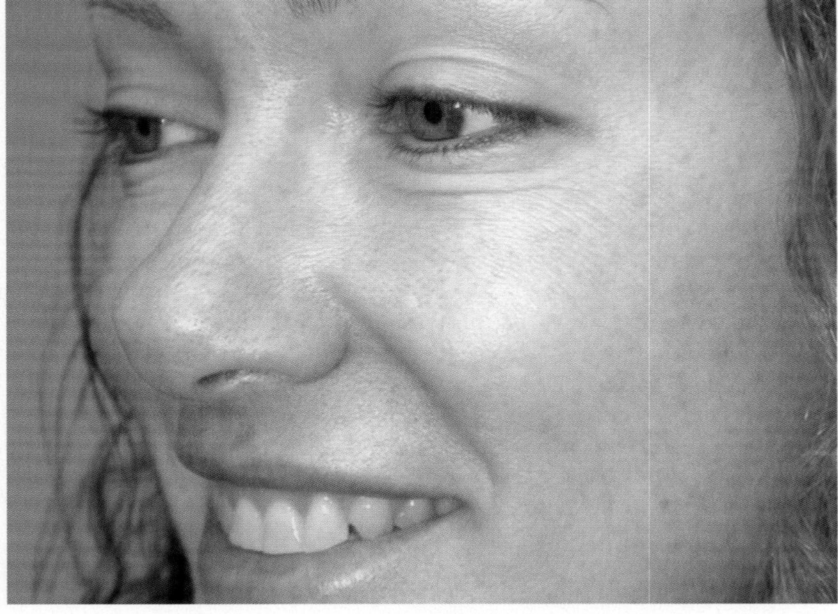

B

Figure 4 Crow's feet before (A) and after (B) botulinum toxin type A.

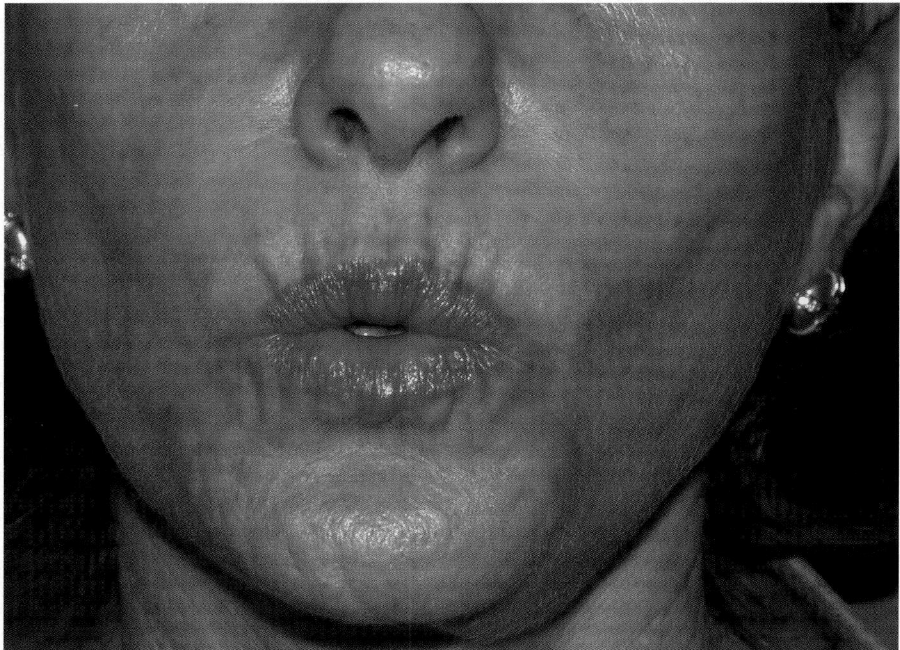

Figure 5 Perioral rhytides.

postoperative BTX-A may help prolong the benefits of surgery by relaxing the muscles that are working to re-establish the depressed brow (3). Because surgical brow lifts may have unpredictable cosmetic outcomes based on postsurgical healing, stabilization of brow musculature is important for a predictable final brow position (43).

Concurrent treatment of BTX-A with periorbital rhytidectomy improves and increases the longevity of the surgical results. Pretreatment of crow's feet with BTX-A allows the muscles to relax, leading to a more accurate estimation of the amount of skin to be resected during surgery and better placement of the incision (44). During lower eyelid ectropion and ''round eye'' repair, the use of BTX-A transiently weakens the lateral fibers of the orbicularis, which can pull on the medial side of the temporal incision and lead to dehiscence after surgery (3).

Soft-Tissue Augmentation

We use BTX-A routinely as adjunctive therapy with soft-tissue augmentation to achieve more effective, longer lasting results. BTX-A often eliminates or reduces the muscular activity responsible for the wrinkles, improves the response, and increases the longevity of the filling agent (45).

In a prospective randomized study of 38 patients with moderate-to-severe glabellar rhytides, BTX-A plus nonanimal stabilized hyaluronic acid (NASHA) led to a better response both at rest and on maximum frown than NASHA (Restylane™) alone (Fig. 14-6) (46). In addition, combination therapy led to a longer duration of response: the median time for return to preinjection furrow status occurred at 18 weeks in the NASHA alone and BTX-A alone groups, compared to 32 weeks in patients treated with BTX-A plus NASHA.

It is important to remember that BTX-A injections, given in conjunction with soft-tissue augmentation, may decrease the amount of filling substances required. In general, we inject BTX-A first, wait 2 to 4 weeks, then inject the filling substances. Waiting before augmentation allows BTX-A to soften the muscle contractions so that fillers can be added to correct the remaining lines.

Laser Resurfacing

BTX-A in conjunction with laser resurfacing leads to superior and longer-lasting outcomes. Lasers address static wrinkles and stimulate new collagen, whereas BTX-A prevents the recurrence of dynamic wrinkles. In addition, the adjunctive use of BTX-A aids the healing of newly resurfaced skin long enough to effect more permanent eradication of wrinkles. As in the case of soft-tissue augmentation, BTX-A should be given up to 2 or 3 weeks prior to laser resurfacing and at least 1 week before, which allows sufficient time for BTX-A to prevent muscle movement at the time of resurfacing.

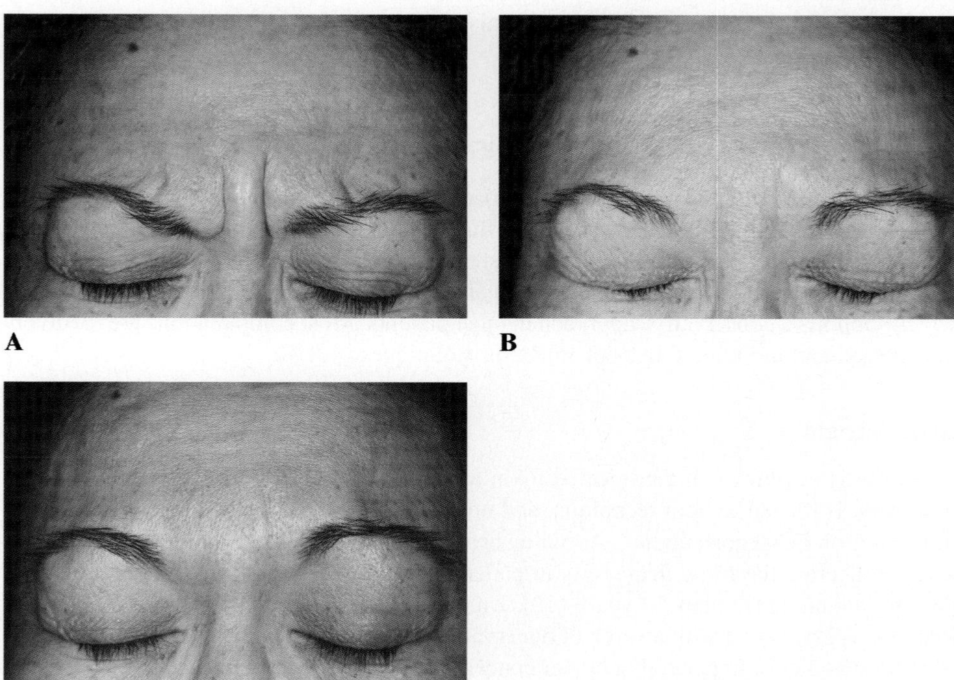

Figure 6 Glabellar rhytides before and after treatment with combined botulinum toxin type A (BTX-A) and nonanimal stabilized hyaluronic acid (NASHA). A: Maximum frown prior to treatment. B: Maximum frown 1 week after BTX injection to glabella. C: Maximum frown 3 months after combined BTX and NASHA treatment.

Regular postoperative injections, given every 6 to 12 months, prolong the effects of resurfacing, especially for the improvement of forehead, glabellar, and canthal rhytides, compared to laser resurfacing alone (47). West and Alster (48) found an enhanced and longer-lasting improvement of forehead, glabellar, and canthal rhytides when BTX-A injections were given postoperatively in conjunction with CO_2 laser resurfacing, compared to patients who received laser resurfacing alone. Lowe et al. (49) found that BTX-A in conjunction with ablative resurfacing in the treatment of crow's feet resulted in significantly higher treatment success rates compared with laser alone.

Broadband Light Therapy

Both BTX-A and broadband light (BBL) therapy are noninvasive procedures associated with little recovery time or epidermal wounding. Results of the first prospective randomized study of BTX-A and BBL therapy (Intense Pulsed Light™, Lumenis, Santa Clara, CA) in 30 patients with moderate-to-severe crow's feet show that both therapies may work synergistically to treat facial aging (27). Patients in the BTX-A plus BBL group experienced a better response at rest and with maximum smile, as well as a slightly improved response to treatment of associated lentigines, telangiectasia, pore size, and facial skin texture, compared to BBL alone. Overall, combined BTX-A and BBL therapy led to a 15% global aesthetic improvement compared to BBL alone. Although further investigation is required, these results certainly are promising for patients with extensive facial aging and photodamage.

SIDE EFFECTS AND COMPLICATIONS

Side effects that may occur with BTX-A injections include transient swelling or bruising at the injection site, mild headache, and flulike symptoms. To minimize ecchymosis, patients are instructed to avoid aspirin, nonsteroidal anti-inflammatory drugs, and vitamin E (50). Smaller doses of BTX-A are less likely to cause problems than larger doses, which supports a conservative approach in most patients. Most complications are relatively uncommon and are related to poor injection techniques (42).

Brow Ptosis

Brow ptosis occurs when the injected toxin affects the frontalis during glabellar or brow treatment, is related to poor technique, and underscores the need to understand the effects of BTX-A on facial musculature. Avoiding brow ptosis begins with proper patient selection and preinjecting the brow depressors in patients with low-set brows or mild brow ptosis, and in patients older than 50 years (42). It is important to remember that each point of injection is associated with an area of denervation due to toxin spread of about 1 to 1.5 cm (diameter 2–3 cm). In general, a higher concentration allows for more accurate placement, greater duration of effect, and fewer side effects. Injecting the glabella and the whole forehead in one session is also more likely to produce brow ptosis (42). Patients must remain upright for 2 hours, exercise the treated muscles as much as possible for the first 4 hours, and strictly avoid rubbing or massaging the injected area for 2 hours following treatment. Mild brow ptosis responds to apraclonidine (Iopidine® 0.5%) alpha-adrenergic agonist ophthalmic eye drops.

Eyelid Ptosis

Ptosis of the upper eyelid is largely technique related and occurs when the injected toxin migrates to the upper eyelid levator muscle, producing a weak paralytic effect as early as 48 hours or as late as 14 days after injection and persisting from 2 to 12 weeks. The incidence of ptosis in our clinic is low (0%–1.0%). We recommend accurate dose dilution and injecting the toxin no closer than 1 cm above the central eyebrow. Patients should remain vertical for 2 to 3 hours after injection and should refrain from manipulating the injection site. Bothersome ptosis can be treated with alpha-adrenergic eyedrops, which causes contraction of Müller muscle, which situated beneath the levator muscle of the upper eyelid (42).

"Mr. Spock" Eyebrow

A quizzical or ''cockeyed'' appearance can occur in the brow when the lateral fibers of the frontalis muscle have not been injected appropriately and the untreated lateral fibers of frontalis pull upward on the brow. To treat, inject a small amount of BTX-A into the fibers of the lateral forehead that are pulling upward carefully; overcompensation can lead to an unsightly hooded brow (42).

Periorbital Complications

Bruising, diplopia, ectropion, or a drooping lateral lower eyelid and an asymmetrical smile (caused by the spread of toxin to the zygomaticus major) are reported complications of BTX-A in the periorbital area. Inject laterally at least 1 cm outside the bony orbit or 1.5 cm lateral to the lateral canthus. Reduce ecchymosis by injecting superficially and avoiding blood vessels, placing each injection at the advancing border of the previous injection.

Immunogenicity

Botulinum toxins are proteins capable of producing neutralizing antibodies and eliciting an immune response, causing patients to no longer respond to treatment (3). Such individuals who initially respond but then fail to respond completely are referred to as ''secondary nonresponders'' and are considered to have neutralizing antibodies to BTX. The rate of formation of neutralizing antibodies has not been well studied, nor have the crucial factors for neutralizing antibody formation been well characterized (5). However, the total protein concentration and number of units injected are critical in determining potential immunogenicity, and some studies suggest that BTX-A injections at more frequent intervals or at higher doses may lead to a greater incidence of antibody formation (5). The protein concentration in the current lots of BOTOX is significantly lower than in previous lots and has been shown to be less antigenic than the original product. Secondary lack of effectiveness to BTX-A (due to the development of immunological resistance) is exceedingly rare in cosmetic patients and must be distinguished from a much more common degree of resistance, which is associated with the need for increased doses, rather than immunologic mechanisms.

FUTURE OUTLOOK

BTX-A is safe and effective treatment for the aging face, particularly when combined with other procedures. Used alone, BTX-A is a convenient and rapid method of reducing facial lines associated with hyperfunctional muscles. More importantly, the side effects are minimal and transient when an experienced clinician performs the injections. Newer approaches using BTX-A in combination with other facial rejuvenation procedures such as surgery, soft-tissue augmentation, and ablative and nonablative laser resurfacing prolong and enhance benefits. With the current level of interest in this treatment modality, multiple new applications for BTX-A therapy can be expected in the future.

REFERENCES

1. Finn JC, Cox SE, Earl ML. Social implications of hyperfunctional facial lines. Dermatol Surg 2003; 29:450–455.
2. Scott AB, Collins CC. Pharmacologic weakening of extraocular muscles. Invest Ophthalmol 1973; 12:924–927.
3. Carruthers A, Carruthers J. Botulinum toxin type A: history and current cosmetic use in the upper face. Semin Cutan Med Surg 2001; 20:71–84.
4. Meunier FA, Schiavo G, Molgo J. Botulinum neurotoxins: from paralysis to recovery of functional neuromuscular transmission. J Phy siol Paris 2002; 96:105–113.
5. Product monograph. BOTOX cosmetic? (botulinum toxin type A for injection) purified neurotoxin complex. Irvine. CA: Allergan Inc., 2002.
6. Sakaguchi G. Clostridium botulinum toxins. Pharmacol Ther 1982; 19:165–194.
7. Schantz EJ. Botulinum toxin: the story of its development for the treatment of human disease. Perspect Biol Med 1997; 40:317–327.
8. Scott AB. Botulinum toxin injection into extraocular muscles as an alternative to strabismus surgery. Ophthalmology 1980; 87:1044–1049.
9. Carruthers JDA, Carruthers JA. Treatment of glabellar frown lines with C. botulinum-A exotoxin. J Dermatol Surg Oncol 1992; 18:17–21.
10. Borodic GE. Botulinum A toxin for (expressionistic) ptosis overcorrection after frontalis sling. Ophthalmol Plast Reconstr Surg 1992; 8:137–142.
11. Blitzer A, Brin MF, Keen MS. Botulinum toxin for the treatment of hyper-functional lines of the face. Arch Otolaryngol Head Neck Surg 1993; 9:1018–1022.
12. Package insert. MYOBLOC? (botulinum toxin type B) injectable solution. San Francisco. CA: Elan Pharmaceuticals, Inc.
13. Package insert. Dysport?: Clostridium botulinum type A toxin-haemagglutinin complex. Maidenhead. Berkshire. UK: Ipsen Limited.
14. Nussgens Z, Roggenkamper P. Comparison of two botulinum-toxin preparations in the treatment of essential blepharospasm. Graefes Arch Clin Exp Ophthalmol 1997; 235:197–199.
15. Odergren T, Hjaltason H, Kaakkola S. A double blind, randomised, parallel group study to investigate the dose equivalence of Dysport and Botox in the treatment of cervical dystonia. J Neurol Neurosurg Psychiatry 1998; 64:6–12.
16. Brin MF, Lew MF, Adler CH, et al. Safety and efficacy of NeuroBloc (botulinum toxin type B) in type A-resistant cervical dystonia. Neurology 1999; 53:1431–1438.
17. Brashear A, Lew MF, Dykstra DD. Safety and efficacy of NeuroBloc (botulinum toxin type B) in type A-responsive cervical dystonia. Neurology 1999; 53:1439–1446.
18. Carruthers JA, Lowe NJ, Menter MA. A multicentre, double-blind, randomized, placebo-controlled study of efficacy and safety of botulinum toxin type A in the treatment of glabellar lines. J Am Acad Dermatol 2002; 46:840–849.
19. Carruthers J, Carruthers A. BOTOX use in the mid and lower face and neck. Semin Cutan Med Surg 2001; 20:85–92.
20. Ramirez AL, Reeck J, Maas CS. Botulinum toxin type B (Myobloc) in the management of hyperkinetic facial lines. Otolaryngol Head Neck Surg 2002; 126:459–467.

21. Sadick NS. Botulinum toxin type B (Myobloc) for glabellar wrinkles: a prospective open-label response study. Dermatol Surg 2003; 29:348–350.
22. Sadick NS. Prospective open-label study of botulinum toxin type B (Myobloc) at doses of 2400 and 3000 units for the treatment of glabellar wrinkles. Dermatol Surg 2003; 29:501–507.
23. Alster TS, Lupton JR. Botulinum toxin type B for dynamic glabellar rhytides refractory to botulinum toxin type A. Dermatol Surg 2003; 29:516–518.
24. Lowe N, Lask G, Yamauchi P. Efficacy and safety of botulinum toxins A and B for the reduction of glabellar rhytids in female subjects, Presented at the American Academy of Dermatology 2002 Winter Meeting, Feb 22–27, 2002, New Orleans, LA.
25. Matarasso SL. Comparison of botulinum toxin types A and B: a bilateral and double-blind randomized evaluation in the treatment of canthal rhytides. Dermatol Surg 2003; 29:7–13.
26. Pribitkin EA, Greco TM, Goode RL. Patient selection in the treatment of glabellar wrinkles with botulinum type A injection. Arch Otolaryngol Head Neck Surg 1997; 123:321–326.
27. Carruthers J, Carruthers A. The effect of full face broadband light treatments alone and in combination with bilateral crow's feet BTX-A chemodenervation. Dermatol Surg 2004. In press.
28. Klein AW. Dilution and storage of botulinum toxin. Dermatol Surg 1998; 24:1179–1180.
29. Hexsel DM, Trindade de Almeida A, Rutowitsch M. Multicenter, double-blind study of the efficacy of injections with botulinum toxin type A reconstituted in 6 consecutive weeks. Dermatol Surg 2003; 29:523–529.
30. Alam M, Dover JS, Arndt KA. Pain associated with injection of botulinum A exotoxin reconstituted using isotonic sodium chloride with and without preservative: a double-blind, randomized controlled trial. Arch Dermatol 2002; 138:510–514.
31. Huang W, Foster JA, Rogachefsky AS. Pharmacology of botulinum toxin. J Am Acad Dermatol 2000; 43:249–259.
32. Carruthers A, Carruthers J, Cohen J. Dose dependence, duration of response and efficacy and safety of botulinum toxin type A for the treatment of horizontal forehead rhytids, Presented at the American Academy of Dermatology 2002 Winter Meeting, Feb 22–27, 2002, New Orleans, LA.
33. Flynn TC, Carruthers A, Carruthers JDA. Surgical pearl: the use of the Ultra-Fine II short needle 0.3-cc insulin syringe for botulinum toxin injections. J Am Acad Dermatol 2002; 46: 931–933.
34. Alam M, Dover JS, Klein AW, Arndt KA. Botulinum A exotoxin for hyperfunction facial lines: where not to inject. Arch Dermatol 2002; 138:1180–1185.
35. Carruthers A, Carruthers J, Said S. Dose-ranging study of botulinum toxin type A in the treatment of glabellar lines, Presented at the 20th World Congress of Dermatology, July 1–5, 2002, Paris, France.
36. Carruthers A, Carruthers J. Botulinum toxin type A for treating glabellar lines in men: a dose-ranging study, Presented at the 20th World Congress of Dermatology, July 1–5, 2002, Paris, France.
37. Carruthers JA, Kiene K, Carruthers JDA. Botulinum A exotoxin use in clinical dermatology. J Am Acad Dermatol 1996; 34(5 pt 1):788–797.
38. Carruthers A, Carruthers J, Cohen J. Dose dependence, duration of response and efficacy and safety of botulinum toxin type A for the treatment of horizontal forehead rhytids, Presented at the American Academy of Dermatology 2002 Winter Meeting, Feb 22–27, 2002, New Orleans, LA.
39. Garcia A, Fulton JE. Cosmetic denervation of the muscles of facial expression with botulinum toxin: a dose-response study. Dermatol Surg 1996; 22:39–43.
40. Lowe NJ, Lask G, Yamauchi P. Bilateral, double-blind, randomized comparison of 3 doses of botulinum toxin type A and placebo in patients with crow's feet. J Am Acad Dermatol 2002; 47:834–840.

41. Keen M, Kopelman JE, Aviv JE, et al. Botulinum toxin: a novel method to remove periorbital wrinkles. Facial Plast Surg 1994; 10:141–146.
42. Klein AW. Complications and adverse reactions with the use of botulinum toxin. Dermatol Surg 2003; 29:549–556.
43. Dyer WK, Yung RT. Botulinum toxin-assisted brow lift. Facial Plast Surg 2000; 8:343.
44. Guerrissi JO. Intraoperative injection of botulinum toxin A into orbicularis oculi muscle for the treatment of crow's feet. Plast Reconstr Surg 2000; 105:2219–2228.
45. Fagien S, Brandt FS. Primary and adjunctive use of botulinum toxin type A (Botox) in facial aesthetic surgery: beyond the glabella. Clin Plast Surg 2001; 28:127–148.
46. Carruthers J, Carruthers A. A prospective, randomized, parallel group study analyzing the effect of BTX-A (BOTOX®) and non animal sourced hyaluronic acid (NASHA, Restylane™) in combination compared to NASHA (Restylane™) alone in severe glabellar rhytides in adult female subjects. Dermatol Surg 2003; 29:802–809.
47. Carruthers J, Carruthers A, Zelichowska A. The power of combined therapies: Botox and ablative facial laser resurfacing. Am J Cosmetic Surg 2000; 17:129-131.
48. West TB, Alster TS. Effect of botulinum toxin type A on movement-associated rhytides following CO_2 laser resurfacing. Dermatol Surg 1999; 25:259-261.
49. Lowe N, Lask G, Yamauchi P. Botulinum toxin type A (BTX-A) and ablative laser resurfacing (Erbium:YAG): a comparison of efficacy and safety of combination therapy vs. ablative laser resurfacing alone for the treatment of crow's feet, Presented at the American Academy of Dermatology 2002 Summer Meeting, July 31–August 4, 2002, New York, NY.
50. Alam M, Arndt KA, Dover JS. Severe, intractable headache following injection with botulinum A exotoxin. J Am Acad Dermatol 2002; 46:62–65.
51. Flynn TC, Carruthers A, Carruthers JDA. Botulinum Toxin A treatment of the lower eyelid improves infraorbital muscles and widens the eye. Dermatol Surg 2001; 27:703–708.

15

Fat Transplantation

Lisa M. Donofrio *Yale University, New Haven, Connecticut, and Tulane University, New Orleans, Louisiana, U.S.A.*

William P. Coleman *Tulane University Health Sciences Center, New Orleans, Louisiana, U.S.A.*

- Changes in the shape of the face throughout life are due largely to the redistribution of fat.
- Any attempt at truly rejuvenating the old face should consist of rebalancing the fat compartments via fat augmentation and microliposuction techniques.
- Fat transfer to the face has experienced a recent resurgence. Better parameters for fat graft harvesting and transfer now exist that preserve the structural integrity of fat tissue and appear to increase long-term viability.

INTRODUCTION

Facial fat distribution is a primary causative factor in what morphologically is denoted as the aging face. In youth the facial contours are full and round, and project forward away from the underlying bony framework. A young face has a preponderance of fat in the upper third of the face, lending it a shape reminiscent of an inverted triangle (Fig. 1). With aging, fat remodeling leads to involution of fat compartments, bony demarcation, and a downward displacement of tissues. Compounding this dysmorphism in even slightly overweight individuals is the pocketing of fat in the lower face, leading to a ''flipping of the triangle'' seen in the young face (Fig. 2). Thus, the topography of an old face is ''hills and valleys,'' with the hills corresponding to areas of fat hypertrophy and the valleys fat atrophy. Any attempt at truly rejuvenating the old face consists of rebalancing the fat compartments via fat augmentation and microliposuction techniques.

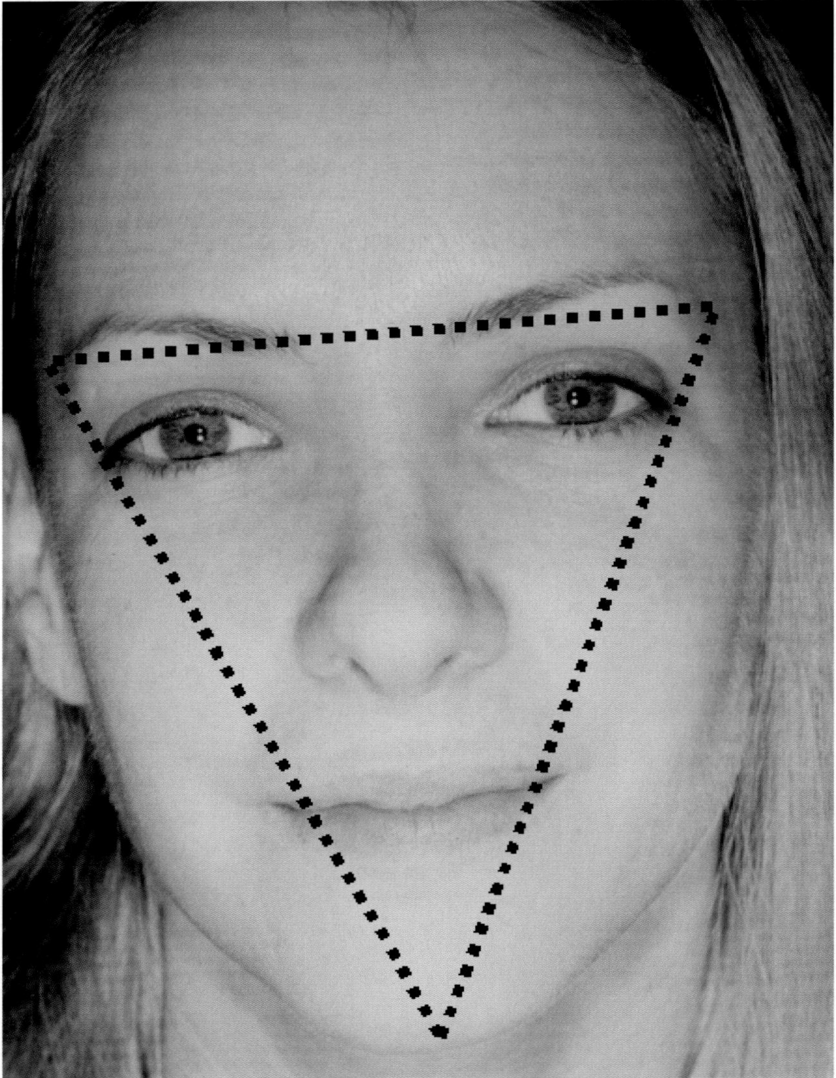

Figure 1 Triangular configuration of a young face.

Fat transfer to the face has experienced a recent resurgence. Better parameters for fat graft harvesting and transfer now exist that preserve the structural integrity of fat tissue and appear to increase long-term viability. Microlipoinjection as described by Pinski and Coleman (1) details the atraumatic extraction and blunt retrograde injection of fat in multiple layers. Lipostructure® is another technique that involves blunt multilayer infiltration of intact fatty parcels, but instead of using fat as a filler of creases and hollows, the Lipostructure technique replaces deep atrophied tissues to support and recontour the face. The technique involves the blunt placement of fat starting in the subperiosteal plane then

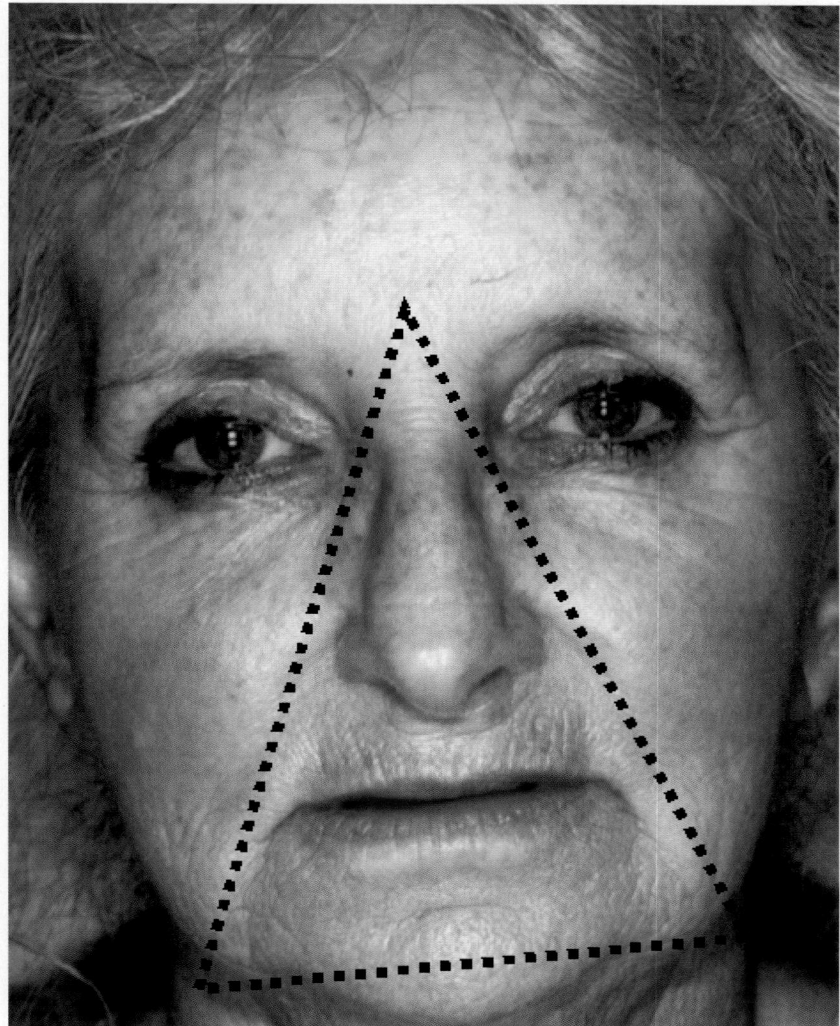

Figure 2 Triangular configuration of an old face.

up through muscle and subcutaneous fat. Although reported retention is high with this technique, there is prolonged bruising and edema (2). The FAMI (fat autograft muscle injection) technique is another approach in which fat is injected into and behind specific facial muscles in an attempt to obtain longer retention (3). Patients who require less down time may benefit from smaller, less aggressive lipoinjection sessions that avoid bone trauma yet adhere to pan-facial structural principles (4). At the same time, or in a different session, microliposuction can be used to trim areas of lipohypertrophy. Microliposuction of the face is not a new concept, but the availability of smaller cannulas affords the procedure more control. By careful planning, both the hypertrophic and atrophic areas of the face can be addressed with a combination of these techniques (Fig. 3).

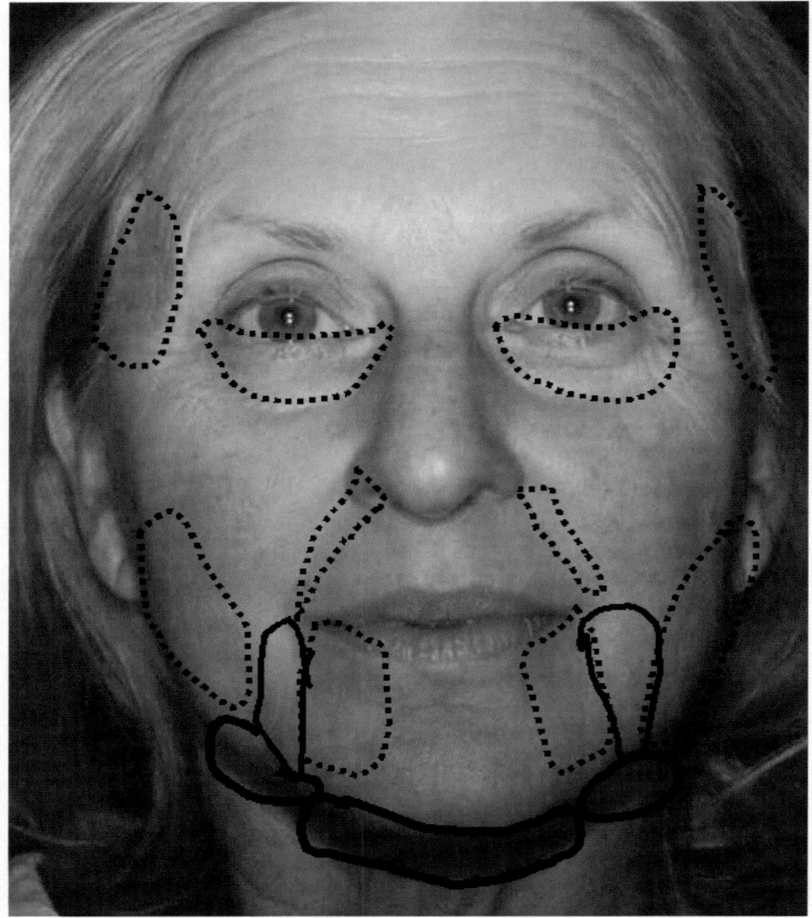

Figure 3 Areas of atrophy (dotted lines) and hypertrophy (solid lines).

PATIENT SELECTION AND SAFETY CONSIDERATIONS

When selecting and counseling patients for lipoaugmentation procedures, it is important to take into account the percentage of body fat and to relate this to a young face. A 30-year-old with 40% body fat will have a very differently shaped face than one with 20% body fat. Therefore, when a 55-year-old woman presents with the desire to look like she did at age 40 years, it is imperative to know how her weight changed over the past 15 years. A young face of an overweight individual will be diffusely rounded and full, whereas an old face of an overweight individual will be bottom heavy with a preponderance of fat in the jowl and submental and medial cheek areas. The restoration of a balanced fat distribution in this person would require microliposuction of these areas, as well as augmentation of the upper and lateral face. Conversely, a 55-year-old who has maintained a stable lean body weight throughout her life in all likelihood will require only diffuse augmentation to reapproximate the facial contours of her youth. Unfortunately, it is precisely these patients in whom finding adequate amounts of fat for harvesting proves most difficult.

Contraindications to lipoaugmentation are the same as for tumescent liposuction and include patients with a history of deep vein thrombosis/pulmonary embolus, sensitivity or true allergy to lidocaine, compromised liver function, coagulopathy, or debilitating illness. If lipoextraction for augmentation is part of a larger liposuction procedure, then total lidocaine dosages less than 55 mg/kg of body weight should not be exceeded (5).

PREOPERATIVE ASSESSMENT

It is prudent during the initial consultation with the patient to construct a map or blueprint of the areas of the face to be augmented/suctioned. Often it is helpful to look at photographs, with the patient, of a time when he or she liked how he or she looked, again taking into account the current total fat mass of the patient and how it affects the current facial contour. Most heavy patients have a history of concurring excessive facial fat accumulation. In the presence of severe solar elastotic damage, these deposits should not be suctioned because the skin envelope may not recontract to the smaller contour. Without accompanying suction, however, augmentation alone will give the heavy-faced patient a rounder fuller face. Individuals with lean body types and faces often forget how much fuller their youthful countenances were and will be unhappy with the outcome if not reminded of this. Unlike a face lift in which the vector of tension is posterior, deep structural filling of the face tents the skin in an anterior and lateral direction, lifting it off of the facial bones. The patient who pulls her skin tightly back, desiring a more ascetic result, should be discouraged from the softer contours of fat transplantation.

Preoperative blood evaluation is left to the discretion of the physician but generally is unwarranted with small-volume lipoextraction. Urine pregnancy tests are performed on all premenopausal women on the day of the procedure. The use of prophylactic antibiotics that cover skin pathogens is controversial; if used, they should be started the day before the procedure and continued for 7 days. Preoperative photographs are essential to follow the progress of the patient and as a baseline reference. Frontal, lateral, inferior oblique, and mimetic muscle animation photographs are all helpful.

ANESTHESIA

The gold standard for safety in any lipoextraction procedure is tumescent anesthesia (6). In its true form, this technique allows for no additional anesthesia and is distinguished from the ''wet technique'' of lipoextraction by the end point of tissue turgidity. Either normal saline or lactated Ringer's solution can be used as the diluent. The final solution is lidocaine 500 mg with 0.5 to 1 mg of epinephrine and 12.5 mEq of sodium bicarbonate per liter. Some favor using lactated Ringer's as the diluent. As a more physiologically supportive medium, the osmolality may enhance the stability of freshly harvested adipocytes. In addition, adding sodium bicarbonate to an already slightly alkaline solution raises the pH further and may offset the acidosis around the fragile oxygen-deprived extracted fat cells. Facial anesthesia can be achieved with sensory nerve blocks using 0.5% to 1% lidocaine with epinephrine. The suborbital nerve as it exits the suborbital foramen can be reached by either an intraoral or transcutaneous route. Likewise, the mental nerve as it exits the mental foramen in the chin can be infiltrated through the mucosal or skin surfaces. Forehead anesthesia requires perineural infiltration of both the supraorbital and supratrochlear nerves. All other areas of the face can be infiltrated directly with 0.05% lidocaine with epinephrine. The lidocaine level should be kept low because lidocaine is harmful to adipocytes (7). The addition of 0.05 mL of sodium bicarbonate to every 4.5 mL of the lidocaine solution lessens the discomfort of injection, as well as alkalinizing the solution for the reasons mentioned earlier. To lessen the anxiety of the procedure, an oral benzodiazepine or clonidine can be given. If, however, the lipoextraction is part of a larger liposuction procedure, then lorazepam and clonidine are the anxiolytics of choice because of their noncompetition with lidocaine for hepatic cytochrome elimination.

FAT EXTRACTION PROCEDURE

Following the infiltration of 0.05% tumescent lidocaine anesthesia, a cutaneous vasoconstrictive ''blanch'' occurs, which typically takes 20 minutes. Aspiration with collection then may occur in three ways. A sterile trap may be attached to a machine-generated aspirator. The concern with this method is the early damage to adipocytes (8). However, recent viability studies have verified this as a legitimate means of harvesting living adipose tissue (9). Manual extraction via a 30- or 60-mL syringe with a locking device makes for a versatile, low-maintenance, fast means of collecting fat. Alternatively, fat harvesting into 10-mL syringes while generating low negative pressures is a preferred method to ensure atraumatic collection of fat. Cannula selection also is important to the production of viable adipocytes. Evidence exists to support the improved viability of fat collected with cannula tips that ''core out'' cylinders of fat replete with in vivo architecture (10). For this reason, we prefer an open-tipped design such as a cobra tip (Fig. 4). Holding the 10-mL syringe with Luer-locked cannula in the dominant hand, the surgeon withdraws

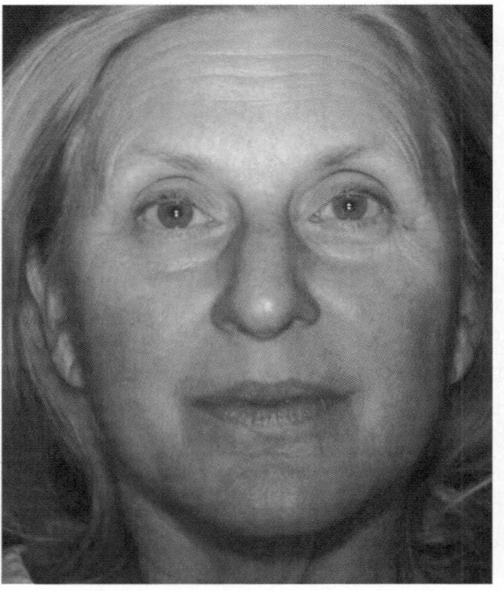

A

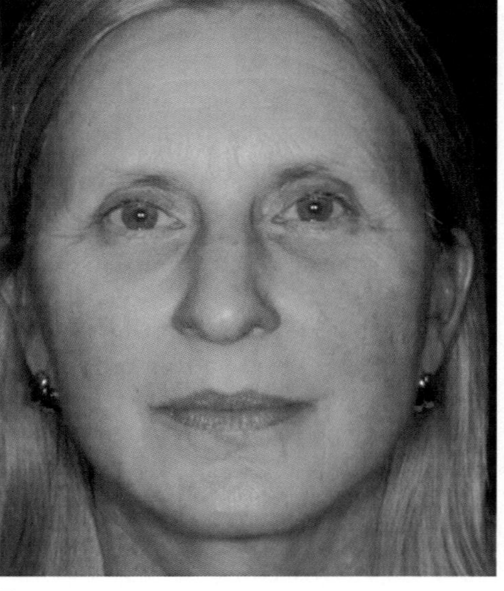

B

Figure 4 Before (A) and after (B) structural augmentation of atrophic areas and microliposuction of hypertrophic areas.

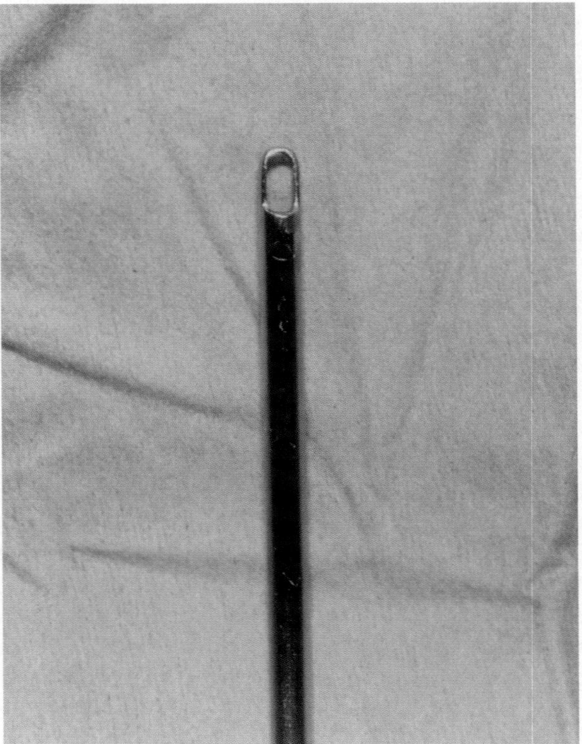

Figure 5 Open tipped extraction cannula (Byron, Tucson, AZ).

1 mL of negative pressure while passing the cannula back and forth within the fat (Fig. 5). The aggressive nature of the tip of this cannula dictates that the operator stay at least 1 cm below the surface to avoid creating dimples in the superficial fat. Most patients appreciate the fat reduction achieved in the donor site, and often this is an opportunity to diminish asymmetries in contour. Every means to avoid contour irregularities should be practiced. For this reason, superficial fat deposits, areas of poor skin tone, and deposits under areas with thin skin need be avoided. Diet- and exercise-resistant fat deposits theoretically should be more tenacious when transplanted. These typically are found on the outer thighs, buttocks. and lower abdomen in women and the flanks in men (11–13).

SMALL-VOLUME FAT TRANSFER

The beginning practitioner may wish to begin with limited volume placement of fat. There is merit to using fat as a ''crease filler.'' Autologous fat is nonallergenic, it has the potential for permanence, and the slightest elimination of shadow can have a great impact on the appearance of the aging face. In addition, fat is a soft, natural-looking filler for lip volume enhancement. In very lean individuals, finding enough fat for extraction can be difficult; often the slightest increase in the projection of the cheek can create the illusion of youth, so any available fat is best used there. Suction of donor site fat in these individuals may require multiple sites. The posterior waist area can be an excellent harvest site, even in thin patients. Once harvested, the fat can be left to settle in the 10-mL syringes via gravity or quickly centrifuged. In either case, the objective is to separate out the tumescent fluid infranate from the fat. Specialty centrifuges are available for this purpose (Byron, Tucson, AZ), but they require that the plunger be removed from the syringes before centrifuging, thus creating an ''open system'' and increasing the risk for contamination. A simpler method is to purchase a centrifuge that can be operated without the top in place and inserting the syringes intact in a criss-cross fashion (Fig. 6). Special Luer-lock caps can be purchased to ensure a tighter seal on the open end of the syringe (Byron, Tucson, AZ). Centrifugation should take place at 3400 rpm for no longer than 20 seconds. Longer centrifugation times can damage the adipocytes (14). The benefits to centrifugation are more densely compacted adipocytes, separation of the triglyceride fraction, and more thorough elimination of lidocaine-containing tumescent fluid. After disposing of the infranate, the fat is transferred to smaller syringes with a female–female Luer device leaving behind any triglycerides. One-milliliter syringes ensure greater control over the placement of small aliquots of fat. All placement of fat should be in a retrograde manner. The nasolabial fold can be filled with 1 to 3 mL of fat using either a 20-gauge needle or a 17- to 18-gauge blunt cannula. Needles may penetrate vessels, so blunt cannulas are preferred. Smaller-gauge instruments may lyse the adipocytes from shear forces and are not recommended. Labiomental creases also respond well to localized filling in this manner. Cheek infiltration is most safely accomplished bluntly, placing 1 to 5 mL in the ''apple'' of each cheek or in the buccal area. Augmentation of the periorbital area is also a wonderful way to rejuvenate the face with small amounts of fat, and this will be discussed later. Any localized defects occurring in the fat, such as atrophic acne scars, traumatic and postsurgical defects, and localized morphea, do well with small-volume fat transfer, but first may require subcison to free up enough space for transplantation (15).

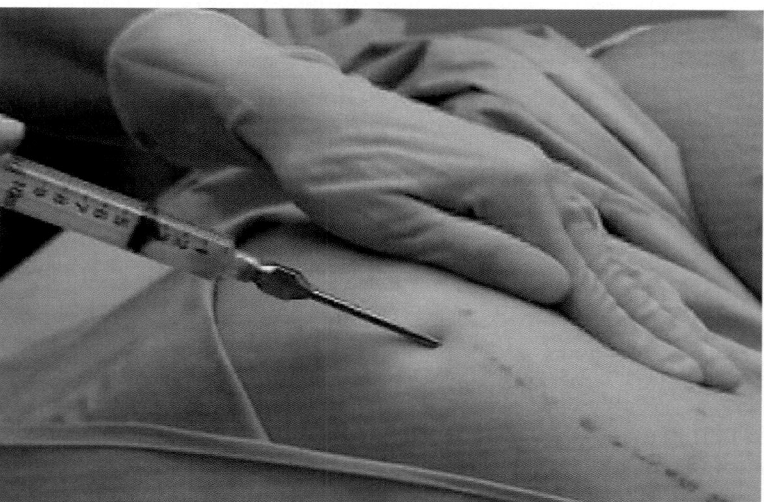

Figure 6 Atraumatic harvesting of fat.

STRUCTURAL AUGMENTATION

Structural augmentation is a deep supportive filling of the face. It most often is done in a pan-facial manner but may be reserved for periorbital or jaw line augmentation alone. Only 1-mL syringes of fat with blunt-tipped 17- or 18-gauge cannulas are used for transplantation with this method (Fig. 7). Incision sites are easily made with an 18-gauge or Nocor® needle (Becton, Dickinson, and Co., Franklin Lakes, NJ). The technique involves weaving small linear strands or tear-shaped droplets of fat in multiple planes of tissue, thus anchoring it and creating a subcutaneous ''scaffolding'' (Fig. 8). It is a dynamic filling technique that accomplishes shifts in neighboring tissues.

MARKING THE FACE FOR STRUCTURAL AUGMENTATION

A striking quality of a youthful face is the absence of shadows. To achieve this in a senescent face, one need fill all areas of shadow, resulting in deflection of light from a rounded surface. When marking the face for augmentation, draw around areas of shadow or areas of flatness that interrupt completion of the facial arcs. The midface should arc gently from the lower tarsus to the jaw line. The jaw line should arc smoothly from ear to ear and from anterior to posterior, forming an obtuse angle with the neck. The temples should be convex and the forehead arced forward. Draw the area of brow filling by having the patient look forward. Lift up on the eyebrow until all or most of the upper lid redundancy is retracted. Mark the lowermost portion as the ''new'' supratarsal crease. Make the lateral border continuous with the temple and the superior border the eyebrow hair. Suborbital markings depend on whether the patient displays the hypertrophic or atrophic variant of aging (16). In the hypertrophic variant, the suborbital fat appears to protrude, lying forward of the cheek. Often there is an exaggerated tear trough at the level of the arcus marginalis in these patients. With the patient glancing up, mark this trough from

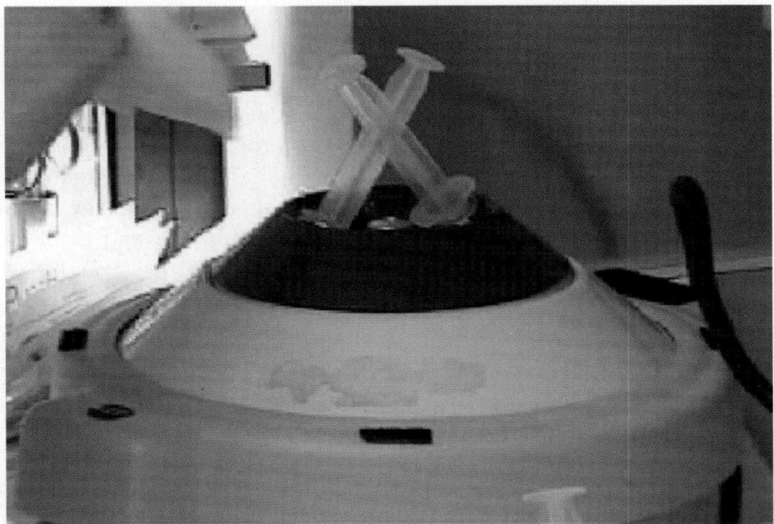

Figure 7 Criss-crossing of 10-mL syringes for centrifugation.

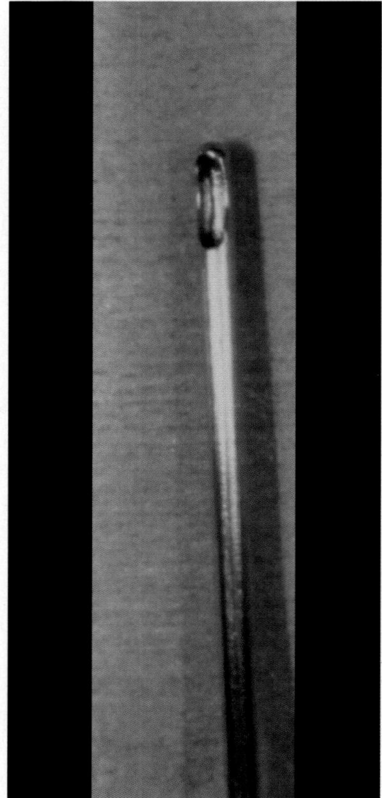

Figure 8 Blunt infiltration cannula (Byron, Tucson, AZ).

medial to lateral. This is the superior border of an inverted triangle that continues down, completing the midface arc. Filling this area advances the cheek forward of the suborbital bulge, thereby changing its relative relationship. The atrophic variant is characterized by a hollowing of the entire area from the tarsus to the orbital ridge and should be drawn in this way, continuing down the cheek if flatness also occurs there. The jaw line should be marked from a line on the anterior border of the mandible, mastoid to mastoid. This connects to a line drawn on the inferior edge of the mandible 1 cm below. In the heavy face, any areas denoted as requiring suction can be designated as such. The goal is to turn the ''hill valley'' topography into a ''gently rolling plain,'' so often it is appropriate to bring the hills down with suction as the valleys come up with augmentation (Fig. 9).

STRUCTURAL FOREHEAD AUGMENTATION

The goal with forehead augmentation is to anteriorly project the forehead away from the calvaria. This serves to lift the brow and reshape the upper third of the face. An additional benefit is the reduction of frontalis muscle-induced horizontal rhytides because subcutaneous fat ''stiffens'' the skin, requiring a greater muscular force to produce the same amount

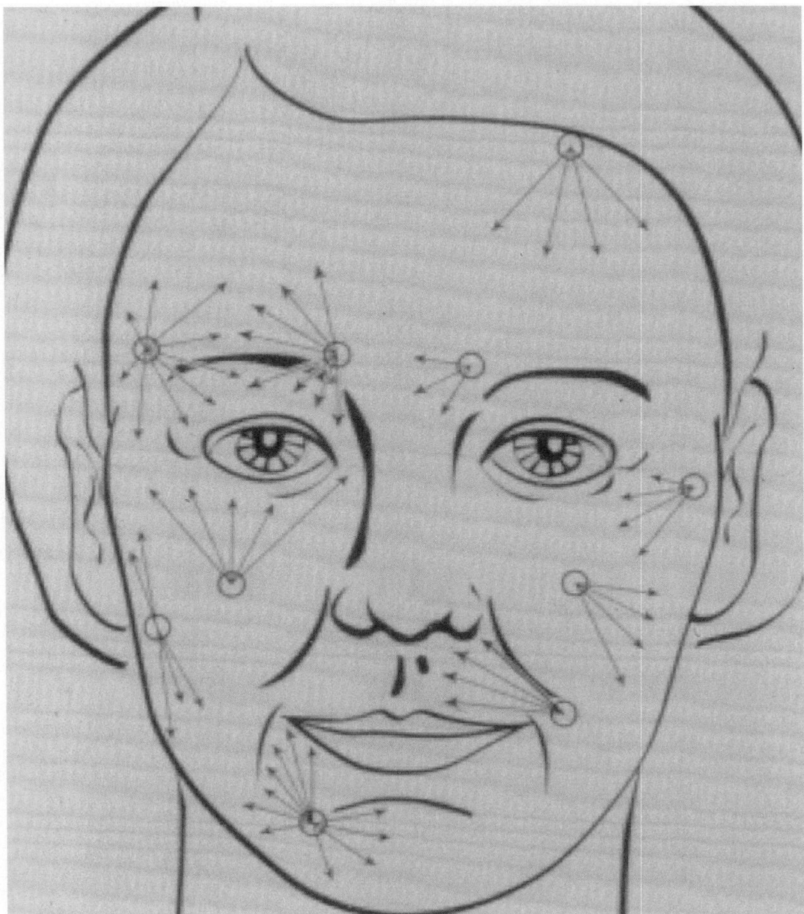

Figure 9 Planned incision sites.

of movement. Incision sites provide easy access to the curvature of the forehead when placed at frequent intervals along the hairline. Placement is subcutaneous and intramuscular, staying in a supragaleal plane. Injection is retrograde and perpendicular, depositing approximately 0.1 mL of fat with each cannula pass. Immediate ridging is common and can be lightly massaged out. Depending on the length of the infiltration cannula, an additional entry site may be needed to fill the glabella and nasal root. The temple can be accessed by a hairline incision or from a site just superior to the zygoma. Typically, the forehead takes 12 to 15 mL of diffusely distributed fat, the glabella 1 mL and the temples 1 to 2 mL each. Extension into the brow area when treating the forehead is a natural progression and is discussed later (Fig. 10).

STRUCTURAL PERIORBITAL AUGMENTATION

A youthful periorbital area is recognizable not merely by the absence of rhydites or loose skin, but also by a distinctive shape that incurs specific dynamic movements and points of

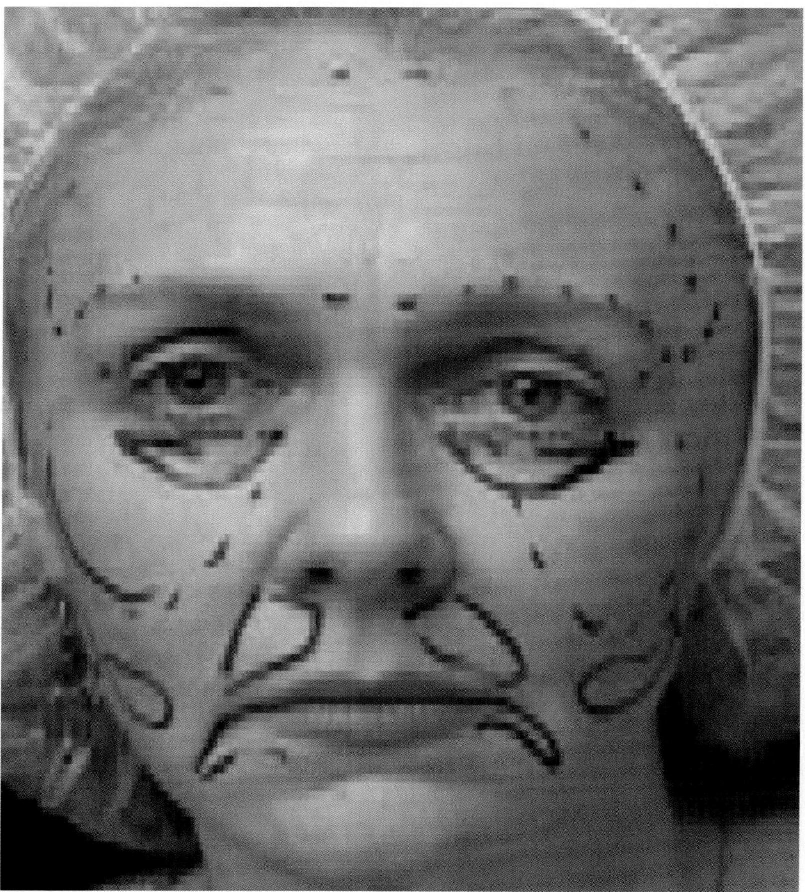

Figure 10 Markings for pan-facial augmentation.

highlight. With aging comes demarcation of the bony orbit and an unmasking of underlying musculature and vascularity. Filling the periorbital tissues with fat softens the contours of the middle third of the face and redrapes excess skin. Brow augmentation usually requires filling from the eyebrow to the supratarsal crease. The direction of infiltration needs to be perpendicular to the crease. Fat is deposited on the withdrawal phase of the movement in less than 0.1-mL droplets, pulling the ''tail'' of the droplet to the level of the brow. The level of infiltration is deep subdermal. Access into the suborbital area is achieved from entry points at the lower nasolabial fold, lateral margin of the orbit, or a tangential incision between the two. Fat in the suborbital area is placed deep to the orbicularis oculi muscle in the case of atrophic suborbital aging. It is easiest to ''slip'' under this muscle via a tangential approach, resulting in less bruising. Also, this avoids the often unmistakable horizontal linear tracts seen when a lateral approach is used. However, it sometimes is necessary to use a lateral entry site when fat placement is needed close to the lash line. It should take 15 to 20 passes to empty a 1-mL syringe of fat in this area, and volumes should not exceed 2 mL per side. The tear trough and nasojugal fold are best filled from an incision site in the nasolabial fold (Fig. 11). Treatment of the hypertrophic suborbital aging pattern requires cheek filling along the orbital rim. The entry is either inferior or tangential, and the level is deep to the zygomaticus muscles. The cannula tip should abut the arcus marginalis as it advances anteriorly into the orbital septum to lend structural support to the lower lid. Anywhere from 1 to 7 mL of fat can be placed in multiple levels: submuscular, intramuscular, and subcutaneous, depending on the breadth of the area to be treated and the amount of anterior projection desired.

STRUCTURAL REPLACEMENT OF THE BUCCAL FAT PAD

Nowhere are aging changes more evident than in the hollowing of the buccal fat pad in the cheek and its uppermost extension into the temple (17). Filling these areas restores a more youthful, healthy contour to the face. Fibrous bands in this area require purposeful placement. Incision sites are for easy access and may be coupled with infiltration of neighboring areas. Infiltration is in the deep subcutaneous tissue, between where the buccinator muscle splits in the lateral cheek. Fat woven in the buccal area must be tapered into contiguous areas, often as far posterior as the anterior auricular sulcus. Injection volumes range from 1 to 5 mL.

STRUCTURAL MANDIBULAR AUGMENTATION

The goal of jaw line augmentation is to create more area in the jaw line by increasing its definition with respect to the neck. This serves to strengthen the appearance of the mandible and to pull up the skin of the neck. The direction of infiltration is either perpendicular to the mandible or parallel along it. For maximum eversion of the neck, a perpendicular

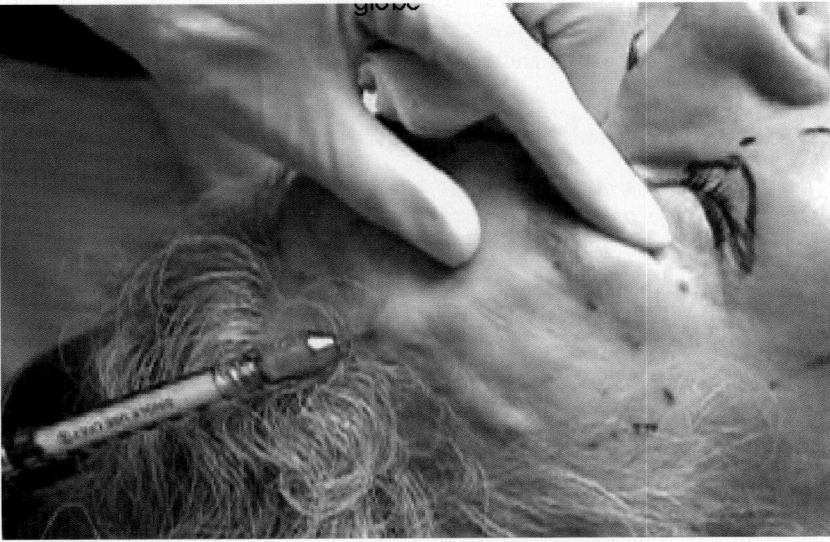

Figure 11 Forehead and brow augmentation. Notice how nondominant hand protects the globe.

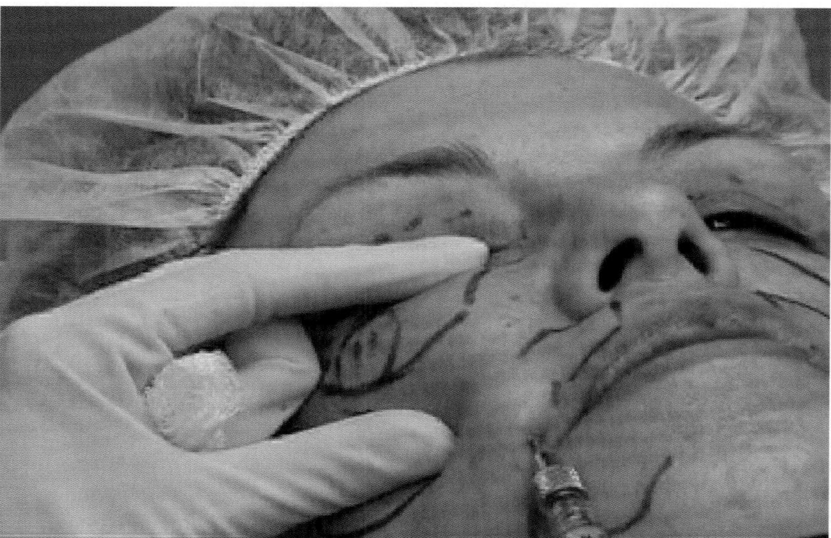

Figure 12 When filling the tear trough, the nondominant hand palpates the orbital rim and protects the globe.

approach is favored (Fig. 12); however, to achieve a smooth contour a second set of parallel passes may be needed. The level of infiltration is superficial, at the dermal subcutaneous junction. A peau d'orange textural change usually signifies the correct level. Infiltration should feel ''snug'' and secure, with a catching of the fibers of the platysmal muscle as it invests superficially. When the jaw line is augmented from ear to ear, it is not unusual to require 18 mL or more of fat. Unlike the Lipostructure™ technique, infiltration of the bony mandible and the masseter muscle is avoided, due to an increased incidence of bulging of fat upon mastication and an overly masculine appearance.

STRUCTURAL PERIORAL AUGMENTATION

One of the hallmarks of an aging face is the involutional change that takes place throughout the perioral area. This can be due in part to fat loss, but mucosal gland atrophy and bony reabsorption also play a role in advancing age. The cutaneous upper lip can be accessed through either an incision at the base of the nasolabial fold or a medial incision at the lateral border of the philtrum. Augmentation of this area pushes it forward and shortens the cutaneous lip. Fat is placed deep to the orbicularis oris muscle just anterior to the mucosa, then woven through the muscle up to the superficial subcutis. Interrupting the attachments of the orbicularis muscle and the skin serves to add tensile strength to the lip and the softening of muscular-induced vertical rhytides. When approaching this area from a medial incision, a finger is placed in the nasolabial fold and fat is deposited right up against it in a perpendicular direction (Fig. 13). Alternatively, fat may be placed parallel to the fold, but the result is not nearly as dramatic. Filling of the chin and lower cutaneous lip occurs in a similar fashion, with a finger abutted against the labiomental crease instead (Fig. 14). The mucosal portion of the lip responds to filling with either a 20-gauge needle

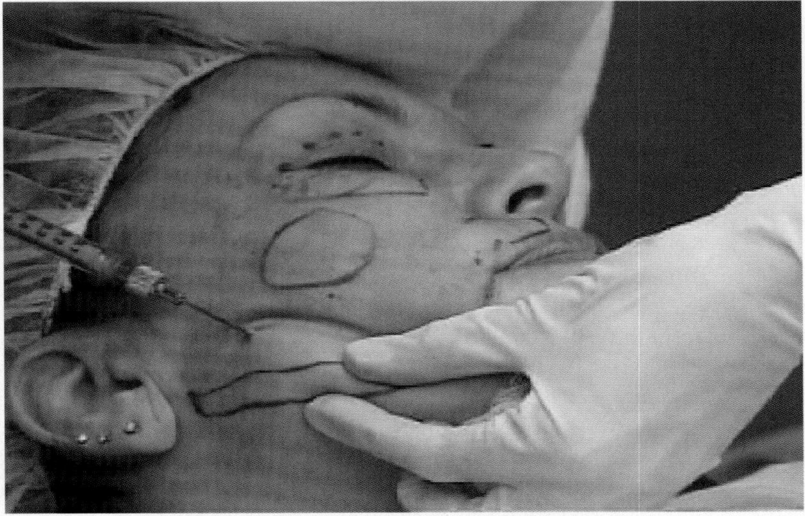

Figure 13 Jaw line augmentation.

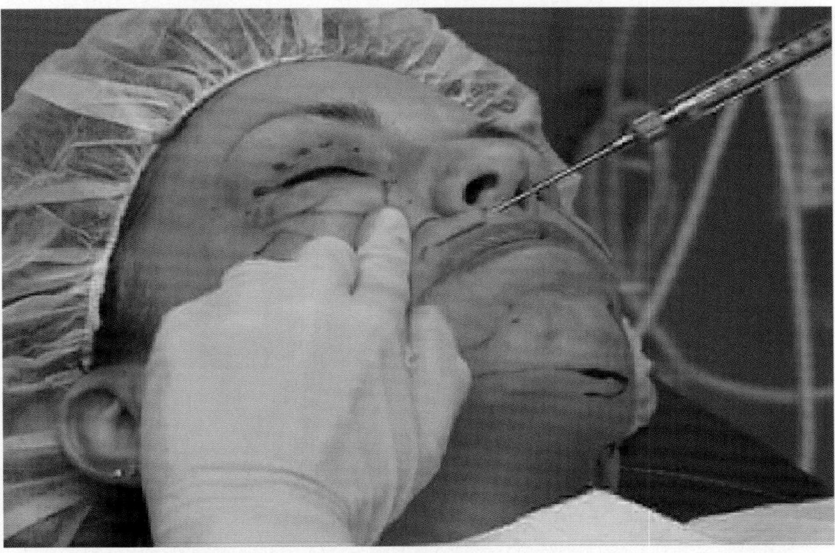

Figure 14 Perioral augmentation occurs perpendicular to folds.

or a blunt infiltration cannula, with the latter incurring more edema (Fig. 15). The entire perioral area can hold 6 to 12 mL of fat.

LIPOCYTIC DERMAL AUGMENTATION AND AUTOLOGOUS COLLAGEN

Fournier was the first to hypothesize the concept of autologous collagen. He noted that fat cells, when mixed with water and frozen, fractionated upon thawing into triglycerides and cellular collagenous debris. This technique was developed further by Pinski and Coleman (1). After fat harvesting in the manner described, fat is left to settle in a syringe and the tumescent fluid decanted off. Sterile water is then added to the syringe, and the mixture passed back and forth through a dual Luer lock with a variable aperture to another syringe. This pulverizes the mixture, which is then frozen in a commercial freezer. Upon thawing, the triglycerides and any watery fraction are disposed of and the emulsion is centrifuged at low rpm. Before injection, any remaining triglycerides are decanted off and the mixture is again passed back and forth through two syringes to homogenize. This material can then be injected through the smallest needle in which it passes, usually 25 gauge, into the deep dermis to fill superficial rhytides. Postinjection massage for areas of irregularity is recommended, as is overcorrection of approximately 50%.

Alternatively, fat can be emulsified right after extraction by passing back and forth through two syringes and then immediately injected into the deep dermis with a 20-gauge needle without prior freezing. This is an excellent way for patients to form their ''own collagen'' in vivo. As the body clears the fat in the dermis, it is replaced by fibrosis, thus accomplishing long-lasting natural augmentation.

MICROLIPOSUCTION

Facial microsuction involves the prudent removal of small amounts of fat from the aforementioned areas of facial fat hypertrophy. Good postoperative skin contraction in these

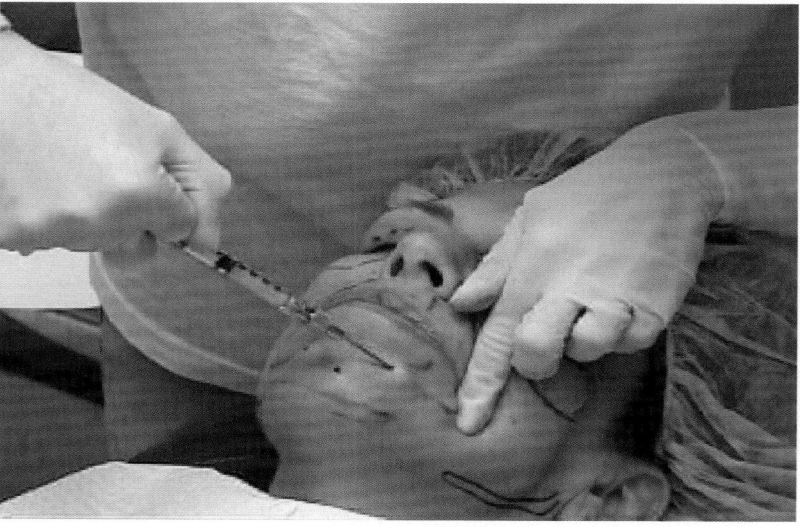

Figure 15 Perpendicular augmentation of labiomental crease.

areas is paramount to a smooth result. The degree of photoaging and skin elasticity must be evaluated before fat removal, even minutely, from these areas. Localized tumescent anesthesia may be accomplished with 0.5% lidocaine, injected via an 18-gauge needle or by 1% lidocaine in sufficient volume to cause turgidity. Suction is accomplished via manual negative pressure on a 10-mL syringe (Fig. 16). The same blunt microcannulas used for transplantation can be used for suction. It is best to always undercorrect to prevent oversuctioning of facial contours and allow for staged skin contraction. Areas amenable to manual suctioning are the area lateral to the nasolabial and labiomental fold, the jowl, and submental areas (Fig. 17). Large neck liposuctions, especially in the lateral and lower neck, respond best to machine-generated suction. Often as little as 0.3 mL of removed fat can make a visual impact on facial morphology. It is unusual to remove more than 2 mL of fat from any area without risking incomplete skin contraction, sagging, or dents.

POWERED LIPOSUCTION

Larger accumulations of fat in the neck respond best to machine-generated suction. Advances in technology have made powered liposuction the ideal method for careful sculpting of areas of excess fat. This approach uses a power-driven cannula that moves 3 to 4000 times per minute in a to-and-fro direction. This not only reduces surgical work but also allows more precise removal of fat. Powered liposuction is ideal for sculpting neck adiposities and can be used conservatively on the lower face as well. A 2-mm cannula is the best

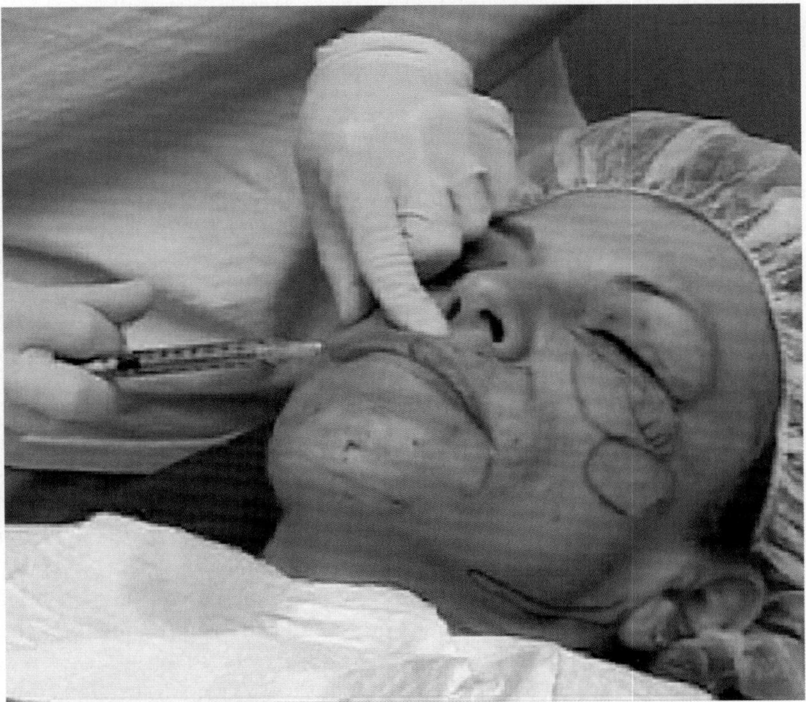

Figure 16 Lip augmentation.

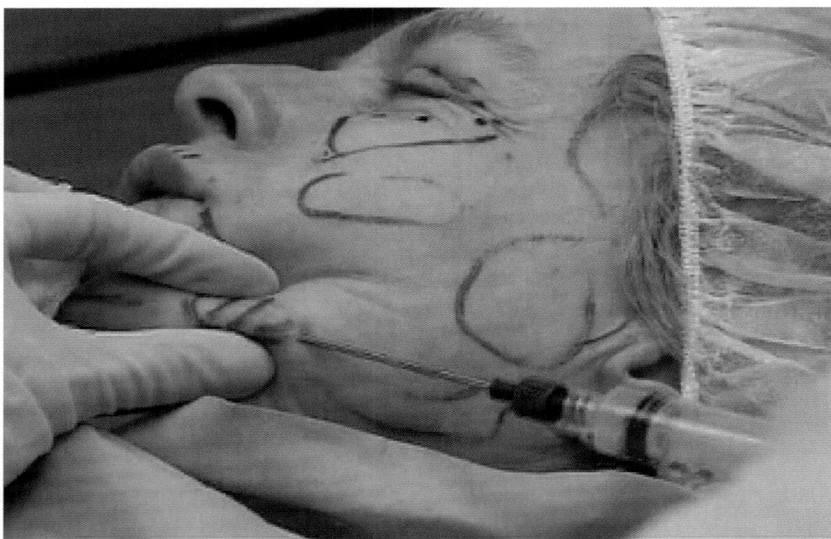

Figure 17 Manual microliposuction of jowl fat.

choice for these areas. The results of liposuction of the neck sometimes can be improved by a submental resection with plication of the platysma muscle, especially in older individuals with redundant submental skin. Postoperative fat transplantation of the lower face and mandibular area enhances the results of these procedures.

POSTOPERATIVE COURSE

The edema that follows blunt infiltration of fat can be profound. For this reason, intramuscular or oral steroids are recommended immediately postoperatively. Either a 7-day tapering dose of prednisone or methylprednisolone or intramuscular triamcinolone can be used. The application of ice packs or cool compresses immediately following the procedure and for 20 minutes every hour is recommended the first and second postoperative days. The patient should be instructed to sleep sitting up or at a 45-degree angle. Anecdotally, some patients find oral Arnica Montana helpful in reducing bruising, but the medical literature fails to substantiate this claim. The ''donor'' sites require absorbable dressings and mild compression for the first 2 days, then an elastic garment such as biking shorts may be worn for comfort. Following facial microliposuction, small amounts of restrictive tape can be applied to enhance contour outcomes and reduce edema in high-movement areas. The application of tincture of benzoin ensures adhesion for up to 3 days. Acetaminophen usually is adequate for pain relief. Nonsteroidal anti-inflammatory agents, vitamin E, and alcohol should be avoided the first week after the procedure, when the risk of capillary leakage and bruising still is high. Inverted exercises such as yoga should be avoided for 1 week, and swimming goggles should not be worn for several days after the procedure. If an antibiotic is started the day before the harvest, it should be continued for 7 days. Most patients undergoing fat augmentation require additional treatments, whether to additionally enhance or maintain their results. These can be scheduled at monthly intervals until the desired correction is achieved. In this way, the patients appear to ''de-age'' over time. Repeat sessions may be accomplished with either fresh fat harvested in the manner described earlier or frozen fat, which will be discussed later.

COMPLICATIONS AND THEIR TREATMENT

Expected sequelae following structural augmentation are ecchymosis, edema, and transient contour irregularities. These typically last 10 to 14 days, but some irregularities can persist for months. In the thin skin of the periorbital area, cannula tracks and fat deposition patterns are commonly apparent after the initial edema has subsided. It often takes 2 months for them to resolve on their own. In the interim, they can be ''blended'' in by passing the cannula at right angles to any linear tracks or ''pushing through'' any apparent globular deposits of fat. Persistent irregularities are uncommon with judicious placement and good technique, but, if encountered, neighboring areas can be filled around any lumps to blend them into the background. Firm hard nodules are representative of fat cysts and require dilute triamcinolone injections, drainage, or even excision to resolve. Ridging and erythema secondary to the fibrosis generated by the dermal implantation of fat are necessary for volume correction to take place but may persist undesirably. Serial intradermal triamcinolone injections usually are required for complete resolution, but this negates the augmentation result. One of the authors (L.D.) has encountered two patients who complained of prolonged pain in the temple and lateral zygomatic area following structural augmentation. Other rarely noted side effects are infection, eruption of herpetic cold sores, and submandibular lymph node enlargement. A review of the literature reveals disconcerting, serious side effects such as middle cerebral artery infarction and blindness (18–24). It is unclear, but these documented occlusive events appear to be related to high-pressure injections of fat and retrograde flow into the internal carotid system (24). For this reason, it is imperative that the fat be transferred with as little syringe pressure as possible, depositing minute amounts during cannula withdrawal.

LONGEVITY OF AUGMENTATION

Long-term retention of fat has been documented by many authors using a multilayer transplantation technique (2,25–31). Theories on longevity of augmentation include replacement fibrosis (32–34), differentiation of stromal progenitor cells into mature adipocytes (35), and viability of transplanted adipocytes through neovascularization (26,36). The authors of these studies note that retention rates appear to be site specific. The periorbital area and cheek have the best retention, followed by the lateral jaw line, forehead, and buccal area. Poorest retention is seen in the lips and perioral area. Poor retention may correlate with high-movement areas or may be the result of using fat as a filler where it anatomically does not belong. A prime example of this is in the nasolabial folds, where direct filling of the fold produces little if any long-term retention, whereas a filling of the adjacent cheek mass to suspend the skin and pull up on the fold gives predictable long-term results. Similarly, redraping of skin over the entire lower face accomplished by structural augmentation in combination with microliposuction produces a better result than direct filling of the labiomental crease alone (Figs. 18 through 21). A comprehensive review of the literature shows that fat graft survival depends foremost on anatomic site,

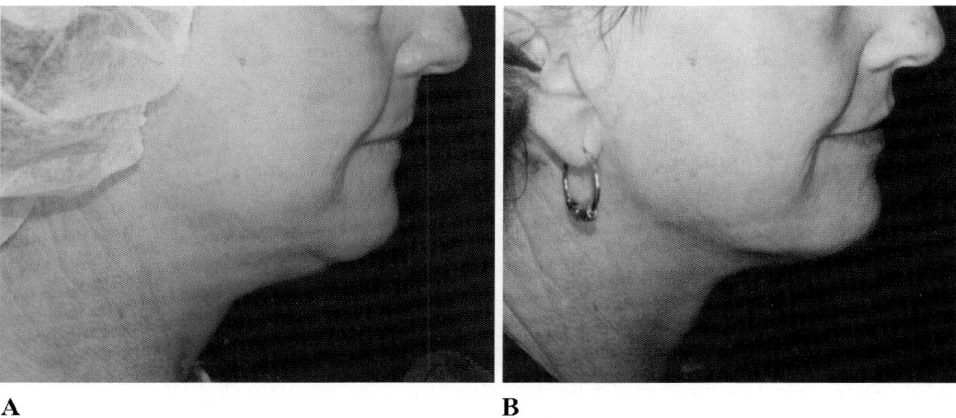

Figure 18 Before (A) and after (B) structural lipoaugmentation to jaw line without any liposuction.

mobility or vascularity of the recipient tissue, or underlying disease, and depends little on collection or reinjection methods (26).

FROZEN FAT

The freezing and storage of aspirated fat is a convenient method for multiple fat transfers without the trouble of extracting fat each time. Many surgeons who routinely augment

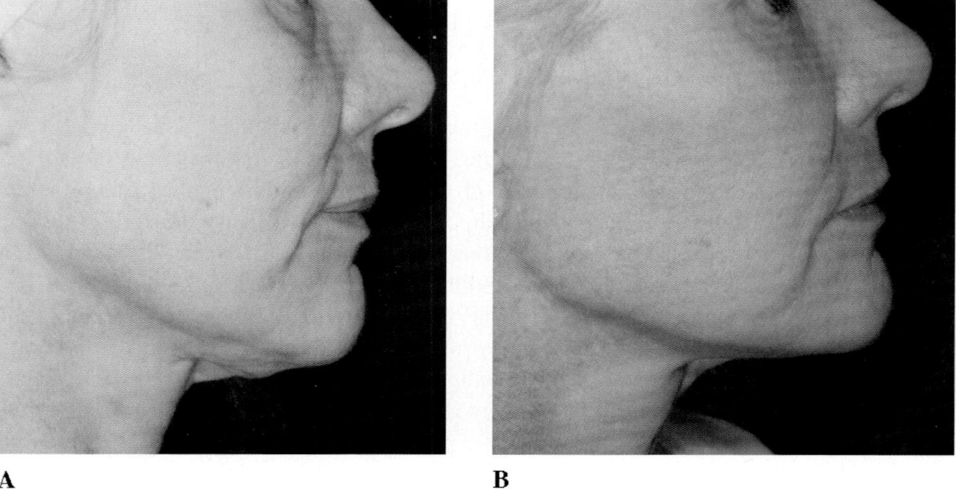

Figure 19 Before (A) and after (B) structural augmentation of jaw line and midface shows redistribution of redundant skin of neck.

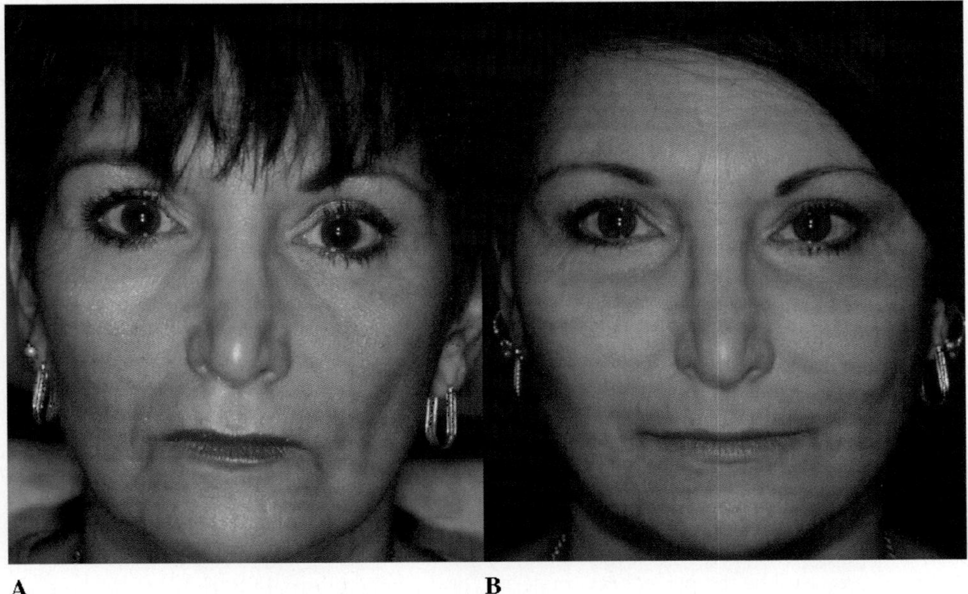

A B

Figure 20 Before (A) and after (B) pan-facial structural augmentation.

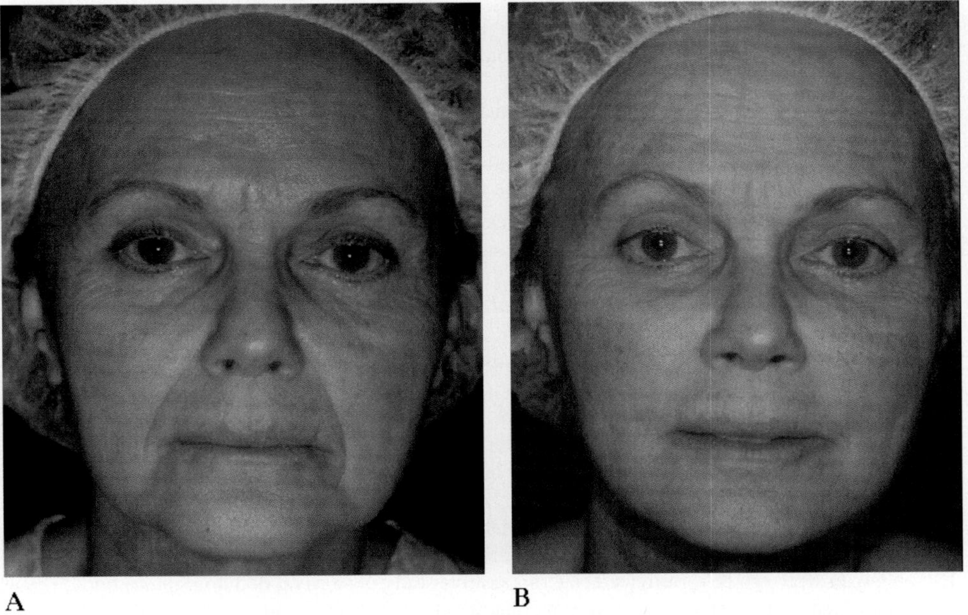

A B

Figure 21 Before (A) and after (B) pan-facial structural augmentation and microliposuction.

with previously frozen fat comment on its tenacity and long-term correction (4,37,38). However, it is uncertain at this time whether freezing fat alters its viability. A review of the literature shows conflicting or poorly designed studies. If freezing fat for future use, the authors recommend the following. Specimens should be meticulously labeled with patient's name, date of procedure, and social security or identifying number. Infranate consisting of settled or centrifuged tumescent fluid should be discarded, but triglycerides, if present, should be left in the syringe to ensure an even freeze. Fat should be slow frozen by placing in freezer at -20°C, double bagged in plastic storage zipper locked bags, and not snap frozen in liquid nitrogen. Freezers for long-term storage need to be monitored and fitted with an alarm that detects changes in temperature. Sterile specimens of fat can be kept frozen for up to 2 years without changing their histological morphology. Fat should be rapidly thawed by placing syringes in an examination glove and tucking it the patient's arm or waistband or under warm tap water. Touch-up procedures with frozen or fresh fat are an excellent way to control overcorrection and be certain that the patient's wishes are continually addressed, especially in the periorbital area where small-volume fat transfers are the only way to ensure a smooth result.

THE FUTURE

Fat may very well be the perfect raw material for the generation of multiple mature tissues. Adipocytes are terminally differentiated cell lineages, incapable of cellular division, but preadipocytes, a pluripotent stem cell found among mature adipocytes, are capable of differentiation into a wide variety of cells (39). The patients with the greatest need for fat augmentation usually are those with little body fat reserve from which to harvest. It is hoped that in these patients, fat can be expanded in culture via a stem cell pathway into abundant mature adipocytes.

REFERENCES

1. Pinski K, Coleman WP. Microlipoinjection and autologous collagen. Dermatol Clin 1995; 13: 339–351.
2. Coleman SR. Long term results of fat transplants: controlled demonstrations. Aesthetic Plast Surg 1995; 19:421–425.
3. Butterwick K, Lack E. Facial volume restoration with the fat autograft muscle injection technique: preliminary experience with a new technique. In: Narins RS, Ed. Safe Liposuction and Fat Transplantation. New York: Marcel Dekker, 2003: 511–525.
4. Donofrio LM. Structural autologous lipoaugmentation: a pan-facial technique. Dermatol Surg 2000; 26:1129–1134.
5. Ostad A, Kageyama N, Moy RL. Tumescent anesthesia with a lidocaine dose of 55 mg/kg is safe for liposuction. Dermatol Surg 1996; 22:921–927.
6. Klein JA. The tumescent technique., anesthesia and modified liposuction technique. Dermatol Clin 1990; 8:425–437.
7. Moore JH, Kolaczynski JW, Morales LM. Viability of fat obtained by syringe suction lipectomy: effects of local anesthesia with lidocaine. Aesthetic Plast Surg 1995; 19:335–339.
8. Niechajev I, Sevcuk O. Long term results of fat transplantation: clinical and histologic studies. Plast Reconstr Surg 1994; 94:496–506.
9. Moscatello DK. Fat transfer: laboratory analysis. Presented at the annual meeting of the American Society for Dermatologic Surgery, Chicago IL, October 31–November 3, 2002.
10. Nguyen A, Pasyk KA, Bouvier TN. Comparative study of survival of autologous adipose tissue taken and transplanted by different techniques. Plast Reconstr Surg 1990; 85:378–386.
11. Lilleth H, Boberg J. The lipoprotein-lipase activity of adipose tissue from different sites in obese women and relationship to cell size. Int J Obes 1978; 2:47–52.

12. Hudson DA, Lambert EV, Bloch CE. Site selection for autotransplantation: some observations. Aesthetic Plast Surg 1990; 14:195–197.
13. Arner P, Engfeldt P, Lithell H. Site differences in the basal metabolism of subcutaneous fat in obese women. J Clin Endocrinol Metab 1981; 53:948–952.
14. Chajchir A, Benzaquen I, Moretti E. Comparative experimental study of autologous adipose tissue processed by different techniques. Aesthetic Plast Surg 1993; 17:113–115.
15. Jacob CI, Dover CS, Kaminer MS. Acne scarring: a classification system and review of treatment options. J Am Acad Dermatol 2001; 45:109–111.
16. Donofrio LM. The technique of periorbital lipoaugmentation. J Dermatol Surg 2003; 29:1–7.
17. Stuzin JM, Wagstrom L, Kawamoto HK. The anatomy and clinical applications of the buccal fat pad. Plast Reconstr Surg 1990; 85:29–37.
18. Dreizen NG, Framm L. Sudden unilateral visual loss after autologous fat injection into the glabellar area. Am J Ophthalmol 1989; 107:85–87.
19. Teimourian B. Blindness following fat injections. Plast Reconstr Surg 1988; 82:361.
20. Feinendegen DL, Baumgartner RW, Schroth G. Middle cerebral artery occlusion and ocular fat embolism after autologous fat injection in the face. J Neurol 1988; 245:53–54.
21. Danesh-Meyer HV, Savino PJ, Sergott RC. Case reports and a small case series; ocular and cerebral ischemia following facial injection of autologous fat. Arch Ophthalmol 2001; 119: 777–778.
22. Egido JA, Arroyo R, Marcos A. Middle cerebral artery embolism and unilateral visual loss after autologous fat injection into the glabellar area. Stroke 1993; 24:615–616.
23. Lee DH, Yang HN, Kim JC. Sudden unilateral visual loss and brain infarction after autologous fat injection into the nasolabial groove. Br J Ophthalmol 1996; 80:1026–1027.
24. Feinendegen DL, Baumgartner RW, Vaudens P. Autologous fat injections for soft tissue augmentation in the face: a safe procedure?. Aesthetic Plast Surg 1998; 22:163–167.
25. Coleman SR. Facial recontouring with liposculpture. Clin Plast Surg 1997; 24:347–367.
26. Sommer B, Sattler G. Current concepts of fat graft survival: histology of aspirated adipose tissue and review of the literature. J Dermatol Surg 2000; 26:1159–1166.
27. Niechajev I, Sevcuk O. Long term results of fat transplantation: clinical and histologic studies. Plast Reconstr Surg 1994; 94:496–506.
28. Fulton J, Suarez M, Silverton K, et al. Small volume fat transfer. J Dermatol Surg Oncol 1998; 24:857–865.
29. Matsudo PK, Toledo LS. Experience of injected fat grafting. Aesthetic Plast Surg 1988; 12: 35–38.
30. Carraway JH, Mellow CG. Syringe aspiration and fat concentration; a simple technique for autologous fat injection. Ann Plast Surg 1990; 24:293–296.
31. Donofrio LM. Structural lipoaugmentation: a pan-facial technique. J Dermatol Surg 2000; 26: 1129–1134.
32. Coleman WP, Lawrence N, Sherman RN, et al. Autologous collagen? Lipocytic dermal augmentation, a histopathologic study. J Dermatol Surg Oncol 1993; 19:1032–1040.
33. Nguyen A, Pasyk KA, Bouvier TN, et al. Comparative study of survival of autologous adipose tissue taken and transplanted by different techniques. Plast Reconstr Surg 1990; 85:378–386.
34. Chajchir A, Benzaquen I. Fat grafting injection for soft-tissue augmentation. Plast Reconstr Surg 1989; 84:921–934.
35. Billings E, May JW. Historical review and present status of free fat graft autotransplantation in plastic and reconstructive surgery. Plast Reconstr Surg 1989; l83:368–381.
36. Peer LA. The neglected free fat graft. Plast Reconstr Surg 1956; 18:233–250.
37. Markey AC, Glogau RG. Autologous fat grafting: comparison of techniques. Dermatol Surg 2000; 26:1135–1139.
38. Jackson RF. Frozen fat: does it work? Am J Cosmet Surg 1997; 14:339–343.
39. De Ugarte DA, Ashjian PH, Elbarbary A, et al. Future of fat as raw material for tissue regeneration. Ann Plast Surg 2003; 50:215–219.

16

Update On Fillers

Rhoda S. Narins *New York University, New York, New York, U.S.A.*

- Be familiar with as many fillers as possible to allow the widest range of use.
- Examine the patient 1 or 2 weeks after treatment to observe your treatment results.
- Bovine collagen and human collagen are the most frequently used commercial fillers, easy to inject, and readily available, but autologous fat transfer is a good alternative for deep furrows.
- Filling substances have greatest utility for the superficial perioral lines, filling in nasolabial folds, and mesolabial or marionette furrows
- New substances will soon become available, including hyaluronic acid, which is part of the normal ground substance of tissue and expands with water absorption after injection.

This is an exciting time for fillers, and many new agents are about to be approved by the U.S. Food and Drug Administration (FDA). Fillers are used for rejuvenation, to treat aging and scars. With scarring and with aging there is loss of connective and subcutaneous tissue, and fillers can replace this lost tissue. Fillers can be used before, between, or in place of face lifts. The latter pulls and removes skin, whereas fillers replace the lost tissue. Fillers work synergistically with surgical procedures to give the best results, but fillers alone can often provide the result the patient wants. Many patients who don't want to undergo a surgical procedure can achieve excellent results noninvasively with fillers combined with botulinum toxin type A (Botox). This is a great means of nonsurgically improving the skin with little or no recovery time. The ''ideal filler'' has yet to be found, but with combinations of the various fillers that soon will be available, excellent results will be expected.

Fillers are used to fill in lines and folds on the face and can mimic a mini–face lift under the right circumstances. Scars from acne, surgery, and trauma can be improved.

Skeletonized hands can be plumped up for a more youthful look. Any of these can be combined with botulinum toxin. The dermatologic surgeon should be comfortable with several fillers to provide patients with the best results.

THE IDEAL FILLER

The ideal filler would give long-lasting and possibly permanent results. It would be easy to use, have viscosity low enough to pass through a small, 30-gauge needle, and be painless to inject. This filler would work for deep folds as well as superficial lines. The ideal filler would be nonallergenic and thus would not need a skin test. It could be used on the same day as the consultation. It would be noncarcinogenic, nonteratogenic, and nonmigratory. Stored at room temperature, this filler should have a long shelf life, and be forgiving and prepackaged. It would be nonanimal in origin so no disease would be transmitted. There would be little or no postoperative morbidity such as swelling, redness, or bruising. There would be no long-term problems such as the development of granulomas. Many fillers have at least some of these attributes.

GENERAL TREATMENT TIPS

1. Use the amount of anesthesia necessary to make the patient comfortable, whether it is a topical cream, local anesthetic, or an anesthetic block. Our clinic almost always uses a block for lip enhancement with fillers.
2. Just prior to injection, wash off the anesthetic cream with water, then dry and mark the area to be injected with povidone-iodine (Betadine). The marking should be dry before commencing treatment.
3. Always aim medially when treating the nasolabial folds so that filler that spreads laterally to the nasolabial fold does not accentuate fullness of the cheek.
4. Examine the patient 1 or 2 weeks after treatment to observe your treatment results and confirm both the physician and patient have achieved the desired result.
5. Use the amount or volume of product necessary to give a good result. If you use too little product, the patient will complain that the filler disappeared too quickly.
6. Be comfortable using several products so that you can treat all kinds of defects including deep hollows, superficial lines and deep folds.
7. Advise patients to avoid ingesting products causing increased bruisability, i.e., nonsteroidal anti-inflammatory drugs such as aspirin, vitamin E, St. John's Wort, and other herbs.
8. Massage the area immediately after injection to smooth out the filler.
9. Use the smallest needle possible so that pain and bruising are reduced. A larger needle may be necessary to undermine an area prior to injection.
10. Make sure the patient is properly positioned and you have good lighting and magnification.
11. ''Subcise'' or undermine the tissue if it is bound down before injecting a filler.

COLLAGEN

Zyderm® and Zyplast®

Zyderm I and II and Zyplast (Inamed, Santa Barbara, CA) have been used successfully as fillers for many years (1–5). Zyderm I has been used since 1976 and was FDA approved in 1981. The products are derived from bovine collagen from an isolated U.S.-raised herd. The material is off-white and opaque. Both come prepackaged in 1–2cc syringes for single use. Zyderm is excellent for superficial etched-in lines and Zyplast fills in the deep folds and lines. For both, a double skin test with Zyderm I is the norm with treatment following the first skin test at 6 weeks, and the second occurring at 2, 3, or 4 weeks. Generally it lasts 4 or 5 months in nasolabial folds and 2 or 3 months in the lips. Generally the duration of action is related to the amount injected. When less than the ideal amount is injected for a particular patient and location, the duration will be shorter than anticipated.

Technique

Zyderm I is injected through a 30–32-gauge needle into the superficial papillary dermis to raise a bleb as it flows along the superficial line, and Zyplast is injected through a 30-gauge needle into the mid dermis or deep dermis to lift up deeper folds using the serial puncture technique. These fillers should spread smoothly into the tissue and be lightly massaged after injection. It is necessary to overcorrect with Zyderm as it is diluted with saline, which is reabsorbed over 24 hours. Zyderm may give a flat yellow look to the skin when placed superficially.

Lips respond with Zyplast flowing along the vermilion border and may also be used to accentuate the filtrum. It is also suggested that it be injected into the musculature of the lip itself. This is called the ''Paris Lip.'' Only Zyderm should be used when treating the glabella region because of one reported case of blindness. For the glabella, Zyderm works best and lasts longest when used in conjunction with botulinum toxin injections. For nasolabial and mesolabial ''puppet'' lines, Zyderm is often layered over Zyplast to get the best correction.

Safety precautions dictate that injections of filling substances into suspected skin infections be avoided. Safety during pregnancy has not been established. Caution is advised in patients who are allergic to beef (a second skin test may be advisable). Zyderm or Zyplast is not recommended for patients on immunosuppressive therapy or in those allergic to lidocaine. Patients are advised to avoid strenuous exercise, extensive sun or heat exposure and alcoholic beverages for 24 hours after the procedure.

Advantages

The advantages of Zyderm and Zyplast are that they have been used successfully for years, come prepackaged with 30-gauge needles, and are easy to use. In addition, they have the ability to treat etched in lines as well as folds and they are formulated with 0.4% lidocaine so that pain is minimal.

Disadvantages

The disadvantages of Zyderm and Zyplast are the need for refrigeration (do not freeze), the possibility of allergic reactions requiring skin testing, the short length of duration of improvement, and the need to use a lot of product in older patients, making treatment very expensive. As with any nonpermanent substance, periodic touch-ups are required.

Complications

At the implant site temporary swelling, erythema, bruising, palpable lumpiness, and visible materia may be experienced. Sensitivity reactions may last 1–9 months and occur in 1–3% of patients. They usually subside within 4–6 months and may be intermittent or continuous. These include erythema, swelling, induration, or urticaria at the implantation site. Treatment may include topical, intralesional, and oral corticosteroids and nonsteroidal anti-inflammatory medication.

Rarely, abscesses or acneiform bumps may appear weeks to months after injection and may result in scar formation (6). These may be treated with intralesional corticosteroids and/or drainage.

Localized necrosis and/or sloughing has been reported in the glabellar and lip areas from direct injection of Zyplast with occlusion of a blood vessel. Scarring usually results. Immediate massage with nitroglycerin cream may be helpful.

One case of blindness was reported after injection into the glabella. For this reason, Zyderm (which is injected more superficially) rather than Zyplast (which is injected deeper and closer to the blood vessels) is recommended for this area.

Cosmoderm and Cosmoplast

CosmoDerm™ I and II and CosmoPlast™ (Inamed) contain purified collagen derived from cell cultures of human fibrocytes. These are the only FDA-approved, commercially available dermal fillers that contain human collagen. The cell line has been tested for viruses, tumorigenicity, retroviruses, etc., and was obtained from the foreskin of a newborn. Because they contain the basic human collagen molecule stripped of antigenic determinants, no skin testing is necessary. This allows use during the consultation visit. The material is whitish and opaque and flows through a 30-gauge needle easily. They are prepackaged in 1-mL syringes and are meant for single use only.

Technique

Injection is similar to Zyderm and Zyplast. CosmoDerm is injected into the superficial papillary dermis, and CosmoPlast is injected into the mid to deep reticular dermis. It is necessary to overcorrect with CosmoDerm as with Zyderm because it is diluted with saline, which is reabsorbed over 24 hours. Care should be used in thin-skinned areas around the eyes and mouth. CosmoDerm is often layered over CosmoPlast for the best results. Do not inject into patients with allergy to lidocaine. Other precautions are similar to those for Zyderm and Zyplast.

Advantages

Advantages are the formulation with lidocaine minimizing patient discomfort, the ability to treat etched in lines, the lack of need for skin testing as there is no allergenicity, and they come pre-packaged in syringes with 30-gauge needles. They are the first same-day single treatment dermal fillers approved in the U.S.

The advantages over the previous collagen products, Zyderm and Zyplast, are the ability to use a filler that has lidocaine in the formulation immediately, as no skin testing is necessary.

Disadvantages

The disadvantages are the need for refrigeration (do not freeze), the cost, the same length of duration as Zyderm and Zyplast and the need for a lot of product in the patient with deeper lines as with Zyderm and Zyplast. Flulike symptoms have been reported in 2–4% of patients.

FAT

Fat is an autologous filling substance that is usually available in large quantities, enabling the dermatologic surgeon to fill in large defects, perform mini–face lifts, and plump up the hands (Figs. 1 and 2). It often lasts for years in the hollows of the cheeks and after repairing surgical defects (Figs. 3 and 4). When used as a mini–face lift, the cheek and under eye hollows as well as the nasolabial and mesolabial marionette lines are injected along with enhancement of the tissue over the zygomas and lateral mandibles, the chin and even the lips. Fat can also be frozen for later use. It can also be used to fill in large cheek hollows with another filler used to augment the nasolabial lines (7–10).

The technique described below is the one used in our clinic and it is based on that of Dr. Sidney Coleman (11). For completeness, many physicians use the FAMI technique described by Dr. Roger Amar in which fat is injected directly into the muscles for better blood supply (12).

Technique

Equipment

Very little equipment is necessary for this surgical procedure. A sterile tray with several 10-cc syringes, a female-female luer-lock adapter, a test tube rack in which the syringes can be placed upright, various needles (including 30-gauge 0.5-in. and 18-gauge, 16-gauge, and 22-gauge spinal needles), a Coleman extraction and injection cannulas, red syringe caps, and gauze pads. Some setup for administration of local anesthesia is necessary, and includes tumescent solution, spinal needles, and a pressure pump with intravenous tubing or 10-cc syringes.

Preoperative Preparation and Anesthesia

The recipient and donor sites are prepped with Betadine, and the patient is placed on the surgical table. A small amount of tumescent anesthetic is injected with a 30-gauge 0.5-in.

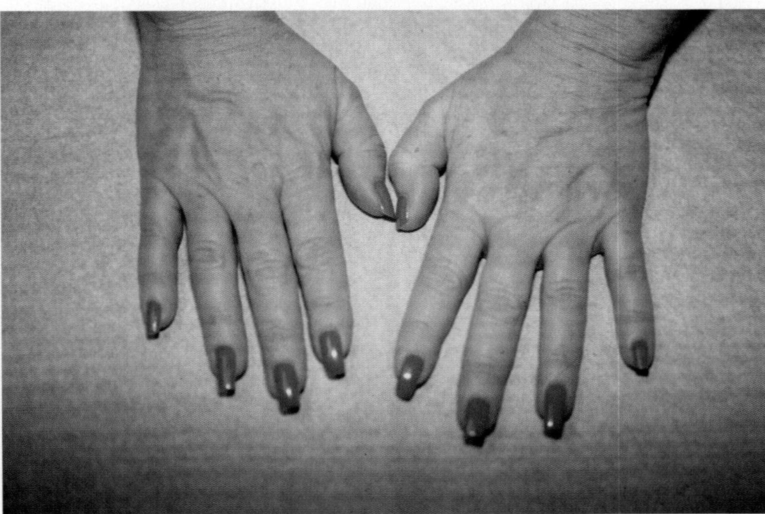

Figure 1 Preoperative fat transfer.

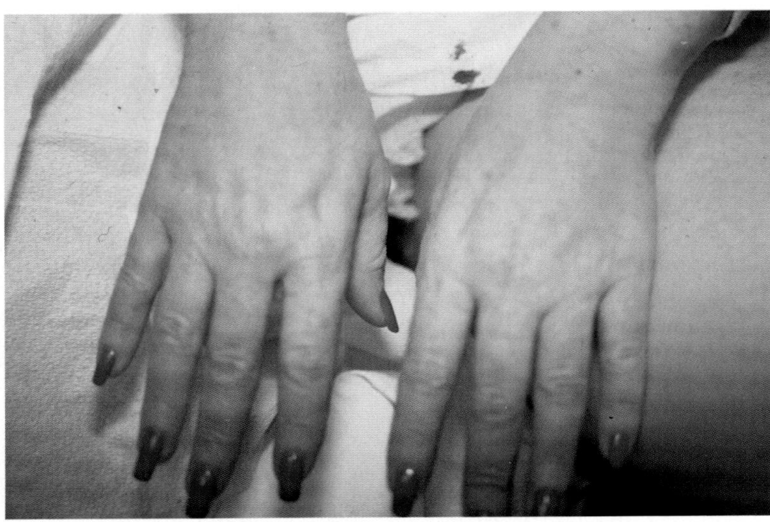

Figure 2 Postoperative fat transfer.

needle using a 3-cc syringe in the ''incision'' area of the donor site. Tumescent anesthesia is injected radially through this incision site using 10-cc syringes and a spinal needle, or using the Klein pump (very low setting) and intravenous tubing with an 18-gauge or 20-gauge spinal needle.

Recipient Site

The incision sites of the recipient areas are injected using a 30-gauge 0.5-in. needle and a 3-cc syringe. A tiny amount of tumescent anesthetic is delivered radially into the reinjec-

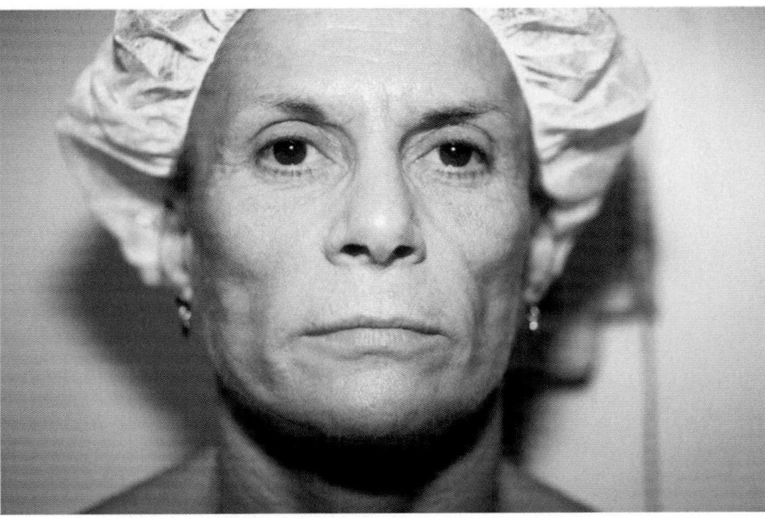

Figure 3 Before fat transfer.

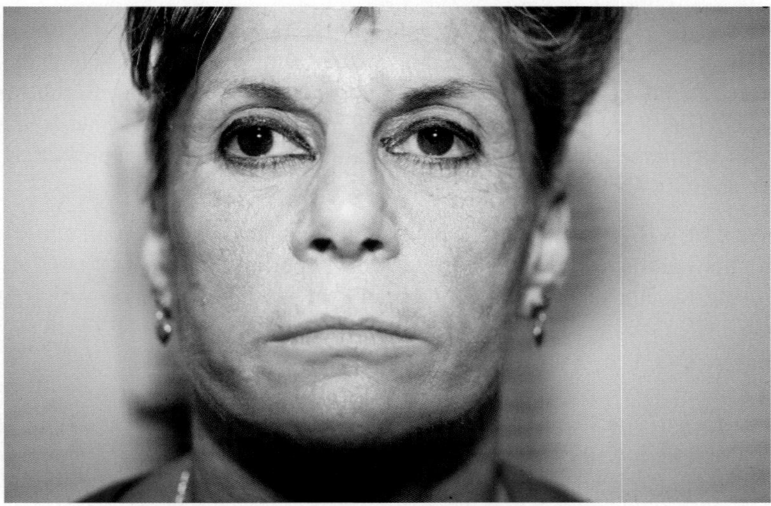

Figure 4 After fat transfer.

tion area using a 30-gauge 1-in. needle or, if the area is large, a 22-gauge spinal needle. In this area, very little anesthesia is needed and it should be delivered under barely any pressure with a syringe so that there is no distortion of the tissue. This slight anesthesia of the recipient area makes reinjection much more comfortable for the patient. Tiny needles are necessary to minimize the risk of bleeding, especially in the fat that is very vascular. When augmenting the nasolabial fold, the commissures of the mouth, lips, puppet lines, and cheeks, one reinjection site can be used on each side just lateral to the lips. If the chin or area anterior to the jowls is being enhanced, two incision sites are used and the fat injected at multiple levels from both incision sites.

Harvesting the Fat

SYRINGE HARVESTING. An incision is made with a 16-gauge needle used as an awl or a 16-gauge NoKor needle. No mark is left from this incision and no suture is necessary. Through this opening, a Coleman extractor attached to a 10-cc syringe can be inserted and used to harvest the fat. Negative pressure is obtained in the syringe by pulling the plunger out and holding it there while the syringe is moved back and forth in the subcutaneous tissue. Fat and fluid fills the syringe that is then placed in the container plunger up so that the fluid can settle to the bottom and the fat can rise to the top. This procedure can be repeated with as many syringes and donor sites as are necessary. The negative pressure on the plunger should be small; pull back 0.5–1 cc and the fat will come out easily.

The infranatant fluid collects at the bottom of the syringe and is easily be expelled by a push of the plunger. A cap is put on the tip of the syringe and the plunger is removed before centrifuging for 1 or 2 minutes. The lock on the tip is removed and any remaining infranatant fluid drains off, and then the oily supranatant fluid is poured off and any remaining supranatant fluid is wicked off with sterile gauze. The plunger is replaced and the fat can then be used for transplantation. The fat appears yellow and clean. The fat that will be used at the time of harvesting is transferred into 1-cc luer lock syringes through a female-female adaptor. The rest of the fat is frozen in the 19-cc syringes with the syringes capped. The patients name, social security number, and the date are carefully placed on each syringe to be saved and they are all placed in the same container that is also labeled with the patients name and the date. This container is then put into alphabetical order in the freezer at −20 °C.

LIPOSUCTION HARVESTING. Fat is harvested by hand as described above and then the typical liposuction with a vacuum machine is performed. Fat for harvesting is not obtained using the liposuction aspirator because of the high pressure, which can injure the fat cells.

Reinjecting the Fat

FRESH FAT. The fat is reinjected through an incision with an 18-gauge NoKor needle using a 1-cc luer lock syringe attached to a Coleman injection cannula using one or two reinjection sites per area. This is to prevent extrusion of the fat through multiple openings. The cannula is inserted to the furthest point, and a tiny aliquot of fat is injected as the syringe is pulled out. This is done at multiple levels of the skin and subcutaneous tissue.

After reinjection, the surgeon should massage the fat in so that it fills the area smoothly. When injecting, the surgeon should keep his hand on the outside of the area so the fat does not get into areas it should not go. Some surgeons over correct as some of the fat may disappear within the first few days after the procedure. We suggest not to overcorrect as our patients want to go back to their normal lives as soon as possible.

When the hands are being injected, one injection site on the back of each hand is used. This is located at the wrist and 5 cc of fat per hand is injected. The patient then contracts to make a fist and the injected fat is massaged to allow an easy spread over the entire hand.

FROZEN FAT. After checking with the patient the day before the procedure to make sure they are coming in for treatment, the amount of fat necessary for reinjection is removed from the freezer a few hours prior to the appointment. The syringes are placed upright in a container and the tray is set up as for fresh fat. The fluid, if there is any is allowed to drain off and the top 0.5–1 cc is not used as it is usually just triglycerides and other fatty acids. It is then pushed through a female-female adaptor into 1-cc luer-lock syringes that are then attached to a Coleman injector, which is a blunt tipped instrument. Local anesthesia is the same as that used for fresh fat reinjection.

Some physicians use a sharp 18-gauge needle to reinject fat monthly with no local anesthetic. We find less frequent intervals necessary when a blunt-tipped instrument is used for injection with a local anesthetic. Increased undermining or subcision with the blunt-tipped instrument appears to add to the result.

Advantages

The advantage of autologous fat is the ability to harvest, use, and then freeze a large quantity of material. This makes it possible not only to fill in deep hollows but also to perform a mini–face lift and fill in surgical areas in other parts of the body as well as plump up the hands to make them more youthful. As it is the patients own fat, there is no problem with allergenicity.

Disadvantages

The disadvantages are the need for a surgical procedure, even though it is performed with local anesthesia, the need for touch-ups in areas of heavy movement (e.g., nasolabial folds and marionette lines), and the need for a local anesthetic prior to injecting the fat.

HYALURONIC ACID GELS: NOT FDA APPROVED

Hyaluronic acids are polysaccharides that occur in all cells in all species and are identical in all living organisms. Hyaluronic acid is part of the normal ground substance of tissue. It is a natural polysaccharide that is an important element in the structural makeup of skin, subcutaneous, and connective tissue as well as in synovial tissue and fluid. These are elastic sugars that bind to water thus increasing hydration and volume and lubricate moving parts helping joints to move smoothly and muscles to glide over each other easily. Common sources include bacterial culture (Restylane), rooster combs (Hylaform), umbilical cord, and others. These implants add volume to the tissue into which they become integrated and in time they are degraded.

Restylane™

Restylane (Q-Med AB, Uppsala, Sweden) is a clear, transparent, viscous hyaluronic acid gel made by that will be distributed by Medicis in the United States and Canada after it is FDA approved. It is a non–animal-stabilized hyaluronic acid. As a nonanimal product made by streptococcal bacterial fermentation, it does not transmit disease and there are no allergic reactions so no skin test is necessary. It is cross-linked and stabilized so it has a long therapeutic effect of 6–12 months. It is biocompatible and biodegradable (13).

Restylane is not yet FDA approved, but clearance for marketing is expected sometime in 2003. It comes in three forms: (1) Fine Lines™, for superficial wrinkles; Restylane, which can be used everywhere; and (3) Perlane™, which is best for deeper folds and lip augmentation (14). The difference in the three products is the size of the molecule. The Fine Lines product is the smallest and Perlane the largest. An FDA phase 3 clinical study showed that Restylane lasts longer than Zyplast and is just as safe, with less product needed to get to the optimum cosmetic result (Figs. 5–7). The study was completed in the spring of 2002 and was submitted to the FDA in June 2002 (15).

Restylane is provided in 0.7-mL prepackaged luer-lock syringes that actually contain 0.8 mL of 20-mg/mL stabilized hyaluronic acid along with a 30-gauge 0.5-in. needle. The product is made for single use only.

The company recommends informing patients to avoid exposure to intense heat after injection. Steam rooms, saunas, and sunbathing should be avoided for 1–3 days. Intense cold should also be avoided. Injection should not be done into infected areas or into blood vessels, although no cases of vascular occlusion have been reported. Restylane has not been tested in pregnant or lactating women.

Technique

Restylane injections are given through a 30-gauge needle intradermally, using serial and/or linear threading injection techniques (Figs. 8 and 9). When using the linear threading technique, the bevel of the needle should be pointed upwards and Restylane should be injected as the needle is withdrawn. A combination of the linear threading and the serial injection technique can be used. Injection should be into the mid-dermis and no overcorrec-

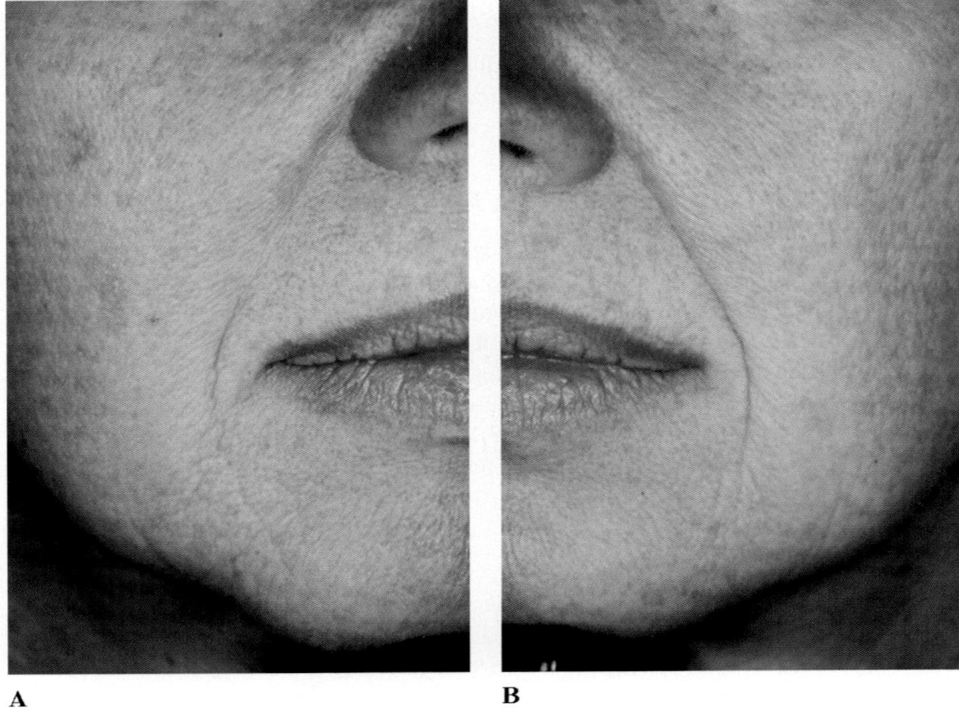

Figure 5 Before treatment with (A) Zyplast and (B) Restylane.

tion is needed. If it is injected too deeply, the longevity of the product will be decreased because of a faster hyaluronic acid turnover rate. If it is injected too superficially, little lumps may be visible. As there is no lidocaine in the syringe, an anesthetic cream or a local anesthetic is needed before treatment to make the injections painless.

Perlane is injected trough a 27-gauge 0.5-in. needle into the deep dermis or superficial subcutaneous tissue. Restylane Fine Lines is injected into the superficial dermis through a 31-gauge 0.5-in. needle and is meant for superficial lines like those around the periorbital region and lips.

If a lot of material is needed for treatment, we recommend an initial treatment followed by evaluation for more injections in 1 or 2 weeks. Periodic touch-ups are required.

Advantages

This is a long lasting, forgiving, nonanimal material that gives a smooth natural result. No skin testing is needed, as there are no allergies, so it can be used immediately. There are different forms for different tissues and since it binds to water, it looks even better in 2 or 3 days than on the day of injection. It comes prepackaged in syringes with needles and does not need refrigeration.

Disadvantages

The lack of lidocaine incorporated with the product means some form of pain prevention is necessary. The occasional postoperative swelling and bruising must also be taken into account. As with any nonpermanent substance, periodic touch-ups are required.

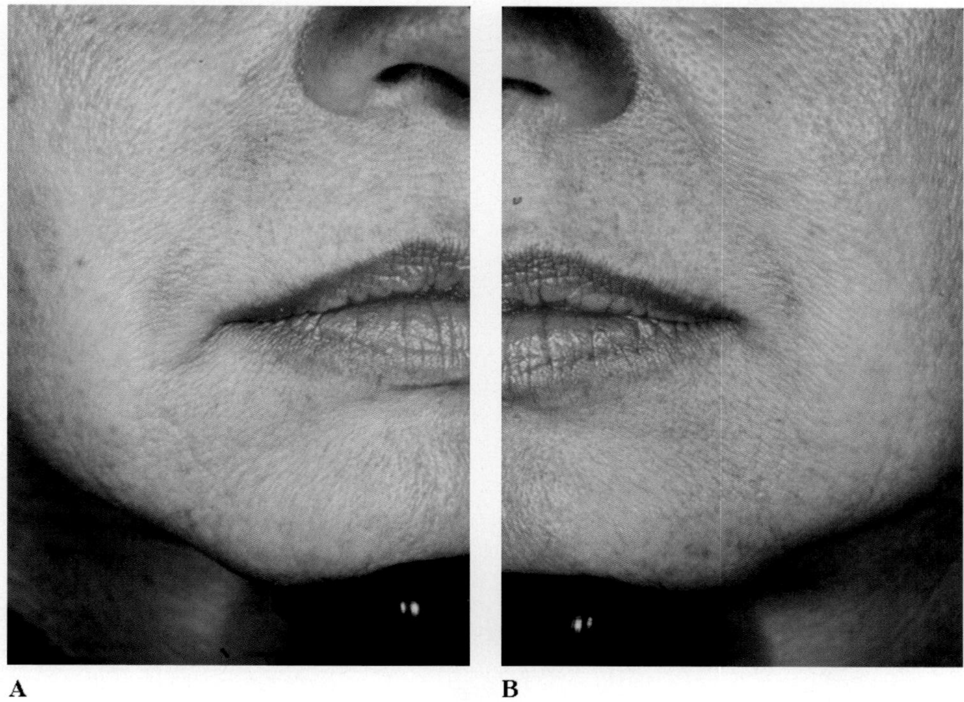

Figure 6 Optimal cosmetic improvement with (A) Zyplast and (B) Restylane.

Complications

At the implant site, patients can occasionally experience swelling, itching, erythema, pain, bruising, palpable lumps, or discoloration that may last for a few days. Rare long-term sequelae have been reported, including swelling, induration, erythema, acneiform nodules, or tenderness. These rare sequelae may appear 2–4 weeks after treatment and are usually self-limited.

Other Hyaluronic Acid Products

None of the hyaluronic acid products are FDA approved at this time. Hylaform® (Biomatrix, Ridgefield, NJ) is a hyaluronic acid gel made by processing the cock's combs of domestic fowl. Restylane is a lower-molecular-weight hyaluronic acid gel with a higher concentration than Hylaform. Hylaform Plus is a new product made for deeper folds. FDA phase 3 clinical trials are underway.

SILICONE: OFF-LABEL USE IN SKIN

The silicone oil that is used today is Silikon 1000 (Alcon Laboratories, Fort Worth, TX). That means the density is 1000 centistokes. The original Dow Corning silicone was 350 centistokes. Its use is off-label for wrinkles and scars. It is a purified product as it has

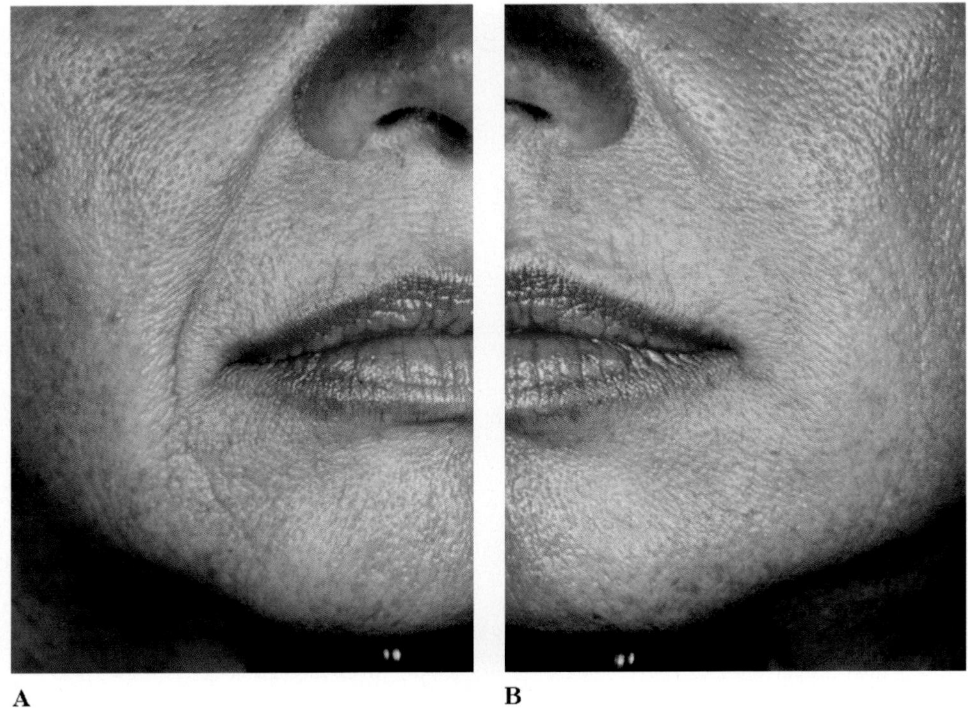

A B

Figure 7 Six months after treatment with (A) Zyplast and (B) Restylane.

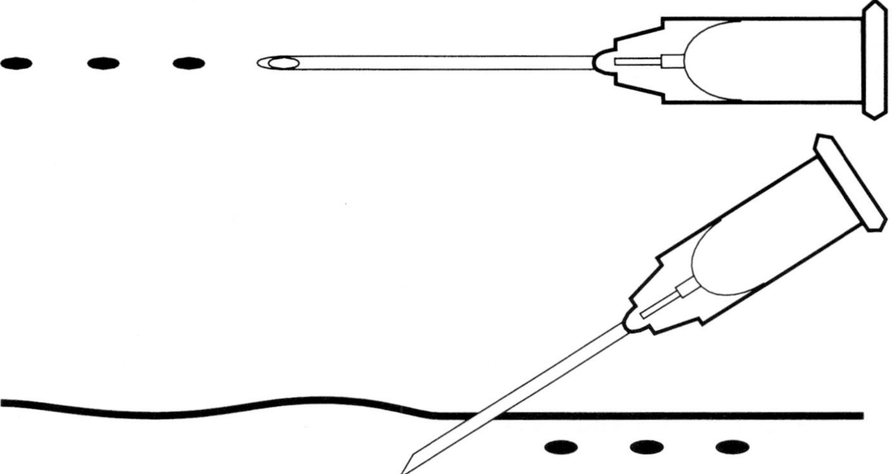

Figure 8 Serial injection technique.

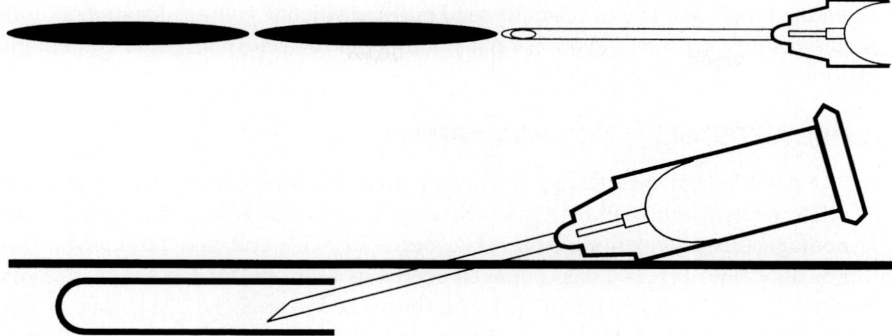

Figure 9 Threading injection technique.

been FDA approved for retinal detachment and has been used for lipoatrophy seen in patients with AIDS. Problems seen in the past were usually due to too much volume injected or adulteration of the fluid with substances such as mineral oil. Initial studies are being done now with Silskin, a similar silicone 100 product, treating wrinkles and aging. FDA phase 3 clinical trials are being planned for the same indication. Silikon 1000 may be used for off-label use, but as it is a device and not a drug, the physician may not advertise its use in the office, the phonebook, a web site or the media.

Silikon 1000 is a sterile, clear, and colorless gel that is relatively inert. There are no preservatives or other ingredients and it is distributed in 10-cc vials with 8.5-cc of sterile silicone oil. The material is drawn into the syringe through a 16-gauge needle. It can be stored at room temperature.

Technique

A microdroplet serial injection technique is used to inject silicone oil. Multiple treatments are necessary at intervals of 4–6 weeks or more. A 1-cc luer lock syringe is used and attached to a 27-gauge needle or the RJ Flo 30-gauge, large-bore needle that patients find more comfortable (order 978-532-0666). Patients must be told that they may not see results for the first two or three treatments.

Advantages

Silicone oil is an ideal filling substance in many ways because it is permanent, needs no skin testing as there are no antibodies to liquid silicone, is stored at room temperature, does not support bacterial growth, can be used to treat many areas, is not painful when an anesthetic cream is used before injection and a modified dental block is used for the lips, and does not cause postinjection morbidity. It is relatively inexpensive and has a long shelf life.

Disadvantages

A microdroplet technique must be used at intervals of 4–6 weeks or more, so it takes several months to get the final result. Granulomas and other side effects are extremely rare when the proper volume of unadulterated purified silicone is used. Treatment of these is with intralesional steroids and occasionally antibiotics to cyclosporine and other immune modulators.

ARTEFILL/ARTECOLL®: NOT FDA APPROVED

Artecoll (Artes Medical, San Diego, CA) is a permanent filler that contains polymethylmethacrylate microspheres (PMMA), which are Plexiglas beads in collagen (i.e., microscopic homogenous polymethylmethacrylate beads in 3.5% collagen suspension, mixed with 0.3% lidocaine) (16,17). The collagen serves as a bridge for the beads. PMMA is commonly called Plexiglas or Lucite and it has been used in artificial eye lenses, dentures, and bone cement. The PMMA is polymerized into 30–40- m spheres that are then suspended in the collagen. The collagen is degraded after injection, leaving the PMMA spheres that remain permanently. The company claims that these spheres cannot migrate as they are encapsulated by 2–4 months by the patient's own tissue that migrates into the spaces between the beads (14,18–20).

U.S. clinical trials for safety and persistence were completed in 2001. The company recommends using a temporary filler first to see if the patient likes the results. Two treatment sessions should be used. Patients should be advised not to make a lot of facial expressions over the first 3 days after treatment, so the substance is not pushed into the subcutaneous tissue. The areas then improve over time and if a patient stretches the skin they may see and feel the whitish implant.

Technique

Press one drop out before injecting. Artecoll is injected deeply using a threading or tunneling technique at the junction between the dermis and subcutaneous tissue through a 27-gauge 0.5-in. needle at the junction between the dermis and the subcutaneous tissue. If it is injected intradermally, the skin will blanch and injection should stop immediately as small nodules can form and prolonged erythema can occur. If the injection is too deep, no resistance is felt. The shape but not the color of the needle should be visualized. Injection should be parallel to the wrinkle as the needle is withdrawn. It is then massaged in very gently and molded with the fingers.

Two treatment sessions should be used as fibrous tissue invades the space between the microspheres. Use 0.5 cc for one nasolabial fold or both frown lines or one lip either upper or lower or both corners of the mouth or both marionette lines. The second treatment should take place after 3–6 weeks. Inject irregularities in the nose epiperiostially. Inject three to five bands of material parallel in nasolabial lines. Inject as bands into the lip along the vermilion border and a band between the dry and wet part of the lips. Do not inject into the muscle of the lip and do not inject as droplets. Add more Artecoll to lips after 3 months if they are soft. Raise a flattened philtrum with two vertical injections upwards from the lip and mold between the fingers.

Advantages

Artecoll gives permanent results (21).

Disadvantages

Skin testing to collagen has to be done prior to treatment. It is contraindicated in people with thin skin, as it can be palpable or visible. Patients can experience swelling, redness, and pain over the first few days. The product must be refrigerated. A temporary filler must be used first. If injected incorrectly, nodules can be seen; these granulomas can appear many years later. Two treatments are required.

Complications

Granulomas, some occurring more than 10 years after injection, have been reported. Long-lasting redness can occur when the injection is too superficial and itching can occur and last for weeks to months.

RADIANCE FN™: OFF-LABEL USE IN THE SKIN

Radiance FN (BioForm Inc., Franksville, WI) is made up of microscopic calcium hydroxy-apatite particles founding bone and suspended in a gel. It has been FDA-approved and used for years in dental reconstruction, bone, bladder, neck, and vocal cord implants. Technically, it comprises calcium hydroxyapatite microspheres suspended in an aqueous polysaccharide gel, similar to Coaptite. The polysaccharide, carboxymethylcellulose stays in place long enough for the body's own tissue to move in and hold it in place. Radiance FN supposedly acts as a scaffolding for bone or for collagen to grow in soft tissue, thus creating volume. Use in the skin is FDA off label.

Technique

Radiance is injected after a block or local anesthesia using a 26-gauge needle subdermally.

Advantages

No skin testing is necessary, as it contains no animal products. Therefore, treatment can be given on the day of consultation. It can reportedly last from 2 to 5 years. One cubic centimeter treats more areas than 1 cc of collagen and it is said to look and feel natural.

Disadvantages

Dental blocks and local anesthesia are necessary because the injections are more painful than Collagen. Swelling can occur for 2 days post-injection and sometimes calcium deposits rise to the surface of the skin and can be easily excised. Granulomas can sometimes occur. It is not to be used for superficial lines but is reported to be good for deeper folds and wrinkles and lip enhancement. If it is injected too superficially, extrusion, infection, firmness and lumps can occur.

Complications

Complications include lumps, extrusion, granulomas, infection and firmness.

CYMETRA™: MICRONIZED ALLODERM®

Cymetra (LifeCell, Branchburg, NJ), technically micronized acellular human cadaveric dermis, is powdered Alloderm. It is supplied in a prepackaged 5-cc syringe of dried material. This reconstituted to 1 cc and is for single use only. The human tissue has been tested, sterilized and treated so it is accepted without rejection. It is a soft implant without allergies that reportedly lasts a little longer than collagen. It should be refrigerated when received to lengthen shelf life.

Technique

Cleanse the area first with soap, water and alcohol. Cymetra is injected into multiple levels after it is rehydrated with saline and, if desired, lidocaine.

For subcision of the nasolabial folds and 18-gauge 1.5-in. needle is used and the material injected as the needle is withdrawn. To inject without subcision using the threading technique, a 23–25-gauge needle is used and 1.5–2 U is injected per side as the needle is withdrawn. For serial injections into the nasolabial folds, a 25–27-gauge 3/8-in. needle is used and 1.5–2 U is injected per side.

When treating the lip, each part is done differently. For the vermilion border, Cymetra is injected using a 22–23-gauge 1.5-in. needle and injecting with the bevel up, tenting the skin while withdrawing the needle. The first injection starts from the Cupid's bow on 1 side to the opposite commissure, and this is then repeated from the other side so that the middle one third of the lip gets double the amount of material. A total of 0.5–1.5 U is used per lip. The next area is the vermilion itself. Here a 23-gauge 1.5-in. needle is used bevel up and tenting the tissue and injecting as the needle is withdrawn. The injection starts one third of the way across the lip to the other side. Again, the middle one third gets twice the amount of Cymetra. Use 1.2 U per lip.

When treating perioral rhytides a 26-gauge 3/8-in. needle should be used immediately subdermal. The skin should be tented and the material injected with the bevel up as the needle is withdrawn. A little bit should also be injected parallel to and just above the white roll in the same manner.

For the triangular depression of the marionette complex, use both the threading and serial puncture technique. The threading technique is done with a 25-gauge 1.5-in. needle threaded with subcision subdermally from below. Injection occurs as the needle is withdrawn with the bevel up and the tissue tented. Each side receives 0.5–1 U Cymetra. Then serial puncture is done using a 25-gauge 3/8-in. needle with immediate subdermal placement.

The malar depression is injected using a 22-gauge 1.5-in. needle threaded subdermally three times horizontally and three times vertically for an even crisscross pattern. The area can be rolled even with a cotton swab or massaged bimanually.

For all areas gentle massage is then done and the patient warned not to massage the area any further and to avoid facial expressions as long as possible, for 6 hours or more. More than one treatment may be necessary for optimal improvement.

Advantages

Advantages include treatment at the consultation, as no skin test is necessary. It can be stored at room temperature and lasts up to 6 months.

Disadvantages

Cymetra must be rehydrated to use. It should be refrigerated. The company recommends it not be used in patients who have a collagen autoimmune disease or in those who are allergic to antibiotics as traces of antibiotics may be present in the injection material. The company also it advises physicians not to use it around the eyes or in the glabella. More than one treatment may be necessary for optimal improvement.

GORE-TEX®

Gore-Tex (W. L. Gore and Associates, Flagstaff, AZ) is a permanent filling substance made of expanded polytetrafluoroethylene (ePTFE) created by the extrusion of Teflon. Nodules of ePTFE are connected by a multidirectional fibril structure to make a polymer. This polymer is biocompatible, soft and pliable and comes in sheets, patches and tubes of varying sizes. It has been used in the body since 1971, including abdominal wall and hernia repairs, and for skin augmentation since 1991. It is inert and nonallergenic with low tissue reactivity and minimal capsule formation. The substance has 20–30- m pores that allow tissue to grow into the material. That anchors the material but sometimes makes it more difficult to remove. The best areas in which to use these implants are the deep furrows that some people have in the nasolabial lines and glabella. It has also been used in the lips. Softform is a tubular form of Gore-Tex (ePTFE) that is already in a trocar, made and prepackaged to be used in the nasolabial folds and the vermilion border of the lips. Fibroblastic material fills these tubes after 6 months. However, one out of 11 patients needed the material removed for various reasons (see Disadvantages).

Technique

The implants are placed in the subcutaneous tissue. A hollow trocar is used to tunnel subcutaneously though the deepest part of the fold after local anesthesia has been given. The implant is then pulled through by dragging back with the trocar, needle, or suture and then trimming the ePTFE. The 3–5-mm incision sites are then sutured. Pre and postsurgical antibiotics are generally used. With Softform, the tubular material is placed in the shaft of a cutting trocar that is then placed in an outer cannula.

Collagen can be layered over this material if more correction is needed.

Advantages

This is a permanent filler that is stored at room temperature.

Disadvantages

A surgical procedure with incision areas is necessary to implant the material. The tissue that grows into it and stabilizes it makes it difficult to remove. Extrusion may occur. Patients must be warned that the material may need to be repositioned and that the implant may be palpable and this can be annoying.

FASCIAN

Fascian™ (Fascia Biosystems, Beverly Hills, CA) is preserved fascia lata in particulate form made from screened human cadavers and was introduced in 1999. Fascia is mostly collagen protein and is thick, dense, and cushy. It takes the body many months or years to absorb this material. Fascian comes in prepackaged 3-cc luer-lock syringes of the dried material. The tissue is tested for various diseases, irradiated, particulated, and vacuum sealed. This treatment is done so it is not rejected and does not cause infection or disease. Fascian particles come in various sizes, < 0.25 mm, < 0.5 mm, and < 2.0 mm; all three need to be rehydrated in 3–5 mL of saline or saline and lidocaine solution before injection. Wait 5–10 minutes and agitate the solution. After injection, the company feels that recollagenization occurs around the graft that acts as a scaffolding. The saline or saline and lidocaine solution is absorbed. It has been reported to last 3–8 months and does not need to be refrigerated. No skin test is required.

Technique

After rehydrating the material with lidocaine and anesthetizing the area with a local anesthetic or anesthetic block, the area to be injected is subcised with a 20-gauge needle and the material is injected with a 16–29-gauge needle, depending on the particle size. Injections are placed subdermal. Do not inject into the dermis as inflammation with erythema and swelling as well as lumpiness can occur. Replace the needle if it gets clogged.

Advantages

Skin testing is unnecessary so treatment can be given immediately. Some physicians prefer using a more temporary substance first. It can be stored at room temperature and may last a little longer than collagen.

Disadvantages

The substance must be rehydrated before use and a local anesthetic or anesthetic block must be used. Trace amounts of polymyxin sulfate, bacitracin, or gentamycin may be present so do not us if a patient has allergies to any of these substances. Fascian should not be used for superficial lines as intradermal injection can lead to lumpiness or inflammation.

NEW-FILL®: NOT FDA APPROVED

New-Fill (Biotech Industry SA, Luxembourg) is polylactic acid (PLA) used in suture material for more than 40 years. It is nontoxic, synthetic, immunologically inactive, and easily absorbable. The New-Fill brand of PLA has been approved in Europe for soft-tissue augmentation of scars and wrinkles. It is very popular for the lipoatrophy associated with HIV disease. It is sold in a kit of two vials each containing 150 mg of powdered product. Five cubic centimeters of sterile water with or without lidocaine is added to reconstitute it for injection. The fluid is absorbed in 1 week and the PLA particles are said to stimulate collagen growth. More than one session may be needed for treatment and the product lasts for 18–24 months. A local anesthetic must be used, as it is painful to inject.

Technique

The product does not need to be refrigerated and no skin test is necessary so it can be used immediately.

Disadvantages

New-Fill PLA needs to be reconstituted. More than one session is needed for treatment and a local anesthetic must be used to minimize discomfort.

Complications

Granulomas have been reported to occur, and are probably technique- and dilution-dependant.

REFERENCES

1. Klein AW, Elson ML. The history of substances for soft tissue augmentation. Dermatol Surg 2000; 26:1096–1105.
2. Knapp TR, Kaplan EN, Daniels JR. Injectable collagen for soft tissue augmentation. Plast Reconstruct Surg 1977; 60:389–405.
3. Cooperman LS, MacKinnon V, Bechler G, Pharriss BB. Injectable collagen: six years' clinical investigation. Aesthetic Plast Surg 1985; 9:145–151.
4. Matti BA, Nicolle FV. Clinical use of Zyplast in correction of age- and disease-related contour deficiencies of the face. Aesthetic Plast Surg 1990; 14:227–34.
5. Stegman SJ, Tromovitch TA. Implantation of collagen for depressed scars. J Dermatol Surg Oncol 1980; 6:450–453.
6. Stegman SJ, Chu S, Armstrong R. Adverse reactions to bovine collagen implant: clinical and histologic features. J Dermatol Surg Oncol 1988; 14(suppl 1):39–48.
7. Illouz YG. The fat cell ''graft,'' a new technique to fill depressions. Plast Reconstr Surg 1986; 78:122–123.
8. Fournier PF. Facial recontouring with fat grafting. Dermatol Clin 1990; 8:523.
9. Asken S. Autologous fat transplantation: micro and macro techniques. Am J Cosm Surg 1987; 4:111.
10. Glogau RG. Microlipoinjection. Arch Dermatol 1988; 124:1340.
11. Coleman SR. Facial recontouring with lipostructure. Clin Plast Surg 1997; 24:347–367.
12. Amar RE. Microinfiltration adipocytaire (MIA) au niveau de la face, ou restructuration tissulaire par greffe de tissu adipeux. Ann Chir Plast Esthet 1999; 44:593–608.
13. Friedman PM, Mafong EA, Kauvar ANB, Geronemus RG. Safety data of injectable nonanimal stabilized hyaluronic acid gel for soft tissue augmentation. Dermatol Surg 2002; 28:491–494.
14. Pollack SV. Some new injectable dermal filler materials: Hylaform, Restylane, and Artecoll. J Cutan Med Surg 1999; 3(suppl 4):29.
15. Narins RS, Brandt F, Leyden J, Lorenc P, Rubin M, Smith S. A randomised, double-blind multicenter comparison of the efficacy and tolerability of Restylane vs Zyplast for the correction of the nasolabial folds. Dermatol Surg 2003; 29:588–595.
16. Lemperle G, Ott H, Charrier U, Hecker J, Lemperle M. PMMA microspheres for intradermal implantation. Part I. Animal Research. Ann Plast Surg 1991; 26:57.
17. Lemperle G, Hazan-Gauthier N, Lemperle M. PMMA microspheres (Artecoll) for skin and soft tissue augmentation. Part II. Clinical investigation. Plast Reconstr Surg 1995; 92:331.
18. McClelland M, Egbert B, Hanko V, Berg RA, DeLustro F. Evaluation of Artecoll polymethylmethacrylate implant for soft-tissue augmentation: biocompatibility and chemical characterization. Plast Reconstr Surg 1997; 100:1466.
19. Lemperle G, Romano JJ, Busso M. Soft tissue augmentation with Artecoll: 10-year history, indications, technique, and potential side effects. Dermatol Surg 2003; 28:573–587.
20. Lemperle G. Artecoll augmentation of wrinkles and acne scars. In: Klein AW, Ed. Tissue Augmentation in Clinical Practice: Procedures & Techniques. 2nd ed. New York: Marcel Dekker, 2003.
21. Carruthers A. Artecoll: an injectable micro-implant for longlasting soft tissue augmentation. Skin Ther Lett 1999; 4:1.

17

Treatment of Vascular Lesions Related to Photoaging

Robert A. Weiss *Johns Hopkins University School of Medicine, Baltimore, Maryland, U.S.A.*

Mitchel P. Goldman *University of California, San Diego, California, U.S.A.*

- The most common vascular lesions related to photoaging are facial telangiectases, but these may occur on other sun-exposed areas such as the chest and legs.
- Telangiectases that are arteriolar in origin are small in diameter, bright-red in color, and do not protrude above the skin surface while telangiectases that arise from venules are wider, blue in color and often protrude above the skin surface.
- Lasers or intense pulsed light are the preferred method of treatment for facial telangiectases although electrosurgery and sclerotherapy are still performed frequently.
- Treatment of telangiectasia of the face by intense pulsed light gives an additional benefit of textural smoothing and reduction of pigmentation.
- Sclerotherapy is the preferred method for leg telangiectases.
- Treatment of poikiloderma of the neck and chest responds best to intense pulsed light.

Photoaging-related telangiectases most often occur on the face, with areas such as chest and legs frequently involved. Telangiectasia related to photoaging may begin as venous, arteriolar, or capillary in origin. Many patients who present for treatment of facial veins also are also concerned about appearance of vascular abnormalities on the leg. We estimate that approximately one of out five patients seen for treatment of facial veins will also have some form of vascular cosmetic blemish on the leg.

The most common vascular lesion related to photoaging is the development of facial telangiectasia. These can be individual and relatively isolated or large groups of matted telangiectases on the cheeks (Fig. 1). The term telangiectasia refers to superficial cutaneous vessels visible to the human eye (1). These vessels measure 0.1 to 1.0 mm in diameter and represent a dilated venule, capillary, or arteriole. Telangiectases that are arteriolar in origin are small in diameter, bright red, and do not protrude above the skin surface. Those that arise from venules are wider, blue, and often protrude above the skin surface. Telangiectasia arising at the capillary loop are often initially fine, red lesions, but become larger and purple or blue with time (2).

Telangiectases have been subdivided into four classifications based on clinical appearance: (1) simple or linear, (2) arborizing, (3) spider, and (4) papular (3). Red linear and arborizing telangiectasia are very common on the face, especially the nose, mid cheeks, and chin. These lesions are also seen relatively frequently on the legs. Papular telangiectasia is frequently not related to photoaging but part of genetic syndromes, such as Osler-Weber-Rendu syndrome, and also are seen in collagen vascular diseases. Cherry hemangiomas are small, round, red to purple dome-shaped vascular ectasias that are also seen scattered anywhere on the face or body. In addition, patients develop enlargement of slightly larger venulectases that appear as purplish vessels on the cheeks, periorbital region, and vermilion. All forms of telangiectasia are thought to occur through the release or activation of vasoactive substances under the influence of a variety of factors, such as anoxia, hormones, chemicals, infection, and physical factors such as ultraviolet (UV) radiation, with resultant capillary or venular neogenesis (3).

Spider telangiectasia of the face is most commonly seen in patients with fair skin (Fitzpatrick type I and II), since these patients are the most susceptible to UV damage. Facial telangiectases are especially common on the nasal alae, nose, and mid cheeks, and are probably due to persistent arteriolar vasodilation resulting from vessel wall weakness induced by UV damage. They are worsened by damage to the surrounding connective and elastic tissue from chronic sun exposure, or rarely from the use of topical steroids. There is a definite familial or genetic component to these lesions. Rosacea may be an accompanying condition (Fig. 2).

Fortunately, the treatment of facial telangiectasia is much more predictable than the treatment of telangiectasia of the legs. The skin heals quickly and is much less likely to scar with a similar depth of injury than on other body locations. Treatment results are often seen much more quickly as healing is much faster on the well-oxygenated skin of the face. Facial vessels also have the advantage of a more uniform depth than the legs. The vascular walls themselves are much thinner and uniform, and hydrostatic pressure plays no major role. Arterial pressure is occasionally a factor as seen in spider angiomata with a small central arteriole. This is important when deciding on a method of treatment as sclerotherapy into a bright red arteriolar fed vessel on the cheek incurs more risks of necrosis than the use of laser or light to shut down the branches and shrink the arteriolar component.

Whereas the cause of telangiectasia on the legs is predominantly hydrostatic pressure, facial vessels appear to result from sunlight-induced damage to the collagen of the vessel wall. Sun exposure damages and weakens collagen with cumulative exposures, resulting in ectasia. In addition, there is a relatively high incidence of rosacea on the face. Rosacea consists of frequent flushing associated with telangiectases, papules, and pustules. As more

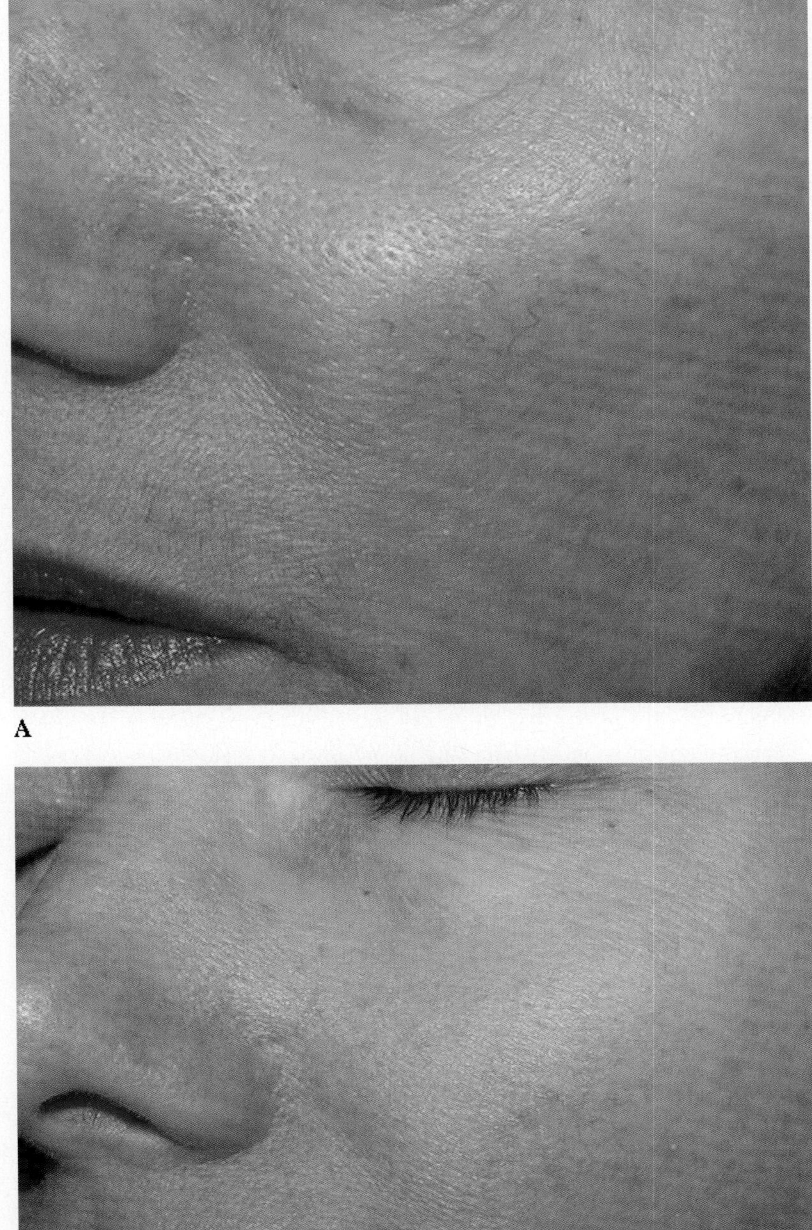

Figure 1 (A) Most common presenting vascular feature of photoaging in the white patient is telangiectasia. In this individual, the telangiectases are in the early stages of photoaging seen in the fourth decade of life. (B) Treatment with IPL reduces the total amount of visible vessels and smoothes the skin. A double-pulse 570-nm filter, 2.4-msec + 6-msec pulse with 10-msec delay, and a fluence of 29 J/cm^2 were used.

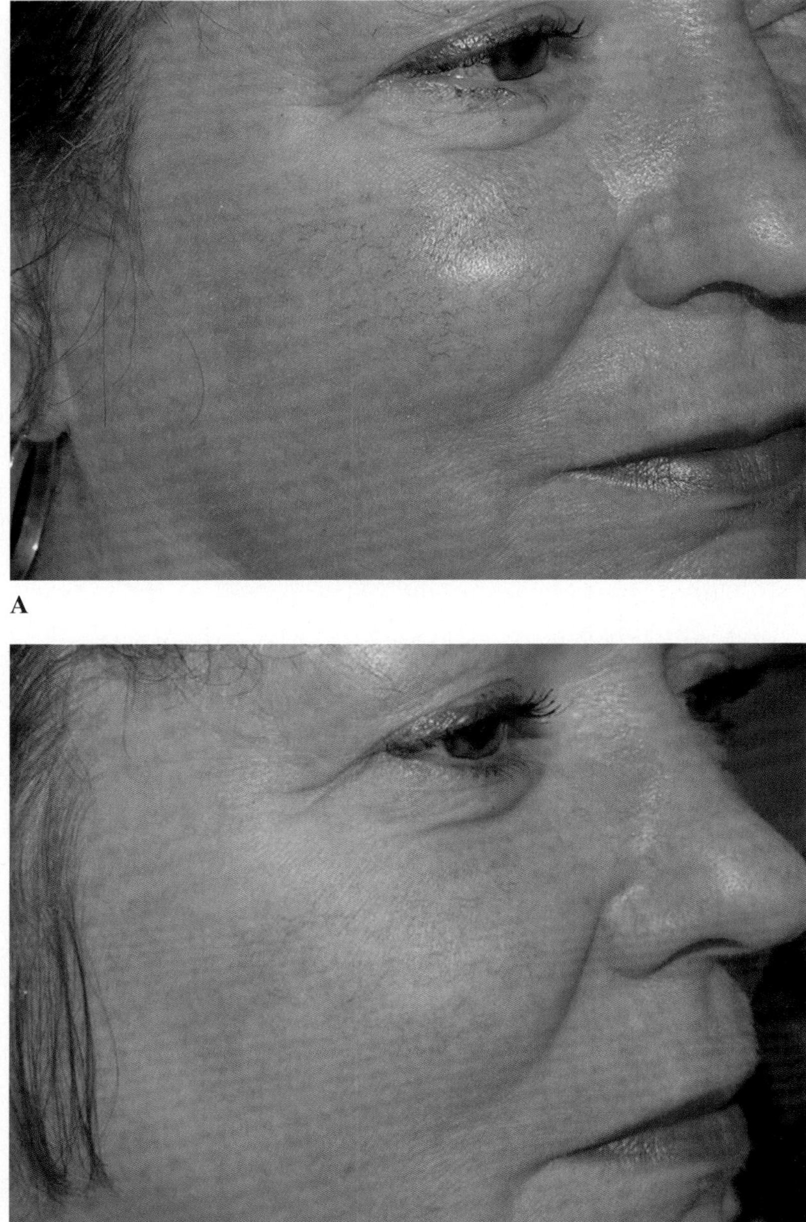

Figure 2 Rosacea is thought to be related to photoaging. Intensity and duration of flushing episodes are reduced following IPL treatment of the face. Before (A) and after (B) three treatments with Vasculight IPL (Lumenis, Santa Clara, CA) using a 550-nm filter, double pulse of 2.4 and 7 msec, delay of 10 msec, and a fluence of 27–29 J/cm^2.

individuals exercise more frequently and vigorously, the incidence of facial flushing has increased. Repeated prolonged facial flushing leads to telangiectasia. Genetic factors also play a large role, and the rosy cheek appearance passes from one generation to the next in individuals susceptible to rosacea. Aging of the skin (accelerated by sun exposure) causes more telangiectasia with collagen breakdown (4). Repeated trauma to the face will also induce localized erythema and ultimately vascular dilatation.

Patients with telangiectasia of various types present for treatment primarily because of cosmetic concerns. Therefore, it is important that the procedure be relatively risk-free without unsightly scarring. Various modalities can be used to treat telangiectasia of the face or other regions. The reader is referred to other sources for a more in-depth discussion of this topic (5,6). What follows are our personal recommendations from 20 years of experience with electrodesiccation, sclerotherapy, and a variety of lasers including the pulse dye laser (PDL), long-pulse dye laser, argon laser, frequency-doubled neodymium: yttrium-aluminum-garnet laser (532-nm Nd:YAG), intense pulsed light (IPL) in all its forms, and a variety of 1064-nm long-pulsed Nd:YAG lasers (1064-nm Nd:YAG).

ELECTROSURGERY

Electrodesiccation is frequently used worldwide to treat facial telangiectasia because the device is readily available at a relatively low cost. Electrodesiccation is a process in which heat is generated from resistance of tissues to the passage of a highly damped current from a single electrode. Dehydration occurs in the tissue immediately adjacent to the needle point, and as cellular fluids are evaporated, tissue destruction results. The vessel must be cauterized or electrocoagulated every 2 to 3 mm with very low amperage current (1–2 A). Some degree of epidermal necrosis occurs due to the nonspecific nature of cauterization. Multiple treatments are typically necessary for successful treatment. Punctate white or pigmented scars may occur if excessive thermal damage occurs. Groove type scars along the nasal alae is the most common adverse effect of electrodesiccation.

Best results are achieved when the lowest effective fluence and the finest electrodes are used. Electrodes that are coated with Teflon so that only the tip of the electrode or one side of the electrode is exposed tend to provide the safest treatment. In addition, use of a bipolar current (with the patient grounded to a plate at a distance from the treated area) allows one to treat with a lower fluence. With bipolar treatment, the current passes through the cannulated vessel for several millimeters with relative selectivity. When performed with care, electrodesiccation is effective, but is best reserved for the smallest of telangiectasia. This technique has been popularized by Kobayashi, who reports excellent results (7).

Serious adverse effects from electrosurgery such as disturbance of pacemakers and implantable cardio-defibrillators are extremely rare. To prevent disruption to electric currents in these devises, short bursts are recommended with minimal power settings. Rare instances of pacemaker interference with skipped beats and reprogramming have been reported in a survey of dermatologic surgeons performing electrocoagulation during cutaneous surgery. An incidence of 0.8 cases/100 years of surgical practice occurred but may not be representative of all patients undergoing electrodesiccation of telangiectasia (8).

SCLEROTHERAPY

Sclerotherapy refers to the injection of a foreign substance into the lumen of a vessel to cause endothelial and mural damage with resulting thrombosis, vessel wall necrosis and subsequent fibrosis. Best results are obtained on superficial vessels of the legs, or vessels greater than 0.4 mm in diameter. Facial telangiectasia are less responsive to sclerotherapy than leg telangiectasia and are also more prone to the complication of cutaneous necrosis. Many facial telangiectases, especially those that are bright red and less than 0.2 mm in diameter, are arteriolar in origin. Injecting a sclerosing solution into these vessels may produce necrosis of the overlying skin. When a sclerosing solution is injected into a high-flow arterial system, complete endothelial and mural destruction does not occur. Superficial and patchy endothelial necrotic cells combine with necrotic red and white blood cells combine to form microemboli and sludge, which lodge in vessels downstream. This manifests as punctate cutaneous necrosis. In addition, arterial vasospasm may also occur, producing ischemia at the point of injection. Therefore, when performing sclerotherapy on facial blood vessels, it is important to warn patients that temporary punctate necrosis is possible. Injection of facial telangiectasia, however, can give excellent results with careful technique.

Other complications common to sclerotherapy of leg veins, such as telangiectatic matting and hyperpigmentation, rarely if ever occur when injecting facial telangiectases (9). The reason for the low incidence of these adverse effects is unknown. Hyperpigmentation occurs from extravasation of red blood cells (RBCs) through a damaged vessel wall under high venous pressure from gravitational effects as well as refluxing blood flow through feeding reticular veins. Hemosiderin within the RBCs is poorly absorbed in some patients and produces the brown pigmentation.

In treating facial veins, venous pressure is not as high as the veins are above the level of the heart but facial telangiectasia are connected to feeding arterioles producing high pressure at least equal to that seen in leg telangiectasia. Telangiectatic matting occurs from the release of angiogenic factors secondary to vessel destruction and resulting inflammation from sclerotherapy. Facial vessel injury is less likely to lead to matting, the reason for which is not understood.

Technique

Our recommendations for ensuring optimal treatment while minimizing the chance for cutaneous necrosis follows. First, a very small volume of sclerosing solution (< 0.1 mL) is injected very slowly (over 10–30 sec) into the vein. One should not try to overfill the entire visible vein with sclerosing solution. This will make it possible for the solution to migrate into deeper vessels or even arteriovenous connections with resulting ulceration. A good rule of thumb is to stop the injection when you do not see the sclerosing solution flowing through the vessel.

A 30-gauge needle will suffice for most vessels, although a disposable 32-gauge needle recently available may aid cannulation of very small vessels. The 32-gauge needles are less painful than 30-gauge needles and decrease the likelihood of inadvertent perivenular injection. The disadvantages of using 32-gauge needles are that they dull after five to 10 injections, and easily bend. One should never hesitate to change needles if a vein cannot be cannulated easily. It is usually not the ''tough skin'' of the patient but a dull needle that makes injection difficult. One-half-inch 30-gauge needles, although 0.3 mm in diameter, are honed to an oblique bevel that permits cannulation of vessels 0.1 mm in diameter or smaller. We do not recommend using needles longer than 0.5 in. as they are too flexible for reliable and accurate cannulation.

Injection pressure is also important. Use of a 3-mL syringe filled with 1 or 2 mL of sclerosing solution (depending on the number of vessels to be treated) is ideal. A 3-mL syringe fits well in the palm of the hand and can be easily manipulated. If telangiectases are injected under excessive force, they may rupture and result in extravasation of solution. Therefore injections should be made with minimal pressure. In addition, the slower the injection, the longer the solution will be in contact with the vessel wall.

Depth of needle insertion is also important. The location of almost all facial telangiectases is in the upper dermis. The most common error in technique is to place the needle tip deep to the vessel. To enter the vessel at a less acute angle almost parallel to the skin surface, the needle should be bent to 145 degrees with the bevel up. If the needle is not within the vessel, the solution will either leak out onto the skin or produce an immediate superficial wheal. At times, gentle upward traction can be applied as the needle is advanced to ensure superficial placement.

When a detergent-type of sclerosing solution (polidocanol, sodium tetradecyl sulfate [STS], sodium morrhuate, or ethanolamine oleate) is injected into a slow flow venular system (which is represented by a blue-green facial venule greater than 0.4 mm in diameter), its destructive action may occur far from the site of injection. STS has less range of action and is a somewhat safer than polidocanol for remote effect. It is not uncommon for the sclerosing effect within veins to continue for several centimeters from the point of injection. For the face, use of an osmotic sclerosing solution, such as hypertonic saline or hypertonic saline/dextrose solutions, may theoretically be safer owing to a more local effect. With the osmotic agent, endothelial and mural fibrosis occurs in a localized area within the concentration gradient of the injected solution. This limits the fear of sclerosing deeper and more distal venular drainage patterns, such as the retro-orbital venous plexus. Unfortunately, osmotic solutions are more painful to inject than detergent solutions and have a higher risk of ulceration with extravasation. A solution of 72% glycerin is also possible to inject with minimal risks. It is important to have an assistant hold pressure on the site of injection for 5–10 min when using an osmotic or glycerin solution.

Complications of Sclerotherapy Treatment of Facial Telangiectasia

Sclerotherapy treatment of facial telangiectasia has been proven to be effective and safe (8). However, there is a potential for sight threatening complications from periocular vascular manipulation.

Inadvertent intra-arterial injection of corticosteroid suspensions in the periocular region has been reported to lead to embolic occlusion in the ophthalmic artery distribution and result in blindness (10). Inadvertent intra-arterial injection is the likely factor permitting steroid particulate emboli to reach the retinal circulation. Severe visual loss has also been reported following intralesional steroid injection into a chalazion, again apparently causing retinal and choroidal embolic occlusion presumably as a consequence of inadvertent intra-arterial injection (11). Since it is not a suspension, STS injection would be less likely to lead to distal embolic phenomena; however, as an intravascular sclerosant agent, it clearly presents a danger if it gains inadvertent access to the arterial system supplying the eye in concentrations that will produce endothelial toxicity. An embolus composed of denatured endothelial cells and blood cell elements could result. Presently accepted standards of injection technique, including careful placement of the needle, repeated aspiration, and careful stabilization of the syringe, do not guarantee that the physician can detect if the bevel is against the vessel wall, within the wall, if the vessel is constricted, or if there has been any intra-arterial placement of the needle (12,13). Therefore, one must keep looking at the injected vessel for signs of extravasation and sclerosant flow.

Although Green (14) advocates sclerotherapy for periocular veins, his technique uses comparatively large volumes (1–3 cc) of STS. He argues that despite numerous and variable connections between the superficial facial and deep orbital venous systems, injection into superficial eyelid veins is ''highly unlikely'' to reach the orbit. Since periorbital venous pressure is quite low, we believe that intravenous eyelid injection could reach the orbit (where there are no venous valves) and hence the ocular adnexa, the central retinal vein, the choroidal vortex veins, or even the cavernous sinus via these vascular channels. Monocular blindness has been reported following STS injection into a venous malformation partially located in the orbit (15).

Surgical Removal: Phlebectomy

Weiss and Ramelet (16) reported surgical removal of the vein through a puncture or minimal incision utilizing a phlebectomy hook. This was shown to be effective in treating and long term removal of periorbital veins (Fig. 3). Surgical removal is performed using local anesthesia. The vein to be removed is injected with just enough 1% lidocaine with epinephrine to produce adequate anesthesia. Use of minimal anesthetic solution allows the vein to remain where it is marked prior to surgery.

After injection of lidocaine, an 18-gauge needle is used to puncture the skin. The Ramelet hook is used to harpoon the vein and lift it out of the puncture site. Minimal probing for the vein helps to minimize bruising and damage to perivascular tissue and nerves. After successful ''hooking'' of the vein, it is gently extracted to the longest possible length. No sutures are necessary. Significant skill is required to master this surgical technique of finesse. We advise learning and becoming very comfortable with ambulatory phlebectomy on leg veins initially. On the legs larger incisions will result in less noticeable and less objection markings than on the face.

LASER THERAPY

Multiple lasers are available for destroying facial telangiectases. These lasers act by selectively heating the vessel to cause its destruction through the absorption of laser energy by oxygenated and deoxygenated hemoglobin. The advantages and disadvantages of presently available lasers are described below.

In contrast to facial veins, sclerotherapy remains the standard procedure for treatment of leg veins. Public interest in laser and light treatment of leg veins is high, and under the right circumstances they can produce excellent results. For leg telangiectasia, however, reverse pressure from associated reticular or varicose veins must be recognized or treatment will be doomed to failure. In many patients, a combination of treatments is necessary as lasers and light sources do not effectively treat associated reticular and varicose veins.

The choice of wavelength(s) and pulse duration is related to the type and size of target vessel treated. Deeper vessels require a longer wavelength to allow penetration to their depth. While pulse duration must be matched to vessel size, the larger the vessel diameter, the longer pulse duration required to effectively thermally damage the vessel. The relative importance of the hemoglobulin absorption peaks in green (541 nm) and red to infrared (800–1000 nm) shifts as the depth and size of blood vessel changes. Absorption by hemoglobin in the long visible to near infrared range appears to become more important for vessels over 0.5 mm and at least 0.5 mm below the skin surface (17).

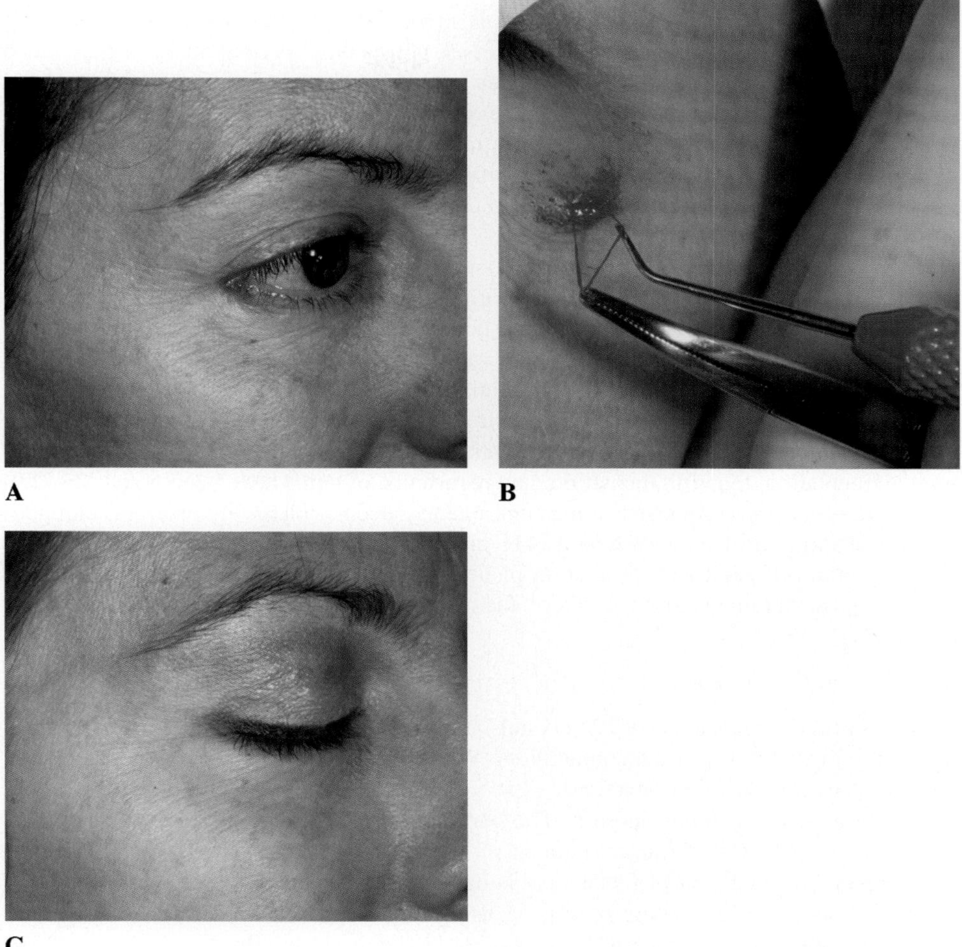

Figure 3 Removal of periocular vein by ambulatory phlebectomy. (A) Before removal. (B) The thin venous strand is removed with a Ramelet hook. (C) Six weeks after removal.

Various devices have been utilized in an effort to enhance clinical efficacy and minimize the adverse sequelae of telangiectasia treatment. While results on facial telangiectasia is excellent, most have also been associated with adverse responses for leg telangiectasia and response rate far lower than those associated with sclerotherapy. This is related both to insufficient vessel destruction to competition from overlying melanin, and the lack of treatment of hydrostatic pressure from the ''feeding'' venous system.

Continuous-Wave Lasers

Carbon Dioxide Laser

Carbon dioxide (CO_2) lasers were used early on in an effort to obliterate telangiectatic vessels by means of precise vaporization without significant damage to adjacent tissue

(18–20). However, because CO_2 laser light is so well-absorbed by water in the overlying epidermis and dermis overlying the blood vessel, nonspecific thermal injury is guaranteed regardless of whether pulsed or continuous wave sources are used (19). All reported studies demonstrate unsatisfactory cosmetic results (18–20). Treated areas show multiple hypopigmented punctate scars with either minimal resolution of the treated vessel or neovascularization adjacent to the treatment site. Because of its nonselective action, the CO_2 laser has no advantage over the electrodesiccation needle.

Argon Laser

Argon (488 nm and 514 nm) and argon-pumped continuous-wave dye lasers (515–590 nm) are well absorbed by hemoglobin and penetrate to the depth of mid dermal vessels, over 1 mm into skin. Treatment parameters vary and laser powers of 0.8–2.9 W, exposure times of 50 msec, 0.2 sec, 0.3 sec, and continuous and spot sizes of 0.1 mm and 1 mm have been used. Though the success rate in treating facial telangiectasia has been reported to be good-to-excellent in 65–99% of patients treated (21–23), pitted and depressed scars, hypopigmentation, hyperpigmentation, and recurrence of veins have been noted (24–27).

The reason these adverse healing consequences occur with the argon laser is competition for absorption of its wavelength (411 nm and 514 nm) from epidermal melanin as well as radial diffusion and dissipation of heat from the target blood vessels secondary to long pulse durations. Both of these factors result in relatively nonspecific thermal destruction

KTP 532-nm Green Lasers

Potassium-titanyl-phosphate (KTP) crystals are highly reliable, convenient to work with, and easily available to laser manufacturers. While the mechanism of these devices vary, each produce millisecond domain pulses at 532 nm. When pulsed in milliseconds, vessel coagulation occurs without purpura. The various lasers available differ in the spot size which ranges from 0.5–4 mm in diameter.

Results of treatment of facial vessels have been excellent (28). Recent results with the KTP laser have been more promising using larger spot sizes (3–5 mm) and longer pulse durations of 10–50 msec at fluences of 14–20 J/cm^2. Using fluences between 12–20 J/cm^2 delivered with a 3–5-mm diameter spot size, a train of pulses is delivered over the vessel until spasm or thrombosis occurs. Cooling appears to be of significant benefit in protecting the epidermis thus allowing use of higher, more effective fluences (29). One study comparing four different 532-nm lasers shows comparable 75–100% efficacy between them (30).

Flashlamp-Pumped Pulsed Dye Laser

The traditional PDL (585 nm, 450 sec pulse duration) is highly effective in treating a variety of cutaneous vascular lesions, including PWS and facial telangiectasia. It is less effective, however, in the treatment of leg veins. The original PDL was developed for the treatment of port wine stains in children, where the average vessel is superficial and has a diameter of 100 m and an average depth of 0.46 mm. While 585-nm light can penetrate 1.2 mm to reach the typical depth of leg telangiectasia (31), the pulse duration is inadequate to effectively damage all but superficial fine vessels, approximately 0.1 mm or smaller in diameter. In general, telangiectasia of the lower extremities treated with the PDL are less responsive and are more prone to post-therapy hyperpigmentation than when treated with sclerotherapy.

In preliminary animal studies in the rabbit ear vein, approximately 50% of vessels treated with an effective concentration of sclerosant demonstrated extravasated RBCs, while after PDL treatment extravasated RBCs were apparent in only 30% of vessels treated (32). Rabbit ear vein treatment with the PDL resulted in a relative decrease in perivascular inflammation, compared to vessels treated with sclerotherapy alone.

In clinical use, the treatment technique involves delivering a series of pulses overlapping 10–20%, tracing the vessels to be treated with a spot size of 2, 3, 5, 7, or 10 mm, or an elliptical delivery spot, treating an area of interlacing telangiectasia with overlapping spots to cover the involved area. Delivery energies range from 5.0–14.0 J/cm^2 depending on the spot size used and are adjusted according to vessel response. The end-point is purpura or vessel spasm.

Initial studies using the 0.45-msec pulse duration FLPD laser demonstrated high efficacy but resulted in purpura that lasted for 1 or 2 weeks (33). In this study 182 patients treated with the 0.45-msec pulse laser at 6–7.75 J/cm^2 with a 5-mm diameter spot size were evaluated. A 76–100% clearance was obtained in 83.5% of patients with the remainder having 51–75% clearance.

A technique to increase efficacy and decrease purpura is to use double and triple pulses (pulse stacking) at subpurpuric fluences. Tanghetti et al. (34) recently used pulse stacking to increase efficacy on photoaging with reduced side effects, but found that multiple treatments with or without pulse stacking had excellent results on the signs and symptoms of photoaging, including telangiectasia.

Long-Pulse Dye Lasers

Based on the theory of selective photothermolysis, the predicted pulse duration ideally suited for thermal destruction of vessels the size of leg telangiectasia (0.1 mm to several millimeters in diameter) is in the 1–50 msec domain (35). Long-pulsed dye lasers with variable pulse durations as long as 40 msec (V-Beam, Candela, Wayland, MA; V-Star, Cynosure, Chelmsford, MA) are now available. Each device uses a rhodamine dye to produce wavelengths of 595 nm. These longer pulse durations and longer wavelengths theoretically improve our ability to treat deeper, larger caliber vessels.

Newer FLPD lasers that extend the pulse duration to 1.5, 3, 6, 10, 20, and 40 msec and use dynamic cooling or continuous air cooling have eliminated most of the pain and have minimized purpura associated with the first generation FLPD lasers. Typical fluences of 10 J/cm^2 with a 10-msec spot size usually result in 90% resolution of facial telangiectases in one treatment with minimal pain and purpura. Improvement in rough texture and pigmentation of photoaging is also seen (Fig. 4).

For leg telangiectasia, the results are not as good even with longer pulsing. In a single treatment of vessels less than 0.4 mm in diameter using the 595-nm, 1.5-msec PDL (Cynosure) and an experimental 595-nm, 4-msec pulsed dye laser clearing rates were not clinically significant with either device, and the rates of both hypopigmentation and hyperpigmentation were significant (36).

In a multiple-treatment study, three treatments were performed 6 weeks apart using the 595-nm, 1.5-msec PDL (Candela) through a transparent hydrogel dressing with a 2 × 7-mm elliptical spot at 20 J/cm^2. One hundred percent of patients had at least 50% clearing, but 50% of treated areas became hyperpigmented and 20% hypopigmented (37).

Copper-Vapor Laser

The copper-vapor laser operates at two specific wavelengths, 578 nm (yellow) and 511 nm (green), and delivers a ''quasi-continuous wave'' composed of pulsed laser light energy

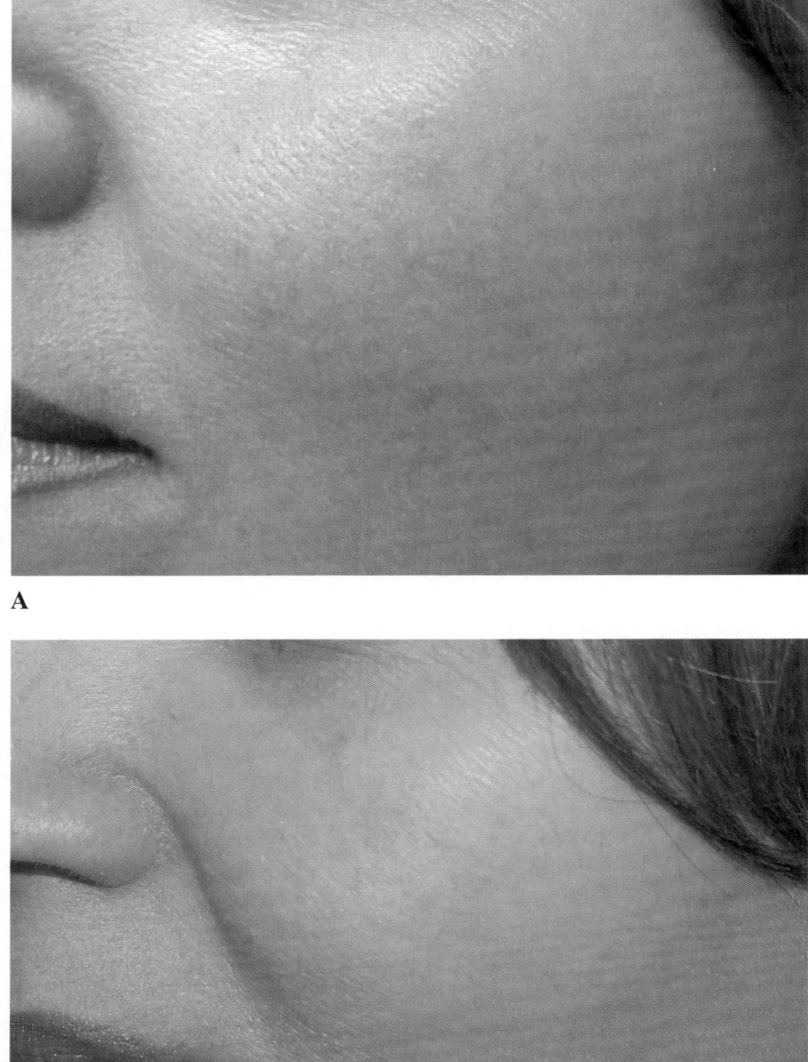

Figure 4 Improvement in telangiectasia, skin texture, and pigmentation with use of the long-pulsed dye laser (V-Star, Cynosure, Chelmsford, MA). Treatment included a 2-msec duration, 2.5 J, 10-mm spot, and three passes. (A) Before treatment. (B) After treatment.

in 20-nsec pulses at a frequency of 15,000 pulses/sec. This train of pulses interacts with tissue in the same manner as a continuous beam because of the accumulation of heat with the large number of pulses delivered. Because of resulting thermal diffusion, it is necessary to electronically gate the pulse to a 20–50-msec duration.

These refinements should allow this laser to work within the thermal relaxation time of telangiectasia. When the laser is used without these refinements, it is somewhat safer and more effective than the argon laser for treatment of facial telangiectasia and has the advantage of leaving very minor superficial crusts overlying treated vessels in contrast to the very visible dark purpuric impact spots of the FLPD laser. A comparison of the copper-vapor laser with the FLPD laser in adults with facial telangiectasia demonstrated no difference in efficacy but crusting with the copper vapor and purpura with the FLPD laser (38).

Long-Pulse Nd:YAG (1064 nm)

Long-pulsed 1064-nm lasers have recently been developed in an effort to target deep relatively large caliber cutaneous vessels. The primary benefit of this wavelength is deep penetration and the absence of absorption in melanin, thus allowing treatment even in deeply pigmented individuals. However, high energies must be used for adequate penetration. Only with sufficient fluence and facilitation of heat dissipation can the posterior wall of a larger diameter (1–2 mm) vessel filled with deoxygenated hemoglobin be reached and heated.

The newer pulsed 1064-nm lasers have pulse durations between 1 and 200 msec (Vasculight™, Lumenis, Santa Clara, CA; Cool Touch Varia™, CoolTouch Corp, Roseville, CA; Lyra™, Laserscope Lyra, San Jose, CA; Coolglide™, Altus, Burlingame, CA). In general, treatment with long-pulse 1064-nm laser light is relatively painful, requiring cooling and topical anesthesia. Large caliber vessels (> 0.5 mm in diameter) respond best. Recent data suggest that by using smaller spots and even higher fluences, even small vessels respond. Our most recent data indicate an approximately 75% resolution of leg telangiectasia at 3 months using 16-msec pulse durations with fluences of 130–140 J/cm^2 (39).

For patient comfort, epidermal cooling is provided with the Coolglide and the Lyra using contact cooling provided with the system. The CoolTouch Varia supplies a cryogen spray which can be programmed both before and after the laser pulse. The concept behind the applying the spray after the cooling pulse is for thermal quenching of the heat released from larger vessels following the laser heating. For the Vasculight, cooling may be provided through cold gel or a contact skin chilling device at 1–4°C.

Larger violaceous vessels of the face may be treated with these devices (Fig. 5). The fluence must be lowered by 30–40% for facial vessels as compared to the legs. A recent study of facial telangiectasia and periocular reticular veins showed excellent results in 17 patients using a cryogen spray-cooled 1064-nm system. Greater than 75% improvement was observed in 97% of the treated sites (40).

Intense Pulsed Light Source

The high-intensity pulsed light source was developed as a device to treat ectatic blood vessels using noncoherent light emanating from a filtered flashlamp (Vasculight(SR, Lumenis) Although Lumenis is the largest and most well known of the IPL device manufactures, other manufactures of pulsed-light devices include Energis Technology (Swansea, UK), which markets an Energis Elite IPL system for hair removal only, and Danish Derma-

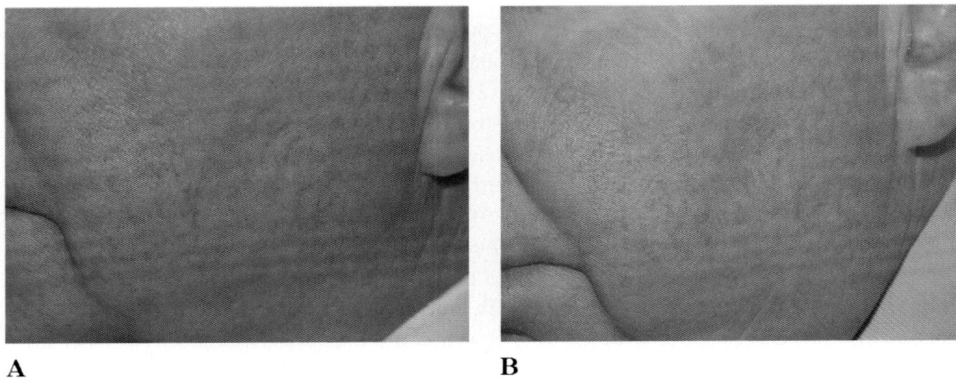

A B

Figure 5 Treatment of larger veins on the face with the 1064-nm Nd:YAG laser (Vasculight, Lumenis, Santa Clara, CA). (A) Before treatment. (B) Two months after one treatment showing 50% improvement.

tologic Development (Hoersholm, Denmark), which markets the Elipse system for hair and vascular indications. The Energis system is a low-output device, with 5–19 J/cm^2 output, spot size of 10 × 50 mm, pulse train length of 15–40 msec, and pulses per train of four or five. There is a fixed delay between pulses of 1.5 msec. By comparison, the Lumenis device is a high-output device with up to 90 J/cm^2 output, spot size of 8 × 35 mm, variable pulse lengths of 2–40 msec, and infinitely variable delay between pulses of 1 to 1000 msec.

Selectivity for IPL is obtained primarily by manipulating pulse durations to match thermal relaxation times of vessels larger than 0.2 mm and use of filters to remove lower wavelengths of visible light. Fluence can be very high, with the unit delivering up to 90 J/cm^2. Sequential pulsing of 1–12-msec duration separated and synchronized with 1–100-msec rest intervals delivers wavelengths of 515–1000 nm. It is most frequently used with the 550-nm and 570-nm filters to deliver primarily the yellow and red wavelengths with some infrared. A device that produces a noncoherent light as a continuous spectrum longer than 550 nm was thought to have multiple advantages over a single-wavelength laser system. These include absorption by both oxygenated and deoxygenated hemoglobin and by larger blood vessels located deeper in the dermis being affected. In reality, the primary advantage has been larger spot size and relatively low incidence of purpura on facial telangiectasia.

For facial telangiectasia, we have found that the 550-nm, 560-nm, or 570-nm lasers produce optimal results. We choose a longer cut-off filter for darker skin types and/or larger blood vessels. Typical pulse durations are 2.4 msec + 4.0 msec (double pulse) with a 10-msec delay between the pulses for pigmentation-predominant photoaging but 2.4 msec + 6.0 msec for telangiectasia-predominant photoaging. The delay time is lengthened to 20–30 msec in patients with darker skin types and in Asian skin, which tends to react to thermal injury greater than white skin. Typical fluences range from 24–38 J/cm^2 and again are related to the sensitivity of the skin and the degree of epidermal cooling. To minimize nonspecific epidermal damage, the crystal is placed on a layer of ice-cold clear gel 2 or 3 mm in thickness for noncooled crystals (floating technique). When using the Quantum IPL with a thermoelectrically cooled crystal, a thin layer of gel is used with the crystal resting directly on the skin with the crystal at maximal cooling (direct contact technique) (Fig. 6).

Studies on the treatment of leg telangiectasia and poikiloderma of Civatte have proven the efficacy as well as limitations of IPL technology. Few studies have evaluated IPL efficacy purely on facial telangiectasia. Most studies with the IPL comment on its photorejuvenation effects that include elimination of lentigos, reduction of pore size, and minimization of fine wrinkles in addition to treatment of telangiectasia. Bitter reported that the IPL used in ''FotoFacial settings'' produced more than 75% improvement in telangiectasia in 38% of patients and more than 50% reduction in telangiectasia in 70% of patients (41). Negishi et al. (42) found a greater than 75% improvement in telangiectasia in 33% of their Japanese settings (similar to Bitter's findings except for a decrease in fluence and a longer delay time between the double pulses). Their study showed 83% of patients had an improvement in telangiectasia of greater than 50%.

Another IPL device (Ellipse Flex, Danish Dermatologic Development) was used in 27 patients with facial telangiectasia. This IPL has a lower cut-off (555 nm) as well as an upper cut-off filter (at 950 nm) with a median wavelength at 705 nm delivered through a 10 × 48-mm crystal light guide. Fluences required to produce a slight bluing of the vessels ranged 13–22 J/cm^2. Pulse durations were 10 msec for vessels less than 0.4mm in diameter and 15 and 30 msec for larger vessels. Patients received one to four treatments, with an average of 2.54 treatments per patient. A total of 83.4% of patients had greater than 50% clearing, and 66.7% had greater than 75% clearance (43).

For leg veins and IPL, the development of the short-pulse–long-pulse protocol using 2.4–3-msec and 7-msec pulses separated by a 10–20-msec delay and a 570-nm filter has yielded the best results for leg veins using the IPL device. Response rates of 74% in two

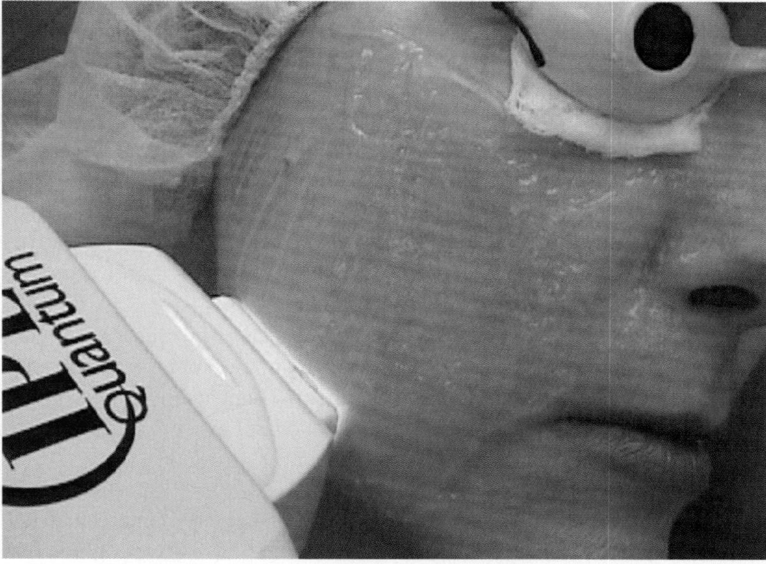

Figure 6 Thin layer of gel with a thermoelectrically cooled crystal used with IPL treatment.

treatments with an 8% incidence of temporary hypopigmentation or hyperpigmentation has been reported (44). By combining a shorter pulse (2.4–3 msec) with a longer pulse (7–10 msec), it is theoretically possible to ablate smaller and larger vessels overlying one another in the dermis. The shorter pulses theoretically are absorbed more selectively by smaller more superficial vessels, while the longer pulses are absorbed by the larger diameter vessels. Additionally, new contact epidermal cooling devices improve treatment results by allowing larger fluences with less risk to the epidermis.

The Role of Cooling

The concept of cooling the skin in an effort to protect the epidermis during laser treatment of dermal targets was first studied by Gilchrest et al. (45) with the use of ice prior to argon laser treatment of port wine stains. There has been a recent resurgence of interest in skin cooling during skin laser therapy in an effort to not only cool and protect the epidermis and to prevent other collateral dermal damage, but also to reduce the discomfort associated with treatment. Because high fluences are required to adequately damage larger telangiectases, cooling appears to be especially important in their treatment in an effort to limit unwanted collateral injury. Several approaches have been taken, including water-cooled chambers applied directly to the skin through which the laser beam is directed, cooling coupling gels, and refrigerated spray cooling devices. Preliminary results suggest that cooling helps to spare epidermal damage, allowing use of higher fluences, thus yielding more damage of the targeted vessels, with a greater degree of clearing per treatment (46,47).

CHEST VEINS AND TELANGIECTASIA

Photoaging on the upper chest of women is very common. A typical appearance shows very rough skin which is a component of poikiloderma (Fig. 7). Most telangiectases on the chest are also a component of poikiloderma, which includes telangiectasia, increased pigmentation, and epidermal and dermal atrophy with textural changes. These changes typically extend down from the lateral neck to the décolletage region. IPL has been reported to be very valuable for treatment of poikiloderma (48). Improvement after a series of treatments obtained typically lasts for several years with rigorous sun protection of the affected areas (49). For larger veins on the breast or chest, there are a number of common problems that may cause these.

Post-traumatic vessels may appear on the breast shortly after an isolated incident of trauma. These vessels can be treated easily, provided that the trauma was remote and that the vessels have not been undergoing any recent change.

Postoperative dilated vessels are most often noticed after breast augmentation with implants. These vessels may be treated, but treatment should not be undertaken for at least 6 months after the implant procedure as spontaneous improvement may occur. Special care is required to avoid puncturing an implant that may have migrated or extruded into an unexpectedly superficial location.

Some patients are concerned about normal vessels that are particularly prominent because of variant anatomy or because of translucent skin. Patients must be specially warned of the risks of resistance to treatment in normal vessels. Also, patients with translucent skin will always be able to see superficial veins more easily as they become more apparent with age; they must understand that maintenance treatment will be necessary.

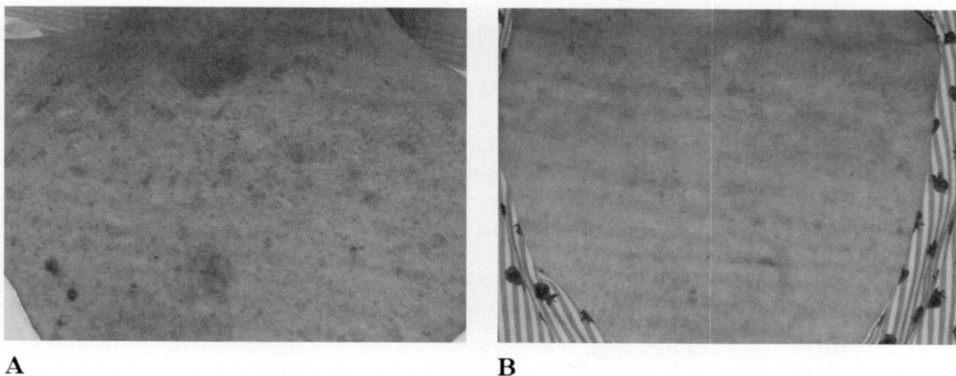

A B

Figure 7 Telangiectasia and pigmentation, a component of poikilodermatous type of photoaging of the chest. (A) Before treatment of décolletage and upper neck regions (B) After one IPL treatment (using the same settings as for telangiectasia of the face). Note disappearance of cherry hemangiomas on the right side of the chest.

Treatment of the Chest

Telangiectases of the chest are treated with the same methods used to treat facial telangiectases, with IPL or lasers as the preferred method owing to improvement of signs of photoaging. For smaller telangiectases on the chest, we have had excellent results with IPL, and others have reported excellent results on with PDLs (49). When treating larger reticular blue breast veins, the concentration and volume of sclerosant should be kept to a minimum as they often drain directly into small-caliber deep vessels.

High grades of compression are not possible in the breast area, but a tight-fitting sport brassiere is recommended for the first 48 hours to minimize inflammation as much as possible. Patients are advised to sleep in a supine position for several days. Bruising is common.

SUMMARY

Treatment of facial venous vascular lesions in adults can be very successful. Almost all the laser devices available in the visible light range produce good results on vascular lesions of the face. Knowledge of lesion type and differences in response by size and location can assist in selecting the procedure that is most likely to be successful. Wavelengths of lasers may be fined tuned for size or color of each telangiectasis. Although electrocautery is used frequently, a more selective method of laser or IPL is usually a better choice. Some larger facial or chest vessels respond well to sclerotherapy or ambulatory phlebectomy. Larger cavernous lesions may require deeper penetration of 1064-nm (infrared) wavelengths or manipulation to reduce the total depth for laser penetration. An additional benefit of treatment of telangiectases due to photoaging may be the smoothing of skin and reduction of irregular pigmentation.

REFERENCES

1. Merlen JF. Telangiectasies rouges, telangiectasies bleues. Phlebologie 1970; 23:167–174.
2. Weiss RA, Goldman MP. Advances in sclerotherapy. Dermatol Clin 1995; 13:431–445.

3. Goldman MP, Bennett RG. Treatment of telangiectasia: a review. J Am Acad Dermatol 1987; 17:167–182.
4. Glogau RG. Aesthetic and anatomic analysis of the aging skin. Semin Cutan Med Surg 1996; 15:134–138.
5. Goldman MP, Fitzpatrick RE. Cutaneous Laser Surgery. 2nd ed.. St.Louis: Mosby, 1999.
6. Weiss RA, Feied CF, Weiss MA. Vein Diagnosis and Treatment: A Comprehensive Approach. New York: McGraw-Hill, 2001.
7. Kobayashi T. Electrosurgery using insulated needles: treatment of telangiectasias. J Dermatol Surg Oncol 1986; 12:936–942.
8. el Gamal HM, Dufresne RG, Saddler K. Electrosurgery, pacemakers and ICDs: a survey of precautions and complications experienced by cutaneous surgeons. Dermatol Surg 2001; 27: 385–390.
9. Goldman MP, Weiss RA, Brody HJ, Coleman WP, Fitzpatrick RE. Treatment of facial telangiectasia with sclerotherapy, laser surgery, and/or electrodesiccation: a review. J Dermatol Surg Oncol 1993; 19:899–906; quiz 909–910.
10. Shafir R, Cohen M, Gur E. Blindness as a complication of subcutaneous nasal steroid injection. Plast Reconstr Surg 1999; 104:1180–1182.
11. Thomas EL, Laborde RP. Retinal and choroidal vascular occlusion following intralesional corticosteroid injection of a chalazion. Ophthalmology 1986; 93:405–407.
12. McGrew RN, Wilson RS, Havener WH. Sudden blindness secondary to injections of common drugs in the head and neck: I. Clinical experiences. Otolaryngology 1978; 86:ORL-51.
13. McGrew RN, Wilson RS, Havener WH. Sudden blindness secondary to injections of common drugs in the head and neck: II. Animal studies. Otolaryngology 1978; 86:ORL-7.
14. Green D. Removal of periocular veins by sclerotherapy. Ophthalmology 2001; 108:442–448.
15. Siniluoto TM, Svendsen PA, Wikholm GM, Fogdestam I, Edstrom S. Percutaneous sclerotherapy of venous malformations of the head and neck using sodium tetradecyl sulphate (sotradecol). Scand J Plast Reconstr Surg Hand Surg 1997; 31:145–150.
16. Weiss RA, Ramelet AA. Removal of blue periocular lower eyelid veins by ambulatory phlebectomy. Dermatol Surg 2002; 28:43–45.
17. Smithies DJ, Butler PH. Modelling the distribution of laser light in port-wine stains with the Monte Carlo method. Phys Med Biol 1995; 40:701–731.
18. Apfelberg DB, Smith T, Maser MR, Lash H, White DN. Study of three laser systems for treatment of superficial varicosities of the lower extremity. Lasers Surg Med 1987; 7:219–223.
19. Landthaler M, Haina D, Waidelich W, Braun-Falco O. Laser therapy of venous lakes (Bean-Walsh) and telangiectasias. Plast Reconstr Surg 1984; 73:78–83.
20. Apfelberg DB, Maser MR, Lash H, White DN, Flores JT. Use of the argon and carbon dioxide lasers for treatment of superficial venous varicosities of the lower extremity. Lasers Surg Med 1984; 4:221–231.
21. Apfelberg DB. Summary of argon laser usage in plastic surgery. Scand J Plast Reconstr Surg 1986; 20:13–18.
22. Apfelberg DB, Maser MR, Lash H. Argon laser treatment of cutaneous vascular abnormalities: progress report. Ann Plast Surg 1978; 1:14–18.
23. Achauer BM, Vander KV. Argon laser treatment of telangiectasia of the face and neck: 5 years' experience. Lasers Surg Med 1987; 7:495–498.
24. Apfelberg DB, Smith T, Maser MR, Lash H, White DN. Dot or pointillistic method for improvement in results of hypertrophic scarring in the argon laser treatment of portwine hemangiomas. Lasers Surg Med 1987; 6:552–558.
25. Dixon JA, Huether S, Rotering RH. Hypertrophic scarring in argon laser treatment of port-wine stains. Plastic and Reconstructive Surgery 1984; 73:771.
26. Lyons GD, Owens RE, Mouney DF. Argon laser destruction of cutaneous telangiectatic lesions. Laryngoscope 1981; 91:1322–1325.
27. Dolsky RL. Argon laser skin surgery. Surg Clin North Am 1984; 64:861–870.

28. Keller GS. KTP laser offers advances in minimally invasive plastic surgery. Clin Laser Mon 1992; 10:141–144.
29. Adrian RM. Treatment of leg telangiectasias using a long-pulse frequency-doubled neodymium:YAG laser at 532 nm. Dermatol Surg 1998; 24:19–23.
30. Goldberg DJ, Meine JG. A comparison of four frequency-doubled Nd:YAG (532 nm) laser systems for treatment of facial telangiectases. Dermatol Surg 1999; 25:463–467.
31. Garden JM, Tan OT, Kerschmann R, Boll J, Furumoto H, Anderson RR. Effect of dye laser pulse duration on selective cutaneous vascular injury. J Invest Dermatol 1986; 87:653–657.
32. Goldman MP, Martin DE, Fitzpatrick RE, Ruiz-Esparza J. Pulsed dye laser treatment of telangiectases with and without subtherapeutic sclerotherapy. Clinical and histologic examination in the rabbit ear vein model. J Am Acad Dermatol 1990; 23:23–30.
33. Ruiz-Esparza J, Goldman MP, Fitzpatrick RE, Lowe NJ, Behr KL. Flash lamp-pumped dye laser treatment of telangiectasia. J Dermatol Surg Oncol 1993; 19:1000–1003.
34. Tanghetti EA, Sherr EA, Alvarado SL. Multipass treatment of photodamage using the pulse dye laser. Dermatol Surg 2003; 29:686–690.
35. Dierickx CC, Casparian JM, Venugopalan V, Farinelli WA, Anderson RR. Thermal relaxation of port-wine stain vessels probed in vivo: the need for 1–10 millisecond laser pulse treatment. J Invest Dermatol 1995; 105:709–714.
36. Alora MB, Herd RH, Szabo E. Comparison of the 595nm long pulse (1.5ms) and the 595m ultra-long pulse (4ms) laser in the treatment of leg veins. Lasers Surg Med 1998; 10(suppl): 38.
37. Grossman MC, Bernstein LJ, Kauvar AB, Laughlin S. Treatment of leg veins with a long pulse tunable dye laser. Lasers Surg Med 1996; 8(suppl):35.
38. Waner M, Dinehart SM, Wilson MB, Flock ST. A comparison of copper vapor and flashlamp pumped dye lasers in the treatment of facial telangiectasia. J Dermatol Surg Oncol 1993; 19: 992–998.
39. Weiss RA, Weiss MA. Early clinical results with a multiple synchronized pulse 1064 nm laser for leg telangiectasias and reticular veins. Dermatol Surg 1999; 25:399–402.
40. Eremia S, Li CY. Treatment of face veins with a cryogen spray variable pulse width 1064 nm Nd:YAG Laser: a prospective study of 17 patients. Dermatol Surg 2002; 28:244–247.
41. Bitter PH. Noninvasive rejuvenation of photodamaged skin using serial, full-face intense pulsed light treatments. Dermatol Surg 2000; 26:835–842.
42. Negishi K, Wakamatsu S, Kushikata N, Tezuka Y, Kotani Y, Shiba K. Full-face photorejuvenation of photodamaged skin by intense pulsed light with integrated contact cooling: initial experiences in Asian patients. Lasers Surg Med 2002; 30:298–305.
43. Bjerring P, Christiansen K, Troilius A. Intense pulsed light source for treatment of facial telangiectasias. J Cosmet Laser Ther 2001; 3:169–173.
44. Weiss RA, Weiss MA, Marwaha S, Harrington AC. Non-coherent filtered flashlamp intense pulsed light source for leg telangiectasias: Long pulse durations for improved results. Lasers Surg Med 1998; 10(suppl):40.
45. Gilchrest BA, Rosen S, Noe JM. Chilling port wine stains improves the response to argon laser therapy. Plast Reconstr Surg 1982; 69:278–283.
46. Chess C, Chess Q. Cool laser optics treatment of large telangiectasia of the lower extremities. J Dermatol Surg Oncol 1993; 19:74–80.
47. Waldorf HA, Alster TS, McMillan K, Kauvar AN, Geronemus RG, Nelson JS. Effect of dynamic cooling on 585-nm pulsed dye laser treatment of port- wine stain birthmarks [see comments]. Dermatol Surg 1997; 23:657–662.
48. Weiss RA, Goldman MP, Weiss MA. Treatment of poikiloderma of Civatte with an intense pulsed light source. Dermatol Surg 2000; 26:823–827.
49. Weiss RA, Weiss MA, Beasley KL. Rejuvenation of photoaged skin: 5 years results with intense pulsed light of the face, neck, and chest. Dermatol Surg 2002; 28:1115–1119.

18

Treatment of Photoaging-Associated Pigmentary Changes

John Z. S. Chen / Roy G. Geronemus *New York University School of Medicine, New York, New York, U.S.A.*

- Judicious use of preoperative and postoperative tretinoin and hydroquinone products can often improve treatment efficacy.
- Strict sun protection reduces the risk of undesirable hyperpigmentation and future recurrence.
- Patient selection is the key to success. The ideal candidate is a fair-skinned individual (Fitzpatrick skin type I–III) with superficial pigmented lesions. A darker-complexioned individual with deep-pigmented lesions should be approached more cautiously.

Chronic exposure to ultraviolet (UV) radiation causes skin changes known as photodamage. In addition to loss of elasticity and changes in the skin texture, alterations in skin color and the appearance of pigmented spots are clinical signs of photoaging. Sun damage can induce alteration of the pattern of melanin deposition in normal and neoplastic keratinocytes or proliferation of melanocytes, with subsequent excess of local melanin. With the former category are ephelides (freckles). Solar or senile lentigines and pigmented actinic keratoses represent sun-induced proliferation of keratinocytes with an excess of melanin as well. Among melanocytic proliferation displaying hyperpigmentation and related to sun exposure are sunburn freckles, the psoralen-UVA–induced freckles or lentigines and variants of malignant melanoma.

Ephelides are multiple-pigmented spots measuring a few millimeters in diameter. They are genetically determined and vary in their color intensity according to sun exposure (1). They follow a distinct photodistribution and are most common in white patients with skin types I or II. Ephelides appear in childhood, increase in number in adults, and seem to regress during old age. The most common sites are the nose, cheeks, shoulders, and extensor aspects of the arms. It is assumed that a somatic mutation of epidermal melanocytes leads to increased melanin production.

Lentigo, the prototype of the so-called age spot, is the most common photoaging-associated pigmentary lesions. It represents a pigmented macule in chronically UV-exposed skin. The face and extensor aspects of the forearms and the dorsal hands are predominantly affected, mainly in whites. The lesions, usually well defined and irregularly shaped, vary in color from yellow-brown to dark brown. The size can range from a few millimeters to several centimeters in diameter.

In this chapter, different options on the treatment of pigmented changes associated with photoaging are discussed.

TOPICAL RETINOIDS

Topical application of tretinoin has been proved to be an effective treatment for photodamage. Several double-blind, vehicle-controlled studies indicated that treatment with either 0.1% or 0.025% tretinoin induced statistically significant improvement in the effects of photoaging, including mottled or blotchy dyspigmentation, compared with vehicle treatment (2,3). There were no significant differences in the overall clinical efficacy of treatment with 0.1% vs. 0.025% concentrations of tretinoin. However, the 0.1% tretinoin cream is far more likely to induce local irritation, such as erythema and scaling than the 0.025% concentration. Thus, it is unnecessary to push tretinoin use to the point that brisk retinoid dermatitis develops to achieve maximum clinical improvement of photoaged skin. On the contrary, equal impressive clinical results may be achieved with sparring but diligent use of tretinoin, an approach that can minimize retinoid dermatitis. A 48-week regimen of treatment once daily with 0.05% tretinoin cream, followed by treatment three times weekly for an additional 24 weeks, maintained and, in some cases, even enhanced the improvements in photoaging skin (4). Topical tretinoin therapy should be continued in order to maintain clinical improvement. Topical tretinoin can be effectively used to treat postinflammatory hyperpigmentation caused by inflammatory conditions such as acne or folliculitis in black patients (5). In our experience, topical tretinoin is more effective when it is combined with other treatment methods, such as chemical peel or laser, in treating pigmentary changes than as a single agent.

SKIN-LIGHTENING/DEPIGMENTING AGENTS

Skin-depigmenting agents are commonly used to treat disorders of hyperpigmentation. Hydroquinone (HQ), a tyrosinase inhibitor, is one of the most commonly prescribed. A 2% HQ formulation is readily available over-the-counter in various cosmetic preparations. Adverse effects are quite limited. Contact dermatitis occurs in a small number of patients and responds well to topical steroids. An uncommon, yet important, adverse effect of HQ is exogenous ochronosis. This disorder is characterized by progressive darkening of the area to where the product containing HQ is applied. Exogenous ochronosis has been reported in black patients and after use of high concentrations of HQ for a prolonged period. However, cases occurring after the use of 2% HQ have also been reported. For this reason, the use of HQ should be discontinued if no improvement occurs within 4 months. HQ-induced ochronosis often responds to topical steroids and chemical peels. For better efficacy, HQ is often compounded into various mixtures. Tretinoin has been used to enhance the efficacy of HQ. The original Kligman formula involves compounding 5% HQ with 0.1% tretinoin and 0.1% dexamethasone in a hydrophilic ointment base. Application of HQ should be strictly limited to the lesions as it may cause hypopigmentation of surrounding normal skin.

Azelaic acid is prescribed as a 20% cream and has been combined with glycolic acid (15% and 20%), and its efficacy has been compared with HQ 4% in the treatment of facial hyperpigmentation in dark-skinned patients. It has been reported that the combination formula was as effective as HQ 4% cream, although with a slightly higher incidence of local irritation (6). Other agent, such as kojic acid, has also been used as skin-lightening agent. Kojic acid is used in concentrations ranging from 1–4%. Although effective as a skin-lightening agent, it causes higher incidence of irritant contact dermatitis. In a study comparing glycolic acid/kojic acid combination with glycolic acid/HQ, no statistical difference in efficacy existed between kojic acid and HQ. However, the kojic acid preparation was found to be more irritating (7).

CHEMICAL PEELS

Background

Chemical peels are defined as the application of a chemical agent to the skin resulting in controlled destruction of the outer layer of skin for the treatment of certain skin diseases or conditions. The destruction of portions of the epidermis and/or dermis with these chemical agents results in an improved clinical appearance of the skin, with fewer rhytides and decreased pigmentary dyschromia. Peels are categorized based on the histological depth of injury produced by the peeling agents: superficial peels penetrate through the epidermis and to upper regions of the papillary dermis, medium peels penetrate to the deeper area of the papillary dermis and upper reticular dermis, while deep peels penetrate to the depth of the mid reticular dermis (8,9). Pigmented lesions of photodamaged skin, such as ephelides and lentigines, can be treated with all of the three different types of peels, provided that the majority of the melanocytic pigment is within the peel depth.

The therapeutic agents for superficial peel are many. Trichloroacetic acid at concentration of 10–25% has been used for many years. Jessner's solution, or Comb's mixture, is a combination of salicylic acid 14%, lactic acid 14%, and resorcinol 14% in 95% alcohol. -Hydroxy acid peels include lactic acid, glycolic acid, tartaric acid, and malic acid. Glycolic acid at concentration of 50–70% can be very effective to smooth out the surface of the skin and lighten pigmentation of sunspots.

Various agents and concentrations may be combined to enhance the depth of the peel. Three combination peels currently being used are carbon dioxide (CO_2) and trichloroacetic acid (TCA) 35%, Jessner's solution and TCA 35%, and glycolic and TCA 35%. These peels are as effective as the other medium depth peels with lower risk of scarring and pigmentary dyschromia.

Deeper peels such as phenol, Baker Gordon formula, or 50% TCA are also very effective when applied locally to each lesion. They are less commonly used today because of the higher risk of scarring and other side effects associated with these deeper peels.

Patients Selection

Patient selection is the key to success. Patients should be well informed and have realistic expectations about the procedure. The ideal candidate is a fair-skinned individual (Fitzpatrick skin type I–III) with intact adnexal structures presenting with superficial pigmentary changes and photodamage. On the other hand, a less then optimal candidate is a darker-complexioned individual with decreased sebaceous gland activity and deeply pigmented lesions or unrealistic expectations. Although chemical peels can be offered to those with darker skin (Fitzpatrick skin type IV–VI), the risk of unwanted pigmentation is much greater in these patients than in those of lighter skin. Other factors that need to be considered include previous use of isotretinoin, history of herpes simplex virus infection, hypertrophic scarring, smoking, pregnancy, or radiation treatment.

Technique

The skin should be cleansed to remove any cosmetic products, skin oils, and keratin debris, followed by gentle scrubbing with alcohol or acetone-soaked gauge pads. A large cotton-tipped applicator or cotton ball is soaked in the peeling solution and wrung out to prevent any dripping during application. The peeling agent is applied carefully to one cosmetic unit at a time to ensure even coverage, starting from the forehead area and proceeding down one cheek and around the face to the other cheek. The areas around the eyes need to be treated separately, by using a semimoist cotton applicator, to ensure that the acid does not get into the eyes. Perioral and perinasal area can be treated last. The patient is instructed to keep the eyes closed to minimize tearing. Reapplication of the peeling agent may be necessary if the frost is uneven or not white enough. The peel is carefully timed from the initial contact of the skin to the time that the acid is washed off. The initial application of glycolic acid is usually 50% solution and is left on for about 3 min. This can be repeated every 4 weeks with either the time being increased by 30 sec or the concentration of the acid being increased to 70%. Eventually, patients will be able to tolerate peel lasting for up to 8 min. The development of frost represents the end stage of the chemical peel and indicates that keratin agglutination has occurred. Depending on the agent used, the white tint may vary from a brighter white in a superficial peel to a grayish white in a deep peel. Neutralization can be achieved by cold water or wet, cool towels applied to the face following the frost. Other neutralizing agents that can be used include bicarbonate spray or soapless cleanser. Some chemical peels, such as salicylic acid and TCA, do not necessarily require a neutralization step since the skin neutralizes the acid itself (10). Glycolic acid peels must be neutralized as soon as erythema appears. Patients should be instructed to rinse the skin under running cold tap water following the application of wet, cool towels.

After the peel, it is important that the patient follow instructions given by the physician to prevent complications. The patient should avoid sun exposure or at least seek sun protection by applying a potent sunscreen and wearing a hat. An ointment, such as petroleum jelly or bacitracin, should be applied to the involved skin.

The patient should be instructed to remain vigilant for any signs of infection. If the patient has a history of cold sores, treating the patient with acyclovir (400 mg by mouth twice daily or an equivalent drug is advisable, beginning 2 days prior to the peel and continuing for 7 days after the peel.

Results

Figure 1 shows the results of a medium-depth chemical peel (solid CO_2 followed by TCA 35%) for treatment of lentigines and other types of photodamage.

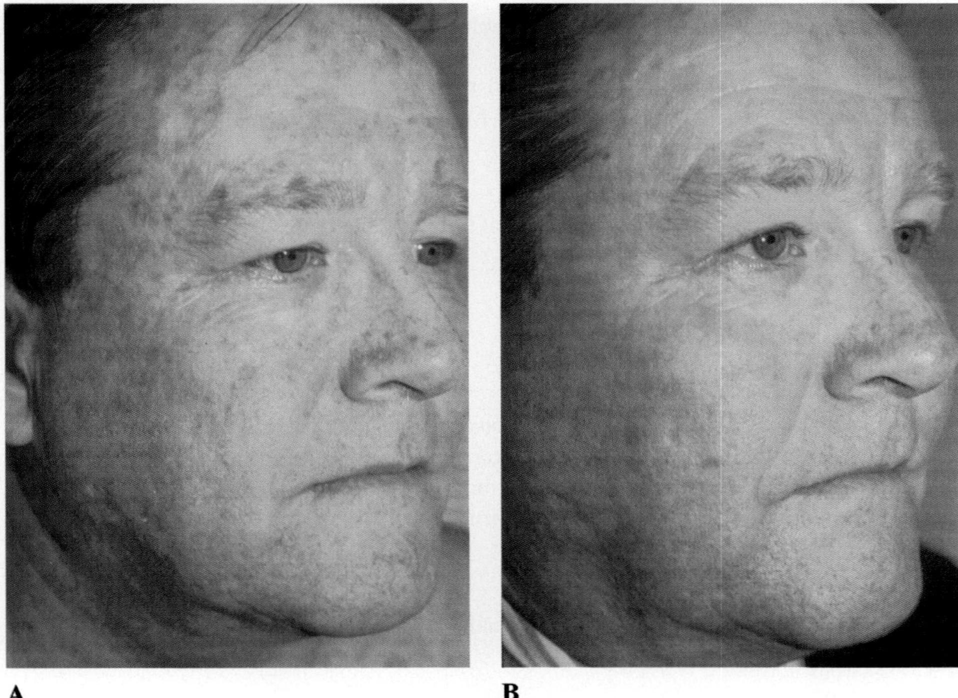

Figure 1 Before (A) and after (B) medium-depth chemical peel (solid CO_2 followed by TCA 35%) for actinic keratoses in a Fitzpatrick type II Glogau photoaging type III male showing resolution of actinic keratoses, lentigines, and old scarring 6 months afterwards. (Courtesy of Harold J. Brody, MD.)

Risks and Common Associated Problems

The development of pigmentary changes, prolonged erythema, infection, and even scarring are potential risks.

Hyperpigmentation is probably the most common side effect of chemical peels. In general, the deeper peels are more susceptible to postinflammatory hyperpigmentation. Hyperpigmentation caused by glycolic peels is usually temporary. Strict sun protection and judicious use of preoperative and postoperative tretinoin and hydroquinone products can reduce the risk of undesirable hyperpigmentation.

Erythema usually subsides in 30–90 days, but sometimes erythema continues for a prolonged period. Prolonged erythema is usually not permanent, and topical hydrocortisone can be used to speed the healing process (11).

If the patient has a history of herpetic outbreaks, treating the patient with acyclovir (400 mg by mouth twice daily) or an equivalent drug is advisable, beginning 2 days prior to the peel and continuing for 7 days after the peel. *Candida* infections also can develop, for which a short course of ketoconazole can be used. Cultures need to be taken, and appropriate antibiotics should be administered.

Properly matching the patient and peeling agent can decrease the risk of scarring. Also, to further decrease the risk of scarring, the patient should be advised to refrain from picking at the healing skin. Patients with a history of keloids should not undertake medium or deep peels because of the higher risk of hypertrophic scarring.

Combined Techniques

Chemical peels can be combined with topical tretinoin and hydroquinone products, dermabrasion, or intense-pulse light treatment.

LIQUID NITROGEN CRYOSURGERY

Background

Liquid nitrogen spray is also effective in light-complexioned patients. For the best cosmetic results, especially on the hands and arms, terminate the liquid nitrogen spray as soon as the lesion blanches. Freezing longer than this may cause hypopigmentation rather than simple elimination of lentigines with a return to normal-colored skin.

Patient Selection

The ideal candidate is a fair-skinned individual (Fitzpatrick skin type I–III) with superficial pigmentary changes and photodamage.

Technique

The spray technique, dipstick applicator method, and cryoprobe method can all be used. In the spray method, the nozzle tip of the spray gun is held about 1 cm away from the treatment site, and liquid nitrogen is sprayed on the lesion until an ice ball is formed. Feathering, the process of gradually and lightly freezing the area surrounding the ice ball to prevent an abrupt edge, can provide better cosmetic results. In dipstick applicator method, a cotton-tipped applicator is dipped into liquid nitrogen from a polystyrene cup. The dipstick applicator is then firmly pressed against the lesion for the desired duration. For cryoprobe method, the cold probe, a metal attachments made of copper, is used to serve as heat-conducting probes for cryotherapy. The probe is firmly pressed against the lesion during the treatment (12).

Lentigines can be treated with one 5–10-sec freeze with feathering completed every 4–6 weeks until resolved. Often, one treatment is all that is required.

Risks and Common Associated Problems

The most common complications include local pain, hypopigmentation or hyperpigmentation, and blister formation. Hemorrhage, infection, change in sensation, and scarring are rare.

LASERS

Background

Based on the principle of selective photothermolysis, several different types of lasers can effectively treat photoaging-associated pigmentary changes with minimal risk of adverse sequelae. Selective photothermolysis states that if a chromophore such as a melanosome is irradiated with a very brief laser pulse light of an appropriate wavelength, the target can be destroyed without causing collateral damage (13). Numerous lasers can specifically target pigmented lesions, including red-light lasers (694-nm ruby and 755-nm alexandrite), green-light lasers (510-nm pulsed dye, 532-nm frequency-doubled neodymium:yttrium-aluminum-garnet [Nd:YAG]) and near-infrared lasers (1064-nm Nd: YAG). The wide range of lasers that can be used to treat pigment is the result of the broad absorption spectrum of melanin. The other less pigment-specific lasers have also been used to treat pigmented lesions, including the argon, krypton, copper, CO_2, and most recently, erbium: yttrium-aluminum-garnet (Er:YAG) lasers. However, with more selective wavelength and appropriate pulse duration when performing laser surgery, the risk of adverse effects can be greatly reduced.

Technique

Red-Light Lasers

The two currently available red-light pulsed lasers for pigmented lesions are the Q-switched ruby and Q-switched alexandrite lasers. The Q-switched ruby laser emits a 694-nm beam with pulse duration of 20–50 nsec. The Q-switched alexandrite laser emits a 755-nm wavelength with pulse duration of 50–100 nsec. The longer wavelengths of these lasers allow deeper penetration of laser light into the dermis. The target chromophore in epidermal-pigmented lesions is the melanosome, which has an estimated thermal relaxation time ranging from 10–100 nsec (14). The pulse duration of both ruby and alexandrite lasers fall within this time period, which means that these lasers emit less heat to surrounding tissues without causing collateral damage. Light absorption by melanin decreases as the wavelength increases, peaking in the UV range and falling significantly in the near infrared region. The wavelength of ruby lasers is better absorbed than that of alexandrite lasers, thus less energy is needed to effectively destroy pigment target. However, in darker-complexioned individuals, it is recommended to use the longer wavelength lasers (e.g., 755 nm of alexandrite) for less absorption by melanin and lower risk of pigmentary changes.

The Q-switched ruby laser light is well absorbed by melanin and minimally absorbed by hemoglobin. Thus, this laser can be used for epidermal and dermal-pigmented lesions while avoiding vascular dermal structures. Epidermal-pigmented lesions usually clear after one or two treatments with the Q-switched ruby laser (15).

The 755-nm Q-switched alexandrite laser is less well absorbed by melanin compared to the 694-nm ruby laser, making the latter less likely to cause postoperative hypopigmentation. A good response has been seen in the treatment of lentigines.

Green-Light Lasers

These lasers produce energy with pulses shorter than the thermal relaxation time of melanosomes. Examples of green-light lasers are the flashlamp-pumped pulsed dye and frequency-doubled Q-switched Nd: YAG lasers. The flashlamp-pumped pulsed dye laser produces a 510-nm wavelength with 300-nsec pulse duration, whereas the frequency-doubled Q-switched Nd:YAG laser produces a 532-nm wavelength with a 5–10-nsec pulse of energy. Both lasers produce excellent results when used to treat epidermal-pigmented lesions such as solar lentigines and ephelides (16). Because the green wavelength of these lasers is also well absorbed by oxyhemoglobin, purpura formation may occur following laser treatment. Purpura occasionally leads to postinflammatory hyperpigmentation.

The flashlamp-pumped pulsed dye laser treatment at fluence of 2–3.5 J/cm^2 results in excellent clearing of epidermal-pigmented lesions. Ninety percent of treated epidermal pigmented lesions can be cleared after three treatments. A typical treatment response includes purpura lasting 5–7 days, followed by subsequent sloughing of the treated lesion at 7–14 days. This laser is not generally available in today's commercial market. Epidermal lesions such as lentigines and ephelides can be lightened considerably by the frequency-doubled Q-switched Nd:YAG at a fluence of 2–5 J/cm^2. However, when treating pigmented lesions, nonspecific vascular injury almost always develops, which leads to formation of purpura.

Nonpulsed, quasi-continuous wave green-light lasers such as the copper-vapor (511 nm), krypton (520–530 nm), and variable pulse with potassium-titanyl-phosphate (KTP) (532 nm) lasers share some characteristics with the above-mentioned pulsed lasers. Because the thermal relaxation time of the melanosome is exceeded when using these lasers, the clinical results can be less predictable and more treatment sessions are usually required to achieve similar results to those seen with pulsed green lasers.

Near-Infrared Lasers

These lasers include the CO_2 laser (10,600 nm) and the Er:YAG laser (2940 nm). In general, photodamage of the epidermis and dermis is responsive to laser resurfacing by these lasers. Lentigines, actinic keratoses, and pigmented seborrheic keratoses can be removed with the stripping of the epidermal layer. Melanin does not absorb these wavelengths well. Thus these lasers are not ideal for the treatment of epidermal-pigmented lesions.

The CO_2 laser emits an invisible infrared beam at a 10,600-nm wavelength, targeting both intracellular and extracellular water. When light energy is absorbed by water-containing tissue, skin vaporization occurs with production of coagulative necrosis in the remaining dermis. Lower fluences (5 J/cm^2 at pulse duration of shorter than 1 msec) limit the thermal damage to the epidermis. Two different CO_2 laser technologies can deliver sufficient energy to vaporize the skin. One involves the use of an ultrashort pulse to deliver the energy to tissue. The second employs a computer-controlled optomechanical shutter system, which scans a continuous wave beam so rapidly that the emitted light is prevented from contacting skin for more than 1 msec.

The Er:YAG laser emits wavelength at 2940 nm. The depth of ablation is about 1 μm, which is shallower than the 20-μm depth for CO_2 laser light. This allows more precise ablation with less residual thermal damage (17). The Er:YAG laser is preferable for treating superficial pigmentary photodamaged lesions with the advantage of faster healing, less postoperative erythema.

Dyschromias, including solar lentigines, often are improved with laser resurfacing, although they generally are not regarded as a primary indication for laser resurfacing treatment. Absolute contraindications include isotretinoin use within the previous 1 year, history of keloids/hypertrophic scars, active cutaneous bacterial or viral infection in the area to be treated, and ectropion (for infraorbital resurfacing). Successful laser resurfacing depends on reepithelialization from normal or intact adnexal structures. Therefore, conditions that result in decreased adnexal structures of the skin, such as ongoing ultraviolet exposure, prior radiation therapy to treatment area, and collagen vascular diseases are relative contraindications.

Mild complications sometimes occur and usually are of minimal consequence. Minor complications include milia formation, perioral dermatitis, acne and/or rosacea exacerbation, and postinflammatory hyperpigmentation. Moderate complications include localized viral, bacterial, and *Candida* infection, delayed hypopigmentation, persistent erythema and prolonged healing. The most severe complications are hypertrophic scarring, disseminated infection, and ectropion. Early detection of complications and rapid institution of appropriate therapy are extremely important.

Results

Examples of treatment response after ruby laser and CO_2 laser resurfacing are shown in Figures 2 and 3, respectively.

THE INTENSE-PULSE LIGHT SOURCE

Background

The intense pulsed light device (IPL) is a broadband light source that emits a continuous spectrum in the range of 515–1200 nm. Low-end cut-off filters are used to eliminate shorter wavelengths depending on the application. The IPL device has been shown to be effective for treating photoaging-associated dyspigmentation with minimal or no downtime (18–20).

Technique

Settings of 550-nm filter, double pulse (2.4 ms), 10-ms delay, and 4-ms pulse are most often used. Fluences can range from 30–44 J/cm. The water-based gel, kept at refrigerator temperature, should be applied to the skin with thickness of at least 1 or 2 mm prior to the treatment.

Results

Figure 4 shows the results of IPL treatment for lentigines and other types of photodamage.

Risks and Common Associated Problems

Side effects include temporary mild crusting lasting 1–3 days, erythema, and mild facial edema. Hypopigmentation and purpura have been reported but are rare.

DERMABRASION

Background

Dermabrasion can be employed to improve hyperpigmentation of facial skin. Superficial dermabrasion usually removes the excess of pigment. It is less frequently being used today for this purpose due to the risk of side effects and the availability of other treatment options.

Technique

The electric hand engines used in dermabrasion produce 15,000–30,000 rpm. Typically, smaller shapes such as cones or pears are used in confined areas around the nose, eyelids, and mouth. Fraises and wire brush wheels are used on the broad flat surfaces of the

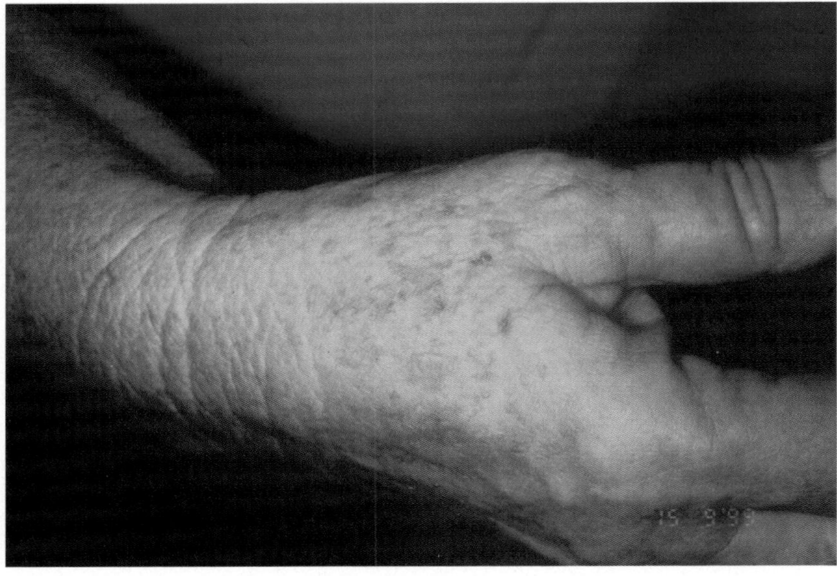

A

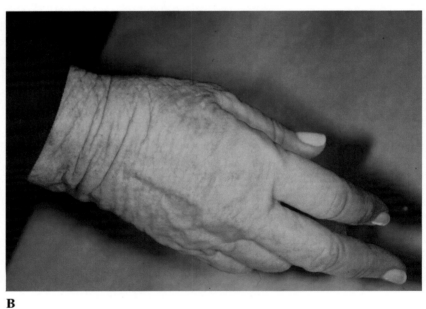

B

Figure 2 Solar lentigines. (A) Numerous lesions on the right dorsal hand before laser treatment. (B) One month after a single Q-switched ruby laser (694 nm, 4.5 J/cm^2, 6.5-mm spot size, and 20-nsec pulse duration) treatment, there was clearing of the treated lesions with some residual erythema.

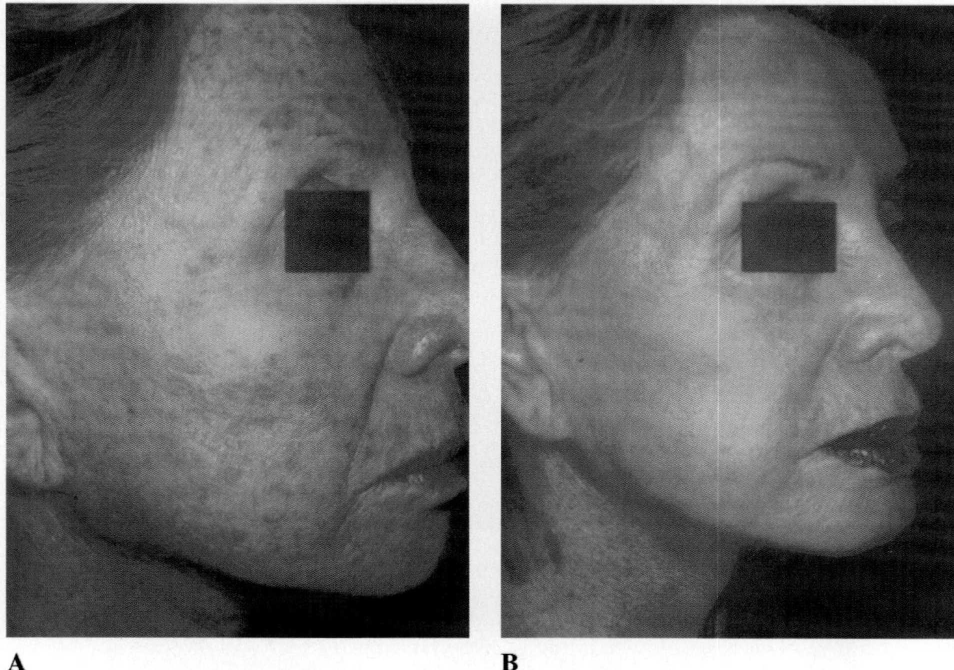

A B

Figure 3 Carbon dioxide laser resurfacing for the treatment of pigmentary changes and chronic photodamaged skin. (A) Before treatment. (B) Six months after full-face UltraPulse laser resurfacing at fluence of 300 mJ/pulse, power of 60 W, and CPG density of 6 with two pulses.

forehead, cheeks, and nonfacial areas. Fraises can be used without spray refrigerant, whereas the wire brush requires a firm frozen surface to safely abrade large areas. Once the area to be abraded is frozen, perform three-point retraction using the two hands of the surgical assistant and nondominant hand of the surgeon. Cotton towels can be used for blotting and retraction. The correct hand position for holding the abrading instrument places the forefingers around the body of the hand engine, while the thumb stabilizes the neck. The direction of rotation of the abrading end-piece can be clockwise or counterclockwise. For right-handed surgeons, counterclockwise rotation directs the momentum of rotation toward the thumb in a stabilizing fashion. Make passes with archiform horizontal strokes perpendicular to the direction of the rotating brush or fraise.

A surgical landmark for abrading into the superficial papillary dermis is the presence of cornrow bleeding produced by an eruption of the small vascular loops in the dermal papilla. As the depth of abrasion moves into the reticular dermis, these vascular channels and the subsequent red dots become larger (21).

Once the dermabrasion is completed, application of a compress with gauze soaked with 1% lidocaine and epinephrine (1:100,000 concentrate of epinephrine) for 5–10 minutes decreases stinging and provides hemostasis. An open or closed wound care regimen then can be initiated. Most open wound care routines use saline or 0.25% vinegar compresses applied four or five times daily followed by an occlusive ointment such as petrola-

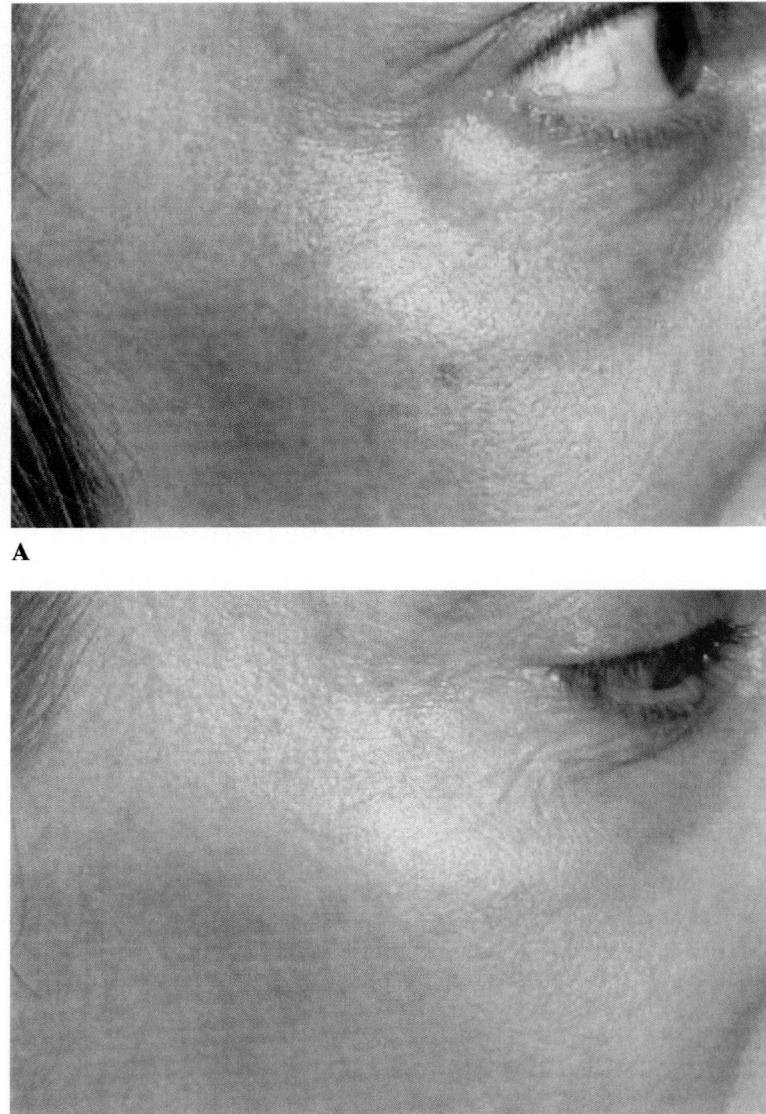

Figure 4 Intense pulsed light photorejuvenation for the treatment of pigmentary changes, lentigines, and vascular changes. (A) Before IPL treatment. (B) After two treatments performed 1 month apart with the Quantum SR Program I (550-nm filter, 2.4-msec double pulse, 10-msec delay, 26 J/cm^2, and close contact). (Courtesy of Robert A. Weiss, MD.)

tum or white Vaseline ointment. Avoid mentholated, scented, or antibiotic topical preparations because they may irritate or sensitize the patient.

Risks and Common Associated Problems

Milia are one of the most common complications of dermabrasion and usually appear 2–4 weeks postoperatively and resolve with daily application of topical tretinoin. Repigmentation often occurs upon sun exposure, usually 3 or 4 weeks after the procedure. Patients must be cautioned against sun exposure and instructed in proper use of sunscreen. Hydroquinones must be instituted at the first signs of hyperpigmentation after dermabrasion to prevent excessive hyperpigmentation.

In patients with skin type IV or V, repigmentation is unpredictable and dermabrasion may worsen the hyperpigmentation (22). These individuals should be approached cautiously and the patients should be fully informed that dermabrasion presents a risk of worsening their problem. Very deeply pigmented African Americans of skin type VI usually repigment evenly and experience very few problems of irregular or mottled postoperative pigmentation.

REFERENCES

1. Brues AM. Linkage of body build with sex, eye color and freckling. Am J Hum Genet 1950; 2:215–239.
2. Weiss JS, Ellis CN, Headington JT, Tincoff T, Hamilton TA, Voorhees JJ. Topical tretinoin improves photodamaged skin: a double-blind vehicle controlled study. JAMA 1998; 259: 527–532.
3. Griffiths CEM, Kang S, Ellis CN, et al. Two concentrations of topical tretinoin (retinoid acid) cause similar improvement of photoaging but different degrees of irritation: a double-blind, vehicle controlled comparison of 0.1% or 0.025% tretinoin creams. Arch Dermatol 1995; 131: 1037–1044.
4. Olsen EA, Katz HI, Levine N, et al. Sustained improvement in photodamaged skin with reduced tretinoin emollient cream treatment regimen: effects of once-weekly and three-weekly applications. J Am Acad Dermatol 1997; 37:227–230.
5. Bulengo-Ransby SM, Griffiths CEM, Kimbrough-Green CK, Finkel LJ, Hamilton TA, Ellis CN, Voorhees JJ. Topical tretinoin therapy for hyperpigmented lesions caused by inflammation of the skin in black patients. N Engl J Med 1993; 328:1438–1443.
6. Schallreuter KU, Wood JW. A possible mechanism of action for azelaic acid in the human epidermis. Arch Dermatol Res 1990; 282:168–171.
7. Nakagawa M, Kawai K, Kawai K. Contact allergy to kojic acid in skin care products. Contact Dermatitis 1995; 32:9–13.
8. Monheit GD. Chemexfoliation: a review. Cosm Dermatol 1998; 1:16–19.
9. Brody HJ. Chemical Peeling and Resurfacing. 2nd ed.: Mosby-Year Book, 1997.
10. Duffy DM. Alpha hydroxy acids/trichloroacetic acids risk/benefit, strategies. A photographic review. Dermatol Surg 1998; 24:181–189.
11. Resnik SS, Resnik BI. Complications of chemical peeling. Dermatol Clin 1995; 13:309–312.
12. Kuflik EG. Cryosurgery updated. J Am Acad Dermatol 1994; 31:925–944.
13. Anderson RR, Parrish JA. Selective photothermolysis: precise microsurgery by selective absorption of pulsed radiation. Science 1983; 29:524–527.
14. Polla LL, Margolis RJ, Dover JS. Melanosomes are a primary target of Q-switched ruby laser irradiation in guinea pig skin. J Invest Dermatol 1987; 89:281–286.
15. Ashinoff R, Geronemus RG. Q-switched ruby laser treatment of labial lentigos. J Am Acad Dermatol 1992; 27(5 Pt 2):809–811.

16. Kilmer SL, Wheeland RG, Goldberg DJ. Treatment of epidermal pigmented lesions with the frequency-doubled Q- switched Nd:YAG laser. A controlled, single-impact, dose-response, multicenter trial. Arch Dermatol 1994; 130:1515–1519.
17. Teikemeier G, Goldberg DJ. Skin resurfacing with the erbium:YAG laser. Dermatol Surg 1997; 23:685–687.
18. Bitter PH. Noninvasive rejuvenation of photodamaged skin using serial, full-face intense pulse light treatments. Dermatol Surg 2000; 26:835–842.
19. Weiss RA, Goldman MP, Weiss MA. Treatment of poikiloderma of Civatte with an intense pulse light source. Dermatol Surg 2000; 26:823–827.
20. Weiss RA, Weiss MA, Beasley KL. Rejuvenation of photoaged skin: 5 years results with intense pulse light of the face, neck and chest. Dermatol Surg 2002; 28:1115–1119.
21. Alt TH. Technical aids for dermabrasion. J Dermatol Surg Oncol 1987; 13:638–648.
22. Stegman SJ. Dermabrasion in cosmetic dermatologic surgery. Cosmetic Dermatologic Surgery 1990; Year Book:59.

19

Treatment of Photoaging in Asian Skin

Henry H. Chan *Queen Mary Hospital, Pokfulam, Hong Kong*

- Asian skin is more likely to develop adverse reactions such as postinflammatory hyperpigmentation following laser surgery and intense pulsed light source (IPL) treatment.
- The ideal nonablative laser used to reduce wrinkles and improve skin texture in Asian patients should have a long wavelength, adequate cooling, and no downtime, be simple less variable, and show long-term improvement.
- A combination approach using both 1320-nm neodymium:yttrium-aluminum-garnet (Nd:YAG) and IPL can be particularly advantageous in the use of nonablative skin rejuvenation in Asians for treatment of wrinkles and pigmentation.
- The photomechanical effect of Q-switched lasers for the treatment of lentigines in Asians may be less desirable than millisecond-domain lasers and light sources.
- Radiofrequency for skin tightening may be used in Asian skin without altering surface pigmentation.

Treatment for photoaging in Asian patients differs from that in white patients in several important respects. Asians with photodamage tend to have more pigmentary problems but less wrinkling than whites. Chung et al. (1) performed photographic assessment of 407 Koreans between the ages of 30 to 92 years and assessed the manifestation of cutaneous damage. Their findings confirmed that pigmentary changes are common features of photoaging in Asians, with seborrheic keratosis being the major pigmentary lesion in men and lentigines the prominent feature in women. Such differences in clinical manifestations also lead to different patient expectations, and treatment goals must be clarified with the patient before the commencement of therapy. Finally, beside lentigines and seborrheic keratosis, acquired bilateral nevus of Ota-like macules, or Hori macules, is another pigmentary condition that is triggered by ultraviolet light. This condition, although rare in whites, occurs in 0.8% of Asian women (2), and its management will be reviewed herein.

THE USE OF LASERS FOR NONABLATIVE SKIN REJUVENATION IN ASIANS

Ablative vs. Nonablative

Laser skin resurfacing has never been particularly popular in Asia, because Asians tend to have less wrinkles. Furthermore, the adverse effects associated with laser resurfacing in Asians such as erythema and postinflammatory hyperpigmentation are particularly troublesome (Fig. 1). Nonablative rejuvenation with its lower risk of adverse effects and downtime has generated much interest in Asia. Many lasers have been used for this purpose, and can be classified into several types. The vascular type (pulse dye lasers and 532-nm Nd:YAG lasers) affects the papillary dermal vessels, and in doing so leads to microvascular

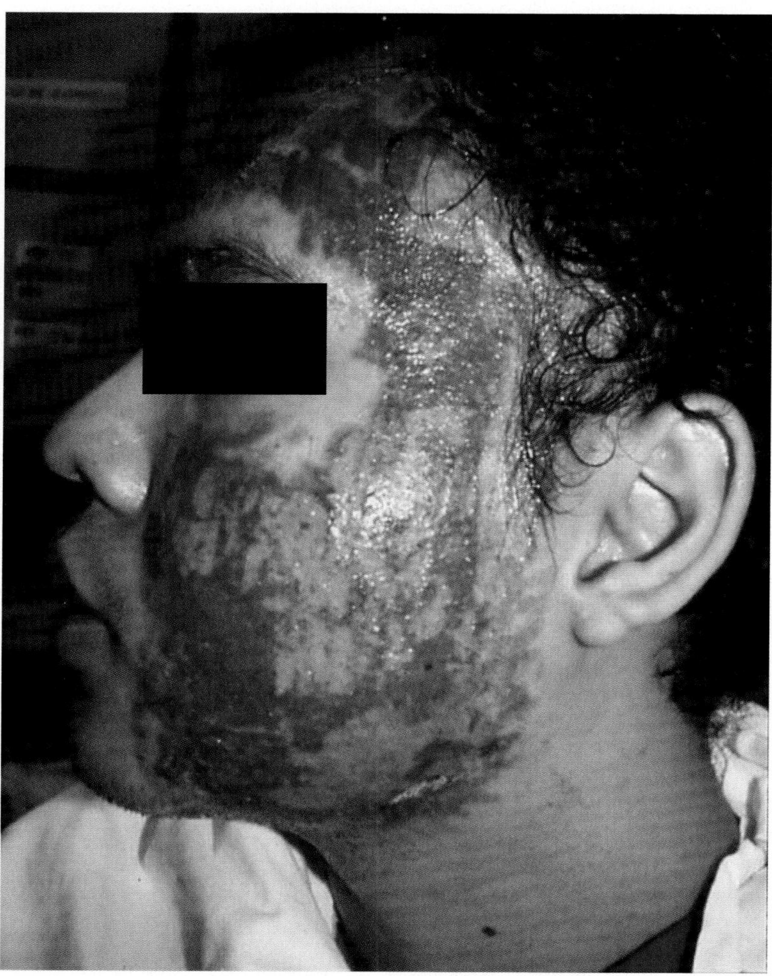

Figure 1 2 days after one ablative laser treatment for acne scarring (three passes with a carbon dioxide laser followed immediately by one pass with a Er:YAG laser).

damage. The subsequent healing process generates new collagen production. The infrared type of lasers (1064–1540 nm) target water, and the photothermal effect that is produced as a result of the laser-tissue interaction causes a raise in the dermal temperature. The consequences are collagen tightening, increased fibroblastic activities, and increased collagen production.

Because Asians, with their higher epidermal melanin content, are more likely than whites to develop adverse reactions, especially postinflammatory hyperpigmentation, the ideal nonablative laser to reduce wrinkles and improve skin texture for Asians should have the following properties:

- Long wavelength
- Adequate cooling
- Simple and less variable
- No downtime
- Long-term improvement

Previous studies that looked at the use of lasers for the treatment of port wine stain in Asians indicated that those with higher epidermal melanin content are at greater risk of adverse effects when vascular lasers are used. Even with the development of skin cooling, adverse effects can develop. A retrospective study evaluated the results of a glass cooling chamber-equipped variable-pulse 532-nm neodymium:yttrium-aluminum-garnet (Nd:YAG) laser (2–10 msec with a 2–4-mm^2 spot diameter and fluence between 8 and 20 J/cm^2; Versapulse, Lumenis, Palo Alto, CA) in the treatment of port wine stain in Chinese patients, and found that the Versapulse 532-nm laser may be only partially effective (3). High fluence is necessary to achieve the desired clinical response, and although contact cooling reduces the risk of epidermal damage, texture changes can still occur. More recently, another study looked at the use of pulsed dye laser (585 nm) in conjunction with cryogen spray cooling in the treatment of port wine stain in Chinese patients and found that complications, especially pigmentary changes, can still occur (4). Although for nonablative skin rejuvenation much lower fluence is used with these vascular lasers, adverse effects, especially pigmentary changes, remain a possibility. Consequently, longer-wavelength lasers with lower risk of epidermal melanin interference are more suitable for Asian patients.

Q-Switched Nd:YAG (1064 nm)

The Q-switched (QS) 1064-nm Nd:YAG laser was one of the first lasers in the infrared spectrum to be used for nonablative skin rejuvenation. Goldberg et al. (5,6) used pinpoint bleeding as the clinical end point for nonablative skin rejuvenation in lighter skin type patients (type I–III), and found clinical as well as histological data to support the use of QS 1064-nm Nd:YAG laser for the treatment of rhytides. However, my experience of using this system for the treatment of nevus of Ota in Asian patients indicates that hyperpigmentation can be common, and it affected 10.5% of patients when higher fluence was used (7). A 1064-nm Nd:YAG laser in the millisecond domain together with long-pulsed 532-nm potassium titanyl phosphate (KTP) laser has been used successfully for nonablative skin rejuvenation in Asians. Lee (8) treated 150 patients (skin type I–V) with the long-pulsed KTP 532-nm (Aura, Laserscope, San Jose, CA) and long-pulsed Nd:YAG 1064-nm (Lyra, Laserscope) lasers, both separately and combined. The fluences that were used varied between 7 and 15 J/cm^2 at –20-msec pulse duration with a 2-mm handpiece, and

6–15 J/cm^2 and 30–50 msec with a 4-mm handpiece for KTP. The Nd:YAG fluences were set at 24–30 J/cm^2 for a 10-mm handpiece and 30 J/cm^2 for a SmartScan Plus scanner (Laserscope). These energies were delivered at 30–65-msec pulse durations. All of the patients were treated monthly for three to six times, and observed for up to 18 months after the last treatment. All 150 patients were found to have a mild to moderate degree of improvement in wrinkling, a moderate degree of improvement in skin tone and texture, and significant degree of improvement in redness and pigmentation. Combined KTP and Nd:YAG laser treatment was superior to treatment using either laser alone (8).

The 1320-nm Nd:YAG Laser

Among all of the long-wavelength lasers that are used for nonablative skin rejuvenation, the 1320-nm Nd:YAG laser is one of the few lasers that have been extensively investigated. Most studies have investigated light-skinned patients. For the dark-skinned group, Trelles et al. (9) studied the use of a 1320 Nd:YAG nm laser among Spanish patients and found histological improvement and fair to significant clinical improvement 4–6 months after twice-weekly treatment for 4 weeks in total (1320-nm Nd-YAG, 30–35 J/cm^2, 30-msec dynamic cooling, 40-msec delay, 5-mm spot size; CoolTouch, Laser Aesthetics, Auburn, CA). No study has investigated its use on Asian skin. More recently, we compared the use of 1320-nm Nd:YAG laser and an IPL in nonablative skin rejuvenation in a Chinese population. Forty-seven patients with Glogau classification type 2 photoaging were recruited and randomized to receive treatment with either the 1320-nm laser or the IPL. All had received treatment at monthly intervals for at least 4 months before assessment. All patients were assessed using a structured questionnaire for the degree of improvement in terms of skin texture, pigmentation, and wrinkle improvement. A cutometer was used for the objective measurement of skin elasticity and firmness. The results indicated that for the subjective degree of improvement, 37% patients who were treated with 1320-nm Nd-YAG laser recorded moderate to significant improvement, as compared to 20% of those who were treated with IPL (Figs. 2–4). However, in terms of pigmentation, all patients who were treated with IPL recorded at least a mild degree of improvement as compared to 33% of patients treated with the 1320-nm Nd-YAG laser. Cutometer assessment indicated significant improvement in the firmness and elasticity of most of the important parameters for 1320-nm Nd:YAG laser treatment, but only some of the parameters for IPL treatment (Tables 1 and 2). This allows one to conclude that the 1320-nm Nd:YAG laser is more effective than the IPL in the improvement of wrinkles. However, in terms of pigment reduction, IPL appears to be superior. A combination approach using both 1320-nm Nd: YAG and IPL treatment can be particularly advantageous in the use of nonablative skin rejuvenation in Asians. While adverse effects such as the blister formation and increased pigmentation may be associated with the use of the 1320-nm Nd:YAG laser, they are uncommon. If an adverse reaction occurs, it is usually mild (minor pitted scarring has been reported). To reduce the risk of complications, the following measures are recommended:

- Perform three passes: two with precooling and one with a postcooling cryogen spray of tetrafluoroethane. The fluence that is used for the first and second precooling passes should be in the range of 16–22 J/cm^2. The fluence for the first and second passes was determined by achieving a peak temperature of 42–45°C. The third pass should be delivered with a fluence of 13–17 J/cm^2 and aim to achieve a temperature of less than 40°C after laser treatment.

- The temperature should be rechecked after 10 treatment spots, as the cutaneous temperature tends to increase.
- Because complications are more likely to develop in the central facial area and in pitted scars, careful temperature monitoring is necessary in these regions.

The 1450-nm Diode Laser

The 1450-nm diode laser is another nonablative laser with a wavelength that lies in the infrared spectrum. A control study that compared 1450-nm diode laser treatment with

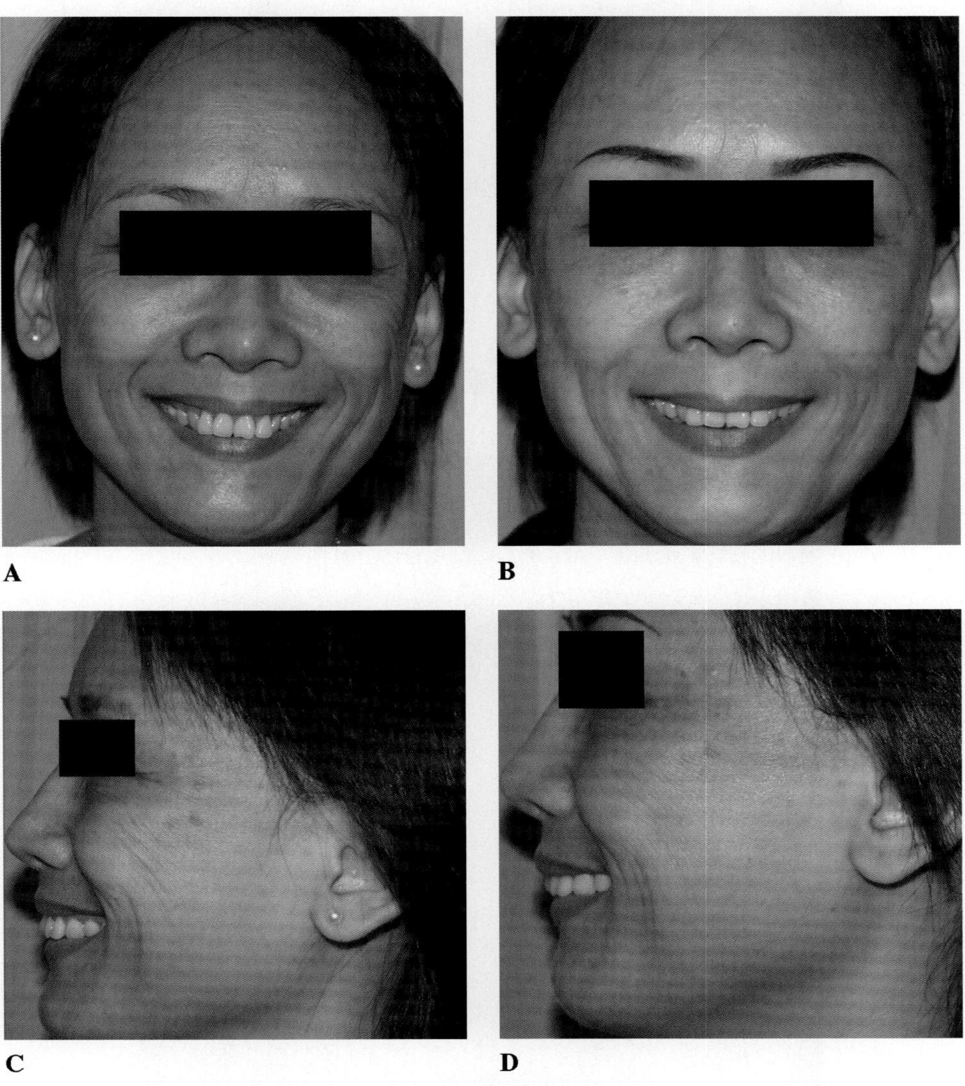

Figure 2 (A and C) Patient with photoaging before treatment. (B and D) After the fifth treatment with the 1320-nm Nd:YAG laser (three passes: (1) precooling, 17–23 J/cm^2; (2) precooling, 16–18 J/cm^2; (3) postcooling, 12–17 J/cm^2).

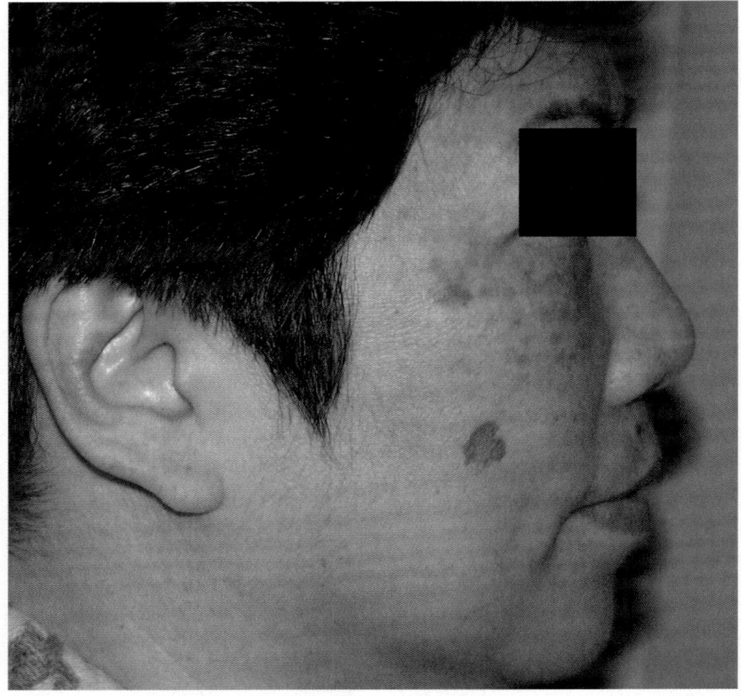

A

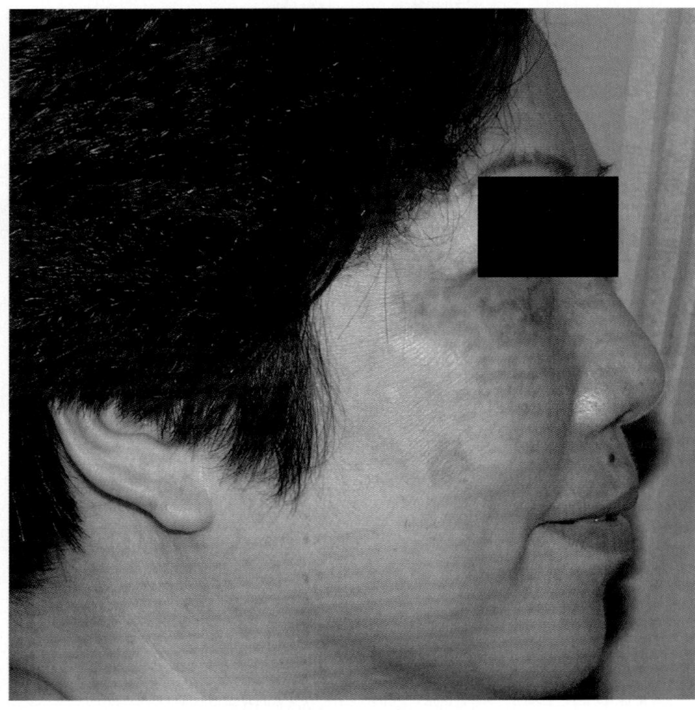

B

Figure 3 (A) Patient with photoaging before treatment. (B) After 6th treatments with Intense pulsed light source (640-nm filter, 28–33 J/cm^2, T1 = 4.2 msec, T2 = 4.8 msec, D1 = 20 msec).

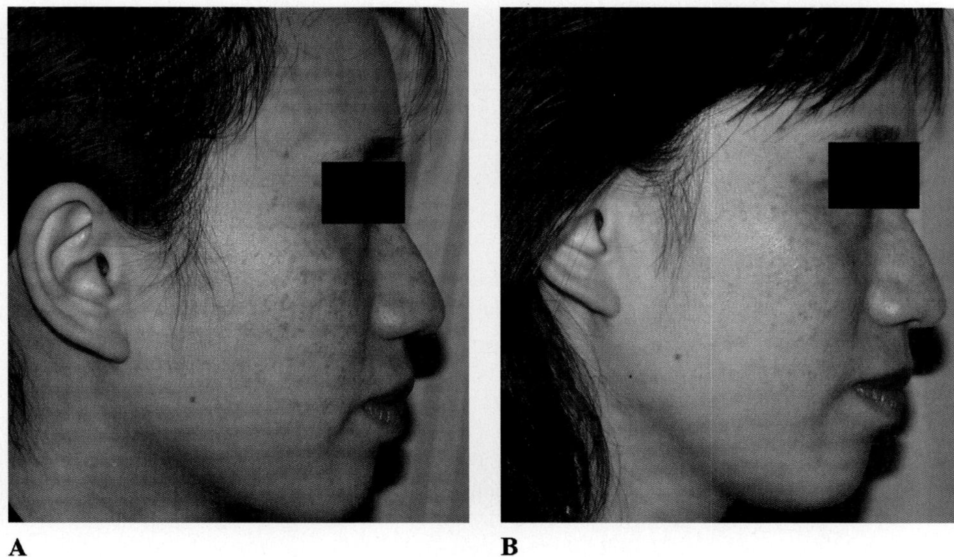

Figure 4 (A) Patient with photoaging before treatment. (B) After six treatments with an intense pulsed light source (560-nm filter, 22–29 J/cm^2, T1 = 2.4 msec, T2 = 4 msec, D1 = 15 msec).

Table 1 Assessment of Viscoelasticity for the 1320-nm Nd:YAG (Cutometer SEM 575, Germany)

		Viscoelasticity parameters				
Area	Treatment	R0	R2	R5	R6	R7
Area beside right eye N = 22	Before treatment	0.603	0.242	0.190	0.058	0.180
	After six treatments	0.653	0.398	0.311	0.075	0.289
	Remark	$P = 0.034$ Elasticity ↑	$P = 0.000$ Elasticity ↑	$P = 0.000$ Elasticity ↑	$P = 0.011$ Elasticity ↑	$P = 0.000$ Elasticity ↑
Forehead N = 22	Before treatment	0.445	0.202	0.167	0.077	0.155
	After six treatments	0.501	0.369	0.277	0.097	0.252
	Remark	$P = 0.000$ Elasticity ↑	$P = 0.000$ Elasticity ↑	$P = 0.000$ Elasticity ↑	$P = 0.014$ Elasticity ↑	$P = 0.000$ Elasticity ↑

Table 2 Assessment of Viscoelasticity for the IPL Quantum (Cutometer SEM 575, Germany)

Area	Treatment	Viscoelasticity parameters				
		R0	R2	R5	R6	R7
Area below left eye (N = 12)	Before treatment	0.532	0.272	0.206	0.083	0.190
	After six treatments	0.588	0.335	0.246	0.065	0.231
	Remark	$P = 0.029$ Elasticity ↑	$P = 0.010$ Elasticity ↑	$P = 0.048$ Elasticity ↑	$P = 0.017$ Elasticity ↓	$P = 0.027$ Elasticity ↑
Area below right eye (N = 12)	Before treatment	0.516	0.288	0.222	0.085	0.204
	After six treatments	0.603	0.387	0.287	0.068	0.269
	Remark	$P = 0.000$ Elasticity ↑	$P = 0.000$ Elasticity ↑	$P = 0.000$ Elasticity ↑	$P = 0.013$ Elasticity ↓	$P = 0.000$ Elasticity ↑

dynamic cooling to treatment with dynamic cooling alone for facial rhytides showed that 13 out of 20 patients had clinical improvement on the laser/cryogen-treated side, whereas none showed improvement on the cryogen-only side (10). Although this laser can theoretically be of particular advantage for dark-skinned patients given its long wavelength, postinflammatory hyperpigmentation is surprisingly common. Hardaway et al. (11) found that postinflammatory hyperpigmentation developed in six out of nine light-skinned patients (skin type I–III). This finding was confirmed by Tanzi et al. (12), who investigated the use of this laser for the treatment of facial rhytides in 25 light-skinned patients (skin type I–III). The incidence of postinflammatory hyperpigmentation was 18%. Although all cases resolved with the use of topical bleaching agents, the average duration even in this light-skinned group was 14 weeks. As most cases tend to develop after the second treatment and the total duration of cryogen spray was 60 msec, it was proposed that the extended cooling duration led to a high rate of postinflammatory hyperpigmentation. Therefore, the 1450-nm diode laser should not be used for nonablative skin rejuvenation in dark-skinned patients until issues of the optimal cooling parameters are resolved.

Erbium Glass Laser (1540 nm)

The 1540-nm erbium glass laser is another long-wavelength infrared system that has been used for nonablative skin rejuvenation. Ross et al. investigated the use of a 1540-nm erbium glass laser with contact cooling by a sapphire cooling hand piece in nine patients who were treated in postauricular sites (13). Various combinations of laser parameters and pulsing were used, and biopsies were performed to assess the degree of improvement. The findings indicated that although selective dermal heating can be achieved, the range of fibroplasia and lack of clinically substantial cosmetic enhancement suggested that the dermal thermal damage achieved might have been too deep. However, others have not made similar observations, possibly because of differences in laser parameters. Using photographic evaluation, a dose-response study indicated the optimal parameter for a 1540-nm erbium glass laser is 24 J/cm^2 delivered in three pulses (8 J/cm^2 per pulse) for the periorbital area and five pulses (40 J/cm^2) for the perioral area (14). The same group of investigators then performed further clinical studies using assessments methods that included clinical ultrasound imaging and profilometric evaluation. Their results confirmed the effectiveness of this laser even after 14 months of follow up (15). The advantage of 1540-nm erbium glass over other lasers in the infrared spectrum is that it is painless. The lack of a clinical end point, however, is a disadvantage. Whether other investigators can confirm the results previously reported remains to be seen.

THE USE OF LASER AND IPL FOR THE TREATMENT OF LENTIGINES IN ASIANS

Lentigines and seborrheic keratosis are common manifestations of photoaging in Asians. Consequently, the effective removal of these lesions is often considered the major goal of therapeutic outcome. Techniques used include photothermal (millisecond domain) or photomechanical (nanosecond domain) treatment of lentigines in dark skinned patients. The question is: Which is more desirable?

For the last decade, several laser systems have been shown to be effective in the treatment of lentigines. These systems include the 510-nm pulse dye laser, the frequency-doubled QS Nd:YAG 532-nm laser, the QS ruby laser, and the QS alexandrite laser (16–18). Like most aesthetic procedures, the risk of adverse effects is important. Dark-skinned patients such as Asians have a higher epidermal melanin content and are more likely to develop complications such as hyperpigmentation. Studies of the use of QS lasers in dark-skinned patients have indicated that the risk of postinflammatory hyperpigmentation (PIH) is approximately 20% (19).

The QS ruby and QS alexandrite laser systems emit light that is well absorbed by melanin. However, the greater depth of penetration can be a disadvantage because there is a potential for permanent follicular melanocytic damage causing leukotrichia when a high fluence is used (20). A low fluence can lead to sublethal damage of the follicular melanocytes. This, in turn, stimulates the follicular melanocytic function, which leads to the development of hyperpigmentation.

Q-Switching vs. Millisecond Pulse Durations

Three years ago, our group performed an in vivo study of 34 patients and compared a QS 532-nm Nd:YAG laser to a long-pulse 532-nm Nd:YAG laser (20). We found that long-pulse 532-nm laser (6.5–8 J/cm^2, 2-mm spot size, 2-msec pulse duration, with slate gray appearance as the clinical end point) could result in a lower risk of PIH when used in the treatment of lentigines in Asians (Table 3). Long-pulsed lasers differ from QS lasers in the sense that they have a photothermal but not a photomechanical effect. Q-switched lasers generate high-energy radiation with a very short pulse duration (in terms of nanoseconds) and produce intense energy that leads to a rapid rise in temperature (1000°C) within the target subcellular chromophore. As the laser pulse duration is shorter than the thermal relaxation time of the target, a temperature gradient is created between the target and its surrounding tissue (21,22). When the temperature gradient collapses, it generates localized shockwaves that cause fragmentation of its targets. This photomechanical reaction leads to the melanosomal disruption that is seen after QS laser irradiation (22–24).

We created controversy when we suggested that the photomechanical effect of QS lasers may not be desirable when used in the removal of lentigines in Asians (20). However,

Table 3 Degree of Clearing

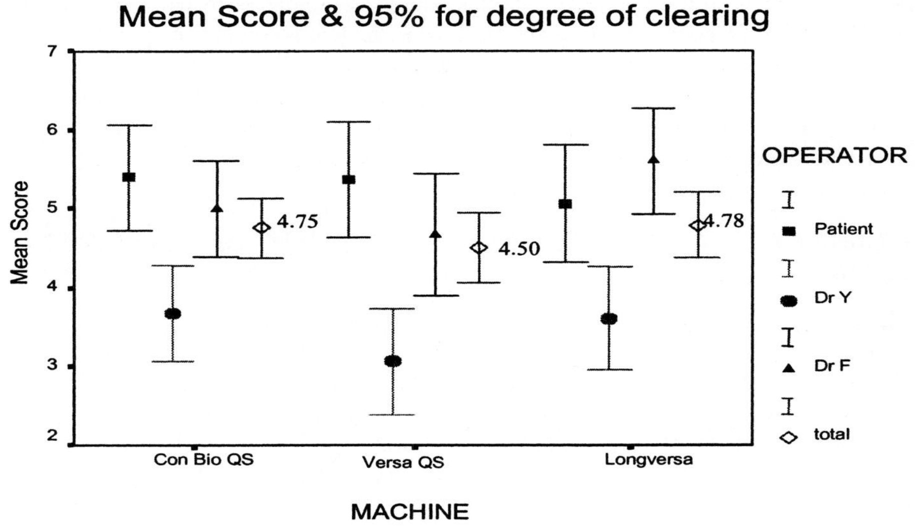

* Con Bio QS vs Versa QS, p = 1.00
Con Bio QS vs Longversa, p = 1.00
Longversa vs Versa QS, p = 1.00

other investigators have recently confirmed our findings (25). The IPL, which emits a broad band of visible light from a noncoherent filtered flashlamp in the millisecond domain, produces photothermal effects. Recent studies that investigated the use of IPL to remove lentigines in Asians confirmed their effectiveness. Interestingly, no case of PIH was observed in the several independent studies (26,27). These observations confirm my hypothesis that the photomechanical effect of QS laser for the treatment of lentigines in Asians is not desirable.

The main concern about the use of the long-pulse laser and IPL for the treatment of epidermal-pigmented lesions is the potential for thermal diffusion from the epidermis to the dermis, which increases the risk of scarring. To prevent such an occurrence, the pulse duration that is chosen should be shorter than the thermal relaxation time of the epidermis, which is estimated to be about 10 msec if the epidermal thickness is 100 μm (28,29).

Importance of Wavelength

More factors may be involved as the photomechanical effect may not be desirable; however, the wavelengths play an important role as well. For a 532-nm(30) Nd:YAG laser, the wavelength is absorbed not only by melanin but also by hemoglobin. Anderson et al. (23) investigated the effect of a QS Nd:YAG 532-nm laser on cutaneous pigmentation and found that at a high fluence, purpuric macule could occur after the immediate white appearance faded. Such purpura correlated with the histological changes of erythrocyte coagulation within the superficial vessels. Interestingly, under electron microscopy, the destroyed erythrocytes demonstrated vacuolation, a change that typically occurs as a result of the photomechanical effect of the QS laser. Damage of the superficial vessels will lead to inflammation, and in Asian skin PIH can occur as a consequence. Interestingly, a 351-nm xenon/fluoride-pulsed excimer laser, one of the first used experimentally for the treatment of pigmented lesion when the concept of selective photothermolysis was proposed, may be of particular advantage when used in Asian skin, given its lack of dermal penetration (the damage is confined to 100 μm within the epidermis). This lack of dermal penetration could reduce the risk of inflammation and subsequent PIH.

Another means to further reduce the risk of PIH when the long-pulse vascular green (such as the 532-nm Nd:YAG) laser is used for lentigines is the use of diascopy or pressure before and during the laser pulse. By compressing the vasculature and removing hemoglobin from the vessel, vascular injury is prevented, and this reduces the risk of purpura. Such an effect can be achieved by attaching a convex contact window to one of these lasers handpiece and push the window into the skin (R. Anderson, personal communication, 2003).

MY EXPERIENCE WITH IPL TREATMENT FOR NONABLATIVE SKIN REJUVENATION IN ASIANS

Intense pulsed light is a polychromatic nonlaser noncoherent light with a spectrum of 400–1200 nm. By emitting a fixed spectrum of wavelengths rather than a fixed wavelength, IPL has several advantages and disadvantages. A fixed spectrum of wavelengths allows penetration of different depths as well as the targeting of multiple chromophobes (31). This can be of particular advantage given the fact that nonablative skin rejuvenation often involves treatment of several skin elements including pigmentation, telangiectasia, and collagen remodeling. The use of a cut-off filter system to confine the emitted radiation to a certain spectrum of wavelengths allows some degree of selectivity, though not to the extent of laser therapy. Another advantage of IPL is that different pulse widths can be set, and one can choose the appropriate parameters that match the thermal relaxation time of the targets. The multiple purposes of IPL systems can be of particular advantage for clinicians with limited resources.

Having stated all of these advantages, the use of IPL also has disadvantages. This particularly applies to dark skinned patients given the higher epidermal melanin content, and therefore increases the risk of adverse effects. Cooling is important, especially when dermal structures such as water or vessels are the main targets. If, however, the removal of epidermal pigment is the main goal, then excessive cooling can reduce the efficacy. The large variation in parameters and the wide spectrum of potential combinations in wavelengths, pulse width, and fluence imply that the user's experience is vital to achieving the desirable clinical outcome.

Negishi et al. (26) were among the first to investigate the use of IPL in Asians. Using an IPL vasculight, they studied its use for skin rejuvenation in 97 Japanese patients and found that 90% experienced a reduction in pigmentation, 83% experienced an improvement in telangiectasia, and 65% experienced an improvement in texture after three treatment sessions. A cut-off filter of a shorter wavelength (550 nm, 28–32 J/cm^2 with a double pulse mode of 2.5–4.0/4.0–5.0 msec and a delay time of 20.0/40.0 msec between pulses) was used, and the epidermal melanin was affected, which led to a greater degree of reduction in pigmentation. The group observed no cases of PIH.

More recently, Huang et al. (32) used the same device and similar parameters (cut-off filter 550–590 nm, fluence 25–35 J/cm^2, with a single-pulse or double-pulse illumination and a pulse width of 4.0 msec) and treated 36 Chinese patients with freckles. Their findings indicated good to excellent results after a mean of 1.4 treatment sessions. The mean number of treatment sessions to achieve good results differed significantly from Negishi et al.'s work, as well as that of others, despite the use of similar parameters (Fig. 5). It is worthwhile to point out that the mechanism of action for IPL with a short-wavelength filter to remove lentigines is, to a certain degree, due to the lack of effective epidermal cooling. As epidermal melanin is affected by the photothermal property of the IPL, it is destroyed and removed. Consequently, to achieve the rapid resolution of lentigines in Asian patients with a more aggressive approach using the IPL, hypopigmentation (sometimes even a barlike appearance) can occur. One major disadvantage with the Vasculight IPL (Lumenis, Santa Clara, CA) is inadequacy in skin cooling. Cold gel is essential to protect the epidermis, and although it can provide some degree of protection, it can only offer parallel cooling and is by no means optimal . Furthermore, if the cold gel is applied to half of the face before IPL treatment, then the temperature of the cold gel cannot possibly be consistent, even with a speedy operator (Fig. 6) Negishi et al. avoided this problem by applying cold gel before each pulse, but the treatment sessions were substantially lengthened (26).

The IPL Quantum (Lumenis, Santa Clara) has also been extensively studied. Kawada et al. (27) examined 60 patients with solar lentigines or freckles and found a significant degree of improvement (50% or more reduction in pigment) in 68% after IPL treatment (560-nm filter, 20–24 J/cm^2, 2.6–5.0-msec pulse duration in double or triple pulses with pulse delays of 20 msec). Negishi et al. used the same device to treat 73 Japanese with photoaging (33). After the fifth treatment, a combined rating of greater than 60% improvement was given to more than 80% of patients for pigmentation, telangiectasia reduction or removal, smoother skin texture, and overall improvement. Furthermore, histological evaluations showed strong staining of type I and III collagen. Unlike Vasculight, the Quantum IPL has less variables and is more user friendly. Most importantly, the integrated contact cooling system of IPL Quantum allows optimal and consistent cooling. However, such optimal cooling can also be a disadvantage when used for the treatment of epidermal pigmentation. Excessive cooling reduces the photothermal effect, and more sessions are required for pigmentation removal. As stated in the earlier part of this chapter, our findings indicated that a combined approach with 1320-nm nonablative laser can be of particular value.

Many other IPL systems are now manufactured, and it is not possible to discuss them all in great detail (31). It is best to discuss systems that I am familiar with or for which there are preliminary data on Asian skin types. Ellipse Flex system (Danish Dermatologic Development, Hoersholm, Denmark) is an IPL system that was developed in Denmark and is only available in Europe and Asia. It consists of a dual-mode filtering system, which means that in addition to cut-off filters, it also consists of a water-filtering system in the applicator. The advantage of the water filtering system is that by removing water as a chromophobe, nonselective photothermal injury is reduced. Another advantage of this system is that it consists of multiple absorption peaks (542, 577, and 630 nm), and therefore further improves selectivity on targets such as melanin and hemoglobin. As water absorption is filtered out, it is more effective for the removal of pigment and telangiectasia than for wrinkle reduction. My experience indicates that it can be effective in pigment removal after three or four treatment sessions (Fig. 7).

Estelux (Palomar, Burlington, MA) is another IPL system that emits radiation from 510–1200 nm. It uses a coolroller to cool the skin surface. Its advantage, according to

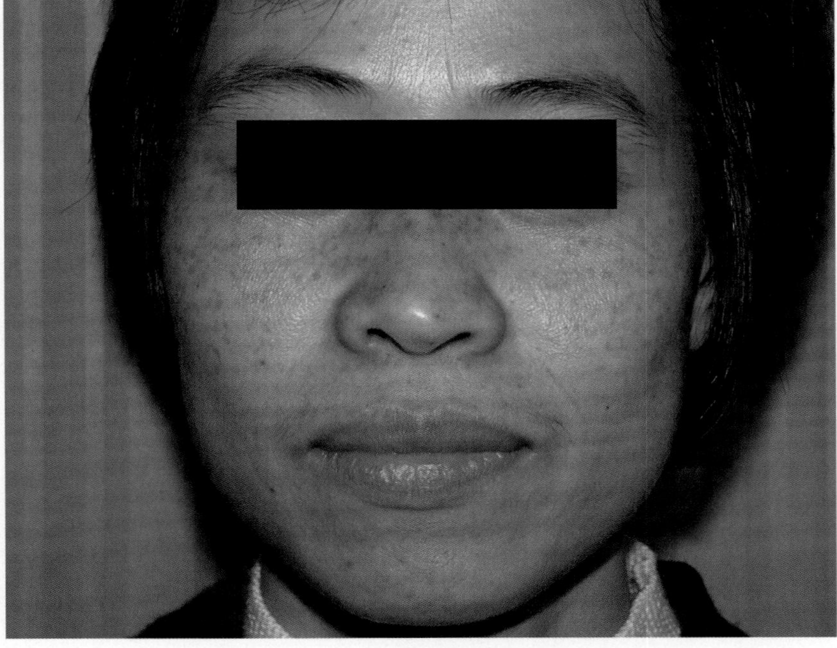

A

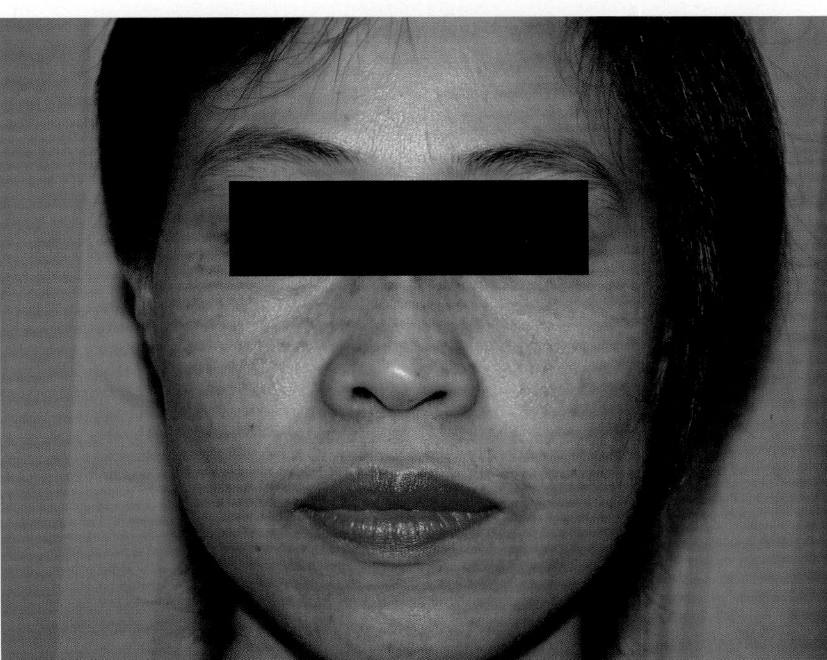

B

Figure 5 (A) Patients with lentigines before treatment. (B) After the eighth treatment with IPL (570-nm filter, 45 J/cm^2, pulse duration of 3.5 msec for T1 and T2, pulse delay of 20 msec). (A and B) Patient with rosacea before treatment.

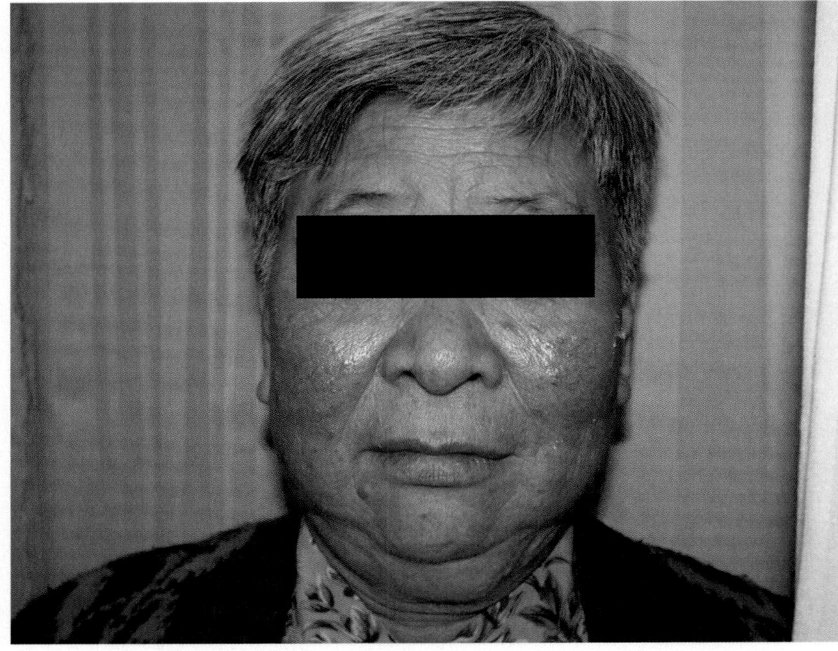

A

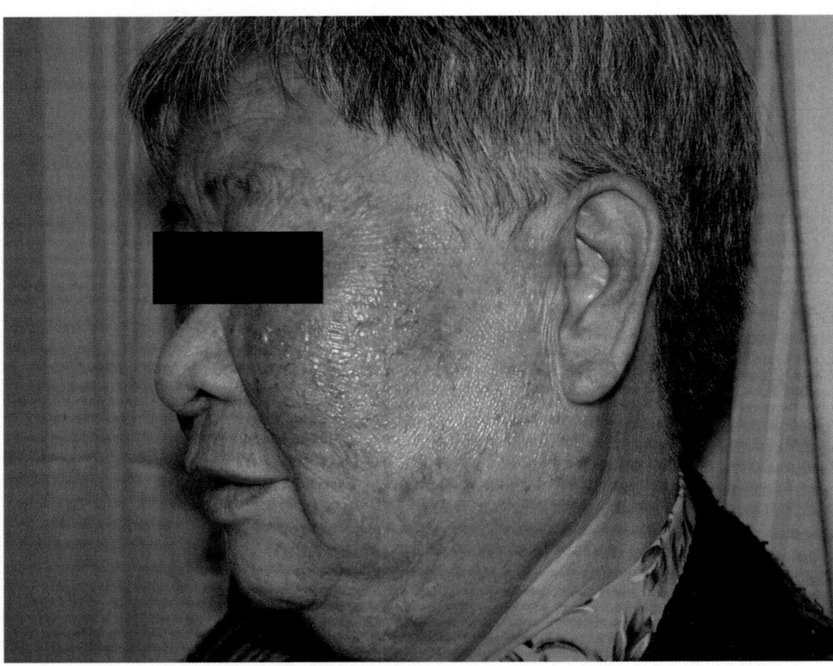

B

Figure 6 Before (A) and 1 week after (B) treatment with IPL (570-nm filter, 35–45 J/cm^2, duration of 3–4 msec for T1 and T2, pulse delay of 20 msec). (C and D) After the fourth treatment with IPL (570-nm filter, 35–45 J/cm^2, duration of 3–4 msec for T1 and T2, pulse delay of 20 msec).

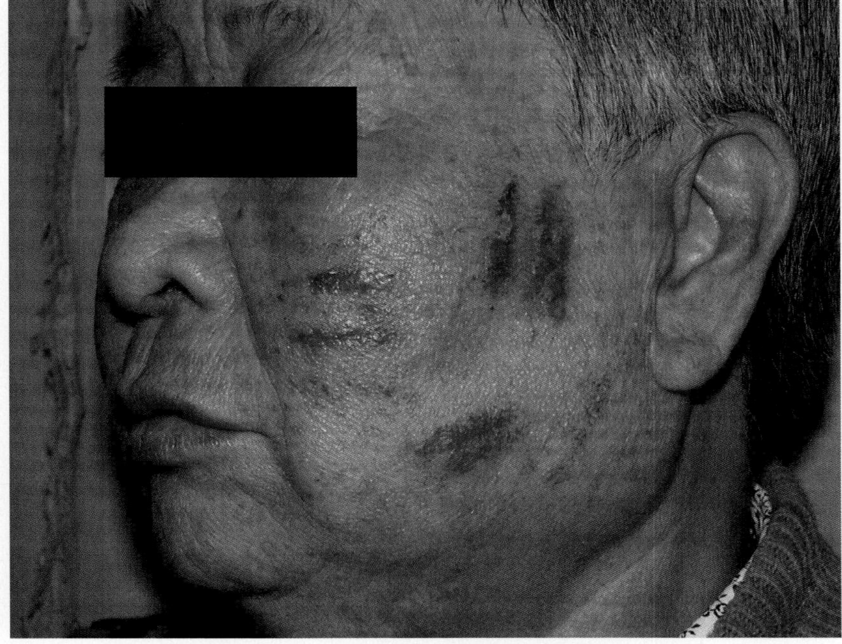

C

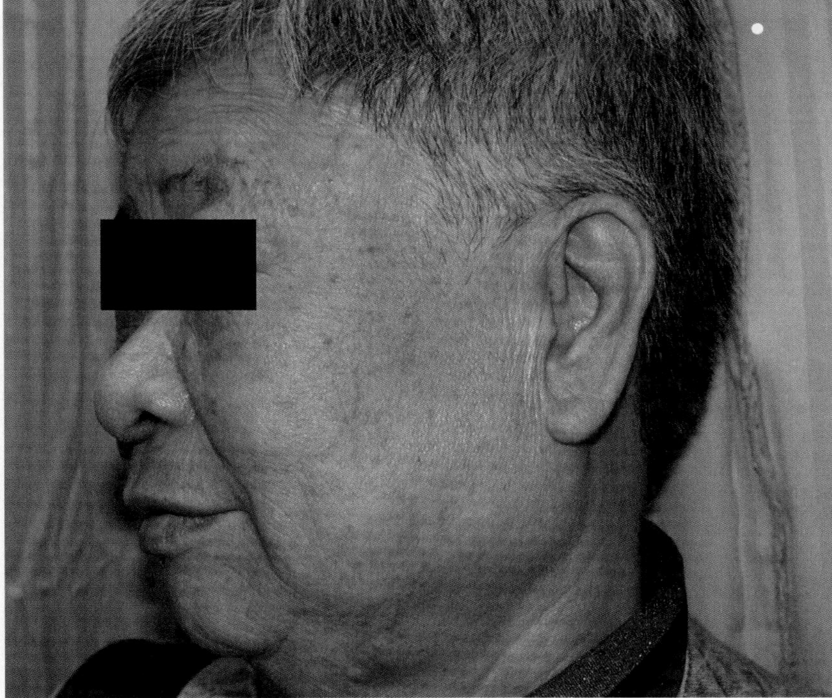

D

Figure 6 Continued.

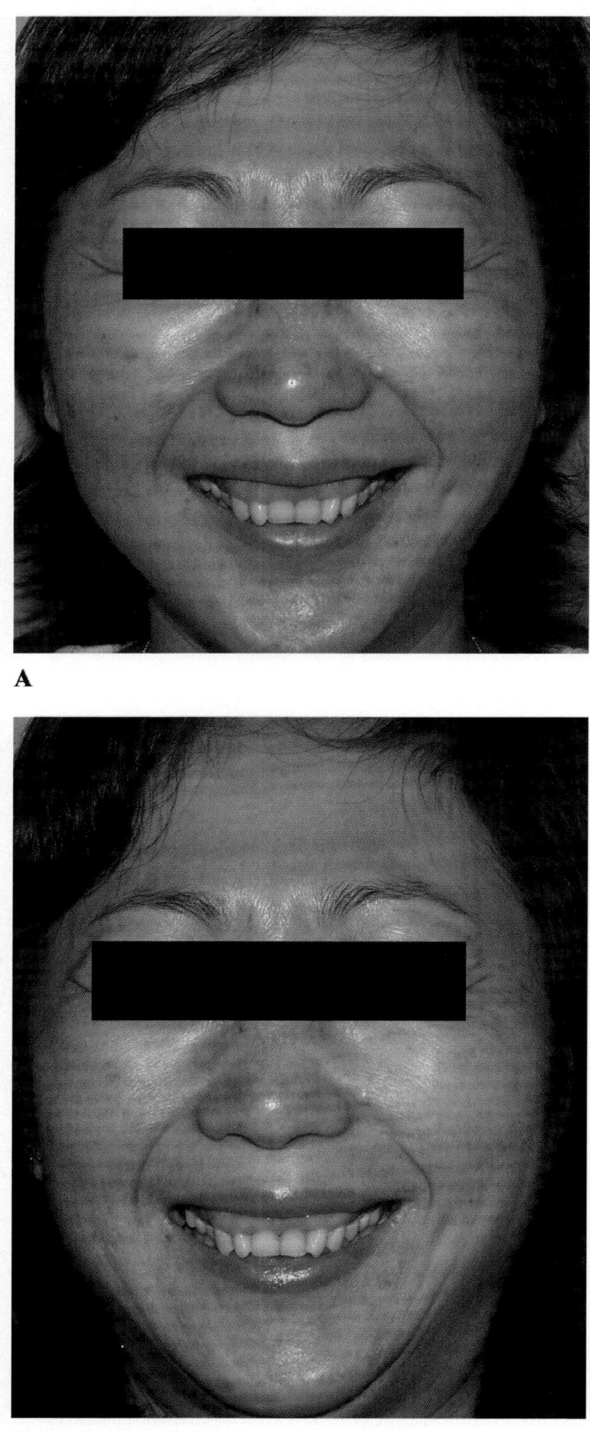

Figure 7 (A) Patients with lentigines before treatment. (B) After one treatment with IPL (Ellipse; VL-2 filter, 2.5-msec pulse time, 10-msec pulse delay, skin type IV, 9 J/cm^2).

the manufacturer, is that by emitting a continuous pulse width that ranges from 10–100 msec, the epidermal temperature rise is lower than multiple pulses, which allows a better safety margin. Further selectivity is achieved by fluence density that varies with wavelength.

Plasmalite is another IPL that emits a continuous light spectrum between 535 and 1000 nm. The system uses a dye-impregnated polymer cut-off filter (535, 550, 560, 580, and 615 nm) and a copolymer matrix filter to block infrared light ($>$ 1000 nm) from the gas-filled flashlamp. A Thai study looked at its use in 201 patients with a wide range of skin conditions, including photoaging, hypertrophic scarring, PIH, freckles, acquired bilateral nevus of Ota-like macules and melasma. Post-treatment hyperpigmentation occurred in eight cases. The response to treatment depended on the condition, and although the device was considered to be moderately effective for photorejuvenation in Asians, it was less effective for epidermal hyperpigmentation. The melasma response was the least satisfactory, with worsening of hyperpigmentation in 16.67% of patients (N. Polnikorn, personal communication, 2002). The main disadvantage of this system is that it is very manual and one must change the lamps when switching from the photorejuvenation mode to the hair-removal mode. Cooling is also inadequate and may lead to the high risk of complication that was observed in this study.

THE USE OF LASER AND IPL FOR NONABLATIVE SKIN REJUVENATION IN ASIANS: A PRACTICAL APPROACH

Although IPL can be effective in the removal of lentigines in Asians, the number of treatment sessions (four to six) that are required to achieve the desired effect raises the issue of cost effectiveness (34). Patients are therefore informed in detail about the advantages and disadvantages of IPL and lasers for the treatment of lentigines. The lack of downtime that is associated with the use of IPL can be attractive to some. The fact that IPL can also lead to the improvement of rhytides is of particular advantage. For those in whom the main concern is lentigines or cost effectiveness, test areas with a laser device are performed. If the outcome for lentigines clearance is satisfactory then the patient is advised to undergo full face treatment. Excellent results may be achieved after one or two sessions. However, if PIH develops at the test sites, then IPL is suggested.

It is necessary to emphasize the importance of pretreatment preparation, including the use of topical bleaching agents such as topical hydroquinone cream, vitamins C and E, and adequate sun block, and it is part of my practice to start patients on these preparations at least 2 weeks before their laser/IPL procedure. I also advise patients to resume such treatment as soon as possible, which is usually 5–7 days after laser/IPL surgery, when the epidermal crusting falls off.

RADIOFREQUENCY AND SKIN REJUVENATION

Radiofrequency differs significantly from laser surgery in the sense that instead of targeting a particular chromophobe, it involves the passage of an electrical current leading to volumetric tissue heating. Tissue is heated depending on the degree of its resistance to electron movement. To protect the epidermis, simultaneous contact skin cooling is necessary. The advantage of radiofrequency is that the operator can control the depth and the amount of energy that is delivered, and skin type will not influence the effect, which is a major advantage when used in the treatment of photoaging in Asians.

Ruiz-Esparza et al. (35) studied the use of a radiofrequency device (ThermaCool, Thermage, Haywood, CA) in performing medical face lifts on 15 patients with treatments areas that included periauricular skin, the temporal area, and the submental regions. Their findings indicated that 14 of 15 patients obtained cosmetic improvement from facial skin tightening with visible results as early as 1 week and generally within 3 months after the procedure without wounding or scarring. Other devices combine the use of radiofrequency with IPL, but limited data are available regarding these devices.

ACQUIRED BILATERAL NEVUS OF OTA-LIKE MACULES (ABNOM OR HORI MACULES)

Acquired bilateral nevus of Ota-like macules (ABNOM), or Hori macules, is an Asian condition that affects about 0.8% of the population (36). Clinically, ABNOM presents as bluish hyperpigmentation that usually affects the bilateral malar regions. Other areas can also be involved, including the temples, the root of the nose, the alae nasi, the eyelids, and the forehead. Unlike in nevus of Ota, the pigmentation in ABNOM occurs in a symmetrical bilateral fashion, has a late onset in adulthood, and does not involve the mucosa. Like other dermal melanocytosis, treatment modalities such as chemical peels and dermabrasion are either ineffective or associated with a higher risk of scarring.

The use of QS lasers has generated much interest. In 1999, Kunachak et al. (37) examined a series of patients who had been treated with a QS ruby laser (fluence 7–10 J/cm^2 at a repetition rate of 1 Hz and spot size of 2–4 mm). Their findings confirmed the effectiveness of the QS ruby laser, with complete clearance observed in over 90% of the patients. There was no recurrence after 6 months to 4.3 years (with a mean of 2.5 years) of follow up. Postinflammatory hyperpigmentation was common, and affected 7% of their patients. The QS 1064-nm Nd:YAG laser is also effective (38,39).

Postinflammatory hyperpigmentation is common, and affects 50–73% of patients. More recently, my group conducted a retrospective analysis of 32 female Chinese patients who underwent treatment with QS alexandrite laser (755 nm, spot size 3 mm, 8 J/cm^2) (40). Topical hydroquinone and tretinoin cream were given to those patients with hyperpigmentation after laser surgery. With a mean of seven treatment sessions (range, two to 11 sessions), and a mean treatment interval of 33 days, two observers identified over 80% of the patients as having more than 50% clearing, and they identified complete clearance in more than 28% of the patients (Fig. 8). Hyperpigmentation occurred in 12.5% of the patients, but in all cases it resolved after treatment with hypopigmenting topical medications. Both our study and those of others indicated a high risk of PIH when laser is used for the treatment of ABNOM. Hence, all patients should be given preoperative and postoperative topical bleaching agents.

In my experience, ABNOM tends to be more resistant to therapy. Consequently, our group, as well as others, have started treating such patients more frequently with repeat laser procedures every 4 weeks. The idea behind such an aggressive approach is to treat the area before epidermal repigmentation occurs. In doing so, more laser energy can reach the dermal target chromophore through a hypopigmented epidermis without the competitive absorption of epidermal melanin. For resistant cases (failure to improve after four treatment sessions), QS alexandrite laser treatment is followed immediately by QS Nd:YAG laser treatment. The fluence should be lower (4–5 J/cm^2 for both lasers), and the repetition rate should be reduced (to no more than 3.3Hz) to reduce the risk of adverse

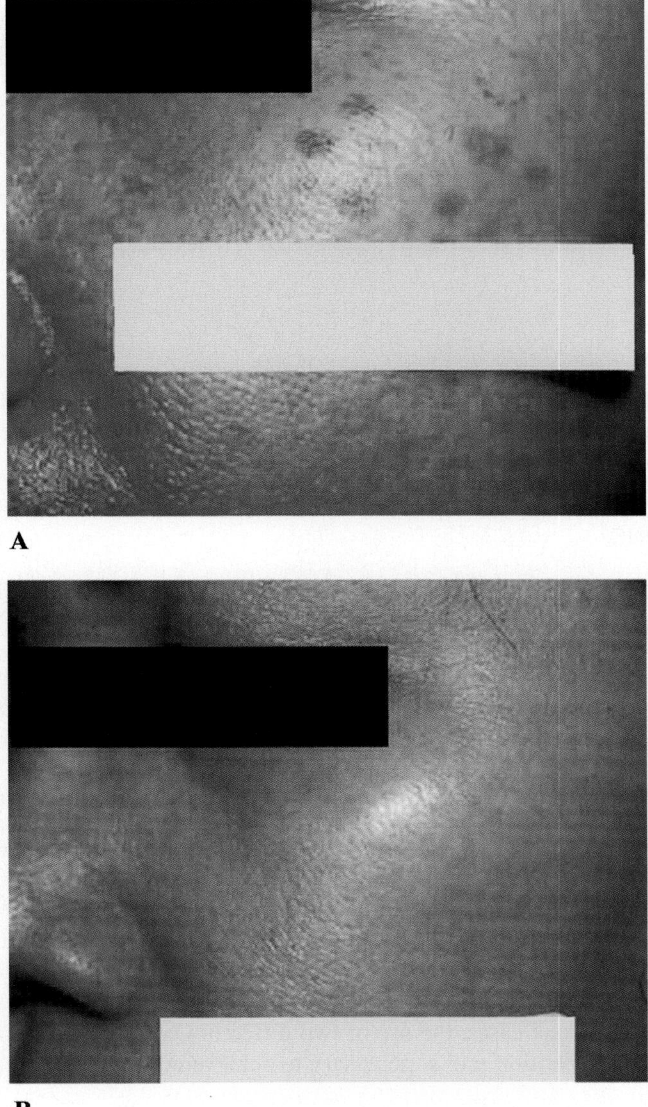

Figure 8 (A) Acquired bilateral nevus of Ota-like macules before laser treatment. (B) After the ninth treatment with QS alexandrite laser (8 J/cm^2).

Table 4 Key Points

◆ Long-wavelength lasers should be used for the improvement of wrinkles and skin texture in Asians.
◆ Long-pulse (532 nm) lasers and IPL are effective for removal of lentigines in Asians and are associated with a lower risk of PIH.
◆ For ABNOM, shorter treatment interval and, if necessary, the use of two different QS lasers in the same treatment interval can lead to an excellent outcome.

effects. Nevertheless, transitory pigmentary disturbance is not uncommon, and patients should be warned of this prior to their treatment. Although there are claims that IPL can be used for the treatment of dermal pigmentation such as tattoos, it is my experience that this approach can be associated with a high risk of scarring.

CONCLUSIONS

Use nonablative lasers targeted for water only for the treatment of wrinkles. Suggestions for treatment are summarized in Table 4. Long-wavelength lasers should be used for the improvement of wrinkles and skin texture in Asians. Both 1320-nm Nd:YAG and 1540-nm erbium glass lasers appear to be effective for such purposes. Unless the issue of the optimal cooling parameters is resolved, the 1450-nm diode laser can be associated with a higher risk of PIH and should not be used for nonablative skin rejuvenation in Asians.

Lentigines Respond to IPL and Long-Pulse 532-nm Laser Treatment

The photomechanical effects of QS lasers can be associated with a higher risk of PIH when used for the treatment of lentigines in Asians. Long-pulse 532-nm Nd:YAG lasers and IPL are effective to remove lentigines, although the latter requires several treatment sessions, which may impact on cost effectiveness. The lack of downtime for IPL and the knowledge that IPL can also lead to the improvement of rhytides are particular advantages. For ABNOM, QS lasers used in a short treatment interval (4 weekly) can lead to good response, but for resistant cases, the use of two different QS lasers in the same treatment session with a low repetition rate is necessary to achieve an excellent clinical outcome.

REFERENCES

1. Chung JH, Lee SH, Youn CS, Park BJ, Kim KH, Park KC, Cho KH, Eun HC. Cutaneous photodamage in Koreans: influence of sex, sun exposure, smoking, and skin color. Arch Dermatol 2001; 137:1043–1051.
2. Sun CC, Lu YC, Lee EF, Nakagawa H. Naevus fusco-caeruleus zygomaticus. Br J Dermatol 1987; 1:545–553.
3. Chan HH, Chan E, Kono T, Ying SY, Ho WS. The use of variable pulse width frequency double neodymium: YAG 532 nm laser in the treatment of port wine stain in Chinese. Dermatol Surg 2000; 26:657–661.
4. Chiu CH, Chan HH, Ho WS, Yeung CK, Nelson JS. Prospective study of pulsed dye laser in conjunction with cryogen spray cooling for treatment of port wine stains in Chinese patients. Dermatol Surg:In press.

5. Goldberg DJ, Whitworth J. Laser skin resurfacing with the Q-switched Nd:YAG laser. Dermatol Surg 1997; 23:903–906.
6. Goldberg DJ, Silapunt S. Q-switched Nd:YAG laser: rhytid improvement by non-ablative dermal remodeling. J Cutan Laser Ther 2000; 2:157–160.
7. Chan HH, Leung RS, Ying SY, Lai CF, Kono T, Chua JK, Ho WS. A retrospective study looking at the complications of Q-switched alexandrite (QS Alex) and Q-switched neodymium: yttrium-aluminum-garnet (QS Nd-YAG) lasers in the treatment of nevus of Ota. Dermatol Surg 2000; 26:1000–1006.
8. Lee MW. Combination visible and infrared lasers for skin rejuvenation. Semin Cutan Med Surg 2002; 21:288–300.
9. Trelles MA, Allones I, Luna R. Facial rejuvenation with a non-ablative 1320 nm Nd:YAG laser: a preliminary clinical and histologic evaluation. Dermatol Surg 2001; 27:111–116.
10. Goldberg DJ, Samady JA. Intense pulsed light and Nd:YAG laser non-ablative treatment of facial rhytids. Lasers Surg Med 2001; 28:141–144.
11. Hardaway CA, Ross EV, Paithankar DY. Non-ablative cutaneous remodeling with a 1.45 microm mid-infrared diode laser: phase II. J Cosmet Laser Ther 2002; 4:9–14.
12. Tanzi EL, Williams CM, Alster TS. Treatment of facial rhytides with a nonablative 1,450-nm diode laser: a controlled clinical and histologic study. Dermatol Surg 2003; 29:124–128.
13. Ross EV, Sajben FP, Hsia J, Barnette D, Miller CH, McKinlay JR. Nonablative skin remodeling: selective dermal heating with a mid-infrared laser and contact cooling combination. Lasers Surg Med 2000; 26:186–195.
14. Levy JL, Besson R, Mordon S. Determination of optimal parameters for laser for nonablative remodeling with a 1.54 microm Er:glass laser: a dose-response study. Dermatol Surg 2002; 28:405–409.
15. Fournier N, Dahan S, Barneon G, Rouvrais C, Diridollou S, Lagarde JM, Mordon S. Nonablative remodeling: a 14-month clinical ultrasound imaging and profilometric evaluation of a 1540 nm Er:Glass laser. Dermatol Surg 2002; 28:926–931.
16. Goldberg DJ. Benign pigmented lesions of the skin: treatment with Q-switched ruby laser. J Dermatol Surg Oncol 1993; 19:376–379.
17. Grekin RC, Shelton RM, Geisse JK, Frieded I. 510-nm pigmented lesion dye laser: its characteristics and clinical uses. J Dermatol Surg Oncol 1993; 19:380–387.
18. Kilmer SL, Wheeland RG, Goldberg DJ, Anderson RR. Treatment of epidermal pigmented lesions with the frequency-doubled Q-switched Nd:YAG laser. A controlled, single impact, dose-response, multicenter trial. Arch Dermatol 1994; 130:1515–1519.
19. Murphy MJ, Huang MY. Q-switched ruby laser treatment of benign pigmented lesions in Chinese skin. Ann Acad Med Singapore 1994; 23:60–66.
20. Chan HH, Fung WKK, Ying SY, Kono T. An in vivo trial comparing the use of different types of 532 nm Neodymium: yttrium-aluminum-garnet (Nd:YAG) lasers in the treatment of facial lentigines in Oriental patients. Dermatol Surg 2000; 26:743–749.
21. Anderson RR, Parish JA. Selective photothermolysis: Precise microsurgery by selective absorption of pulsed radiation. Science 1983; 220:524.
22. Carome EF, Clark NA, Moeler CE. Generation of acoustic signal in liquids by ruby laser-induced thermal stress transients. Appl Phys Lett 1964; 4:95–97.
23. Anderson RR, Margolis RJ, Watenabe S. Selective photothermolysis of cutaneous pigmentation by Q-switched Nd:YAG laser pulses at 1064, 532, and 355 nm. J Invest Dermatol 1989; 93: 28–32.
24. Dover JS, Margolis RJ, Polla LL. Pigmented guineas pig skin irradiated with Q-switched ruby laser pulses: morphologic and histologic findings. Arch Dermatol 1989; 125:43–49.
25. Rashid T, Hussain I, Haider M, Haroon TS. Laser therapy of freckles and lentigines with quasi-continuous, frequency-doubled, Nd:YAG(532nm) laser in Fitzpatrick skin type IV: a 24 month follow up. J Cosmet Laser Ther 2002; 4:81–85.

26. Negishi K, Tezuka Y, Kudshikata N, Wakamatsu S. Photorejuvenation for Asian skin by intense pulsed light. Dermatol Surg 2001; 27:627–632.
27. Kawada A, Shiraishi H, Asai M, Kameyama H, Sangen Y, Aragane Y, Tezuka T. Clinical improvement of solar lentigines and ephelides with an intense pulsed light source. Dermatol Surg 2002; 28:504–508.
28. Anderson RR, Parish JA. The optics of human skin. J Invest Dermatol 1981; 77:13–19.
29. Trelles MA, Verkruysse W, Pickering JW. Monoline argon laser (514 nm) treatment of benign pigmented lesions with long pulse lengths. J Photochem Photobiol 1992; 16:357–365.
30. Margolis RJ, Dover JS, Polla LL. Visible action spectrum for melanin-specific selective photothermolysis. Lasers Surg Med 1989; 9:389–397.
31. Raulin C, Greve B, Grema H. IPL technology: a review. Lasers Surg Med 2003; 32:78–87.
32. Huang YL, Liao YL, Lee SH, Hong HS. Intense pulsed light for the treatment of facial freckles in Asian skin. Dermatol Surg 2002; 28:1007–1012.
33. Negishi K, Wakamatsu S, Kushikata N, Tezuka Y, Kotani Y, Shiba K. Full-face photorejuvenation of photodamaged skin by intense pulsed light with integrated contact cooling: initial experiences in Asian patients. Lasers Surg Med 2002; 30:298–305.
34. Chan HH, Murad A, Kono T, Dover J. Clinical application of lasers in Asians. Dermatol Surg 2002; 28:556–563.
35. Ruiz-Esparza J, Gomez JB. The medical face lift: a noninvasive, nonsurgical approach to tissue tightening in facial skin using nonablative radiofrequency. Dermatol Surg 2003; 29:325–332.
36. Sun CC, Lu YC, Lee EF, Nakagawa H. Naevus fusco-caeruleus zygomaticus. Br J Dermatol 1987; 1:545–553.
37. Kunachak S, Leelaudomlipi P, Sirikulchayanonta V. Q-Switched ruby laser therapy of acquired bilateral nevus of Ota-like macules. Dermatol Surg 1999; 25:938–941.
38. Kunachak S, Leelaudomlipi P. Q-switched Nd:YAG laser treatment for acquired bilateral nevus of Ota-like maculae: a long-term follow-up. Lasers Surg Med 2000; 26:376–379.
39. Polnikorn N, Tanrattanakorn S, Goldberg DJ. Treatment of Hori's nevus with the Q-switched Nd:YAG laser. Dermatol Surg 2000; 26:477–480.
40. Lam AY, Wong DS, Lam LK, Ho WS, Chan HH. A retrospective study on the efficacy and complications of Q-switched alexandrite laser in the treatment of acquired bilateral nevus of Ota-like macules. Dermatol Surg 2001; 27:937–941.

20

Treatment of Photoaging in African American and Hispanic Patients

Susan C. Taylor *College of Physicians and Surgeons, Columbia University, New York, New York, U.S.A.*

Nicole M. DeYampert *St. Luke's-Roosevelt Hospital Center, New York, New York, U.S.A.*

- Photoaging among African Americans and Hispanics is less pronounced than that seen in white-skinned individuals.
- Fine wrinkling, pigmentary inconsistencies, skin textural changes, and benign cutaneous growths are the most commonly observed characteristics of photoaging in this population.
- The therapeutic modalities used to address photoaging in African Americans and Hispanics are often less invasive than those that address the needs of individuals with photodamaged white skin.
- A variety of modalities are used to improve the appearance of aging African American and Hispanic skin and include topical, oral, and resurfacing agents, as well as fillers and neuromuscular relaxers.
- Postinflammatory hyperpigmentation and scarring are possible adverse events that must be considered when selecting therapeutic modalities to address aging in this population.

There appears to be a racial and ethnic differential in the development of photaging with African Americans and Hispanics, with Fitzpatrick skin phototypes IV–VI displaying less susceptibility. Although hereditary factors may be involved, these differences are most likely related to the protective properties of widespread epidermal melanosomal dispersion and increased melanin content in these racial and ethnic groups (1). Photoaging among African Americans and Hispanics does occur, but it is more pronounced in individuals with lighter skin hues (2). Additionally, the characteristics of photoaging tend to occur at a more advanced age in African Americans as compared to whites (3). Unlike white skin, where deep wrinkles, furrows, yellow skin discoloration, discrete solar lentigines, flat seborrheic dermatoses, ephelides, and cellular atypia manifested as actinic keratosis are present, these characteristics of photoaging are less apparent in the African American and Hispanic populations (4). The features of photoaging that are most often apparent in the racial and ethnic groups include fine wrinkling, pigmentary inconsistencies, skin textural changes, and the development of benign cutaneous growths. In addition, characteristics of intrinsic aging are apparent in racial and ethnic skin and manifest as loss of support of the skin with gravity-dependent sagging, laxity of skin, and prominence of the lines of facial expression. To improve the appearance of the maturing African American or Hispanic patient, treatment strategies designed to address both the components of extrinsic and intrinsic aging are necessary. The selection of appropriate treatment modalities will depend on the extent of damage, with less invasive techniques and treatments often sufficing in this patient population.

PHOTOAGING VS. INTRINSIC AGING

Although there are genetic differences in intrinsic aging of the skin, this type of aging seemingly should not differ significantly with race or ethnicity. Intrinsically aged skin is characteristically smooth, without pigmentary changes but with prominent lines of expression. Histologically, intrinsic aging displays atropy of both the epidermal and dermal layers of the skin as well as flattening of the epidermal rete ridges (5). A loss of skin elasticity occurs with gravitational forces, leading to sagging of the skin. This sagging is most apparent in dependent portions of the skin, especially the neck and jawline areas. Sagging of the malar fat pads toward the nasolabial folds is a characteristic feature in African Americans (6). Lines of expression become apparent in areas of repetitive muscle movements such as the forehead, glabella, and periocular and perioral areas. Bone resorption in the face adds to skin laxity and facial fat atropy may result in concavity in the temple and central cheek areas.

In contrast, photoaging is characterized in white skin by a constellation of changes, which include wrinkling, coarseness, sallow complexion, and laxity of the skin coupled with generalized mottling, solar lentigines, flat seborrheic keratosis, ephelides, and telangiectasias (4). In racial and ethnic skin, fine wrinkling of the skin may appear in those individuals with lighter skin hues, especially in those Hispanics who have lighter skin. Crow's feet or periorbital lines are seen more often that lipstick lines or fine perioral lines in African Americans. Inconsistent pigmentation is noted in African Americans and Hispanics, and appears as uneven hyperpigmentation or, in some cases, an overall darker facial complexion as compared to the skin on non–sun-exposed sites.

HISTOLOGIC DIFFERENCES IN PHOTOAGING IN AFRICAN AMERICANS AND WHITES

Montagna et al. (7) performed the only racial comparative study of the morphology of the skin of black and white women. Histological analysis of the skin of the malar eminences of the faces of 19 black and 19 white women was performed. Although histological evaluation of the skin of some of the 19 black women analyzed revealed an entirely normal epidermis, in others vacuoles and dyskeratosis were present in the keratinocytes of the malpighian layer. These alterations were reported to be similar to those observed in white skin. However, white epidermis showed frequent focal areas of atropy and/or necrosis, and mild atrophy was observed in only one of the 19 black women (age range of these subjects was 22 to 50 years). Since characteristics of photoaging are observed at later ages in blacks, it would be valuable to obtain this data from black women older than 50 years in whom the epidermal changes of atropy and necrosis might be observed. Furthermore, in the one patient in whom these changes were observed, they were characterized as mild, which is consistent with clinical observation.

Elastosis was not observed in the specimens of any of the black subjects in contrast to variable amounts of moderate to extensive elastosis seen in whites. However, dermal changes were observed in the older black subjects. There was an increase in the number and thickness of elastic fibers in the reticular dermis. Elastic fibers, configured in single strands in younger black subjects, appeared in thicker braidlike configurations in those 50-year-old subjects. In addition, it was reported that the amount and distribution of elastic fibers in the skin of a 45-year-old light-skinned black woman resembled those in white women, as did the staining pattern of the elastic fibers. Areas of elastic fibrolysis were small in this light-skinned black woman. These data support the clinical observation that photoaging is more prominent in lighter-skinned African Americans, but even in this group the characteristics are mild. Finally, most of the older white women in the study had wrinkles besides the lateral canthi (crow's feet), and on the corners of the mouth; none the 19 black women ages 50 years and younger had obvious wrinkles.

The Montagna data revealed that entire epidermis of blacks contained greater numbers of melanosomes, and that the distribution of melanosomes was similar regardless of age. This distribution was felt to account for protection from severe photodamage. Melanophages in black dermis were more numerous and larger that in white dermis. Melanophages were observed to become progressively smaller in the deeper dermis and additionally, small melanosome-containing macrophages were seen in the dermis of black skin. We have clinically observed pigmentary abnormalities associated with photoaging in the darker racial and ethnic groups. Although age related differences in the number of dermal melanophages or in the amount of melanin contained within the melanosomes were not reported in this study, one might suspect that they do occur and this would support the observation of increased pigmentation associated with advancing age in blacks.

Resorbtion of elastotic tissue and replacement with collagen fiber bundles and other elastotic fibers is felt to cause shrinking of the dermal volume of the skin. In the Montagna study, this reduction was reported to occur less precipitiously in the facial skin of young and middle-aged black women. This finding of resorption would explain in part the development of facial concavity and laxity of the skin observed in women of color.

Histological studies of photoaging in the Hispanic population are not available. It may be surmised that photoaging in darker Hispanics may be similar to that in African Americans.

When analyzing the characteristics of aging common to African American and Hispanic skin, four distinct components are apparent: inconsistent pigmentation, fine wrinkling, sagging and volume loss. Pigmentation disorders may be addressed with sun protection products, topical creams, peeling agents or microdermabrasion. The often mild and superficial rhytids can be ameliorated with chemical peeling agents, topical agents, botulinum toxin, fillers as well as more aggressive modalities such as lasers or dermabrasion. Sagging of the skin is addressed with botulinum toxin, fat transfer or surgical lifting. The loss of volume of the skin can be ameliorated with dermal fillers substances such as collagen, hyaluronic acid or autologous fat transfer.

TOPICAL TREATMENTS IN AFRICAN AMERICAN AND HISPANIC PATIENTS

A hallmark of photoaging in black and Hispanic skin is inconsistent pigmentation, which is characterized by mottled and confluent hyperpigmentation as well as a general darkening of the sun-exposed skin. One would expect that lasers that selectively target and destroy epidermal pigment, 510-nm pigmented lesion dye laser, 511-nm copper-vapor laser, 514-nm argon laser, 694-nm ruby laser, and the 755-nm alexandrite, would be appropriate for the treatment of hyperpigmentation associated with photoaging in individuals with skin of color (6). Laser-stimulated melanogenesis leading to hyperpigmentation as well as laser-induced melanocyte injury leading to hypopigmentation, known adverse events associated with laser therapy, most likely limit laser therapy as a frequently used therapeutic modality for the treatment of the pigmentation inconsistencies (8). Consequently, we rely on topical therapy for photoaging associated pigmentation abnormalities. As previously discussed, photoaging in black and Hispanic skin is not as severe as compared to white skin. Therefore, superficial rhytids, when present, are also ameliorated with topical agents obviating the need for more aggressive therapeutic modalities such as laser resurfacing.

Broad Spectrum Sunscreens

The characteristics of photoaging are primarily due to the effects on the epidermis and dermis of ultraviolet (UV) irradiation. Ultraviolet radiation has been demonstrated to decrease collagen production and up-regulate metalloproteinases, enzymes which degrade collagen (9). These effects lead to wrinkling of the skin. Ultraviolet irradiation also increases the number of melanocytes that are actively producing melanin, each melanocyte is stimulated to produce more melanin and increased melanosome transfer from melanocytes to keratinocytes occurs (10). Along with dermal pigment incontinence, this most likely accounts for the pigmentary inconsistencies observed in photoaged black and Hispanic skin.

Both the pigmentary aspect of photoaging and wrinkling may be decreased or prevented by blocking both ultraviolet UVA and UVB radiation. This is achieved with the daily application of broad-spectrum sunscreens. Active ingredients in sunscreens that block UVB include para-aminobenzoic acid, octyl methoxycinnamate, and octyl salicylate. Protection from the entire range of UVA may require several active ingredients. Ultraviolet A-2 radiation is blocked by oxybenzone and titanium dioxide, while UVA-1 radiation is blocked by avobenzone and zinc oxide. For individuals with darker skin to achieve full protection, chemical sunscreens containing an ingredient from both groups is necessary. The physical blocker, titanium dioxide, which blocks UVB and UVA-2, provides the best protection from ultraviolet radiation of the sunscreens which are available. Although micronized products are available, they often impart a whitish or purplish appearance to darker skin which is not cosmetically acceptable to many patients.

Retinoids

It has been well demonstrated that retinoids prevent and treat photoaging in individuals with white skin. Histological examination of white skin treated with either 0.1% or 0.025% tretinoin cream revealed resolution of cellular atypia, a more compact stratum corneum, less clumping of melanin in basal cells and a more orderly differentiation of keratinocytes (11). Ultrastructurally, there was evidence of hyperproliferation of keratinocytes. In addition, retinoids have been demonstrated to increase collagen synthesis and partially restores type I collagen.

The findings of a study by Bulengo-Ransby et al. (12), who evaluated the efficacy of tretinoin for the treatment of hyperpigmented lesions in 68 black subjects, provide insight into the effects of retinoids for photoaging in this patient population. Histologic examination of black skin treated for 40 weeks with topical tretinoin revealed significant increases in the degree of compaction of the stratum corneum, the thickness of the granular-cell layer, epidermal thickness, mitotic figures, and spongiosis as compared with vehicle. Epidermal melanin content was noted to decrease in the tretinoin group as compared to the vehicle group. There was clinical lightening of the hyperpigmented lesions after 40 weeks of treatment and a clinically minimal but statistically significant lightening of the subject's normal skin as well. This study demonstrates that tretinoin is effective for the treatment of hyperpigmentation in blacks and also induces histological changes associated with improvement in other parameters of photoaging.

Hydroquinones

The use of topical products containing hydroquinones is effective therapeutic modality for the treatment of a variety of pigmentary disorders including the pigmentary inconsistencies associated with photoaging. Hydroquinones target the function and proliferation of melanocytes as well as the structure, function and degradation of melanosomes. Direct melanocyte injury, inhibition of enzymatic oxidation (via tyrosinase) of tyrosine to dihydroxyphenylalanine (DOPA) and the subsequent synthesis of melanin, formation of abnormally melanized melanosomes, and increased degraded of the melanosome packages after transfer into adjacent keratinocytes have been demonstrated in vivo with hydroquinone (13).

Hydroquinone has been used for the treatment of various types of dyschromias, in particular postinflammatory hyperpigmentation, melasma, and UV-induced dyschromia. Sanchez and Vazquez (14) among others demonstrated significant improvement in melasma using 3% hydroquinone in the treatment of 46 women with melasma. Ruiz-Maldonado and Orozco-Covarrubias (15) recommended 2–4% hydroquinone for treatment of postinflammatory hyperpigmentation for 3–6 months duration. Glenn et al. (16) demonstrated that 6% hydroquinone solution produced a statistically significant lightening in various pigmentary disorders as compared to 3% hydroquinone.

As with most pigmentary disorders, the pigmentation associated with photoaging requires the application of the hydroquinone twice daily directly to the area of involvement for approximately 3 months. Although in general well tolerated, allergic and irritant contact dermatitis may develop with exposure to hydroquinones. Finally, hydroquinone use infrequently results in the development of ochronosis.

Other Depigmenting Agents

Azelaic acid and kojic acid are alternative depigmenting agents that can be used in individuals who are allergic to hydroquinones. Hyperactive cells display increased uptake of azelaic acid, which is toxic to the cells. Kojic acid is a fungal metabolite found in *Aspergilline oryzae*. Kojic acid induces skin depigmentation through suppression of free tyrosinase, mainly due to chelation of its cooper. Kojic acid may have a high sensitizing potential. Unlike hydroquinone, there is no risk of exogenous ochronosis with azeleic or kojic acid.

Combination Therapy

Fleischer demonstrated that the combination of 2% 4-hydroxyanisole (Mequinol) and 0.01% tretinoin was found superior to either active component for the treatment of solar lentigines and related hyperpigmented lesions (17). In the combination group, moderate improvement or better was achieved in 52% on the forearms and 56% on the face, compared to the tretinoin-alone group, which demonstrated 24% and 33% improvement. Adverse events included redness, burning, stinging, and desquamation of the skin.

Taylor demonstrated that the combination of hydroquinone 4%, tretinoin 0.05%, and fluocinolone acetonide 0.01% resulted in complete or near-complete clearing of melasma in 641 subjects after 8 weeks of treatment (18). Adverse events included redness, desquamation, burning, and dryness of the skin

ORAL TREATMENTS FOR PHOTOAGING IN HISPANIC PATIENTS

Hernandez-Perez et al. (19) reported the use of oral isotretinoin as an adjunct treatment for cutaneous aging in 60 Hispanic patients from San Salvador, El Salvador. The parameters assessed included improvement in wrinkles, discoloration, thickness, oiliness, size of follicular pores, and general improvement of the skin. Subjects were evaluated by two medical observers and via a patient self-assessment for a minimum of 6 months after the end of the study. The 50 subjects were divided into two groups: group A received a 2-month course of thrice-weekly isotretinoin (dose range, 10–20 mg) following cosmetic surgery, whereas group B received cosmetic surgery alone.

The patients in both groups underwent a vast array of cosmetic and surgical procedures. These procedures included chemical peels, topical α-hydroxy acid products and tretinoin, botulinum toxin, collagen injections, blepharoplasty, liposuction, fat transfer, and/or face lift. Of the patients in group A who received isotretinoin, self-assessment revealed improvement in wrinkles, thickness and color of the skin, size of pores, as well as general improvement in the skin as compared to group B. The skin was reportedly smooth and lighter in color, with improved skin tone and elasticity. The physician parameters assessed likewise demonstrated significant improvement in the skin of group A patients as compared with group B. Adverse events were minimal, with mucocutaneous xerosis reported in less that 10% of cases. There were no reports of excessive scar tissue or exuberant healing. The overall study design, with various surgical and cosmetic procedures, makes it difficult to truly distinguish the effects of the procedures from that of the oral isotretinoin. Nonetheless, given the data supporting the positive effect of topical retinoid on photoaging, it seems likely that oral retinoids may have a very similar effect.

LASER TREATMENT FOR PHOTOAGING IN BLACK AND HISPANIC PATIENTS

Pigmentation changes, both hyperpigmentation and hypopigmentation, are an unpredictable and common adverse event associated with laser treatments. Lasers stimulate melanocytes directly and the thermal damage produces an inflammatory response, which also stimulates melanocytes and promotes melanogenesis. It was demonstrated with laser resurfacing that nearly 100% of patients of patients with skin phototype IV experienced hyperpigmentation when evaluated 3 months after laser treatment (20). Preoperative, intraoperative, and postoperative treatment strategies are used with variable success to minimize this adverse event. These include minimizing thermal damage by using low fluences, down-regulating melanocytes with preoperative use of sunscreen and hydroquinone agents, and postoperative sunscreen and topical corticosteroids. Hypertrophic and keloidal scarring is also potential complication in individuals with darker skin. Systemic diseases that have the potential to adversely affect the results of laser and other cosmetic procedures are another consideration in this patient population. These diseases include sickle cell anemia, thalassemia, and glucose 6-phosphate dehydrogenase deficiency (8). These hemolytic disorders are more prevalent in African American, Mediterranean, and Southeast Asian patients. They may impact normal coagulation and impede postoperative healing. The possibility of these dramatic adverse events, coupled with the often mild to moderate photodamage in many blacks and Hispanics, has resulted in the infrequent use of lasers in photaging in this population.

Laser Resurfacing in Hispanic Patients

Ruiz-Esparza et al. (21) performed a study evaluating the safety of laser skin resurfacing with the carbon dioxide laser in 36 Hispanics with skin phototypes II–V. The patients had rhytides and acne scars. The age range of the subjects was 29–78 years. Subjects were followed up monthly for 6 months and assessed via photography and patient self-assessments. Daily pretreatment with a broad-spectrum sunscreens, sun avoidance, and 2% topical hydroquinone was instituted for 29 of the subjects. A carbon dioxide laser (UltraPulse 5000 c; 250–300 mJ/cm^2, density of 3 to 4, spot size of 2mm, and a repetition rate of 2 per second) was used. Two to four passes on the rhytides and four to seven on the acne scars were done. The minimal mechanical trauma technique was used. Aquaphor and a dressing were applied for 48 hours. Healing occurred in 6 or 7 days in all patients treated for rhytides and 14 days for those with acne scars.

All patients were reportedly satisfied with the cosmetic improvement obtained, with 32 subjects reporting 60–100% improvement at 6 months and three reporting 50% or less improvement. No cases of persistent erythema, hyperpigmentation, or hypopigmentation were seen at 90 days or at the completion of the study. There were two cases of focal erythema at the angles of the jaw that was interpreted as incipient hypertrophic scarring. A class-1 topical corticosteroid was applied for 2 weeks with resolution of the erythema and no scar formation. Hyperpigmentation was seen in nine patients. Faint ill-discernible mild hyperpigmentation was seen in seven subjects. Two cases of focal pigmentation on the cheeks were seen but resolved after the 3-month follow-up visit. Two cases of milia formation were seen. The investigators reported that an even pigmentation was obtained in all patients, even those with Fitzpatrick type V skin.

Laser Ablation of Benign Growths

Dermatosis papulosa nigra (DPN) occur frequently in African Americans. The lesions may appear during the second or third decade of life. They progress in size, location, and number until the sixth or seventh decades of life. Although there is no direct evidence that DPN, histologically similar to seborrheic keratosis, is a manifestation of photoaging or intrinsic aging, a correlation may be made with the development of photoaging-associated seborrheic keratosis in Asians. There are several modalities for the treatment of DPN and these include laser ablation using the carbon dioxide, erbium:yttrium-aluminum-garnet laser, or 532-nm diode lasers. However, as expected, associated with these modalities is the risk of postinflammatory hyperpigmentation.

Spoor (22) reported his experience treating DPN in 34 African American, Hispanic, and Asian patients with the 532-nm diode laser. A 700-μm spot size was used for the majority of the lesions, an energy density of 8 J/cm^2 (8–16 J/cm^2), a power of 3.0 W, and a repetition rate of 4 Hz. A cooling gel was applied immediately prior to the treatment.

The treatment end point was either a darkening of the lesion or a popping sound indicating implosion of the lesion. The DPN exfoliated after several weeks. Adverse events were reportedly minimal. Postinflammatory hyperpigmentation was not reported. Overall, the 532-nm diode laser was felt to be a rapid, effective, and well-tolerated treatment that avoided the need for infiltrative anesthetics.

SURGICAL OPTIONS FOR PHOTOAGING IN BLACKS AND HISPANICS

Superficial Excision

Dermatosis papulosa nigra as a manifestation of photoaging has been discussed. There are several surgical modalities that are used to remove DPN. These modalities include electrodessication and scissor excision. The principle is to subject darker skin to minimal trauma or damage. Superficial excision using a sharp Gradle scissor to remove the base of the lesion may offer a clear benefit. Electrodessication of DPN until an ashen or gray color develops, with low settings, is another appropriate method. The lesions will spontaneous exfoliate after a period of 4–10 days. Anesthetic may or may not be used for these procedures. Postinflammatory hyperpigmentation or hypopigmentation are potential adverse event for these procedures. Postoperative treatment of postinflammatory hyperpigmentation with a topical hydroquinone product will alleviate the discoloration within a short period. Finally, cryotherapy of DPN is not recommended in darker-skinned individuals owing to the possible development of long-lasting postinflammatory hypopigmentation.

Facelifts

As skin laxity and sagging are additional components of aging in black and Hispanic subjects, the performance of surgical procedures such as facelifts are often appropriate. Special considerations in this patient population includes keloidal and hypertrophic scarring and postinflammatory hyperpigmentation.

RESURFACING MODALITIES

Salicylic Acid Chemical Peeling Agents

Chemical peeling agents are used to resurface the skin of individuals of color. Peeling agents address textural, superficial wrinkling, and pigmentary skin changes associated with photaging. Grimes (23) investigated the clinical efficacy and safety of superficial salicylic acid peels in 20 African Americans and five Hispanics with skin phototypes V and VI. Eleven patients had pigmentary abnormalities, including postinflammatory hyperpigmentation and melasma; five had textural changes with rough, oily skin and enlarged pores; and nine had acne vulgaris. The average age of the subjects was 34 years. The patients were pretreated with hydroquinone 4% for 2 weeks prior to undergoing a series of five salicylic peels, performed at 2-week intervals. Moderate to significant improvement was observed in 88% of subjects and mild clearing occurred in 12%. The series of salicylic acid peels in combination with 4% hydroquinone expedited and facilitated the resolution of postinflammatory hyperpigmentation and melasma. There was also a decrease in overall facial pigmentation, which was cosmetically acceptable for the patient. There were no side events in 84% of the patients. One patient experienced crusting and hypopigmentation

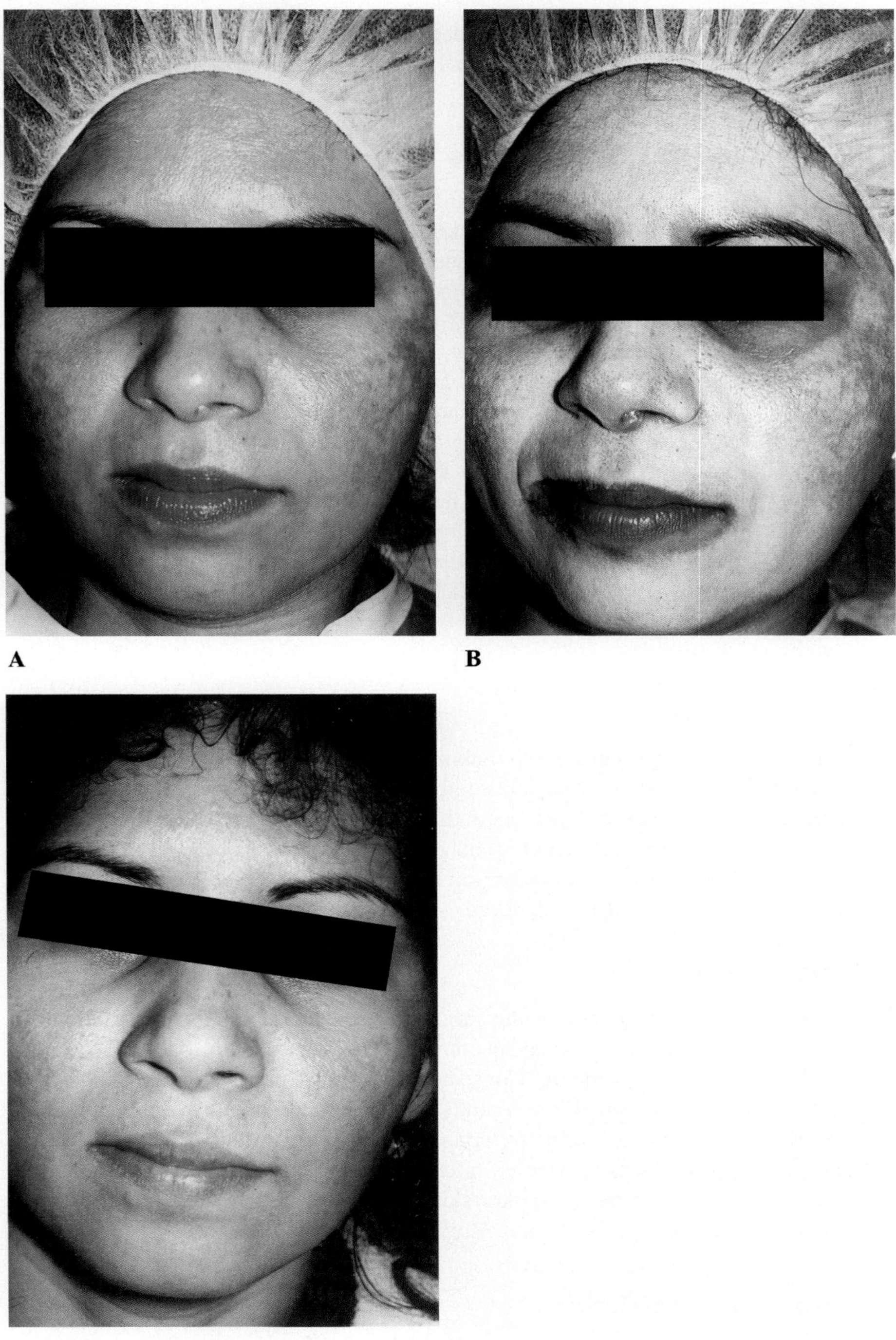

Figure 1 (a) Melasma in a Hispanic woman prior to treatment. (b) TCA peel placed on a Hispanic woman for melasma. (c) One year after treatment for melasma with a TCA peel (Courtesy of Dr. Maritiza Perez, New York, NY).

which resolved in seven days. Three patients had transient dryness and hyperpigmentation that resolved within 7–14 days. Neither residual hypopigmentation nor hyperpigmentation occurred.

Glycolic Acid Chemical Peeling Agents

Burns et al. (24) studied the treatment of postinflammatory hyperpigmentation in 19 African American female patients of Fitzpatrick skin phototypes IV–VI. Serial glycolic peels in addition to topical therapy with hydroquinone and tretinoin were investigated. The nine control group patients used a topical regimen consisting of daily use of a sun-protection-factor 15 sunscreen and the application of 2% hydroquinone and 10% glycolic acid gel twice daily with 0.05% tretinoin cream at night. The 10 peel patients used the same topical regimen and, in addition, received six serial glycolic acid peels (50–60%). The results revealed a trend in the subjects in the peel group toward greater and more rapid improvement then those in the control group. Five patients in the control group and all patients in the peel group experienced mild erythema and desquamation. All patients in the peel group experienced focal erythema and mild burning during the peels. Focal superficial vesiculation developed in seven patients but resolved within 3 days without scarring or hyperpigmentation. The study suggested that serial glycolic acid peels enhance the efficacy of the topical regimen when treating postinflammatory hyperpigmentation in black patients. In addition, the use of glycolic acid peels to minimize wrinkling due to photoaging has been well described.

Other Peeling Agents

Jessner's or modified Jessner's peels are combination peels containing resorcinol, salicylic acid, and lactic acid. They are often used in combination with other peeling agents. Trichloroacetic acid peels are medium-depth peels that range in concentration from 10–40%. These peels are used to treat fine winkles and pigmentary abnormalities. However, these peels must be used with caution on blacks and Hispanics with darker skin because of the risk of postinflammatory hyperpigmentation.

Microdermabrasion

Microdermabrasion is another therapeutic modality used for resurfacing of the skin. It uses micronized aluminum oxide crystals in combination with a vacuum suction to remove various levels of the stratum corneum. Consequently, it may improve fine wrinkles, skin texture, and pigmentary abnormalities. A study by Rubin and Greenbaum (25) observed a normalization of the stratum corneum, epidermal thickening, and increased collagen deposition in the papillary dermis after six microdermabrasion sessions. Microdermabrasion appears to be well tolerated on darker skin. The results tend to be similar to those achieved with glycolic acid peels or topical retinoids.

SOFT-TISSUE AUGMENTATION

Soft-tissue augmentation serves to treat wrinkles and areas of volume loss. There are a variety of filler substances, but the most frequently used are bovine-derived and human-derived collagen and fat. Filler substances are particularly useful in the treatment of areas of volume loss in individuals with darker skin.

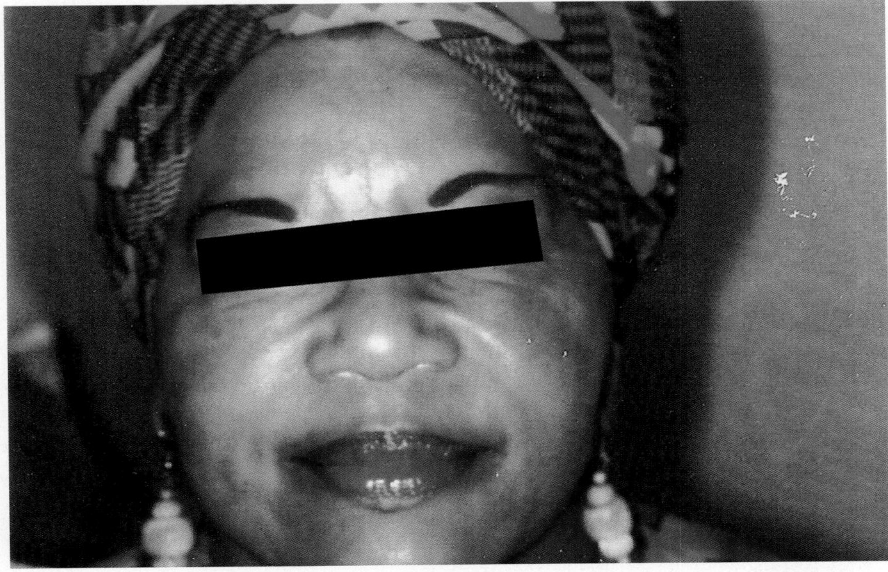

A

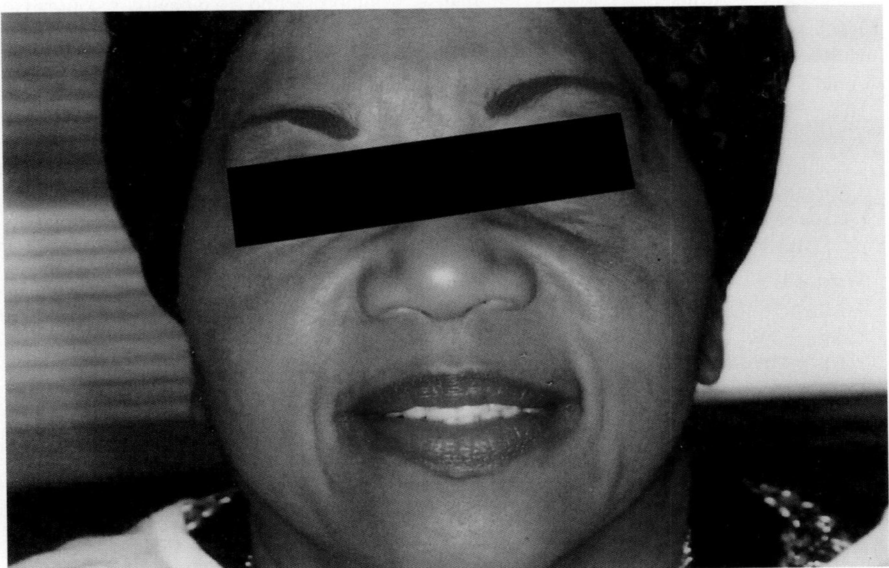

B

Figure 2 (a) African-American woman with sagging malar folds. (b) African-American woman after fat transfer (Courtesy of Dr. Zakia Rahman and Dr. Maritiza Perez, New York, NY).

BOTULINUM TOXIN

The use of botulinum toxin is well established for the treatment of wrinkling associated with facial motion and aging. Botulinum toxin is injected into muscles of the glabellar, forehead, and/or periorbital areas to temporarily paralyze the appropriate muscles and smooth the wrinkle. It is an effective therapeutic modality for individuals of all racial and ethnic backgrounds.

SUMMARY

Photoaging among African Americans and Hispanics is less pronounced that that seen in white-skinned individuals. Therefore, therapeutic modalities used to address fine wrinkling, pigmentary inconsistencies, skin textural changes, and benign cutaneous growths are often less invasive than those that address the needs of individuals with photodamaged white skin. A variety of modalities are used to improve the appearance of aging African American and Hispanic skin. These include topical, oral, and resurfacing agents, as well as fillers and neuromuscular relaxers.

REFERENCES

1. Kaidbey KH, Agin PP, Sayre RM, Kligman A. Photoprotection by melanin: a comparison of black and Caucasian skin. J Am Acad Dermatol 1979; 1:249–260.
2. Halder RM. The role of retinoids in the management of cutaneous conditions in blacks. J Am Acad Dermatol 1998; 39:S98–S103.
3. Halder RM, Grimes PE, McLaurin CI, Kress MA, Kenney JA. Incidence of common dermatoses in a predominantly black dermatology practice. Cutis 1983; 32:388.
4. Castanet J, Ortonne JP. Pigmentary changes in aged and photoaged skin. Arch Dermatol 1997; 133:1296–1299.
5. Fenske NA, Lober CW. Structural and functional changes of normal aging skin. J Am Acad Dermatol 1986; 15:571.
6. Matory WE. Aging in people of color. In: Matory WE, Ed. Ethnic Considerations in Facial Aesthetic Surgery. Philadelphia (PA): Lippincott-Raven, 1998:151–170.
7. Montagna W, Carlisle K. The architecture of black and white facial skin. J Am Acad Dermatol 1991; 24:929–937.
8. Jackson B. Lasers in skin of color. Cosm Dermatol 2003; 16(suppl 3):57–60.
9. Fisher GJ, Wang ZQ, Datta SC, Varani J, Kang S, Voorhees JJ. Pathophysiology of premature skin aging induced by ultraviolet light. N Engl J Med 1997; 337:1419–1428.
10. Hermanns J, Petit L, Martalo O, Pierrad-Franchimont C, Cauwenbergh G, Pierard G. Unraveling the patterns of subclinical pheomelanin-enriched facial hyperpigmentation: effect of depigmenting agents. Dermatology 2000; 201:118.
11. Griffiths CE, Kang S, Ellis CN, Kim KJ, Finkel LJ, Ortiz-Ferrer LC, White GM, Hamilton TA, Voorhees JJ. Two concentrations of topical tretinoin (retinoic acid) caused similar improvement of photaging but different degrees of irritation: a double-blind, vehicle-controlled comparison of 0.1% and 0.025% tretinoin creams. Arch Dermatol 1995; 131:1037–1044.
12. Bulengo-Ransby SM, Griffiths CEM, Kimbrough-Green CK, Finkel LJ, Hamilton TA, Ellis CN, Voorhees CN. Topical tretinoin (retinoic acid) therapy for hyperpigmented lesions caused by inflammation of the skin in black patients. N Engl J Med 1993; 328:1438–1443.
13. Jimbow K, Obata H, Pathak M, Fitzpatrick T. Mechanism of depigmentation by hydroquinone. Journal Invest Dermatol 1974; 62:436–449.
14. Sanchez JL, Vaquez M. A hydroquinone solution in the treatment of melasma. Int J Dermatol 1982; 21:55–58.

15. Ruiz-Maldonado R, Orozco-Covarrubias M de la Luz. Postinflammatory hypopigmentation and hyperpigmentation. Semin Cutan Med Surg 1997; 16:36–43.
16. Glenn M, Grimes PE, Pitt E, Chalet M, Kelley AP. Evaluation of clinical and light microscopic effects of various concentrations of hydroquinone [abstr]. Clin Res 1991; 39:83A.
17. Fleischer AB, Schwartzel EH, Colby SI, Altman DJ. The combination of 2% 4-hydroxyanisol (mequinol) and 0.01% tretinoin is effective in improving the appearance of solar lentigines and related hypopigmented lesions in two double-bline muticenter cinical studies. J Am Acad Dermatol 2000; 42:459–467.
18. Taylor SC, Torok H, Jones T, Lowe N, Rich P, Tschen E, Menter A, Baumann L, Wieder JJ, Jarratt MM, Pariser D, Martin D, Weiss J, Shavin J, Ramirez N. Efficacy and safety of a new triple-combination agent for the treatment of facial melasma. Cutis 2003; 72:67–72.
19. Hernandez-Perez E, Khawaja HA, Alvarez TYM. Oral isotretinoin as part of the treatment of cutaneous aging. Dermatol Surg 2000; 26:649–652.
20. Sriprachya-anont S, Marchell NL, Fitzpatrick RE, Goldman MP, Rostan EF. Facial resurfacing in patients with Fitzpatrick skin type IV. Laser Surg Med 2002; 30:86–92.
21. Ruix-Esparza J, Gomez JMB, De La Torre OLG, Fanco BH, Vazquez EGP. UltraPulse laser skin resurfacing in Hispanic patients. Dermatol Surg 1998; 24:59–62.
22. Spoor TC. Treatment of dermatosis papulosa nigra with the 532 nm diode laser. Cosmetic Dermatol 2001; 14:21–23.
23. Grimes PE. The safety and efficacy of salicylic acid chemical peels in darker racial-ethnic groups. Dermatol Surg 1999; 25:18–22.
24. Burns RL, Prevost-Blank PL, Lawry MA, Lawry TB, Faria DT, Fivenson DP. Glycolic acid peels for post inflammatory hyperpigmentation in black patients: A comparative study. Dermatol Surg 1997; 23:171–174.
25. Rubin MG, Greenbaum SS. Histologic effects of aluminum oxide microdermabrasion on facial skin. J Aesthetic Dermatol Cosm Surg 1999; 1:14.

21

Legal Considerations in the Treatment of Photoaged Skin

David J. Goldberg *Skin and Laser Surgery Specialists of NY/NJ, Mount Sinai School of Medicine, and Fordham University School of Law, New York, New York, U.S.A.*

- The performance of cosmetic treatments for photoaged skin has led to an increase in potential legal considerations.
- The most common legal considerations in the treatment of photoaged skin are those of physician negligence.
- An understanding of the elements in a cause of action in negligence may lessen the likelihood of a successful lawsuit against a physician treating photoaged skin.
- Scarring and pigmentary changes are the most common complications that occur in the cosmetic treatment of photoaged skin.

The treatment of photoaged skin has evolved from a field with a primary medical orientation to one that is increasingly geared toward the cosmetic patient. Although legal considerations can arise in the performance of any medical procedure, they are increasingly seen in the field of cosmetic treatments of photoaged skin. Although many medical-legal issues can arise with these patients, the most common will be those that involve physician negligence.

The first part of the chapter will discuss the elements of negligence and the evolution of a medical malpractice cause of action following treatment of photoaged skin. The second part of the chapter will describe various hypothetical complications and the likelihood of a successful malpractice case evolving from such postoperative complications.

NEGLIGENCE AND STANDARD OF CARE

Any analysis of physician negligence must first begin with a legal description of the elements of negligence. There are four required elements for a cause of action in negligence: duty, breach of duty, causation, and damages. The suing plaintiff must show the presence of all four elements to be successful in her claim (1).

The duty of a physician performing cutaneous antiphotoaging techniques is to perform that procedure in accordance with the standard of care. Although the elements of a cause of action in negligence are derived from formal legal textbooks, the standard of care is not necessarily derived from some well-known textbook. It is also not articulated by any judge. The standard of care is defined by some as whatever an expert witness says it is, and subsequently what a jury will believe. In a case against any physician treating either medical or cosmetic manifestations of photoaged skin, the specialist must have the knowledge and skill ordinarily possessed by a specialist in that field, and have used the care and skill ordinarily possessed by a specialist in that field in the same or similar locality under similar circumstances. A dermatologist, plastic surgeon, or internist performing cutaneous laser surgery, as an example, will all be held to an equal standard. A failure to fulfill such a duty may lead to loss of a lawsuit by the physician. If the jury accepts the suggestion that the physician mismanaged the case and that the negligence led to damage of the patient, then the physician will be liable. Conversely, if the jury believes an expert who testifies for the defendant doctor, then the standard of care, in that particular case has been met. In this view, the standard of care is a pragmatic concept, decided on a case-by-case basis, and based on the testimony of an expert physician. Any physician treating photoaged is expected to perform procedures in a manner of a reasonable physician. He need not be the best in his field; he need only perform the procedure in a manner that is considered by an objective standard as reasonable.

It is important to note that where there are two or more recognized methods of diagnosing or treating the same condition, a physician does not fall below the standard of care by using any of the acceptable methods, even if one method turns out to be less effective than another method. Finally, in many jurisdictions, an unfavorable result due to an ''error in judgment'' by a physician is not in and of itself a violation of the standard of care if the physician acted appropriately prior to exercising his professional judgment.

Evidence of the standard of care in a specific malpractice case includes laws, regulations, and guidelines for practice, which represent a consensus among professionals on a topic involving diagnosis or treatment, and the medical literature including peer-reviewed articles and authoritative texts. In addition, obviously, the view of an expert is crucial. Although the standard of care may vary from state to state, it is typically defined as a national standard by the profession at large.

Most commonly for litigation purposes, expert witnesses articulate the standard of care. The basis of the expert witness, and therefore the origin of the standard of care, is grounded in the following:

1. The witness's personal practice and/or
2. The practice of others that he has observed in his experience; and/or
3. Medical literature in recognized publications; and/or
4. Statutes and/or legislative rules; and/or
5. Courses where the subject is discussed and taught in a well-defined manner.

The standard of care is the way in which the majority of the physicians in a similar medical community would practice. If, in fact, the expert herself does not practice like the majority of other physicians, then she will have a difficult time explaining why the majority of the medical community does not practice according to her ways.

It would seem then that in the perfect world, the standard of care in every case would be a clearly definable level of care agreed on by all physicians and patients. Unfortunately, in the typical situation the standard of care is an ephemeral concept resulting from differences and inconsistencies among the medical profession, the legal system, and the public.

At one polar extreme, the medical profession is dominant in determining the standard of care in the practice of medicine. In such a situation, recommendations, guidelines, and policies regarding varying treatment modalities for different clinical situations published by nationally recognized boards, societies, and commissions establish the appropriate standard of care. Even in some of these cases, however, factual disputes may arise because more than one such organization will publish conflicting standards concerning the same medical condition. Adding to the confusion, local societies may publish their own rules applicable to a particular claim of malpractice.

Thus, in most situations the standard of care is neither clearly definable nor consistently defined. It is a legal fiction to suggest that a generally accepted standard of care exists for any area of practice. At best there are parameters within which experts will testify. Unfortunately, owing to the increased reliance on cosmetic-based technology for the treatment of photoaged skin and unrealistic expectations by the public, physicians may sometimes run the risk of being held to an unrealistic and unattainable standard of care. In the end it is the physician community that establishes that standard of care.

GUIDELINES OF CARE

American physicians have in recent years put forth substantial efforts toward standard setting, specifying treatment approaches to various conditions. Specialty societies such as the American Academy of Dermatology, the American Society for Dermatologic Surgery, and the American Society for Lasers in Medicine and Surgery have developed clinical practice guidelines. The Institute of Medicine has defined such clinical guidelines as ''systemically developed statements to assist practitioner and patient decisions about appropriate health care for specific clinical circumstances.'' Such guidelines represent standardized specifications for performing a procedure or managing a particular clinical problem.

Clinical guidelines raise thorny legal issues (2). They have the potential to offer an authoritative and settled statement of what the standard of care should be for a given medical or cosmetic photo aging condition. A court would have several options when such guidelines are offered as evidence. Such a guideline might be evidence of the customary practice in the medical profession. A doctor acting in accordance with the guidelines would be shielded from liability to the same extent as one who can establish that she or he followed professional customs. The guidelines could play the role of an authoritative expert witness or a well-accepted review article. Using guidelines as evidence of professional custom, however, is problematic if they are ahead of prevailing medical practice.

Clinical guidelines have already had an effect on settlement, according to surveys of malpractice lawyers. A widely accepted clinical standard may be presumptive evidence of due care, but expert testimony will still be required to introduce the standard and establish its sources and its relevancy.

Professional societies often attach disclaimers to their guidelines, thereby undercutting their defensive use in litigation. The American Medical Association (AMA), for example, calls its guidelines ''parameters'' instead of protocols intended to significantly impact on physician discretion. The AMA further suggests that all such guidelines contain disclaimers stating that they are not intended to displace physician discretion. Such guidelines, in such a situation, could not be treated as conclusive.

OTHER CONSIDERATIONS

Plaintiffs usually will use their own expert, as opposed to the physician's expert to define the standard of care. Although such a plaintiff's expert may also refer to clinical practice guidelines, the physician's negligence can be established in other manners as well. These methods include (1) examination of the physician defendant's expert witness; (2) an admission by the defendant that he or she was negligent; (3) testimony by the plaintiff, in a rare case where he is a medical expert qualified to evaluate the allegedly negligent physician's conduct; and (4) common knowledge in situations where a layperson could understand the negligence without the assistance of an expert (3,4).

Some physicians are located within either hospitals or certified ambulatory care centers. In such situations, a plaintiff may seek hospital committee proceeding minutes about the allegedly negligent physician. The plaintiff may request production of a committee's minutes or reports, set forth ''interrogatories'' about the committee process and/or outcome, or seek to depose committee members about committee discussions. If the plaintiff is suing a physician, whose work was reviewed by the committee, the discovery process may seek to confirm the negligence of the professional or to uncover additional evidence substantiating the plaintiff's claims. Such ''discovery'' requests are often met with a claim that information that is generated within or by a hospital committee is not discoverable. Courts have ruled that the discovery protection granted hospital quality review committee records prevents the opposing party from taking advantage of a hospital's careful self-assessment (5). The suing plaintiff must utilize her own experts to evaluate the facts underlying the incident. It is felt, by the courts, that such immunity of committee proceedings protects certain communications and encourages the quality review process. External access to committee investigations, it is argued, stifles candor and inhibits constructive criticism felt to be necessary for a quality review process. Constructive and objective peer criticism might not occur in an atmosphere of apprehension that one doctor's suggestion will be used as a denunciation of a colleague's conduct in a malpractice suit.

When a plaintiff seeks discovery of a facility or hospital incident report, rather than a committee proceeding, policy considerations are somewhat different. Incident reports kept in the medical records, and possible filed by a staff member, are often more directly related to a single claim for malpractice than would general committee investigations. Courts are usually less willing to protect such incident reports.

APPLICATION OF NEW TECHNOLOGY

Because the field of cutaneous photo aging has evolved rapidly over the past decade, physicians are quick to try new innovations and experimental concepts. Such innovations partially explain the excitement of this growing field. New laser and laserlike procedures may fall into a regulatory gaps not covered by the strict regulations for the device itself. Licensing through the Food and Drug Administration (FDA) carefully regulates medical devices such as lasers (6). Most human experimentation is governed by regulations of the Department of Health and Human Services. The regulations require that an institution sponsoring research must establish an Institutional Review Board. Such an organization will evaluate research proposals before any experimentation begins to determine whether human subjects might be ''at risk'' and, if so, how to protect them.

It is not usually difficult to determine whether a new technology laser is being used experimentally. It is, however, very difficult to determine whether an actual given procedure is experimental. Physicians who treat photoaged skin often view themselves as artists in addition to scientists, custom tailoring a treatment for a particular condition. Such approaches can lead to a bad result with variable outcomes in the courts. A laser surgeon who chooses to use a carbon dioxide laser rather than a liposuction cannula to perform a liposuction procedure, with a resultant complication leading to tissue necrosis and sepsis, would have problems suggesting that his medical experimentation conformed to reasonable standard of care. However, another surgeon who chooses, after appropriate informed consent, to use the same laser rather than a scalpel for excision of a nevus, with resultant significant scarring, might be considered an innovator rather than an experimenter. Such a physician would be no more liable for straying from her duty than the surgeon who might use a standard scalpel, with the same complication, for the same procedure.

In fact, most clinical innovation falls between standard practice and experimental research. Much of this innovation is unregulated by the government. The National Commission for the Protection of Human Subjects of Biomedical and Behavioral Research has suggested that any ''radically new'' procedure should be made the object of formal research at an early stage in order to determine whether such a procedure is safe and effective. It could be argued that some of the cutaneous laser procedures that have evolved, using already FDA-cleared laser devices, might be considered radical; most clearly are not.

NEED TO PROVE BREACH OF DUTY OF REASONABLE CARE AND DAMAGES

It is clear then that in order for the plaintiff to win her negligence cause of action against a physician, she must establish that her physician had a duty of reasonable care in treating her and had in fact breached that duty. However, that breach must also lead to some form of damages. A mere inconvenience to the plaintiff, even in the setting of a physician's breach, will usually not lead to physician liability in a cause of action for negligence.

It is often difficult to predict in any given malpractice cause of action what the ultimate outcome will be. The following teaching hypotheticals are designed to be suggestive of potential malpractice cases and the likely results. Any connection between these scenarios and actual malpractice cases is fortuitous.

Teaching Hypothetical 1

JH is a 48-year-old woman with class I rhytides and extensive solar telangiectases. She has used a variety of antirosacea medications and has undergone three sessions of electrocautery for treatment of her telangiectases. These treatment modalities have led to minimal clinical improvement. Her niece had seen a local plastic surgeon for a rhinoplasty procedure and was extremely happy with the cosmetic results. Because of this physician's expertise in cosmetic surgery, and her niece's recommendation, JH sought cosmetic treatment from this physician. The plastic surgeon had been performing rhinoplasty for more than a decade. However, only 1 month prior to treatment, the doctor spent a weekend learning ''laser skin resurfacing.'' It was his understanding that carbon dioxide lasers seal small blood vessels while leading to skin rejuvenation. He correctly assumes that this laser will thermally destroy many of the telangiectases on the face of JH. The plastic surgeon discusses with JH associated risks of cutaneous laser resurfacing, such as scarring and postinflammatory pigmentary changes following the procedure. The physician chooses to rent his laser from a local rental company. This company also rents such lasers as potassium titanyl phosphate (KTP) lasers, Q-switched lasers, and ''hair removal'' lasers. Since the physician has only learned to use the carbon dioxide laser, he chooses to treat his patient with this laser.

The full-face procedure is undertaken without any difficulty. Because of the extensive thermal wound, JH is required to stay in her house for 10 days following the procedure. This is not terribly difficult for her since she has a home-based job and needn't leave her house on a daily basis. The telangiectases respond nicely to treatment. Unfortunately, the postresurfacing erythema lasts for over 6 months. JH had marital difficulties before the laser surgery. Her husband was never supportive of her undergoing the procedure. Because of the prolonged erythema, JH is reluctant to leave her house. This reclusive behavior represents the final strain to her marriage. Her husband leaves her and ultimately files for divorce. Soon thereafter, JH finds out that her telangiectases could have been treated with a KTP laser without any significant ablative wound. There would also have been no delayed erythema following the laser procedure.

JH files a lawsuit against her plastic surgeon. She claims negligence in his use of the carbon dioxide laser to treat her telangiectases. Did he breach the standard of care? If so, will he liable for negligence? The plastic surgeon has a duty of care to JH. His duty is no more or less than that of any dermatologist or other physician performing the identical procedure. His limited weekend training will not be an adequate defense. His lack of knowledge about KTP lasers will also not support his choice of a carbon dioxide laser to treat his patient's telangiectases. Thus, it would appear that he breached his duty of care. He chose to use a laser that is not ideal for the treatment of telangiectases. Is he then liable? His liability would only result if the breach caused ''damages.'' JH will be hard pressed to prove that her already failing marriage and resultant divorce represented damages caused by the inappropriate use of the carbon dioxide laser in the treatment of telangiectases. She is not likely to win the case even though her plastic surgeon chose an inappropriate laser to treat his patient.

Teaching Hypothetical 2

Dr. Doc is a well-known dermatologist with over 5 years of experience using a variety of lasers. For the last 2 years, he has been successfully treating solar lentigines with a variety of lasers and light sources. He recently evaluated an unusual rare Fitzpatrick type V-complected individual (PC) with multiple lentigines. He explains to her that the ideal laser responsive photoaging patient is a light-skinned individual. Because of her complexion, and the potential risk of laser-induced postinflammatory pigmentary changes, Dr. Doc tries to use unusual laser parameters. He also uses a very cold gel on her skin prior to treatment. It is his understanding that such an approach is safer in darker-complected individuals. He also provides PC with a laundry list of general risks such as postlaser scarring and textural changes. She is treated monthly for 2 consecutive months without difficulty. Unfortunately, 2 months after a second session, a hypertrophic scar developed at the site of an post–laser-induced herpes simplex infection that appeared to be activated 1 week after a laser treatment. PC had not had a herpetic outbreak in 30 years and, when asked about such proclivity prior to the first laser procedure, she denied any history of herpes simplex infection. PC learns from a friend that most cutaneous laser surgeons provide their cutaneous laser resurfacing patients with a course of oral antiviral agents, even if they provide no personal history of herpes simplex infections. She reasons, and her attorney agrees, that the same logic should apply to other laser procedures of the skin.

Is Dr. Doc liable? It is clear that there is permanent damage to JH. If this damage resulted from the laser procedure, Dr. Doc might be liable. However, unfortunately for JH, it will be hard to prove that Dr. Doc breached the standard of care. Just because physicians routinely provide their resurfacing patients oral antiviral agents does not mean that such medications are required after all laser procedures. The fact that PC denied a history of oral herpes simplex would only bolster Dr. Doc's defense. The difficulty in treating solar lentigines in darker-complected individuals will have no impact on this cause of action in negligence.

Teaching Hypothetical 3

Dr. Good is a well-trained dermatologist. In fact, she not only learned to use lasers during her residency training, but also undertook a 1-year laser fellowship in 1993. In 1995 she began to perform cosmetic cutaneous laser resurfacing for photoaged skin. In her patient handouts she describes the potential benefits of ablative laser resurfacing as compared to deeper peeling agents. One advantage, she suggests, is the lack of obvious phenol-induce delayed hypopigmentation seen with these deeper peels. Dr. Good provides a consent form to her patients that does mention the risk of scarring and *temporary* pigmentary changes following the laser procedure. In 1996, she performed full-face carbon dioxide laser resurfacing on a 55-year-old Fitzpatrick type II, class III rhytide individual. The patient, BB, followed all the appropriate wound care instructions and returned to Dr. Good's office three times during the 6 months after her laser resurfacing procedure. Both doctor and patient were thrilled with the results and the patient was discharged. Unfortunately, 1 year after the procedure, BB began to notice significant loss of pigmentation (Fig. 1). This problem progressively worsened over the next year. BB was unable to go out of the house without makeup. She became a recluse. Soon thereafter, reports begin to appear in the medical literature about the possibility of delayed post–carbon dioxide laser-induced hypopigmentation. BB brings suit against Dr. Good. BB's attorney produces Dr. Good's promotional materials suggesting the safety of this procedure, the consent form that made no mention of delayed permanent hypopigmentation, and copies of the recent journal articles documenting this problem.

Will Dr. Good lose in this negligence cause of action? It would seem that she breached her duty by not mentioning the risk of permanent post–laser-induced hypopigmentation. Certainly, the alleged breach of her duty is the cause of the permanent damage to BB's face. However, Dr. Good can correctly defend her actions by stating that, *at the time of the incident*, the standard of care was not to warn about delayed carbon dioxide laser-induced permanent hypopigmentation. Dr. Good cannot be held responsible for laser-induced complications that were not known, nor described, at the time of the laser procedure.

Teaching Hypothetical 4

Dr. Laser is well experienced in erbium:yttrium-aluminum-garnet (Er:YAG) laser resurfacing. He uses this laser for superficial resurfacing; all of his patients re-epithelialize in 5–7 days. He routinely places his patients on 1 week of oral antiviral therapy. Recently Dr.

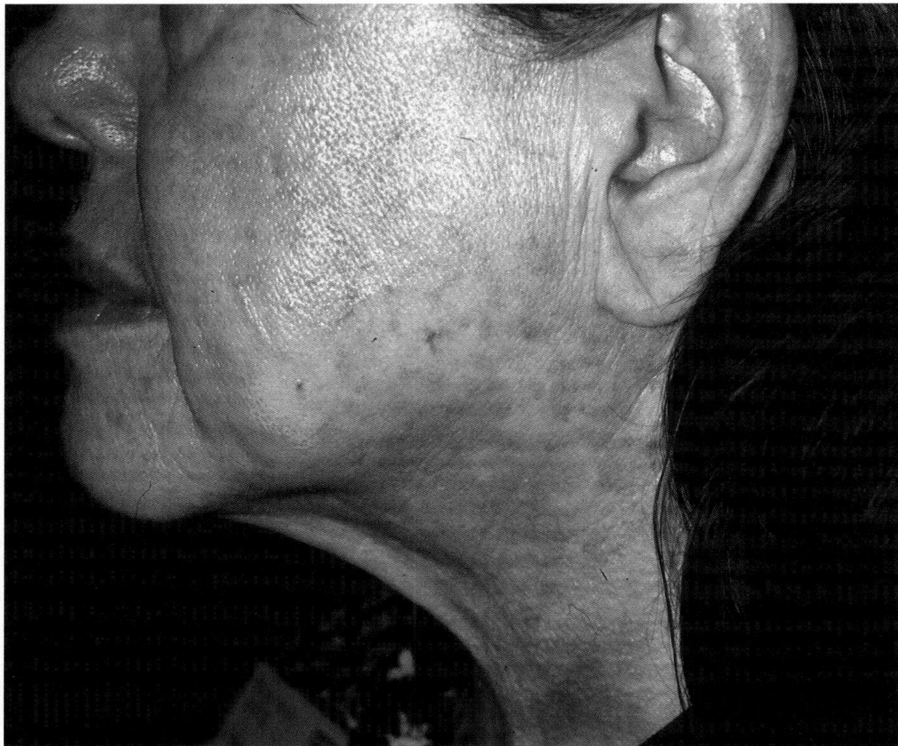

Figure 1 Delayed hypopigmentation after laser resurfacing.

Laser has become disenchanted with this laser's efficacy in the treatment of deeper class III rhytides. He begins to rent a carbon dioxide laser for his more severely wrinkled patients. He continues to give these patients 1 week of oral antiviral treatment despite the fact that re-epithelialization usually takes 10 days in these patients. SG represents one such class III rhytide patient. Dr. Laser performs the carbon dioxide laser procedure, provides a 7-day oral antiviral treatment to his patient, and sees her in the office at day 3 following the laser procedure. At day three, SG appears to be doing well and Dr. Laser advises her to return 3 weeks after the procedure. At the 3-week follow-up visit, she is well healed except for four erosive areas on her lip and upper forehead. Dr. Laser reassures her and suggests that she continue to use moist dressings. Two weeks later the erosions are still not healed and SG seeks evaluation by an expert in the field. This new physician performs a viral culture and determines that she has a herpes simplex infection. He re-treats her with antiviral therapy. She eventually heals but is left with hypertrophic scarring (Fig. 2).

SG files a negligence cause of action against Dr. Laser for performing a procedure that led to her scars, but admits that she signed a consent form that warned her about the risks of laser-induced scarring. When challenged in court about the positive herpes simplex infection, Dr. Laser responds by reminding the jury that he did use 7 days worth of antiviral treatment in this patient, something he traditionally did in his Er:YAG laser-treated pa-

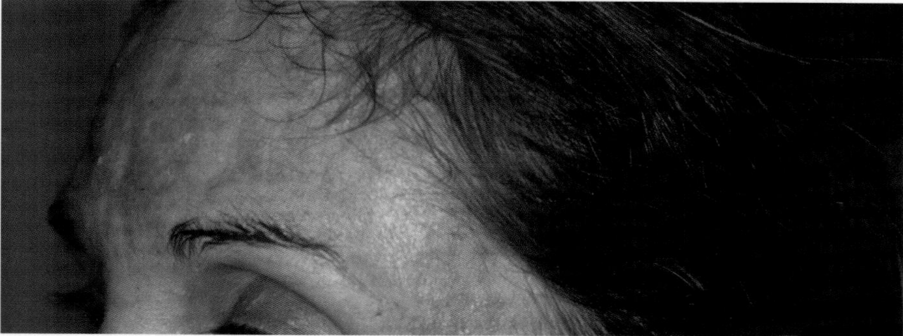

Figure 2 Hypertrophic scarring after laser resurfacing.

tients. Unfortunately for Dr. Laser, he is likely to lose his case. It will be argued, by SG's expert, that it is not the use of antiviral agents that defines the standard of care after laser resurfacing. Instead he will contend the standard of care dictates that antiviral agents be used until full re-epithelialization has occurred. Dr. Laser's duty was not to simply provide his patient with antiviral agents; his duty was to provide such agents for the full 10 days of re-epithelialization. The breach in this duty led to the scars on the face of his patient. Dr. Laser may be found culpable in a negligence malpractice cause of action.

Teaching Hypothetical 5

Dr. Jan, a well-known and respected dermatologist, purchased an old carbon dioxide laser from his medical school roommate, a colon-rectal surgeon in the local community. Dr. Jan undertook extensive training in carbon dioxide laser resurfacing and had a good knowledge of facial anatomy, wound healing, and the use of several good pulsed char-free carbon dioxide lasers. His laser, purchased at a bargain-basement price, was a continuous-wave carbon dioxide laser. Dr. Jan performed 20 full-face laser-resurfacing procedures with this machine. All of his patients were happy with the results. When challenged at a recent meeting about the use of such a continuous-wave laser for resurfacing, Dr. Jan responded by suggesting that he was expert at this technique. In addition, he noted that before the use of pulsed resurfacing lasers, some physicians used such continuous lasers for facial resurfacing.

Recently, Dr. Jan treated his 21st patient, a 55-year-old woman with class II rhytides and photodamage. The technique was performed in an identical manner to that of the previous procedures. Unfortunately, his patient had a protracted course of healing with resultant significant hypertrophic scarring.

The scarred plaintiff brought a lawsuit alleging malpractice by Dr. Jan. The plaintiff's expert, a well-respected cosmetic surgeon, testified that Dr. Jan's use of a continuous-wave nonpulsed carbon dioxide laser represented a deviation in the standard of care. The expert contended that a reasonable medical practitioner would not use a continuous wave laser for cosmetic laser resurfacing. Dr. Jan, testifying on his own behalf, set forth numerous manuscripts from 20 years ago indicating that such lasers could be used for such procedures. He contended that such papers proved that his practice was in accordance with the standard of care, even if such a technique was not used by most.

Dr. Jan's argument that he is performing within the standard of care is a fallacious one. It may be true that laser resurfacing, with a continuous-wave laser, was the standard of care at the time the provided medical literature was written. However, it is uniformly accepted that the standard of care, timewise, is defined at the time a procedure is performed. Dr. Jan cannot claim that his procedure is in accordance within the standard of care, at the time of the procedure, simply because he may have complied with the standard established many years before the actual performance of the procedure. The scarring produced by the continuous-wave laser may very well represent a breach of the standard of care. He is likely to lose in this negligence cause of action.

Teaching Hypothetical 6

Dr. RF recently purchased one of the new nonablative radiofrequency devices. He knows that such devices when used on the forehead can provide some tissue tightening in lifting eyebrows. He also knows that the machine has been FDA cleared for treating periorbital rhytides. Furthermore, he understands that many physicians have successfully used the machine to tighten early jowls and dropping necks. He has heard about some experimental work that has used this machine to try to lift early sagging breast tissue. Dr. RF decides that if tissue tightening is the goal of this technology, he will try to perform a nonsurgical abdominoplasty with the radiofrequency device. He assumes that because abdominal skin is so much thicker than the photoaged skin he characteristically treats that significantly higher treatment parameters should be used. He treats his patient at very high energies. She has extensive blistering following the procedure, which leads to keloidal scarring. Dr. RF has a duty of reasonable care to his patient. His treatment was a breach of that duty and led to significant scarring. He is likely to lose his medical malpractice case.

FUTURE TRENDS

Physicians treating photoaged skin are using exciting ever-changing technology. They are increasingly learning to perform a variety of new procedures. Because such new technology is ever changing, it is important that physicians be aware of their duty of reasonable care. Should they breach that duty, they may be found liable in a medical malpractice cause of action.

In the future, an increased number of modalities for the diagnosis and treatment of photoaged skin will become available. With this development, there may be an associated increase in the number of legal considerations. An understanding of this trend will help both the patient who seeks treatment for photoaged skin and the physician who treats it.

REFERENCES

1. Furrow BF, Greaney TL, Johnson SH, Jost TS, Schwartz RL. Liability in Health Care Law. 3rd ed.. St. Paul: West Publishing, 1997.
2. Hyams AL, Shapiro DW, Brennan TA. Medical practice guidelines in malpractice litigation: an early retrospective. J Health Polit Policy Law 1996; 21:289.
3. *Lamont v Brookwood Health Service, Inc.*, 446 So.2d 1018 (Ala.1983).
4. *Gannon v Elliot*, 19 Cal.App.4th 1 (1993).
5. *Coburn v Seda*, 101 Wash.2d 270 (1984).
6. Federal Food, Drug, and Cosmetic Act, 21 USCA §301.

Index